METHODS IN PHARMACOLOGY

a series of monographs
edited by Arnold Schwartz

METHODS IN PHARMACOLOGY

Volume 1

edited by **ARNOLD SCHWARTZ**

Division of Myocardial Biology
Baylor College of Medicine
Houston, Texas 77025

APPLETON-CENTURY-CROFTS
Educational Division
MEREDITH CORPORATION
New York

Softcover reprint of the hardcover 1st edition 1971

7110-1

Library of Congress Catalog Card Number: 70-92660

ISBN 978-1-4615-7427-9 ISBN 978-1-4615-7425-5 (eBook)
DOI 10.1007/978-1-4615-7425-5

Dedication

This first volume of METHODS IN PHARMACOLOGY is respectfully dedicated to the memory of Sir Henry Hallett Dale (June 9, 1875 – July 23, 1968) whose monumental contributions to Pharmacology depended so much on the *variety* of methods he employed.

Contributors

JULIUS C. ALLEN
Division of Myocardial Biology
Baylor College of Medicine
1200 Moursund Avenue
Houston, Texas 77025

AMIR ASKARI
Department of Pharmacology
Cornell University Medical College
1300 York Avenue
New York, New York 10021

RICHARD J. BING
Professor of Medicine, USC
Huntingdon Memorial Hospital
100 Congress Street
Pasadena, California 91105

ZACK R. BLAILOCK
Major USAF, MC FV 3165671
Department of Pharmacology
12th USAF Hospital (PACAF)
APO San Francisco 96326

EDWARD BRESNICK
Department of Pharmacology
Baylor College of Medicine
1200 Moursund Avenue
Houston, Texas 77025

GEORGE CAMOUGIS
New England Research and Development Laboratories
100 Grove Street
Worcester, Massachusetts 01605

C. COWAN
Department of Medicine
Wayne State University School of Medicine
1400 Chrysler Freeway
Detroit, Michigan 48207

ROBERT E. EDMANDS
Krannert Heart Research Institute
Marion County General Hospital
960 Locke Street
Indianapolis, Indiana 46207

SETSURO EBASHI
Department of Pharmacology
Faculty of Medicine
University of Tokyo
Bunkyo-ku, Tokyo
Japan

E. N. FAWAZ
Department of Pharmacology
American University of Beirut School of Medicine
Beirut, Lebanon

GEORGE FAWAZ
Department of Pharmacology
American University of Beirut School of Medicine
Beirut, Lebanon

JAMES J. FISCHER
Department of Radiology
Yale Medical School
333 Cedar Street
New Haven, Connecticut 06510

JAMES R. FOUTS
Department of Pharmacology
The University of Iowa College of Medicine
Iowa City, Iowa 52240

KALMAN GREENSPAN
Head, Section of Physiology
Krannert Heart Research Institute
Marion County General Hospital
960 Locke Street
Indianapolis, Indiana 46207

S. GUDBJARNASON
Department of Medicine
Wayne State University School of Medicine
1400 Chrysler Freeway
Detroit, Michigan 48207

WILLI HALLE
Laboratory of Circulation Research
German Academy of Sciences
Berlin-Buch
Germany DDR

S. HARIGAYA
Department of Pharmacology
Faculty of Medicine
University of Tokyo
Bunkyo-ku, Tokyo
Japan

CARL JOHNSON
Division of Myocardial Biology
Baylor College of Medicine
1200 Moursund Avenue
Houston, Texas 77025

ARNOLD M. KATZ
Department of Medicine
Mount Sinai School of Medicine of the City University of New York
New York, New York 10029

KWANG SOO LEE
Department of Pharmacology
State University of New York
Downstate Medical Center
450 Clarkson Avenue
Brooklyn, New York 11203

JOSEPH V. LEVY
Research Laboratories
Presbyterian Medical Center
Clay and Webster Street
San Francisco, California 94115

GEORGE E. LINDENMAYER
Cardiology Branch
National Heart and Lung Institute
National Institutes of Health
Bethesda, Maryland 20014

HIDEO MATSUI
Department of Biochemistry
Faculty of Medicine
University of Tokyo
Tokyo, Japan

K. NAGANO
Department of Biochemistry
Tokyo Medical and Dental University School of Medicine
Yushima, Bunkyo-ku
Tokyo, Japan

M. NAKAO
Department of Biochemistry
Tokyo Medical and Dental University School of Medicine
Yushima, Bunkyo-ku
Tokyo, Japan

Y. OGAWA
Department of Pharmacology
Faculty of Medicine
University of Tokyo
Bunkyo-ku, Tokyo
Japan

WILLIAM W. PARMLEY
Department of Medicine
Harvard Medical School
Boston, Massachusetts 02115

P. S. PURI
Department of Medicine
Wayne State University School of Medicine
1400 Chrysler Freeway
Detroit, Michigan 48207

ARNOLD SCHWARTZ
Division of Myocardial Biology
Baylor College of Medicine
1200 Moursund Avenue
Houston, Texas 77025

EDMUND H. SONNENBLICK
Department of Medicine
Harvard Medical School
Boston, Massachusetts 02115

LOUIS A. SORDAHL
Division of Myocardial Biology
Baylor College of Medicine
1200 Moursund Avenue
Houston, Texas 77025

HUBERT C. STANTON
Shell Development Company
P.O. Box 4248
Biological Science Research Center
Modesto, California 95353

LASZLO SZEKERES
Institute of Pharmacology
University of Szeged Medical School
Dóm tér 12
Szeged, Hungary

BERTIL H. TAKMAN
New England Research and Development Laboratories
100 Grove Street
Worcester, Massachusetts 01605

GEORGES UNGAR
Department of Anesthesiology
Baylor College of Medicine
1200 Moursund Avenue
Houston, Texas 77025

ALBERT WOLLENBERGER
Laboratory of Circulation Research
German Academy of Sciences
Berlin-Buch
Germany DDR

Preface

The death of Sir Henry Hallett Dale two years ago brought to a close an era which was characterized by tremendous pharmacologic advancements. During this period, the employment of what present investigators might consider "primitive" techniques yielded information which has become classic. For example, in a paper by Barger and Dale, published in 1910*, one finds not only a beautiful example of a structure-activity study and suggestions of the importance of membranes, but also the concept of *specific receptor* sites introduced by the statement that "the relation of the receptive mechanism to the base (i.e., drug base) may well be one of solid solution of adsorption, and, therefore, more analogous to that of an enzyme to its substrate . . ." The search for drug receptors continues today at an accelerated pace. Hopefully, fundamental knowledge of receptors and the nature of drug-receptor interactions will lead to a rational approach to drug design.

In acquiring skills in the scientific approach to drug mechanism and evaluation, the modern pharmacologist, whether senior investigator or student, frequently is required to employ techniques which are characteristic of other biologic areas. However, it is not enough simply to be grounded in physiology or biochemistry. A pharmacologist, for example, is not "a biochemist who throws a drug or two in his flask," but is rather an individual who should approach a problem by using sound pharmacologic principles, as well as whatever biologic, physical, or chemical techniques that can assist in supplying the answer. It is becoming increasingly obvious that an understanding of the complexities of drug actions and toxicities is vital for the growth and welfare of our society. The design of better drugs to combat specific ailments is a major objective of health-oriented institutions. Never before has there been a greater need for excellent departments and institutes of pharmacology in medical colleges and in allied health schools.

The purpose of METHODS IN PHARMACOLOGY is to acquaint the student, as well as the professional investigator, with the multitude of proven techniques that can be employed in pursuit of the objectives mentioned above, and, in general, to provide the pharmacologist with methods to investigate the action of drugs on both

*Chemical structure and sympathomimetic action of amines. **J. Physiol.**, 41:19-59, 1910.

the organic and molecular levels. Some of the methods require only simple devices, while others utilize expensive equipment that may not be readily available. However, the theory, importance, and usefulness of each procedure is discussed in detail. The authors of each of the methods were selected because of their proven skill and competence in a particular area of pharmacology. The methods are written in a relatively simple, yet detailed, form so that, with the proper equipment and practice, an individual can produce meaningful data even if previously unacquainted with the general techniques. Sufficient references are included for further background study and documentation. Typical examples of results are also included for comparative purposes. Limitations and pitfalls are frequently given.

No attempt was made to cover the entire field of pharmacology. Certain specific topics were selected for this first volume, primarily to present a relatively wide scope of available techniques. Heavy emphasis is placed on cardiac tissues because cardiovascular pharmacology is probably among the most active of the subdisciplines. Editorial prejudice is freely admitted. It is expected that future volumes will include other important areas such as neuropharmacology, renal pharmacology, gastrointestinal pharmacology, and so forth.

The editor recognizes that *some* of the techniques in the volume appear, in one form or another, in other specialized volumes, as well as in published papers. Nonetheless, most of the techniques either have not been published or have not been presented in the detail expressed in this text.

Arnold Schwartz

Contents

Methods in Pharmacology

Volume 1

CHAPTER 1

Nerve and Nerve-Muscle Preparations (As Applied to Local Anesthetics)

George Camougis* and Bertil H. Takman

Astra Pharmaceutical Products, Inc.
Worcester, Massachusetts

INTRODUCTION

This chapter discusses both general and specific aspects of the testing and evaluation of local anesthetic agents. Previous reviews on the testing of local anesthetics (Carney, 1951; Weatherby, 1964) have described testing procedures with major emphasis on whole animal studies. In addition, other reviews have discussed methodology (Gray and Geddes, 1954; Adriani, 1960; de Jong and Wagman, 1963; Barlow, 1964; Truant and Takman, 1965; Turner, 1965). Some of these discussions are brief, others are specialized, and finally others do not stress quantitative methods sufficiently. This chapter will include in vivo, in vitro, toxicity, physical chemical, and analytical methods of evaluating local anesthetics. Whenever possible, quantitative techniques will be stressed. Clinical testing will not be mentioned, except for brief references in the discussion.

*Present address: New England Research and Development Laboratories, Worcester, Massachusetts.

The authors are grateful to Dr. R. N. Boyes, Dr. M. Lebeaux, Mr. J. B. Keenaghan, Mr. J. R. P. Tasse, Miss Georgette Kilpatrick, and Mrs. Kathleen W. Newcomer for their assistance.

The principles of evaluating local anesthetics are substantially similar to those required to evaluate any potentially useful drug. Therefore, the pharmacology, toxicology, and various aspects of the chemistry of the compound in question must be studied. The depth of these studies is determined by many factors, but in the main it will depend upon a judgment of the potential usefulness of the drug. The techniques and methods discussed in this chapter are intended to provide sufficient information so that the results from the studies will provide a sound basis for evaluating the potential of a given drug for clinical use. In that sense, the methods taken together are rather more than a simple screen. While the basic principles are general, the local anesthetics as a specific class of compounds require rather specific methods for their sound evaluation. This chapter deals with those specifics.

IN VIVO METHODS

The main subdivisions of local anesthesia (also, called regional anesthesia) in clinical practice are (1) *conduction* anesthesia, (2) *infiltration* anesthesia, and (3) *surface* or *topical* anesthesia. Therefore, the methods that have been developed for use with whole animals are designed to test these three types of block. Each will be discussed in sequence.

Conduction Anesthesia

Conduction (also block) anesthesia depends upon the application of a local anesthetic on a peripheral nerve trunk, a nerve plexus, or the spinal cord so that nerve impulses cease to propagate through the treated region. Experimental study of conduction anesthesia goes back to the last century when Corning (1885) produced spinal blocks in dogs with cocaine. Table 1 includes a survey of in vivo techniques used to evaluate conduction anesthesia in animals. It becomes apparent from the table that many tests in many animals have been worked out. Therefore, selection of a proper technique requires the consideration of many factors. By experience many laboratories have found that perineural block in small laboratory animals offers the advantages of simplicity, economy, and relatively good reproducibility. More specifically, we will discuss conduction anesthesia in the sciatic nerve of the albino rat.

Six animals in one cage is a convenient number to use. Ideally the animals should weigh about 125 to 175 grams. The animals are identified by clipping the ears in a conventional way. An assistant suspends the animals in a prone position by grasping the base of the tail and thoracic cage. The anesthetist extends a hind limb to its full length and locates the depression for needle insertion by palpation with the left index finger. The site of injection is the area under the skin at the junction of the *biceps femoris* and *gluteus maximus* muscles. The sciatic nerve is blocked in the midthigh region with 0.2 ml of the drug solution administered by a 24- to 25-gauge, ¼-inch needle attached to a 0.25-ml tuberculin syringe. This is

TABLE 1

A Survey of Methods of Evaluating In Vivo Local Anesthesia

Method	Species	References
	CONDUCTION ANESTHESIA	
Plexus anesthesia	Frog	Sollmann, 1918a Bülbring & Wajda, 1945
Spinal block	Frog	Sollmann & Hanzlik, 1928 Bieter et al., 1932
Sciatic block	Rat	Truant, 1958 Truant & Wiedling, 1958/1959 Åstrom & Persson, 1961b
Sciatic block	Guinea pig	Shackell, 1935 Luduena & Hoppe, 1952
Spinal block	Rabbit	Bieter et al., 1936 Luduena & Hoppe, 1951 Luduena, 1957
Peridural block	Cat	Sechzer, 1965 Truant, 1965
Spinal block	Cat	Sechzer, 1965
Spinal block	Dog	Dvorak & Manson, 1930
	INFILTRATION ANESTHESIA	
Infiltration of tail	Mouse	Bianchi, 1956
Cutaneous wheals	Guinea pig	Büllbring & Wajda, 1945 Luduena & Hoppe, 1956
Cutaneous wheals	Dog	Meeker, 1925
	SURFACE ANESTHESIA	
Cutaneous anesthesia	Frog	Sollmann, 1918b Munch et al., 1933
Corneal block	Guinea pig	MacIntosh & Work, 1941 Chance & Lobstein, 1944 Truant & Wiedling, 1958/1959
Corneal block	Rabbit	Sollmann, 1918c Rose, 1931 Sinha, 1936 Wiedling, 1952 Truant & Wiedling, 1958/1959
Sneeze reflex	Rabbit	Nieschulz et al., 1958 Åström & Persson, 1961b
Pubic reflex	Rabbit	Cited by Truant & Takman, 1965
Urethral block	Dog	Langston et al., 1967
	MISCELLANEOUS METHODS	
Withdrawal reflex	Earthworm	Block et al., 1964 Suskevich et al., 1967
Mobility	Goldfish & tadpole	Adams et al., 1926 Meyer, 1937
Vocalization	Mouse	Jones et al., 1965
Pseudohernia	Guinea pig	Loewe, 1936
Vagus block	Rabbit	Copeland, 1924
Sciatic nerve–respiratory response	Rabbit	Schmitz & Loevenhart, 1924 Hirschfelder & Ridges, 1933
Corneal healing time	Rabbit	Castrén & Lavikainen, 1963

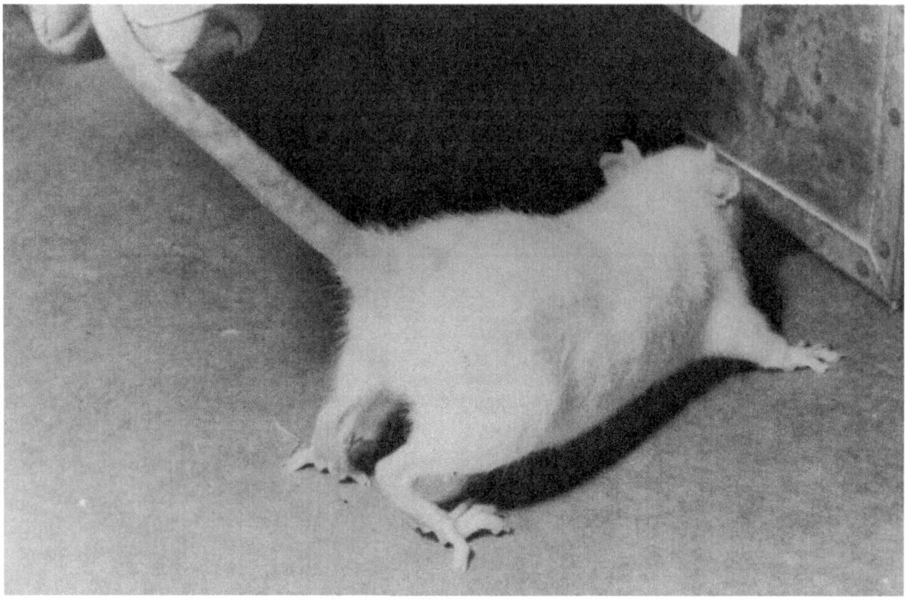

FIG. 1. Appearance of the hind limbs of a rat before injection of a local anesthetic. Note the extension of the digits and the normal, elevated position of the hock.

done by using both hands, the left index finger to feel for the depression, and the right hand for holding the syringe, inserting the needle, and pushing the plunger.

The actual design of the experiment may vary. Usually a 1 or 2 percent solution of a test drug in 0.9 percent NaCl is used as a test solution. One leg may be used for a control drug (e.g., procaine or lidocaine) while the other is used for the test drug. Depending upon the experience of the anesthetist, it may be desirable to do control injections with plain saline in one leg. In such a case one cage (six legs) can be used for the test drug and another cage for the control drug. Saline injections should cause no impairment of function. Small volumes of dyes can also be used for practice in performing anesthesia.

Immediately after the injection, the anesthetist repeatedly checks the digits of the foot and the walking behavior. In the normal foot the digits are wide apart (Fig. 1), while in the blocked leg the digits of the foot are close together (Fig. 2). Also the successful block is evidenced by a dragging of the leg and an inability of the animal to use the leg in walking up the inclined cover of a cage made of wire mesh. An appropriate data sheet is prepared with information on the test compound, the animal, the leg number, and the block data. The block data should include time of injection, time of block, time of recovery, and miscellaneous remarks. After the time of block for each leg is noted (and this requires great skill if the drug blocks quickly), the anesthetist examines each animal every 5 to 10 minutes in order to note the time of recovery. From the data, averages for onset time and duration are calculated, plus the frequency of block is noted. For

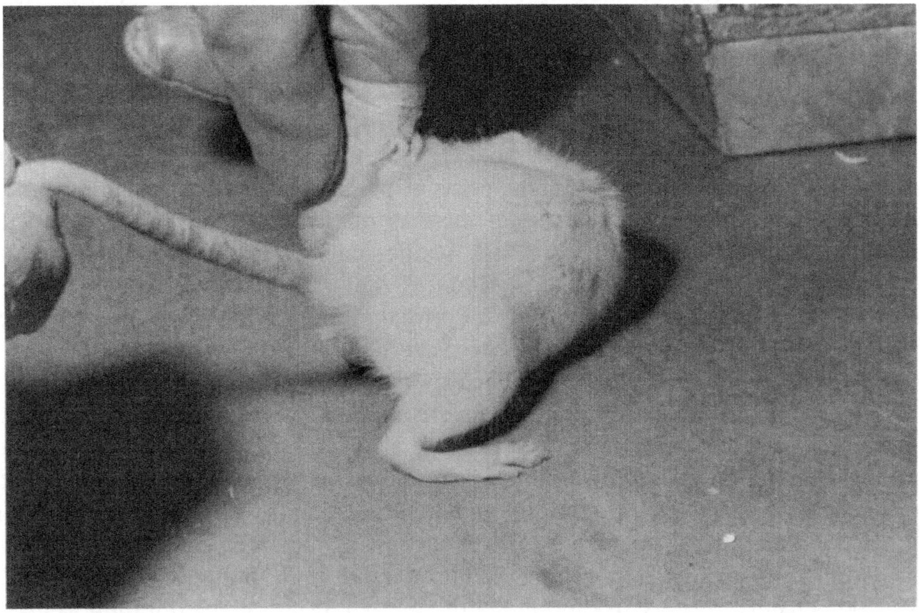

FIG. 2. Appearance of the right hind limb of the same rat shown in Figure 1 after an injection of 0.2 ml of a 2 percent xylocaine solution. Note how the digits are now together, and that the hock is no longer elevated above the substrate.

example, Xylocaine (lidocaine, Astra) 2 percent has the following typical values: onset, 3 minutes; duration, 80 to 100 minutes; frequency, 12/12 (100 percent). Quantitative comparisons between test and control drugs can be made readily. The reader may find other discussions of this method from the pertinent references of Table 1.

Infiltration Anesthesia

With this type of anesthesia, the local anesthetic is deposited around the fine nerve endings by injection under or into the skin. Infiltration anesthesia differs from surface anesthesia in that the latter is produced by direct application of the drug to the epidermal or other surface. Infiltration anesthesia also had its beginnings in the last century when von Anrep (1879) tested cocaine in cutaneous wheals. Since then subcutaneous and intracutaneous (or intradermal) wheals have been favorite methods of testing local anesthetics (Table 1). The technique that will be described is essentially that of Bülbring and Wajda (1945).

Fully grown guinea pigs weighing 300 to 400 grams are used for this test. The backs are shaved with electric shears, care being taken not to abrade the skin. With the use of a 26-gauge, ⅜-inch needle equipped with an intradermal bevel attached to a 0.25-ml tuberculin syringe, injection of the anesthetic solution is made by inserting the needle at an acute angle between the inner and outer layers of skin. The needle needs to be injected only a couple of millimeters into the skin. If it is inserted too far, subcutaneous injections may result. A volume of 0.1 ml is injected, causing a circular wheal to appear on the surface of the skin. Usually three such wheals are made on each side of the back. The wheals are identified further by drawing a circle around each one with a marking pencil. In testing for anesthesia, the investigator pricks the area of the wheal with a needle. If the animals are unanesthetized, a slight prick will cause an obvious twitching reflex. After effective infiltration anesthesia, there is no twitching response, even with repeated pricking. As in the case with sciatic blocks, the animals are tested at convenient intervals. The times of injection, effective block, and recovery are noted on the data sheet. Average values for onset and duration and the frequency (percentage of wheals effectively blocked) are determined.

Again, the design of the particular experiment will dictate the further details. Usually a 1 to 2 percent solution in saline is used; however, concentrations of 0.5 percent of most local anesthetics will produce effective blocks. It is good practice to inject the test drug and control drug in the same animal because sensitivity differences do occur from animal to animal. Four animals with a total of 24 wheals provide a good quantitative basis for comparison. Xylocaine 2 percent will give the following values: onset 2 to 3 minutes; duration, 70 to 90 minutes; frequency, 12/12 (100 percent). A concentration of 0.5 percent will decrease the duration to about one third.

The intradermal wheal test in guinea pigs is valuable in two more respects. Firstly, if the drug has local irritating properties, it will produce erythema and edema. If, after the first examination, the drug appears irritating, the animals can be reexamined 24 hours later, since a good local reaction will have developed by that time. Secondly, this test provides a good basis for evaluation of the actions of epinephrine or other vasoconstrictors injected with the local anesthetic. Local anesthetic drugs in general cause vasodilation. By comparison of the blocking data with and without epinephrine added to the test solutions, a judgment can be made on the actions of vasoconstriction. A marked prolongation of duration indicates strong vasodilation by the local anesthetic drug. An epinephrine concentration of 1:100,000 is a good standard. This concentration added to the usual Xylocaine solution will prolong the duration of block by approximately 100 percent. Epinephrine will also prolong the duration of sciatic nerve blocks in rats. However, the difference is not as marked as in the case of the guinea pig wheals.

Surface Anesthesia

When local anesthetic drugs, either in solution or as crystals, are applied to moist surfaces, they will cause anesthesia. This is because the drug penetrates the surface and blocks the nerve endings. Niemann isolated cocaine and discovered its numbing action on the mucous membranes of the oral cavity, while Koller in 1884 noted its value as a local anesthetic for ophthalmology (Truant and Takman, 1965). Following the pioneering work of Sollmann (1918c), block of the rabbit corneal reflex has come to be a standard test method for evaluating local anesthetics (Table 1).

Albino rabbits are used in these tests. They are placed in rabbit stocks and the upper and lower eyelashes are carefully clipped. An assistant holds open the conjunctival sac, thus making a pocket. The anesthetist, using a 1-ml syringe with a 22-gauge needle, injects the anesthetic solution into the eye pocket. A standardized volume of 0.5 ml is used in our laboratory. The assistant then holds the sac so that the corneal surface is in contact with the solution for 60 seconds. After the exposure period, the corneal surface is touched with a glass rod with a blunt end (Fig. 3). A blunt pencil can also be used. If the eye is anesthetized, the touch of the rod will not elicit the corneal reflex (blinking). Care should be taken not to touch the clipped lashes or the eyelids. Also it is best not to approach the cornea along the direct line of vision. These procedures will assure that the animal is responding only to tactile stimulation of the corneal surface. After the anesthesia wears off, the slightest touch will cause the animal to blink. In actual practice, the anesthetist also tests for the blinking reflex before the solution is placed in the eye.

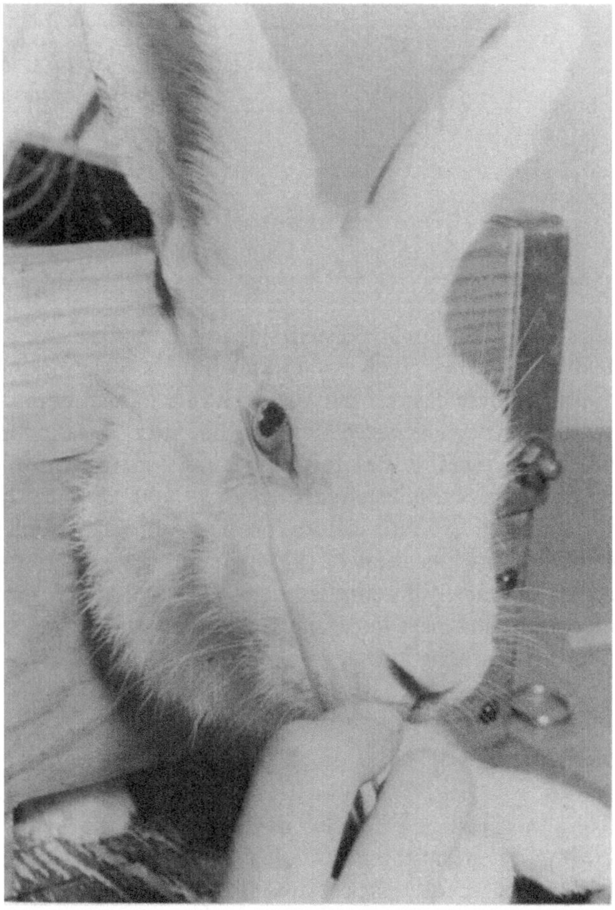

FIG. 3. Technique for stimulation of the rabbit cornea. The rabbit is placed in a stock and the eyelashes clipped. Stimulation is accomplished by mechanical contact of the blunt end of a bent glass rod with the corneal surface.

TABLE 2

A Survey of Various In Vitro Methods Used in Evaluating Local Anesthetics

Preparation	Species	References
Nerve-muscle	Frog	Sollmann, 1917 Meeker, 1925 Sinha, 1936 Ehrenberg, 1948 Skou, 1954a
Isolated nerve	Crab	Dettbarn, 1962
Isolated nerve	Frog	Gasser & Erlanger, 1929 Bennett et al., 1942 Bennett & Chinburg, 1946 Mauro et al., 1958 Truant, 1957, 1958 Rud, 1961 Condouris, 1961 Jefferson, 1963 Ritchie et al., 1965a, 1965b Camougis et al., 1967
Isolated nerve	Rabbit	Ritchie & Greengard, 1961 Ritchie et al., 1965a, 1965b
Isolated nerve	Rat	Condouris & Lagomarsino, 1966
Giant axon	Squid	Narahashi et al., 1967
Single nerve fiber	Frog	Kato, 1934 Tasaki, 1953 Honrubia & Lorente de Nó, 1962 Dettbarn, 1962 Friess & Minzghor, 1965 Hille, 1966

Usually four to six animals are tested side by side. One eye is used for the control solution while the other receives the test solution. The anesthetist tests each eye every 5 minutes. In some cases it may be desirable to test more often. Times of injection, block and recovery are noted. Finally the onset, duration, and frequency values are calculated. Typical values for Xylocaine 2 percent are: onset, 2 to 3 minutes; duration, 20 to 25 minutes; frequency, 6/6 (100 percent). In contrast, the more potent tetracaine will produce a duration of about 60 minutes and an onset of 1 minute following an application of 0.25 percent concentration on the rabbit cornea. However, the potency difference is not as exaggerated in other tests. That is why the complete evaluation of a local anesthetic requires several tests. More will be said about this in the discussion.

Miscellaneous Methods

A number of other tests have been developed for the evaluation of local anesthetics (Table 1). In general the techniques of the earlier papers cited have not been used widely. More recent papers include a technique of abolishing the withdrawal response of an earthworm dipped into 0.0125 N HCl to a depth of 0.25 inch (Block et al., 1964). This method has been used to test a series of new local anesthetics (Kornet, 1966). The technique has been recently modified by Suskevich et al. (1967). Another recent paper (Jones et al., 1965) reports on a quantitative method of evaluating local anesthetics based on the vocalization of mice in response to electrical stimulation. And finally, another report discusses a method of evaluating a local anesthetic by studying its effect on the healing of corneal erosion in the rabbit (Castrén and Lavikainen, 1963). This latter test is a good example of specialized methods developed to test a specific property or action.

IN VITRO METHODS

The critical evaluation of local anesthetics, especially those of clinical value, presented a problem very early. Methods of applying drugs directly to exposed nerves or isolated nerve-muscle preparations were developed in an effort to measure the direct actions of local anesthetics. One has only to read Sollmann (1917) to see how extensive were these early attempts. After electronic instrumentation came into use, direct visualization of the action potential permitted improved measurements of block (Gasser and Erlanger, 1929). Finally various techniques for block of single fibers were developed (Kato, 1934). The developments of in vitro techniques are summarized in Table 2.

Nerve-Muscle Preparation

The isolated nerve-muscle preparation was one of the earlier in vitro methods of testing local anesthetics. The contraction of the muscle after stimulation of the nerve trunk served as the end point for evaluating block of conduction. Only the motor fibers can be tested in this preparation, a limitation that is stressed by Sollmann (1917). Since the magnitude of the response is important, control of the stimulus becomes critical. Sollmann (1917) used an induction coil with the stimulus set considerably above threshold. Later Ehrenberg (1948) and Skou (1954a) used electronic stimulators. Ehrenberg (1948) determined the rheobase, and thus could evaluate the condition of the preparation. All three investigators used the frog.

The nerve-muscle preparation has some advantages over the in vivo methods. In general, whole animal studies are more variable because of many factors, while the isolated preparation can give reliable and accurate data. Also, the isolated preparation permits investigations of physical chemical factors such as the change in pH of the anesthetic solution (Skou, 1954a). Since the details of setting up this preparation are well known in general physiology, they will not be described in this chapter. It is our opinion, however, that the nerve-muscle preparation should be used only if the equipment for studying the action potentials of isolated nerves is not available. The advantages of the isolated nerve preparation outweigh the problems of expense and increased complexity inherent in electrophysiologic methods. Moreover, coping with increasing costs and technical complexity is now a routine matter in most research laboratories.

Isolated Nerve Preparation

In recent years the isolated nerve preparation has largely replaced nerve-muscle preparations. Isolated nerves from various animals have been used, but the frog nerve has been used most extensively (see Table 2).

PREPARATION OF THE NERVE.—A large frog (usually *Rana pipiens*) is sacrificed by severing the vertebral column between the skull and vertebrae with a pair of pointed scissors. A long, slender probe is used to crush the brain and the spinal cord. The skin around the entire body in the region immediately posterior to the forelimbs is cut, and the abdomen and hind legs are skinned by peeling the skin in a posterior direction. The carcass is placed on a dissection board dorsal side up, and the legs are extended and fixed by placing a pin through one of the digits. The fat, muscles, and other tissues are cut in the posterior end of the body so as to expose the nerves extending posteriorly from the cord. The muscles of the thigh are cut and retracted so as to expose the nerve. Finally, the *gastrocnemius* muscle is removed and the *peroneus* muscle is extended laterally from the *tibiofibula*. Then the urostyle is finally severed from the sacral vertebra.

The entire sciatic nerve with branches should now be exposed. A thread with a loop next to the nerve is tied around the nerve in the region of the sacral vertebra. The nerve is then cut anterior to the thread. During the isolation procedure the nerve is kept moist with frog Ringer and manipulated by means of the thread. The connective tissue and the nerve branches are cut carefully as the isolation progresses posteriorly. The nerve is finally cut near the distal end of the *tibiofibula,* and the isolation procedure is complete. The isolated nerve is next extended on a paper towel or filter paper previously soaked with frog Ringer solution. The connective tissue remaining on the nerve during the isolation process is now removed. With the nerve anchored by the thread, the connective tissue is peeled back toward the distal end of the nerve. Any remaining branches are cut at their point of bifurcation. The distal end of the nerve is tied with a length of thread. The *sciatic-peroneal* nerve preparation is now ready for mounting for recording.

MOUNTING THE NERVE FOR RECORDING.—The details for mounting the nerve for recording will depend upon the electrode assembly, nerve chamber, and method of applying the anesthetic. These, in turn, vary considerably from laboratory to laboratory. The essentials, however, are extremely simple. Electrodes for stimulation are placed on one end of the nerve (usually the proximal end) while recording electrodes are placed at the distal end. The anesthetic solution is applied between the two sets of electrodes. Since an average *sciatic-peroneal* nerve preparation is about 8 to 10 cm long, there is sufficient length for many convenient arrangements of electrodes and the technique of applying the local anesthetic. We will describe the method used routinely in our laboratory.

The electrode assembly consists of a series of Ag-AgCl electrodes mounted along a thick strip of Plexiglas. Two electrodes extend beyond the others and serve to guide the nerve into a loop so that it can be immersed at that point into a trough containing the anesthetic (Fig. 4). The nerve is attached by means of the

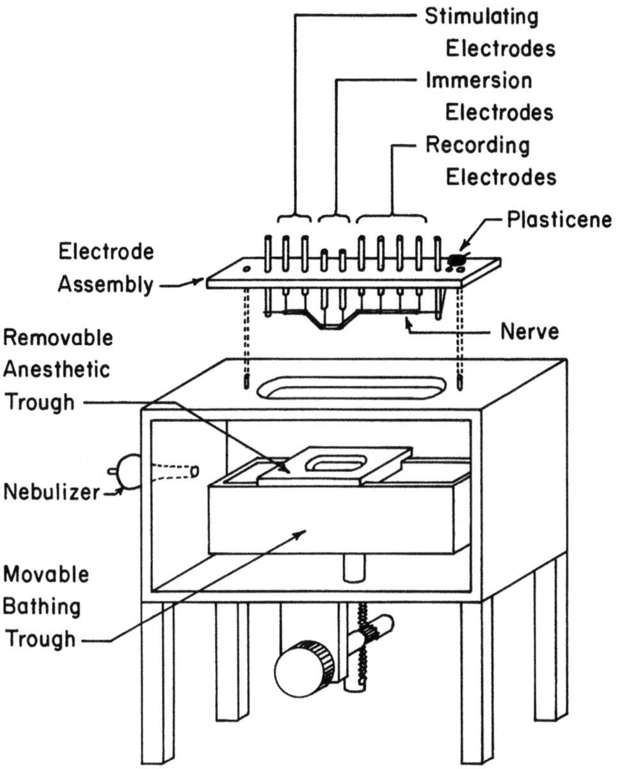

FIG. 4 Diagram of electrode assembly and nerve chamber showing the bathing trough mounted on a rack and pinion, the removable anesthetic trough, and the nebulizer.

threads to terminal posts situated at the two ends of the Plexiglas. The distal end of the nerve is guided along as many of the looped ends of the electrodes as its length permits before it is secured with the thread. It is useful to secure the thread by passing it through a hole in the Plexiglas and securing it in place with Plasticine. Then the tension on the nerve can be readily adjusted. The amount of tension is adjusted so that it is sufficient to prevent the displacement of the nerve away from the electrodes by the surface tension as the nerve is immersed and removed from a trough containing the bathing fluid. The electrode assembly is equipped with two holes which permit it to fit over a nerve chamber. The tops of the electrodes protrude outside, above the chamber, while the lower parts with the nerve are inside the chamber (Fig. 4).

A movable trough operated by a rack and pinion can then be made to move relative to the stationary electrode assembly. This bathing trough contains frog Ringer solution. A smaller, anesthetic trough also made of Plexiglas is then fitted on the bathing trough and is oriented just under the downwardly diverted section of nerve. This section, situated between the two sets of electrodes, is the area to be blocked. The front of the chamber is fashioned as a door, thus permitting it to be closed after making various manipulations inside, such as placing the anesthetic trough. The nerve chamber has a DeVilbiss No. 42 nebulizer inserted at one end for moistening the inside. A nerve that is kept in such a chamber and is periodically bathed in the Ringer solution will last up to 24 hours or longer.

ELECTROPHYSIOLOGIC TECHNIQUE.—Recording action potentials from peripheral nerve is so routine today that many descriptions can be found in the literature, even in elementary textbooks. However, the equipment available is diverse, and it is rare that any two laboratories will have exactly the same assemblage of basic units.

Again, the essentials are very simple; what are required are units for stimulation, amplification, and visual display of the action potential. It is difficult to describe a typical setup other than in general terms. For that reason, specific units will be discussed.

The stimulus pulse is applied through leads connected to two electrodes at the proximal (thick) end of the nerve (Fig. 4). This pulse is provided by a Grass (Model S4) Stimulator coupled with a Grass (Model SIU-4A) Stimulus Isolation Unit (Fig. 5). The operation of these units involves the use of a number of dials and/or switches. Each will be listed with a typical setting:

STIMULATOR		STIMULUS ISOLATION UNIT	
Power	"On"	Mono/Bi	"Mono"
Pulses/DC	"Pulses"	+1/+2	+1
Mono/Bi	"Mono"	Multiplier	0.1
Polarity	+1		
Stimulus	"On"		
Frequency	Varies; usually 3 or 10		
Multiplier	1		
Delay	2-3 msec		
Multiplier	1		
Duration	5 msec		
Multiplier	0.01		
Volts	Varies; 1.5 to 15		
Multiplier	0.1 (not critical)		

The system is coupled to the nerve with a shielded, two-lead cable in the following manner:

1. Connect receptacle No. 1 of the Stimulus Isolation Unit (SIU) to the first stimulation electrode (i.e., that situated nearest to the terminal post).
2. Connect receptacle No. 2 of SIU to the second stimulation electrode. This electrode is the cathode.

The nerve may now be stimulated by placing the mode switch of the stimulator to "Repeat." Best results are obtained when the preparation and electrode assembly are inside a shielded cage that is properly grounded.

The amplification and display system consists of a Tektronix 53/54 E Plug-In Unit and a Tektronix (Type 535) Oscilloscope (Fig. 5). The system is coupled to the nerve by means of a three-lead cord in the following manner:

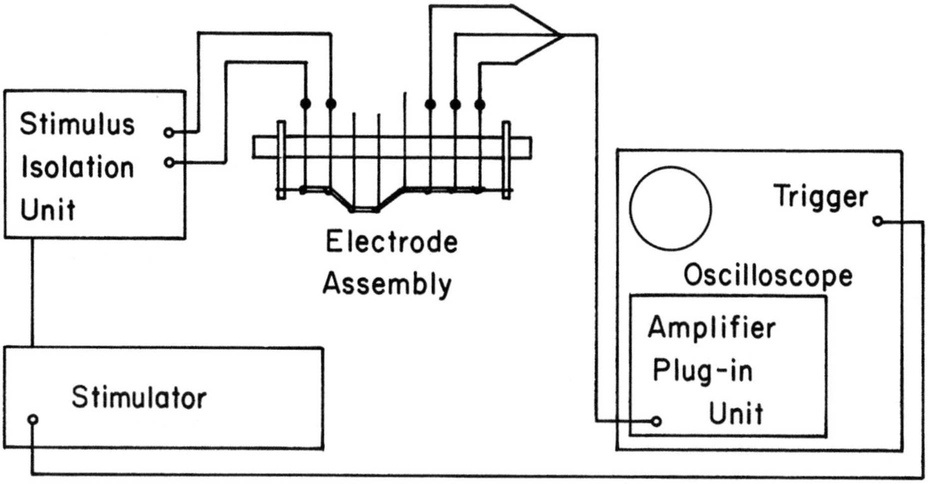

FIG. 5. Block diagram of the electrophysiologic apparatus used for testing the isolated nerve preparation.

1. Black lead (Connection No. 1)–Connected to the third-to-last electrode which makes contact with the nerve; this is the ground lead
2. White lead (Connection No. 2)–Connected to the second-to-last electrode which makes contact with the nerve; this is an active lead
3. Red lead (Connection No. 3)–Connected to the last recording electrode which makes contact with the nerve; this is an active lead

The use of the display system again involves the use of various switches and dials. Each of these is listed with a typical setting:

TEKTRONIX OSCILLOSCOPE	TYPE 535
Power	"On"
Main sweep	
Trigger slope	Ext
Trigger mode	AC fast
Trigger stability and trigger level	Appropriate settings for stable triggering
Time/cm	1
Multiplier	1
Horizontal position	Appropriate for good display

PLUG-IN UNIT	TYPE 53/54E
mv/cm	1 or 0.5
Variable mv/cm	Adjust as necessary
Verticle position	Appropriate for good display
Filters	10 KHz; 8 Hz

Stimulation of the nerve should produce a display on the oscilloscope. Adjusting the voltage setting on the stimulator will cause the action potential to increase and decrease correspondingly on the scope. After pinching the nerve between the last two recording sites, the action potential should be monophasic and appear entirely above the base line. This action potential represents the A spike of the compound action potential.

A good preparation should have an amplitude of about 5 to 10 mv. Its threshold will be a few tenths of a volt. The voltage is adjusted to a value slightly above that required for a maximum A spike. Finally, by varying the stimulus frequency over a range of 1 to 100 pulses/sec and noting the amplitude of the action potential, one can judge the condition of the nerve. A good nerve will not decrease its amplitude to any degree over this frequency range. If the nerve shows high-frequency failure (the so-called Wedensky effect), it may have an abnormal sensitivity to local anesthetics. Therefore, it is advisable to discard nerves with low amplitude action potentials and/or a tendency to decrease their amplitude at high stimulus frequencies (> 50 to 100 pulses/sec). The method described has been developed by Truant; further information can be seen in Mauro, Truant, and McCawley (1948), Truant (1957), and Truant and Wiedling (1958/1959). Rat nerves may also be used (Condouris and Lagomarsino, 1966). However, the relatively shorter length and greater thickness of the rat sciatic nerve compared to the frog is a disadvantage (Camougis, personal observations). Also, it offers no particular advantages for routine testing of local anesthetics.

The instrumentation may vary, as mentioned earlier. Other arrangements that we have used have included the following Tektronix units:

1. Type 535 Oscilloscope, Type 53D/54D Plug-In Unit, and Type 122 Preamplifier
2. Type 532 Oscilloscope and Type 53/54E Plug-In Unit, or Type 53D/54D Plug-In Unit and Type 122 Preamplifier
3. Type 502 Oscilloscope without preamplifier or with a Type 122 Preamplifier

Also the preamplifiers of the Grass Instrument Company used in conjunction with many types of cathode ray oscilloscope are excellent. Recently, inexpensive units of stimulator, amplifier, and oscilloscope have appeared (IMPScope [EV-3], Heath Company; PB3 Scope, Phipps & Bird, Inc.). We have had no experience with these instruments. For stimulation we have also used combinations of the Tektronix 160 series (160A, 161, and 162) and the Bioelectric Instruments Isolator, ISA 129. This combination works very well but is less versatile.

NEUROPHARMACOLOGY.—The test drug is usually made up in a concentration of 5 to 20 mM in frog Ringer of the following composition:

COMPOUND	G/LITER
NaCl	6.5
KCl	0.14
$CaCl_2$	0.12
$NaHCO_3$	0.2
NaH_2PO_4	0.01
Glucose	2.0

If it is known that the compound is unusually strong (e.g., like dibucaine), corresponding dilutions are made. Conversely, if the compound is not very potent, concentrations above 20 mM should be tested; such compounds, however, may have little clinical value. The pH of the test solution is routinely kept between 7.0 and 7.5. Isolated frog nerves will retain their excitability for hours over a pH range of 5 to 9.

Before application of the drug, the amplitude of the A spike is adjusted so that it is 5 cm high on the oscilloscope screen. It is observed periodically for several minutes to ascertain its stability. Then the drug trough is placed on the bathing trough so that it is just under the diverted, center section of the nerve (Fig. 4). This length of nerve must be standardized; 1 cm is a good length, and it is convenient to place the immersion hooks at that interval on the Plexiglas sheet. With the drug trough in position, the nerve is immersed in the anesthetic solution and a time clock is started. At one- or two-minute intervals the amplitude of the A spike is read and plotted on graph paper. For practical purposes, the accuracy of the oscilloscope reading is about 2 percent. Stimulus frequency may be standardized to one frequency (e.g., 10 or 30/sec), or two frequencies may be tested at each time interval.

In our laboratory 30 and 100 pulses/sec are the two standard frequencies. In that way two blocking curves are drawn on the graph paper, since high-frequency failure after drug treatment is usually apparent. After about five minutes of treatment, the drug trough is removed and the nerve is immersed in the Ringer solution of the bathing trough. The nerve is taken out of the bath and the amplitudes are measured at periodic intervals, and thus the recovery process is recorded in graphic form. A block and recovery curve of an isolated nerve treated with Xylocaine is shown in Figure 6.

The details of a given experiment, as always, will depend upon the information desired. In general, the solutions should be sufficiently concentrated to reduce the amplitude of the A spike by 60 to 80 percent (i.e., 20 to 40 percent remaining) within three to five minutes. Then the kinetics of block can be compared between the two drugs. We use Xylocaine as a routine standard although other local anesthetics have also been used. One method of comparing the potencies is to compare the amount of block after a given time of treatment. Another is to compare the times required to achieve a given amount of block, usually 50 percent. Finally, a method that uses a time constant as a measure of rate of block may be employed (Ritchie et al., 1965b). In all of these methods, it will be necessary that the blocking curves be neither too fast nor too slow. Final concentrations for quantitative comparisons can be decided upon rather quickly after a little experience with the drugs being tested. One of the problems with testing local anesthetics is that an isolated nerve shows progressive sensitization to successive treatments. Therefore, a pair of nerves from the same frog are tested together, each nerve receiving three blocks. Nerve I receives test drug, control drug, and test drug in that sequence, while Nerve II receives control drug, test drug, followed by control drug. Careful study of the graphs from the six blocks will reveal the relative potency, the relative reversibility, and the time course for recovery after block. These are all valuable parameters for the sound evaluation of the test drug.

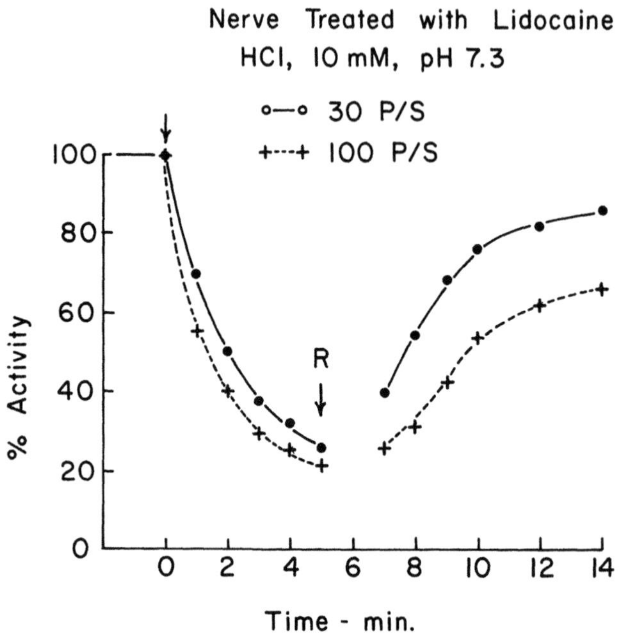

FIG. 6. Block and recovery curves for an isolated frog sciatic nerve treated with a 10 mM solution of lidocaine and stimulated at 30 and 100 pulses per sec. R indicates wash with frog Ringer.

Specialized Techniques with Isolated Nerves

DESHEATHED NERVES.—The nerve is dissected and isolated in the manner described previously. The subsequent steps involved in desheathing call for handling, positioning and, in some instances, exerting tensions on portions of the nerve. Care should be exercised, and these operations should be accomplished by grasping nerve branches along the nerve or the very end of the nerve itself. The nerve is extended on a small (3- by 5-inch) glass plate. The thread at the anterior (central) end of the nerve is fixed in clay. The remains of a nerve branch are found along the first third or so of the nerve. This branch is stretched toward the fixed end of the nerve until the sheath is ruptured at the junction with the main nerve trunk. The sheath in this area is teased away from the nerve fibers and severed. Then, by means of fine forceps, the severed sheath is grasped and pulled over itself toward the distal end of the nerve. The nerve is desheathed over a distance of about one third to one half of its length. However, it may be desheathed to the distal end. The nerve is kept continuously moistened with Ringer during the desheathing process.

The procedure beyond this point is similar to that with the intact nerve. The desheathed nerve is positioned on the electrode assembly so that the desheathed portion will be diverted downward into the anesthetic trough. As a general rule, it takes a local anesthetic of 0.1 to 0.2 times the concentration used on the intact nerve to produce the same degree of block in the desheathed preparation. The desheathed nerve preparation is not recommended for routine screening. Its value lies in its usefulness in testing compounds that give poor block and are suspected of having poor penetration properties. Such compounds can then be tested directly on the excitable fibers. The desheathed nerve was used by Skou (1954a) to test the potencies of several local anesthetics. Condouris (1961) used desheathed bullfrog nerves to study the mechanism of action of cocaine in nerve block. Ritchie and his associates used desheathed nerves from both rabbits and frogs to test the hypothesis that the cationic species of a local anesthetic is the active form (Ritchie and Greengard, 1961; Ritchie, Ritchie, and Greengard, 1965a, 1965b). Camougis et al. (1967) used the desheathed frog nerve in an effort to determine the ionic form of tetrodotoxin responsible for conduction block. Thus the preparation is useful for investigations on the mechanisms of action of excitation block.

EQUILIBRIUM BLOCKS.—It must be remembered that the procedures with isolated nerves already discussed give information on the rates of block; i.e., one plots the change in amplitude as a function of time. Therefore, a comparison of the potency of two drug solutions can be misleading if the penetration rates of the drugs are not similar. Comparison of the blocking data under equilibrium conditions is obviously desirable in certain cases. Equilibrium block with local anesthetics is not studied generally; this is a brief account of a technique developed in our laboratory (Camougis and Newcomer, unpublished information).

Again, the procedure for setting up the isolated nerve for recording is as reported earlier. The nerve need not be diverted downward on the immersing electrodes, as the anesthetic trough is not used. Instead, after the period of control observations, the entire nerve is immersed in the bathing trough (Fig. 4), which is filled with the anesthetic solution. The period of immersion is standardized at 4 minutes. Then the trough is lowered away from the nerve, the nerve is stimulated in air for 1 minute, and the amplitude of the action potential noted. The trough is raised again, the nerve immersed for 4 more minutes, and the procedure repeated over a period of about 30 minutes. Equilibrium is established by this time, and the action potential will not diminish further. The nerve is washed and allowed to recover for at least 1 hour before the next higher concentration is applied. Progressively increasing concentrations result in progressively increasing equilibrium blocks, thus producing a good concentration-effect relation. Several pairs of nerves may be used and the data treated statistically with standard methods

One disadvantage with the method just described is that it is time-consuming. At the suggestion of Dr. Arne Brändström (AB Hässle, Gothenburg, Sweden), we developed a technique for continuous equilibrium blocks. The bathing trough is filled with exactly 125 ml of Ringer at the usual pH. The entire nerve is immersed in the solution, and then the solution is lowered away from the nerve and a reading of the amplitude of the action potential is taken. This is repeated until the amplitude is stable, and the amplitude is adjusted to a convenient height to represent 100 percent on the oscilloscope screen. Then 0.1 or 0.2 ml of a 200 mM drug solution is added to the bath and thoroughly mixed. The nerve is reimmersed

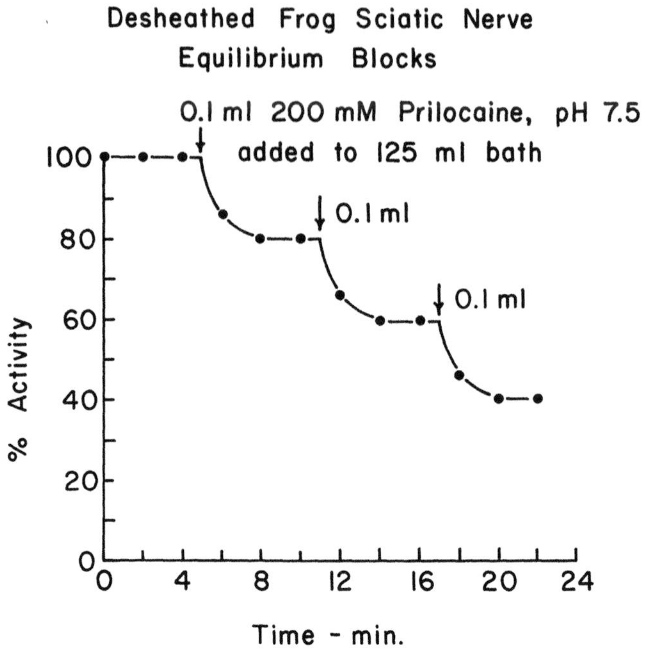

FIG. 7. Graph showing equilibrium blocks of a desheathed frog sciatic nerve after successive treatments with 0.1 ml of 200 mM prilocaine added to 125 ml of Ringer in the bathing chamber.

and amplitude readings are taken at two-minute intervals until two consecutive readings are constant. Equilibrium is usually achieved within a few minutes. Subsequent 0.1- or 0.2-ml aliquots of drug are added periodically, and the new equilibrium blocks are noted. The procedure is repeated until a reasonable degree of block is achieved (50 to 70 percent). The nerve can be recovered and blocked again. If the nerve is blocked to over 90 percent with a potent drug, recovery is poor and another series of blocks cannot be carried out. This procedure may be used with intact or desheathed nerves. Figure 7 shows the results of continuous equilibrium blocks with prilocaine.

SINGLE NERVE FIBERS.—Techniques for studying single nerve fibers were developed soon after electronic instrumentation came in use. Table 2 lists a number of papers in which single-nerve-fiber techniques are used in conjunction with studies on excitation block by various chemicals. The procedure to be described is the one that is used at Astra.

The nerves in the thigh area of the frog are exposed as previously described except that the *gastrocnemius* muscle is not removed. The junction formed by the *tibial* and *peroneal* nerves is traced medially as far as possible, and the *peroneal* nerve is severed at its origin. The sciatic trunk is then severed in the hip area and ligated with thread. The nerve is then dissected from the thigh area and from the *gastrocnemius* muscle, which may then be removed from the carcass. The nerves of

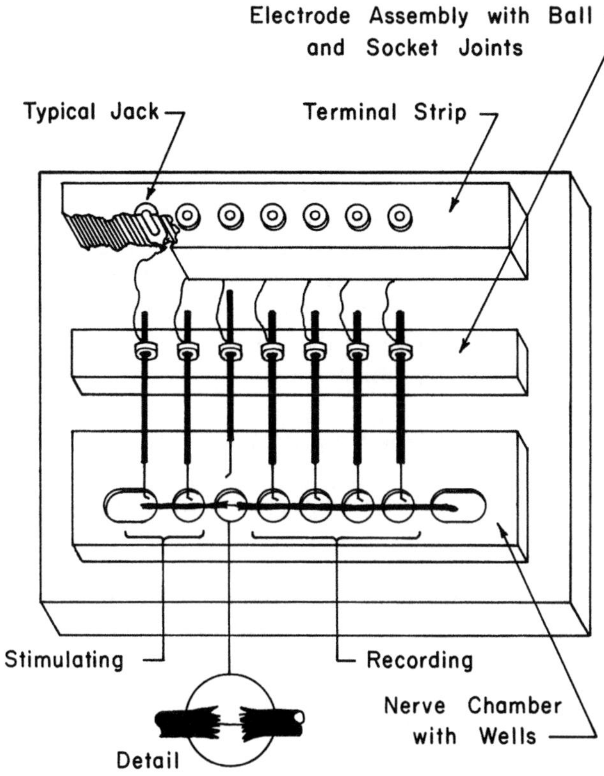

FIG. 8. Diagram of the nerve chamber and electrode assembly for the single nerve fiber preparation.

the lower leg are now exposed, and the *peroneal* nerve is dissected from the leg. All nerves are then cleansed and bathed in frog Ringer solution. The nerve is desheathed along about 40 percent of its length, as previously described. Should a major branch bifurcate below the desheathed area, the desheathing is continued. The branch is then retracted toward the median end of the nerve, separated from the main trunk, and severed. This will insure that the single fiber will not be in this small branch. Working under the microscope, a bundle of nerve fibers which constitute approximately one third of the nerve mass is grasped with a pair of tweezers in the desheathed area. A dissecting needle is placed into the remaining bundle, leaving a small group of fibers in between the needle and tweezers. The instruments are separated from one another until a number of individual fibers appear between them. The pair of tweezers is replaced by a second dissecting needle. The needles are placed along the sides of a selected fiber, and the remaining fibers are withdrawn and severed.

The nerve must then be transferred to a bioelectric couple which consists of a series of wells prepared in a Plexiglas sheet and a number of movable electrodes (Fig. 8). The junctions between all wells are covered with petroleum jelly to prevent electrical continuity of the Ringer between wells. The third well is then half-filled with frog Ringer solution. The distal ends of the nerve are brought together. This is accomplished in such a manner that, when the nerve is picked up by the ends, the severed sections will coincide, and consequently no tension will be placed on the single fiber as it is raised from the dissection glass. The single fiber portion of the nerve is lowered into the well containing Ringer solution. The anterior portion of the nerve is fixed across the first two wells, whereas the posterior portion is fixed across the remaining wells. Petroleum jelly is once more applied to the junctions between wells. Each well is then supplied with Ringer solution. An Ag-AgCl electrode is placed next to the nerve in each well.

The stimulating system is the same as described in Section B. The same settings are appropriate for this preparation as well, and the stimulating leads are connected to the two wells containing the anterior part of the nerve. The display system consists of the following units:

1. A Tektronix Type RM 122 Low-Level Preamplifier and its Tektronix Type FM 125 Power Supply
2. A Tektronix Type 535 Oscilloscope equipped with a Tektronix Type 53 D/54D Plug-In Unit

The system is coupled to the biologic system by means of a three-lead cord connected to the recording electrodes. The use of this system again involves the use of various switches and dials. Each of these is listed with typical settings:

LOW-LEVEL PREAMPLIFIER	TYPE 122
Low freq. resp.	0.2 Hz
High freq. resp.	10 KHz
Voltage gain	1,000
Power	"On"
PLUG-IN UNIT	TYPE 53D/54D
Input selector	A(AC)
mv/cm	10
mv/cm (Multiplier)	2
OSCILLOSCOPE	TYPE 535
Power	"On"
Main sweep	
Trigger slope	Ext
Trigger mode	AC fast
Trigger stability and trigger level	Appropriate for good triggering stability
Time/cm	1 msec
Multiplier	1
Horizontal position	Appropriate for good display

Other instrumentation combinations may be used, as with the multifiber preparations. For example, the Tektronix Type 502 Oscilloscope may be used with a Tektronix Type 122 Preamplifier. With the single fiber, the electrical signal from the preparation is much weaker than with the whole nerve. Consequently more amplification is used. This in turn causes a much "noisier" baseline, and some skill is required to get meaningful results from this preparation. The drug solution may be applied to any well. However, for routine investigations it is applied to a well between the electrode pairs other than that in which the single fiber is located. If the drug is applied to the single fiber, care must be exercised because of the possibility of mechanical injury to the fiber. Also, strong drug solutions must be avoided because irreversible blocks occur readily. See Tasaki (1953) for a similar technique in preparing single fibers.

Miscellaneous Methods

The methods to be mentioned in this section are not used routinely to evaluate local anesthetics. Consequently they will be discussed only briefly. It is felt that they should be listed in order to give the interested reader somewhat more perspective in available in vitro methods.

Nerve ganglia in both frogs and crayfish have been studied. Aceves and Machne (1963) used the spinal ganglia of frogs for intracellular studies on the actions of local anesthetics and calcium on excitation. In this way, both the action potentials and the membrane potentials could be studied. Camougis (1967, 1968) studied the actions of various anesthetic drugs on the spontaneous electrical activity of isolated crayfish ganglia. While the pharmacology of this preparation is relatively unknown, the technique does have the possibility of detecting potential central excitation. For example, cocaine is unique in stimulating the ganglia when compared to conventional local anesthetics.

Local anesthetics have been tested on various muscle preparations. Bianchi and his associates have studied the actions of local anesthetics on coupling systems (Bianchi and Bolton, 1967) and on oxygen consumption (Novotny and Bianchi, 1967) in frog skeletal muscle. Giering and Truant (1957) reported that lidocaine produced sensitization to epinephrine in the in vitro rat uterus. Similar sensitization did not occur with the other local anesthetics tested. Finally, Åström (1964) demonstrated that some local anesthetics have a nonspecific antagonism to epinephrine-induced contractions of isolated strips of rabbit aorta.

Other studies have included various cells and tissues. Brändström et al. (1964) studied the hemolytic actions of a homologous series of local anesthetics, and concluded that the hemolysis is related to the distribution coefficient. Kalyanpur and Ryman (1966) studied the actions of several local anesthetics on intermediary metabolism in *E. coli,* brain slices, and tissue homogenates. Rand and Wilson (1967) used several in vitro preparations and concluded that the local anesthetic and adrenergic blocking activities of a series of guanidine compounds were unrelated.

The papers cited are only examples of many techniques. Local anesthetics depress the excitability of tissues generally, and one could predict the additional studies on myoneural junction block, myocardial tissue block, and actions on the autonomic system. However, a further survey is beyond the intentions of this chapter.

TOXICITY METHODS

The toxicology of local anesthetics has aspects that are both general and specific. Their general toxicology is outside the scope of this chapter, since the underlying mechanisms of metabolism, distribution, excretion, etc., are common to all drugs. In this section, attempts will be made to focus on toxicologic problems that are of more specific interest in the evaluation of local anesthetics. The two major considerations are the danger of systemic toxicity resulting in respiratory and even cardiac arrest, and the possibilities of local irritation at the site of administration. These considerations are of such overriding importance that it is highly desirable to have acute toxicity and irritation data before any extensive tests are made with all the other methods.

Acute Toxicity

MICE.—Initial determinations of acute toxicity should be done with mice because of the advantages of simplicity, economy, and the existence of much published information. Intravenous injections should be given first choice; however, additional data from intraperitoneal plus subcutaneous injections give valuable information on the drug. Concentrations, the weight of the animals, the limits on the volumes injected, and the rates of injection should be standardized. The techniques for the administration of drugs by various routes in mice are widely known and will not be described. Pertinent papers referring to local anesthetics are listed in Table 3. The most useful data are the LD_{50} values, the lethal doses for 50 percent of a group of mice. Specific methods for determination of the LD_{50} can be found in Turner (1965). Each laboratory should do a series of tests with a standard (usually procaine or lidocaine), since Wiedling (1964) has shown clearly how the LD_{50} values from a variety of sources may vary.

The first step in evaluating the acute toxicity data is simply to compare the LD_{50} values. Additional insight can be gained by comparing the LD_{50} values from several routes of administration. The smaller the ratios between the intravenous, intraperitoneal, and subcutaneous values, the greater is the rate of uptake of the drug into the vascular compartment. Good examples of rapid uptake with tetracaine in contrast to some other local anesthetics can be seen both in rabbits (Åström and Persson, 1961a) and in mice (Åström et al., 1964) with different routes of administration. Another important consideration is how the animals die. Conventional local anesthetics in toxic doses kill by causing respiratory failure. Still higher doses will cause cardiac failure. This cause of death is ascertained by quickly opening up the thoracic cavity soon after death and noting the presence or absence of heartbeat. Symptoms prior to death may include mydriasis, emesis, salivation, and convulsions.

Vasoconstrictors added to the local anesthetic may provide additional information. However, the results must be interpreted with caution. The conflicting

TABLE 3

A Survey of Various Methods Used in Evaluating the Toxicity of Local Anesthetics

Method	Species	References
Acute toxicity	Mice	Rider, 1930 Wiedling, 1952, 1960 Luduena & Hoppe, 1952 Hint & Richter, 1958 Richter, 1958 Truant, 1958
Acute toxicity	Rabbit	Truant, 1958 Åström & Persson, 1961a
Loss of righting reflex	Rabbit	Åström & Persson, 1961b Åström, 1965
Acute toxicity	Cat	Truant, 1958
Acute toxicity	Dog	Truant, 1958
Acute toxicity	Monkey	Truant, 1958
Use of vasoconstrictors with local anesthetics	Various	Avant & Weatherby, 1960 Luduena et al., 1960 Åström et al., 1964 Åström & Persson, 1965 Åkerman, 1966
Irritation, ear	Rabbit	Wiedling, 1960
Irritation, back and abdomen	Rabbit	Hoppe et al., 1950 Luduena & Hoppe, 1952 Tait et al., 1958 Truant, 1958
Irritation, eye	Rabbit	Draize et al., 1944 Hoppe et al., 1950 Tait et al., 1958

results of several investigators are discussed by Wiedling (1964). Both Avant and Weatherby (1960) and Åström et al. (1964) found that only with tetracaine out of several common local anesthetics did the addition of epinephrine cause a significant decrease in toxicity after subcutaneous injections. Meanwhile, Luduena et al. (1960) found that L-nordefrin increased the toxicity of mepivacaine when injected subcutaneously in mice, but reduced the toxicity in guinea pigs or rabbits. With intravenous injections, Åström et al. (1964) found that all the local anesthetic solutions tested tended to be more toxic when epinephrine was added, and that this increase appeared to be accounted for on the basis of the added toxicity from the epinephrine. Such findings, however, may have no clinical relevance, since there is no clinical counterpart to the increase in toxicity on the addition of vasoconstrictors (Wiedling, 1964). This is explained by the difference in size between laboratory animals and human patients. In spite of the problems outlined, skillful use of epinephrine in acute toxicity tests with local anesthetics, especially in subcutaneous injections, can provide added insight into the absorption of the test drug.

RABBITS.—Since sublethal toxic doses have greater clinical significance, laboratory tests to study such doses are important. Again, many tests exist with many animals. The rabbit has been found to be very useful for testing sublethal doses. One valuable test is to make repeated injections in the rabbit and thus study its tolerance to the possible cumulative effects of a given drug.

The rabbit (weight, 2.5 to 4.0 kg) is placed in a rabbit stock, and the region around the marginal ear vein is wiped with alcohol. An injection is made into the marginal ear vein using a sterile syringe and needle. Usually a 5-ml syringe equipped with a 20-gauge, 1-inch B bevel needle is used. The dose administered depends upon the toxicity of the drug. Normally a 2 or 4 percent solution is used, and sufficient volume is given so that the dose per injection is 5 mg/kg or 10 mg/kg. The injection is given over a 1-minute period. After an injection the animal is placed on the floor and observed. The behavior and gross physiologic functions of the animal are observed and recorded. If the first dose is nontoxic, the animal is injected again 15 minutes later with the same dose. This may be done up to about 10 times at 15-minute intervals. If no toxic symptoms appear, then that dose given over 60 seconds and repeated for that specific number of times at 15-minute intervals is well tolerated. The next step is to increase the dose by a reasonable amount. Then with a fresh rabbit the procedure is repeated. Toxic symptoms that appear commonly include depression, convulsions, rigid extension of limbs, gasping for breath, and loss of the righting reflex. A large dose may kill the animal before the second injection. Death is usually caused by respiratory or cardiac arrest. Xylocaine usually will not produce any severe toxic symptoms with doses up to about 5 mg/kg. With doses of 5 to 10 mg/kg severe depression will occur, and repeated doses above 10 mg/kg are usually lethal in the rabbit.

Another method is to determine the convulsive dose for 100 percent of the animals (CD_{100}). Then the animals are injected intravenously with the CD_{100} at periodic intervals. The cumulative effects of the drugs can then be determined by noting the incidence of death or the prolongation of the convulsic period. Using this method, Truant (1958) concluded that meprylcaine had a more rapid disposition after injection than procaine.

A third variation of testing tolerance in rabbits is to study the loss of the righting reflex (LRR) after repeated doses. Doses sufficient to cause a brief LRR are selected for the first injection. The duration of the LRR is timed after each injection. Again, doses, rates of injection, and the interval between injections are standardized. Data from several animals with each drug are pooled and appropriate statistical analysis can be made. Using injection intervals of 15 minutes to study the LRR, Åström (Åström and Persson, 1961b; Åström, 1965) was able to conclude that prilocaine is detoxified faster than lidocaine.

Irritation

The rabbit has been used extensively for irritation studies. The ears, back, abdomen, and eyes have all been used as sites of study (Table 3). We have found that the rabbit back is a reliable and simple place to study irritation. The technique that will be described is the one we use routinely; it is essentially the same test reported by others (Table 3).

The rabbit is placed in a rabbit stock and its back is shaved with hair clippers equipped with a No. 40 or Angora hair blade. The hair is shaved from the neck to the rump for two inches on either side of the vertebral column. Care should be exercised not to irritate the skin (clipper burn), and those animals that do not shave cleanly should be discarded. Several circles about 3 cm in diameter are then drawn along both sides of the spine with a soft-tip marking pen. Four or five such circles on either side are a convenient number. Since the texture of the epidermis and hair varies from neck to rump, the circles should be grouped as near to the middle of the back as conveniently possible. The circles will be the sites of the wheals, and they are identified from front to rear and right (R) and left (L) with numbers (e.g., L1, L2, L3, L4, L5; R1, R2, R3, R4, R5). The injections are made near the center of the circles in a manner already described for the guinea pig wheals. It is important to use sterile needles, syringes, and solutions because microbial contamination may produce an inflammatory response. It is unnecessary to swab the sites of injection with germicides. A volume of 0.1 ml is used for each wheal. After the injections are made, the animals are returned to their cages; they are examined about 24 hours later.

In observing the results of the irritation tests, the investigator looks for reactions characterized by erythema, edema, and in extreme cases a central zone of discoloration. This central zone is clearly visible and will oftentimes become necrotic. One of the problems with this irritation test is the comparative difficulty of quantitation. An experienced observer is required for the proper assessment of various degrees of tissue reaction. Truant (1958) and Tait et al. (1958) scored the irritation on scales of 0 to 4, each grade corresponding to specific criteria of irritation. Recently Lebeaux and Camougis (unpublished information) developed a method of scoring that is based on the following:

ERYTHEMA

absent	0
slight	1
moderate	2
marked	3

EDEMA

absent	0
slight	1
moderate	2
marked	3

SIZE OF REACTION (DIAM.)

5 mm or less	1
5 mm to 10 mm	2
greater than 10 mm	3

CENTRAL ZONE OF DISCOLOR

absent	0
present	1

Thus a score of 0 to 10 is possible for a given wheal. The scores of all the wheals for a given solution are added, and the average is called the "mean irritation score." The detailed design of the irritation test may vary. As mentioned, 8 to 10 wheals may be made on one animal. Two wheals may be made with saline controls, while a control anesthetic solution and a test anesthetic solution are used for the remaining wheals. Usually the concentrations are in the range of 0.5 to 2.0 percent. The procedure should be repeated in several animals. An average irritation score for the several animals is thus obtained. Paired data can be treated with routine statistical methods.

Two other points are worth mentioning in regard to irritation testing. Weatherby (1940) and Hoppe et al. (1950) describe a technique in which trypan blue is used for better visualization of the toxic reaction. Subsequent studies that use this technique include those of Luduena and Hoppe (1952), Luduena et al. (1960), and Tait et al. (1958). The second point is the quantitative technique described by Hoppe et al. (1950) and Luduena and Hoppe (1952). A graphical method is used to analyze irritation data; the concentration is plotted against the degree of irritation. From the graph a Threshold Irritant Concentration for an irritation score of 4 (TIC_4) is determined by Luduena and Hoppe (1952). This allows for convenient comparisons of the concentrations of various drugs required to achieve the same degree of irritation.

PHYSICAL-CHEMICAL METHODS

When there is need for a chemical method (analytic, physical-chemical, or biochemical) as an adjunct to a biologic study, it is wise to remember that the pitfalls in the design of this part of the study can be as treacherous and difficult to recognize as any part of the biologic experimentation. Therefore, it is a wise move to discuss the technical as well as the theoretical chemical aspects with an expert—or at least to make an effort to understand the specific chemical area of interest to the investigation, not just superficially, but by intensive and critical reading of pertinent literature.

Besides being of value in the characterization of a molecule, physical-chemical data are used in efforts to achieve correlation between local anesthetic activity and structure, or structure-related parameters. As it may be necessary to have knowledge of more than one elementary physical-chemical property to be able to compose a more complex function to which one wants to correlate some biologic variable, it is often found that rather extensive experimental work must be undertaken to provide for necessary physical-chemical data for the study. For example, calculation of the thermodynamic distribution coefficient necessitates the measurement of both apparent distribution coefficient and pK_a (Löfgren, 1948, p. 110).

Determination of pK_a

The strength of an anesthetic base can be determined in several ways. Most local anesthetics have pK_a values between 7 and 10, and this is well inside the range that allows the use of methods based on measurement of the pH of a water solution containing the base and an appropriate amount of a strong acid (Löfgren, 1948). Therefore, variation on this theme is probably the most common approach to obtain information on pK_a values for the dominating basic function of most local anesthetics. If the water solubility of the base form of the anesthetic is very low, the measurements can be performed in alcohol-water mixtures (cf. Büchi and Perlia, 1962, p. 124). For weak basic functions–e.g., the *p*-amino group of procaine or the ring nitrogen of dibucaine–no valid information can be obtained by this method. It is possible to use instead a spectrophotometric procedure in the cases where the base and its conjugate acid give rise to sufficiently different absorption spectra; see, e.g., Büchi and Perlia (1962, p. 127).

Distribution Coefficients

In principle, distribution coefficients are determined by equilibrating a compound between two phases, one being water (i.e., a buffer solution) and the other a suitable water-immiscible organic solvent or lipid. When equilibrated, the concentration in the two phases is determined and the distribution coefficient can be calculated. The use of distribution coefficients in local anesthetic research is, of course, related to our efforts to gain information on the way an agent will be distributed in different compartments of the body, particularly in nerve. It is obvious that also the rate with which the agent will penetrate into a compartment will be of great importance (see later).

Dwelling on the distribution coefficients first, it seems a priori natural to try to find an organic phase as close to natural body lipids in its properties as possible. Fish oils and oleyl alcohol, besides a number of more conventional organic solvents, have been recommended as such solvents. Brändström (1964b) found, in a study of the distribution coefficients for a series of five tetracaine homologues comparing four different solvents as lipid phase, that the obtained groups of distribution coefficients for each lipid phase formed an almost parallel family of curves when plotted against the number of carbon atoms of the varied part of the molecule. This indicates that the choice of organic phase is not of absolute importance if the interest is the comparison of the magnitudes of the distribution coefficients; at least this seems to be true for a homolgous series, and sufficiently so for closely related compounds.

A few experimental methods of distribution coefficient determinations are given in the following as examples. Löfgren (1948, p. 107) determined distribution coefficients for lidocaine and several of its homologues and analogues by titration of the remaining drug in the buffer phase after equilibrium. A number of dibucaine homologues were investigated by Büchi and Perlia (1962, p. 142) using a polarographic method for the concentration determinations. Büchi, Cordes, and Perlia (1964) later used Lofgren's method for a number of procaine analogues. A rapid and versatile method, particularly suitable for screening, was designed by Brandstrom (1963) using an automatic titrator.

Other Techniques

Diffusion and surface-related phenomena must obviously be close to the attention of the investigator of local anesthesia. Rud (1961) and Büchi and Perlia (1962, p. 145) have studied diffusion of local anesthetics and give references to earlier work and various techniques. Skou's work on surface and interfacial activities and penetration of monomolecular lipid layers (1954b, 1954c, 1954d) gives great emphasis to experimental detail besides being of theoretical interest. For references to later work on various types of model systems in this area of research, the reader is referred to Ritchie and Greengard (1966). Adsorption of local anesthetics on active charcoal has been described by Büchi and Perlia (1962, p. 230). Sekera and Vrba (1960) used displacement adsorbability comparing a series of local anesthetics to methylene blue. The distribution rate for lidocaine between octanol and water has been described by Brändström (1964a); in a dynamic system, the velocity of penetration into a lipid layer obviously can be of greater importance than the distribution coefficient itself. Association of similar molecules into aggregates sometimes can take place. Rohmann et al. (1959) as well as Büchi and Perlia (1962, p. 101) have studied this phenomenon on two homologous series.

ANALYTIC METHODS

The need for analytic methods usually arises after the preliminary screening, and even the specialized pharmacology, have been completed. Attention becomes focused on one or, at most, a few specific compounds. The need to understand the metabolism of the drug becomes dominant. Progressing even further, the analytic procedures are necessary to support clinical testing in humans. A number of methods are currently in use for studying the metabolism of local anesthetics. Several of these methods will be discussed in this section. Earlier discussions of analytic methods applied to local anesthetic research can be found, among others, in Adriani (1962) and in Buchi and Perlia (1962, p. 74).

With few exceptions, the direct analytic determination has to be preceded by isolation steps. It is often extremely important to pay attention to the stability of the studied drug, not only during the period of the analytic determination but also during the time between sampling and determination. Especially with biologic samples is carefulness to be recommended; needless to say, the same goes for drawing analogies from earlier experiences with the same drug in a different animal species. As an example, some findings can be cited in a study of the determination of tetracaine in blood (Porush et al., 1965). Fifteen minutes after the addition of tetracaine to human blood in vitro at 37°C, only 39 percent could be recovered, and after 60 minutes, the agent was completely decomposed. From dog blood the recovery at the same times was 87 and 79 percent, respectively. Similar findings for procaine have been reported (Kisch et al., 1943). The variation in stability for different drugs is indeed wide. For example, human blood containing lidocaine or prilocaine can be kept for a few weeks at room temperature without any observed loss (Keenaghan et al., 1968).

Titration Methods

Titrimetric methods in the determination of local anesthetics of amine type are as a rule only applicable when the agent is present in fairly high concentration. Usually such methods cannot be used in determinations of the drug in biologic tissue samples or blood. They can, however, be of value in checking purity or concentration of commercial or pharmaceutical preparations and in determination of pK_a values and distribution coefficients. The variations in technique to be used in a particular case depend on the purpose and the characteristics of the agent under study. Sufficiently strong bases can be determined in water or water-alcohol mixtures (Löfgren, 1948, p. 29; Bullock and Grundy, 1955); weaker bases have to be analyzed in nonaqueous solution–e.g., titration with perchloric acid in glacial acetic acid, using the latter as solvent.

Spectrophotometric Methods

Colorimetric or spectrophotometric methods offer better possibilities for determination of low concentrations in most cases. Anesthetics that possess suitable absorption maxima, usually in the ultraviolet region, may, after necessary separation procedures, be assayed directly (Porush et al., 1965). However, it is sometimes possible to modify the anesthetic molecule in a way that will give rise to a derivative with absorption in the visible range and/or with a higher extinction coefficient than the drug itself. This procedure can be utilized, for instance, for compounds with aromatic primary amino groups, e.g., procaine, which can be transformed into azo compounds (Brodie et al., 1948). In another technique, the anesthetic is first precipitated as a water-insoluble salt with ammonium reineckate. The precipitate is then redissolved in acetone and the amount of drug determined colorimetrically or spectrophotometrically (Örtenblad and Jonsson, 1951). In the case of organic bases, there is also the possibility of forming a complex with a dye containing an acid group–such as methyl orange, tropaeolin 00, bromothymol blue–so that the complex can be quantitatively extracted into an organic solvent. Sung and Truant (1954) modified the methyl orange technique of Brodie and Udenfriend (1945) for determining the disposition of lidocaine in animals and human volunteers. Hollunger (1960a, 1960b) used the same method to study the metabolism of lidocaine in rabbit tissue. Whereas the gas chromatographic method (see below) offers certain advantages, the methyl orange method is still very useful, as evidenced by an extensive, recent study on the metabolism of lidocaine and mepivacaine in rodents (Heinonen, 1966). Using this method, one has to make sure that no other amino compounds that may interfere by forming complexes with the methyl orange are present. The following procedure is that used at Astra for the analytical determination of Xylocaine and Citanest:

ANALYTIC PROCEDURE:

1. Into a round-bottom, glass-stoppered, 50-ml centrifuge tube, pipette 1 to 4 ml of sample (giving 2 to 30 μg of compound).
2. Add 0.5 ml of trichloroacetic acid (TCA) and mix thoroughly.
3. Add 0.5 ml of 10 N sodium hydroxide and mix thoroughly.
4. Add 10 ml of ethylene dichloride (EDC), shake mechanically for 10 minutes, and centrifuge (about 1,500 rpm) for 5 minutes.
5. Remove aqueous phase by aspiration.
6. Add 5 ml of phosphate buffer, shake 5 minutes, centrifuge, and remove aqueous phase by aspiration.
7. Repeat buffer wash (step 6), carefully removing all traces of water.
8. Transfer 7.5 ml of the EDC phase to a 15-ml glass-stoppered centrifuge tube containing 0.25 ml of isoamyl alcohol, and mix.
9. Add 1 ml of supersaturated methyl orange reagent.
10. Shake mechanically for 3 minutes, centrifuge for 5 minutes, and remove excess methyl orange reagent by aspiration.
11. Pipette 5 ml of the organic phase into calibrated Coleman tubes containing 1 ml of the sulfuric acid-ethanol reagent. Mix well.
12. Read optical density (OD) at 530 mμ in a Coleman-Junior Spectrophotometer, using water for the zero setting.
13. A blank, consisting of the sample without the drug, must also be run through the same procedure.

CALCULATIONS:

Read concentration of sample (OD of sample minus OD of blank) directly from a standard curve (OD vs. concentration).

REAGENTS:

1. Reagent grade ethylene dichloride.
2. 15 percent trichloracetic acid.
3. 10 N sodium hydroxide.
4. Phosphate buffer: to 735 ml of a 0.5 M solution of KH_2PO_4, add approximately 265 ml of 0.5 M $Na_2HPO_4 \cdot 7H_2O$, bringing to a pH of 6.22.
5. Reagent grade isoamyl alcohol.
6. Methyl orange reagent:
   a. Dissolve 1 g of methyl orange in 200 ml of distilled water. Wash twice with 200 ml of EDC, discarding the organic phase.
   b. Saturated boric acid solution: 48 g of boric acid dissolved in 800 ml of warm distilled water.
   c. Just before use, mix equal volumes of the saturated boric acid solution and the 0.5 percent methyl orange solution.
7. Sulfuric acid-ethanol reagent: 2 percent sulfuric acid in absolute ethanol.

Chromatographic Methods

Paper and thin-layer chromatography have found use in qualitative as well as quantitative analyses for local anesthetics. These methods complement quantitative methods, which do not discriminate between different kinds of compounds, no matter how sensitive they are quantitatively. The techniques are useful, especially where the available amounts of drug do not easily permit the direct use of IR spectroscopy or other, similar instrumental methods for identification. Examples of studies using paper chromatography of local anesthetics include Procházka (1966), Büchi and Perlia (1962, p. 89), Gurrieri and Musumeci (1960), Hannig and Karau (1959), and Wagner (1953). For thin-layer methods see Gänshirt (1965), Sunshine and Fike (1964), Šaršunová (1963), and Büchi and Fresen (1966).

Gas-liquid chromatography (GLC) has become more and more important as a quantitative as well as a qualitative analytical procedure. It is, when the thermostability of the anesthetic allows its use, a very sensitive method, often useful down to concentrations of 0.1 μg/ml, or lower. Mixtures of two local anesthetics can be determined quantitatively at the same time; by judicious use of an internal standard, the reproducibility can be made quite satisfactory. Examples of GLC technique applied to local anesthetics have been described by Koehler and Hefferren (1964), Vessman (1964), Beckett et al. (1965, 1966), Svinhufvud et al. (1965), Katz (1966), Pratt et al. (1967), and Keenaghan (1968). It can be advantageous to prepare derivatives of the sample substance, from the viewpoint of obtaining compounds that either are more thermostable or have a lower boiling point, thus making it possible to apply GLC methods to their analyses. Derivatives can also be of value in GLC to help in establishing the identity of drugs (cf. Beckett et al., 1967). It is also worth adding that, as a rule, some other separation technique has to precede the chromatographic procedure, most often an extraction step.

Tracer Technique and Autoradiography

The use of tracer and autoradiographic technique, as with other analytical methods, is based on the need to understand the physiologic disposition of a drug. Such techniques are receiving widespread use in general pharmacology and toxicology, and the reader with a deep interest in this field should consult specific research papers. This section will discuss briefly how tracer techniques and autoradiography have been used to study local anesthetics.

Caution is essential in the interpretation of the obtained results. As the radioactivity will be observed where the radioactive isotope resides at the time of measurement, it is, of course, important to know if it is still part of the original local anesthetic molecule or part of a metabolic product. Therefore, the techniques give maximum information when they are combined with proper separation and identification methods. This combination of methods can facilitate the correct mapping of the metabolic pathway, and supplies the necessary quantitative data for a correct understanding of the metabolic fate of the drug.

Geddes (1965) combined tracer and paper chromatography techniques to study the metabolic breakdown of ^{14}C-labeled prilocaine; this study involved both in vitro and in vivo experiments. Hansson et al. (1965) studied the excretion and biotransformation of ^{14}C-labeled mepivacaine in mice and rats. The study included separation by thin-layer chromatography of mepivacaine and its metabolites. The uptake and release of ^{14}C-prilocaine by isolated guinea pig atria was studied by Lahrtz et al. (1967). They checked the absence of labeled metabolites by paper chromatography.

Another approach has been to do autoradiography with tissues or even whole animals cut in sections. Bromage et al. (1963) studied the penetration of ^{14}C-labeled lidocaine into the neuraxis after injection into the extradural space of dogs. Autoradiograms of sections of the spinal cord showed a relatively greater accumulation of radioactive material along the periphery of the tissue mass. Kristerson, Nordenram, and Nordqvist (1965) exposed the sciatic nerve of the rabbit to ^{14}C-labeled mepivacaine in solution. Subsequent autoradiograms of the nerves revealed the highest concentration of local anesthetic to be in the sheath. Thus the technique is sensitive enough to give a quantitative indication of drug accumulation. In another study, Kristerson, Hoffmann, and Hansson (1965) did whole-body autoradiographic studies of the distribution of ^{14}C-labeled mepivacaine in mice cut in sagittal section. By varying the time interval between injection and sacrifice, a good understanding of the dynamic changes in drug distribution was possible.

DISCUSSION

In the final analysis, the main objective in testing and evaluating compounds with local anesthetic activity is to find a clinically useful agent. Fulfillment of this objective requires at least two things. Firstly, "clinically useful" must be defined for that particular laboratory, and, secondly, a prediction of what will happen with the clinical trials is required. Defining what is clinically useful is very difficult because considerations in addition to scientific and medical questions often play a role in the formulation of policy within which such a definition may be made. Nevertheless, there are some universal agreements as to what constitutes a useful local anesthetic. For example, good agreement can be found among a review article (Gray and Geddes, 1954), a medical reference book (Bonica, 1953), and a pharmacology textbook (Truant and Takman, 1965). For our purposes we can list the requirements of a useful local anesthetic agent as follows:

1. Adequate potency
2. Complete reversibility
3. Rapid onset
4. Excellent frequency

5. Suitable duration
6. Minimal local irritation
7. Minimal systemic toxicity
8. Good solubility
9. Good chemical stability

The reader will note quickly that even such a list allows considerable latitude for the interpretation of a given property. For example, what is "rapid onset"? It is here that we must rely on the careful comparison between the test and control drugs. A drug is useful clinically if it offers advantages over existing drugs.

The next question is, how can we predict the results of clinical trials? The answer is, of course, that we cannot predict accurately, for the very rationale of good clinical pharmacology is to provide a feedback of information to the research laboratory. Adriani (1960) points out the difficulty of predicting results in humans from animal data. Ekenstam (1966) has pointed out that the electronic computer may have future use in evaluating local anesthetics, as demonstrated by Koeltzer and Wehr. In the meanwhile, reliance on animal data plus experience and judgment provide the only answer. We have found that those agents that are used clinically generally produce good results with animals. However, all agents that give good blocks in animals need not prove to be useful clinically. It is here that the toxicity and chemical data must be examined critically.

Once selection of a compound or a small number of compounds has been made because of favorable data from the preliminary tests, secondary testing can be carried out. As mentioned briefly, skillful use of vasoconstrictors is important in evaluating both the pharmacology and the toxicology of the compounds (Adriani, 1960; Avant and Weatherby, 1960; Luduena et al., 1960; Åström et al., 1964; Åström and Persson, 1965; Åkerman, 1966). Cardiovascular effects, especially changes in blood pressure, should be investigated carefully (Truant, 1958; Truant and Wiedling, 1958/1959; Wiedling, 1960; Åström and Persson, 1961b). Acute and subacute toxicology consistent with standard procedures for all drugs are carried out if the compounds are to go to the clinic. Finally, the chemical stability and other pharmaceutical questions must be considered before going to the clinical trials.

While the clinical pharmacology of any drug is today a highly specialized area of drug research, it might be useful to outline some of the literature pertaining to local anesthetics. The earlier literature included tests with humans for infiltration blocks (Sollmann, 1918d; Meeker, 1925; Rider, 1930; Sinha, 1936), conduction block (Sinha, 1936), and surface anesthesia (Sollmann, 1919; Schmitz and Loevenhart, 1924; Meeker, 1925). However, these are not to be considered clinical tests but an extension of animal testing to human subjects. Nevertheless, such tests have played a definite role in evaluating local anesthetics in the past. It is debatable whether they would be useful today. Recent papers on the clinical testing of local anesthetics in humans include evaluation of conduction block (Löfström and Thulin, 1965), intradermal infiltration (Padfield, 1967), and dental anesthesia (Cowan, 1964). An extensive investigation of both local anesthesia and toxicity in both volunteers and patients is reported by Eriksson

(1966). The reader interested in the clinical pharmacology of local anesthetics should read Adriani (1960), Löfström (1966), and Bromage (1967). It is essential that investigators involved actively in the pharmacology of local anesthetics understand some of the clinical aspects of local anesthesia.

In conclusion, we will make one final point. Ekenstam (1966) states that it has often been emphasized that modern local anesthetics possess such good properties that only minor progress can be made at high expense. We agree with him that such a statement appears premature. We have need today for compounds with short durations, very long durations, and greater margins of safety. Certainly there is sufficient opportunity for the imaginative chemist to synthesize novel compounds with local anesthetic properties. The control of pain is a human enterprise that warrants optimism and our best efforts.

REFERENCES

Aceves, J., and Machne, X. 1963. The action of calcium and of local anesthetics on nerve cells, and their interaction during excitation. J. Pharmacol. Exp. Ther., 140:138-148.

Adams, R., Rideal, E. K., Burnett, W. B., Jenkins, R. L., and Dreger, E. E. 1926. Chemical constitution, physiological action and physical properties in a series of alkyl paraaminobenzoates. J. Amer. Chem. Soc., 48:1758-1770.

Adriani, J. 1960. The clinical pharmacology of local anesthetics. Clin. Pharmacol. Ther. 1:645-673.

— 1962. The Chemistry and Physics of Anesthesia. 2nd ed. Springfield, Ill., Charles C. Thomas.

Åkerman, B. 1966. On felypressin (Octapressin®) as an adjunct to lidocaine and prilocaine–an experimental study in animals. Acta Pharmacol., 24:377-378.

Åström, A. 1964. Influence of some local anesthetics upon the adrenaline contraction of isolated strips of rabbit aorta. Acta Physiol. Scand., 60:30-38.

— 1965. Factors affecting the action of Citanest® in vivo. Acta Anesth. Scand. Suppl. 16, pp. 23-27.

— and Persson, N. H. 1961a. The toxicity of some local anesthetics after application on different mucous membranes and its relation to anesthetic action on the nasal mucosa of the rabbit. J. Pharmacol. Exp. Ther., 132:87-90.

— and Persson, N. H. 1961b. Some pharmacological properties of o-methyl-α-propylamino propionanilide, a new local anesthetic. Brit. J. Pharmacol., 16:32-44.

— and Persson, N. H. 1965. Influence of adrenaline on the action of some local anesthetic agents tested in rats. Acta Pharm. Suec., 2:397-402.

— Persson, N. H., and Örtengren, B. 1964. The effect of adrenaline on the toxicities and absorptions of L67 (Citanest®) and some other local anesthetics studied in mice and rabbits. Acta Pharmacol., 21:161-171.

Avant, W. E., and Weatherby, J. H. 1960. Effects of epinephrine on toxicities of several local anesthetic agents. Proc. Soc. Exp. Biol. Med., 103:353-356.

Barlow, R. B. 1964. Introduction to Chemical Pharmacology, 2nd ed. London, Methuen.

Beckett, A. H., Boyes, R. N., and Appleton, P. J. 1966. The metabolism and excretion of lignocaine in man. J. Pharm. Pharmacol. (Suppl.), 18:76-81S.

— Boyes, R. N., and Parker, J. B. R. 1965. Determination of lignocaine in blood and urine in human subjects undergoing local analgesic procedures. Anesthesia, 20:294-298.

— Tucker, G. T., and Moffat, A. C. 1967. Routine detection and identification in urine of stimulants and other drugs, some of which may be used to modify performance in sport. J. Pharm. Pharmacol., 19:273-294.

Bennett, A. L., and Chinburg, K. G. 1946. The effects of several local anesthetics on the resting potential of isolated frog nerve. J. Pharmacol. Exp. Ther., 88:72-81.

— Wagner, J. C., and McIntyre, A. R. 1942. The determination of local anesthetic-potency by observation of nerve action-potentials. J. Pharmacol. Exp. Ther., 75:125-136.

Bianchi, C. 1956. A simple new quantitative method for testing local anesthetics. Brit. J. Pharmacol., 11:104-106.

Bianchi, C. P., and Bolton, T. C. 1957. Action of local anesthetics on coupling systems in muscle. J. Pharmacol. Exp. Ther., 157:388-405.

Bieter, R. N., Harvey, A. McG., and Burgess, W. W. 1932. Spinal anesthesia in summer frogs. J. Pharmacol. Exp. Ther., 45:291-298.

— Cunningham, R. W., Lenz, O. A., and McNearney, J. J. 1936. Threshold anesthetic and lethal concentrations of certain spinal anesthetics in the rabbit. J. Pharmacol. Exp. Ther., 57:221-244.

Block, B. P., Potts, D. J., and Finney, R. S. H. 1964. A simple method for the evaluation of local anesthetic activity using earthworms. J. Pharm. Pharmacol. (Suppl.), 16:85-88T.

Bonica, J. J. 1953. The Management of Pain. Philadelphia, Lea & Febiger.

Brändström, A. 1963. A rapid method for the determination of distribution coefficients of bases for biological purposes. Acta Chem. Scand., 17:1218-1224.

— 1964a. A method for the determination of distribution velocity of bases for biological purposes. Acta Pharm. Suec., 1:145-158.

— 1964b. The use of distribution coefficients in predicting lipid concentration of drugs. Acta Pharm. Suec., 1:159-164.

— Malm, L., and Persson, N. H. 1964. Physico-chemical aspects of the haemolytic effect of local anaesthetics. Acta Pharm. Suec., 1:139-144.

Brodie, B. B., Lief, P. A., and Poet, R. 1948. Fate of procaine in man following its intravenous administration and methods for the estimating of procaine and diethylaminoethanol. J. Pharmacol. Exp. Ther., 94:359-366.

— and Udenfriend, S. 1945. The estimation of basic organic compounds and a technique for the appraisal of specificity. Application to the Cinchona alkaloids. J. Biol. Chem., 158:705-714.

Bromage, P. R. 1967. Physiology and pharmacology of epidural analgesia. Anesthesiology, 28:592-622.

— Joyal, A. C., and Binney, J. C. 1963. Local anesthetic drugs: Penetration from the spinal extradural space into the neuraxis. Science, 140:392-393.

Büchi, J., and Fresen, J. S. 1966. Dünnschichtchromatographische Untersuchungen an homologen und analogen Lokalanästhetica-Reihen. Pharm. Acta Helv., 41:551-574.

— and Perlia, X. 1962. Beziehungen zwischen den physikalisch-chemischen Eigenschaften und der Wirkung von Lokalanästhetica. Aulendorf i. Wurtt, Editio Cantor.

— Cordes, G., and Perlia, X. 1964. Beziehungen zwischen den physikalisch-chemischen Wirkung einiger Procain-Analoge. Arzneimittelforschung, 14:161-169.

Bülbring, E., and Wajda, I. 1945. Biological comparison of local anesthetics. J. Pharmacol. Exp. Ther., 85:78-84.

Bullock, K., and Grundy, J. 1955. Lignocaine hydrochloride and its solutions: purity, tests, stability and assay. J. Pharm. Pharmacol., 7:755-773.

Camougis, G. 1967. Unmasking of a photoinhibitory response in the crayfish caudal ganglion following partial anesthesia. Comp. Biochem. Physiol., 21:231-236.

— 1968. Neuropharmacology of invertebrates: Quantitative studies with an isolated CNS preparation. *In* Efron; D. H., ed. Psychopharmacology, A Review of Progress 1957-1967. Washington, D.C., U.S. Government Printing Office. 1969.

— Takman, B. H., and Tasse, J. R. P. 1967. Potency difference between the zwitterion form and the cation forms of tetrodotoxin. Science, 156:1625-1627.

Carney, T. P. 1951. Benzoates and substituted benzoates as local anesthetics. *In* Medicinal Chemistry. Suter, C. M., ed. New York, John Wiley & Sons, Inc.

Castrén, J. A., and Lavikainen, P. 1963. Animal experiments with a new surface anesthetic. Acta Ophthal., 41:674-677.

Chance, M. R. A., and Lobstein, H. 1944. The value of the guinea-pig corneal reflex for tests of surface anesthesia. J. Pharmacol. Exp. Ther., 82:203-210.

Condouris, G. A. 1961. A study of the mechanism of action of cocaine on amphibian peripheral nerve. J. Pharmacol. Exp. Ther., 131:243-249.

— and Lagomarsino, W. E. 1966. Adrenalectomy in rats and its influence on local anesthesia of peripheral nerves. J. Pharmacol. Exp. Ther., 152:417-424.

Copeland, A. J. 1924. A preliminary report on cocaine, butyn, tutocain, and other local anesthetics. Brit. Med. J., 2:41-44.

Corning, J. L. 1885. Spinal anesthesia and local medication of the cord. New York J. Med., 40:483-485.

Cowan, A. 1964. Minimum dosage technique in the clinical comparison of representative modern local anesthetic agents. J. Dent. Res., 43:1228-1249.

de Jong, R. H., and Wagman, I. H. 1963. Physiological mechanisms of peripheral nerve block by local anesthetics. Anesthesiology, 24:684-727.

Dettbarn, W. D. 1962. The active form of local anesthetics. Biochim. Biophys. Acta, 57:73-76.

Draize, J. H., Woodard, G., and Calvery, H. O. 1944. Methods for the study of irritation and toxicity of substances applied topically to the skin and mucous membranes. J. Pharmacol. Exp. Ther., 82:377-390.

Dvorak, H., and Manson, M. H. 1930. Technique of spinal anesthesia in the dog. Proc. Soc. Exp. Biol. Med., 28:344-347.

Ehrenberg, L. 1948. The time-concentration curve of local anesthetics. Acta Chem. Scand., 2:63-81.

Ekenstam, B. A. 1966. The effect of the structural variation on the local analgetic properties of the most commonly used groups of substances. Acta Anaesth. Scand. Suppl. 25, pp. 10-18.

Eriksson, E. 1966. Prilocaine: An experimental study in man of a new local anesthetic with special regards to efficacy, toxicity and excretion. Acta Chir. Scand. Suppl. 358.

Friess, S. L., and Minzghor, K. R. 1965. Blockade of excitable nodes of Ranvier by stereoisometric phenylacetate esters of tropine and ψ-tropine series. III. Arch. Biochem., 111:61-66.

Gänshirt, H. 1965. Pharmaceutical products. *In* Thin-layer Chromatography. Stahl., E., ed. New York, Academic Press, Inc.

Gasser, H. S., and Erlanger, J. 1929. The role of fiber size in the establishment of a nerve block by pressure or cocaine. Amer. J. Physiol., 88:581-591.

Geddes, I. C. 1965. Studies of the metabolism of Citanest C^{14}. Acta Anaesth. Scand. Suppl. 16, pp. 37-44.

Giering, J. E., and Truant, A. P. 1957. Lidocaine sensitization of the in vitro rat uterus to action of epinephrine. Fed. Proc., 16.

Gary, T. C., and Geddes, I. C. 1954. A review of local anesthetics. J. Pharm. Pharmacol., 6:89-114.

Gurrieri, S., and Musumeci, S. 1960. Identificazione di piccole quantita di cocaina nella novocaina a mezzo della cromatografia su carta. Boll. Sedute Accad. Gioenia Sci. Nat. Catania, [5] 5:489-496.

Hannig, E., and Karau, W. 1959. Zum papierchromatographischen Verhalten des Falicains neben anderen gebräuchlichen Lokalanaesthetica. Pharmazie., 14:153-156.

Hansson, E., Hoffman, P., and Kristerson, L. 1965. Fate of Mepivacaine in the body: II. Excretion and biotransformation. Acta Pharmacol., 22:213-223.

Heinonen, J. 1966. Influence of some drugs on toxicity and rate of metabolism of lidocaine and mepivacaine: Experimental study on mice and rats. Ann. Med. Exp. Biol. Fenn. (Suppl. 3), 44:7-43.

Hille, B. 1966. Common mode of action of three agents that decrease the transient change in sodium permeability in nerves. Nature, 210:1220-1222.

Hint, H. C., and Richter, A. W. 1958. A simple intravenous infusion technique for mice. Method and some applications. Acta Pharmacol., 14:153-157.

Hirschfelder, A. D., and Ridges, A. H. 1933. Bloodless method for recording respiration and quantitative determination of alterations of sensation in small animals. Proc. Soc. Exp. Biol. Med., 30:958-962.
Hollunger, G. 1960a. On the metabolism of lidocaine I. The properties of the enzyme system responsible for the oxidative metabolism of lidocaine. Acta Pharmacol., 17:356-364.
— 1960b. On the metabolism of lidocaine II. The biotransformation of lidocaine. Acta Pharmacol., 17:365-373.
Honrubia, V., and Lorente de Nó, R. 1962. On the effects of anesthetics upon isolated, single frog nerve fibers. Proc. Nat. Acad. Sci. U.S.A., 48:2065-2067.
Hoppe, J. O., Alexander, E. B., and Miller, L. C. 1950. Use of the trypan blue and rabbit eye tests for irritation. J. Amer. Pharm. Ass. 39:147-151.
Jefferson, G. C. 1963. The assessment of conduction anesthesia. J. Pharm. Pharmacol., 15:92-99.
Jones, W. R., Kerley, T. L., and Weaver, L. C. 1965. Quantitative evaluation of conduction anesthetics in albino mice. J. Pharm. Sci., 54:1680-1681.
Kalyanpur, S. G., and Ryman, B. E. 1966. Some effects of local anaesthetics on cell metabolism. Biochem. Pharmacol., 15:691-701.
Kato, G. 1934. The Microphysiology of Nerve. Tokyo, Maruzen.
Katz, J. 1966. Stability of local anesthetics after autoclaving: Determined by gas chromatography. Anesthesiology, 27:835-837.
Keenaghan, J. B. 1968. The determination of lidocaine and prilocaine in whole blood by gas chromatography. Anesthesiology, 29:110-112.
— Boyes, R. N., and Gipson, E. M. 1968. Stability of lidocaine and prilocaine in human whole blood. (personal communication).
Kisch, B., Koster, H., and Strauss, E. 1943. The procaine esterase. Exp. Med. Surg., 1:51-65.
Koehler, H. M., and Hefferren, J. J. 1964. Gas-liquid chromatography of local anesthetics and related compounds. J. Pharm. Sci., 53:745-747.
Kornet, M. J. 1966. New local anesthetics. I. Esters of 1,2-diethyl-3-hydroxymethylpyrazolidine. J. Med. Chem., 9:493-495.
Kristerson, L., Hoffmann, P., and Hansson, E. 1965. Fate of mepivacaine in the body: I. Whole-body autoradiographic studies of the distribution of ^{14}C-labelled mepivacaine in mice. Acta Pharmacol., 22:205-212.
— Nordenram, Å., and Nordqvist, P. 1965. Penetration of radio-active local anaesthetic into peripheral nerve. Arch. Int. Pharmacodyn., 157:148-151.
Lahrtz, H. G., Lüllmann, H., and van Zwieten, P. A. 1967. Accumulation and release of ^{14}C-prilocaine by isolated guinea pig atria. Europ. J. Pharmacol., 1:177-187.
Langston, J. B., Yeager, P. A., Simrell, W. D. and Hogg, M. 1967. Evaluation of a topical anesthetic for use in urology. Invest. Urol., 5:149-154.
Loewe, S. 1936. Pseudohernia, a visible manifestation of local anesthetic action. J. Pharmacol. Exp. Ther., 56:238-251.
Löfgren, N. 1948. Studies on Local Anesthetics. Xylocaine: A New Synthetic Drug. Stockholm, Ivar Haeggströms.
Löfström, B. 1966. Evaluation of local anesthetics in man. Acta Anaesth. Scand. Suppl. 25, pp.23-26.
— and Thulin, L. 1965. Procedures for objective evaluation of nerve blocks. Acta Anaesth. Scand., 9:213-221.
Luduena, F. P. 1957. Experimental spinal anesthesia. Arch. Int. Pharmacodyn., 109:143-156.
— and Hoppe, J. O. 1951. 2-Phenyl-4-thiazolidone derivatives as local anesthetics. J. Amer. Pharm. Ass., 40:132-137.
— and Hoppe, J. O. 1952. Local anesthetic activity, toxicity and irritancy of 2-alkoxy analogs of procaine and tetracaine. J. Pharmacol. Exp. Ther., 104:40-53.
— and Hoppe, J. O. 1956. 2-Alkoxy benzoate and thiobenzoate derivatives as local anesthetics. J. Pharmacol. Exp. Ther., 117:89-96.

— Hoppe, J. O., Coulston, F., and Drobeck, H. P. 1960. The pharmacology and toxicology of mepivacaine, a new local anesthetic. Toxic. Appl. Pharmacol., 2:295-315.
MacIntosh, F. C., and Work, T. S. 1941. Some aminoethanol derivatives possessing local anesthetic activity. Quart. J. Pharm., 14:16-25.
Mauro, A., Truant, A. P., and McCawley, E. L. 1948. Electrophysiological methodology for studies in neuropharmacology. Yale J. Biol. Med., 21:113-120.
Meeker, W. R. 1925. The potentiation of novocaine solutions. J. Lab. Clin. Med., 11:139-162.
Meyer, K. H. 1937. Contributions to the theory of narcosis. Trans. Faraday Soc., 33:1062-1064.
Munch, J. C., Pratt, H. J., and De Ponce, A. M. 1933. Quantitative applications of the modified Türk test. J. Amer. Pharm. Ass., 22:1078-1080.
Narahashi, T., Anderson. N. C., and Moore, J. W. 1967. Comparison of tetrodotoxin and procaine in internally perfused squid giant axons. J. Gen. Physiol., 50:1413-1428.
Nieschulz. O., Hoffman, L., and Popendiker, K. 1958. Zur Pharmakologie des N-(4-phenoxymethyl-γ-phenylpropyl)-morpholin, eines aminoathers mit lokalanaesthetischer wirkung. Arzneimittelforschung., 8:539-544.
Novotny, I., and Bianchi, C. P. 1967. The effect of Xylocaine on oxygen consumption in the frog sartorius. J. Pharmacol. Exp. Ther., 155:456-461.
Örtenblad, B., and Jonsson, K. 1951. A rapid colorimetric method for the assay of Xylocaine ® and the determination of some other organic bases, using ammonium reineckate. Acta Chem. Scand., 5:510-518.
Padfield, A. 1967. The intradermal local analgesic action of prilocaine. A controlled double-blind comparison with lignocaine and procaine. Anaesthesia, 22:556-561.
Porush, I., Shimamura, A., and Takahashi, L. T. 1965. Determination of tetracaine in blood. J. Pharm. Sci., 54:1809-1810.
Pratt, E. L., Warrington, H. P., and Grego, J. 1967. The gas chromatographic determination of mepivacaine in blood with a note on other local anesthetics. Anesthesiology, 28:432-437.
Procházka, Ž. 1966. Partition chromatography. *In* Laboratory Handbook of Chromatographic Methods. Mikeš, O., ed. London, Van Nostrand.
Rand, M. J., and Wilson, J. 1967. The relationship between adrenergic neurone blocking activity and local anaesthetic activity in a series of guanidine derivatives. Europ. J. Pharmacol., 1:200-209.
Richter, A. W. 1958. Estimation of the i.v. mean lethal dose for mice by a constant infusion titration. Acta Pharmacol., 15:37-42.
Rider, T. H. 1930. Local anesthetics derived from dialkylamino propandiols. I. Phenylurethans. J. Pharmacol. Exp. Ther., 39:457-467.
Ritchie, J. M., and Greengard, P. 1961. On the active structure of local anesthetics. J. Pharmacol. Exp. Ther., 133:241-245.
— and Greengard, P. 1966. On the mode of action of local anesthetics. Ann. Rev. Pharmacol., 6:405-430.
— Ritchie, B., and Greengard, P. 1965a. The active structure of local anesthetics. J. Pharmacol. Exp. Ther., 150:152-159.
— Ritchie, B., and Greengard, P. 1965b. The effect of the nerve sheath on the action of local anesthetics. J. Pharmacol. Exp. Ther., 150:160-164.
Rohmann, C., Eckert, T., and Heil, G. 1959. Über Einen Zusammenhang von Molekül-Assoziation und Wirkung bei Oberflächenanästhetika. Arch. Pharm., 292:255-260.
Rose, C. L. 1931. Studies in the pharmacology of local anesthetics; V. A discussion of the present methods of evaluating local anesthetics. Anesth. Analg., 10:159-164.
Rud, J. 1961. Local Anesthetics. An electrophysiological investigation of local anesthesia of peripheral nerves, with special reference to Xylocaine. Acta Physiol. Scand. Suppl., 178, Vol. 51.
Šaršunová, M. 1963. Dünnschichtchromatographie ohne Bindemittel in der Arzneimittelanalyse. Pharmazie, 18:748-750.

Schmitz, H. L., and Loevenhart, A. S. 1924. A comparative study of local anesthetic properties of p-amino benzoyl di-iso-propyl amino ethanol hydrochloride ("Isocaine"), cocaine, procaine and butyn. J. Pharmacol. Exp. Ther., 24:167-177.
Sechzer, P. H. 1965. The effect of organophosphates on nerve conduction. Arch. Int. Pharmacodyn., 157:432-441.
Sekera, A., and Vrba, Č. 1960. Studies on local anesthetics. XXV. (Physicochemical properties of drugs V). J. Amer. Pharm. Ass., 49:394-398.
Shackell, L. F. 1935. Tests of local anesthetics by sciatic nerve block in the intact guinea pig. Anesth. Analg., 14:20-22.
Sinha, H. K. 1936. The local anesthetic actions of certain pyrazoline and quinoline compounds. J. Pharmacol. Exp. Ther., 57:199-220.
Skou, J. C. 1954a. Local anaesthetics. I. The blocking potencies of some local anaesthetics and of butyl alcohol determined on peripheral nerves. Acta Pharmacol., 10:281-291.
— 1954b. Local anaesthetics. IV. Surface and interfacial activities of some local anaesthetics. Acta Pharmacol, 10:305-316.
— 1954c. Local anaesthetics. V. The action of local anaesthetics on monomolecular layers of stearic acid. Acta Pharmacol., 10:317-324.
— 1954d. Local anaesthetics. VI. Relation between blocking potency and penetration of a monomolecular layer of lipoids from nerves. Acta Pharmacol., 10:325-337.
Sollmann, T. 1917. Comparative activity of local anesthetics. I. Paralysis of the motor nerve fibers. Direct application to the sciatic nerve of the frog J. Pharmacol. Exp. Ther., 10:379-397.
— 1918a. Comparative activity of local anesthetics. II. Paralysis of sensory nerve fibers. J. Pharmacol. Exp. Ther., 11:1-7.
— 1918b. Comparison of activity of local anesthetics. III. Anesthesia of frog skin. J. Pharmacol. Exp. Ther., 11:9-15.
— 1918c. Comparison of activity of local anesthetics. IV. Anesthesia of rabbit's cornea. J. Pharmacol. Exp. Ther., 11:17-25.
— 1918d. Comparative efficiency of local anesthetics. V. Anesthesia of the human skin. General conclusions. J. Pharmacol. Exp. Ther., 11:69-80.
— 1919. Comparative activity of local anesthetics. VI. Difficulty soluble anesthetics on mucous membranes. J. Pharmacol. Exp. Ther., 13:429-431.
— and Hanzlik, P. J. 1928. Experimental Pharmacology. Philadelphia, W. B. Saunders Company.
Sung, C. Y., and Truant, A. P. 1954. The physiological disposition of lidocaine and its comparison in some respects with procaine. J. Pharmacol. Exp. Ther., 112:432-443.
Sunshine, I., and Fike, W. W. 1964. Value of thin-layer chromatography in two fatal cases of intoxication due to lidocaine and mepivacaine. New Eng. J. Med., 271:487-490.
Suskevich, J., Campbell, A. H., and Lord, G. H. 1967. A modification of a method for the evaluation of topical anaesthesia in the earthworm. J. Pharm. Pharmacol., 19:456-459.
Svinhufvud, G., Örtengren, B., and Jacobson, S. E. 1965. The estimation of lidocaine and prilocaine in biological material by gas chromatography. Scand. J. Clin. Lab. Invest., 17:162-164.
Tait, C. A., Reese, N. O., and Davis, D. A. 1958. A comparative study of hexyclaine, procaine and lidocaine with specific attention to tissue irritation. Southern Med. J., 51:358-366.
Tasaki, I. 1953. Nervous Transmission. Springfield, Illinois, Charles C Thomas, Publisher.
Truant, A. P. 1957. Local anesthetic studies on isolated frog sciatic nerves. Fed. Proc., 16:341.
— 1958. Studies on the pharmacology of meprylcaine (Oracaine), a local anesthetic. Arch. Int. Pharmacodyn., 115:483-497.
— 1965. Local anesthetic and toxicologic properties of Citanest. Acta Anaesth. Scand. Suppl. 16, pp. 23-27.
— and Takman, B. 1965. Local anesthetics. *In* Drill's Pharmacology in Medicine, 3rd ed. DiPalma, J. R., ed. New York, McGraw-Hill Book Company.

— and Wiedling, S. 1958/1959. A contribution to the pharmacological and toxicological evaluation of a new local anesthetic, dl-N-methylpipecolyl-2,6-xylidide. Acta Chir. Scand., 116:351-361.
Turner, R. A. 1965. Screening Methods in Pharmacology. New York, Academic Press, Inc.
Vessman, J. 1964. Gas chromatography of high boiling amines. Acta Pharm. Suec., 1:183-198.
Von Anrep, B. 1879. Über die physiologische Wirkung des Cocain. Pfluger Arch. Ges. Physiol., 21:38-77.
Wagner, G. 1953. Die papierchromatographische Identifizierung und quantitative Trennung einiger Lokalanaesthetica. Arch. Pharm., 286:232-241.
Weatherby, J. H. 1940. A method for the qualitative estimation of chemical irritation. J. Lab. Clin. Med., 25:1199-1204.
— 1964. Local Anesthetics. *In* Evaluation of Drug Activities: Pharmacometrics. Lawrence, D. R., and Bacharach, A. L., eds. New York, Academic Press, Inc.
Wiedling, S. 1952. Contributions to the pharmacology and toxicology of Xylocaine. Acta Pharmacol., 8:117-133.
— 1960. Studies on α-n-propylamino-2-methylpropionanilide—a new local anesthetic. Acta Pharmacol., 17:233-244.
— 1964. Xylocaine: The Pharmacological Basis of its Clinical Use, 2nd ed. Stockholm, Almqvist and Wiksell.

CHAPTER 2

Myocardial Metabolism and Blood Flow

S. Gudbjarnason, P. S. Puri, C. Cowan and R. J. Bing

Department of Medicine, Wayne State University School of Medicine and Harper Hospital, Detroit, Michigan

ANALYSIS OF THE MYOCARDIAL ENZYME PROFILE

Introduction

Quantitative and qualitative alterations in the enzyme profile of cardiac muscle have been observed following infarction (Gudbjarnason et al., 1968; Gudbjarnason and Priver, 1968), congestive heart failure (Gudbjarnason et al., 1964), and cardiac hypertrophy (Fox and Reed, 1969). The enzyme profile or pattern is a characteristic for a particular organ, and significant changes in the enzyme profile of a tissue may indicate alterations in cellular metabolism. Changes in enzyme profile may then reflect altered substrate availability, altered energy requirements, altered biochemical environment, and tissue injury accompanied by permeability changes or even proliferation of different cell types, such as fibroblasts and leukocytes. It must also be pointed out that alterations observed in enzyme activity, as measured in tissue extracts in vitro, do not necessarily reflect

The original studies cited in this chapter were supported by U.S. Public Health Service Grant No. HE-05043, Michigan Heart Association, The John A. Hartford Foundation, and United Foundation of Detroit.

accurately the alterations in the tissue in vivo, since numerous factors can influence the activity of an enzyme, such as concentrations of the substrate, product, cofactors and coenzymes, allosteric regulators, inhibitor, activator, conformational changes, etc. This procedure differs from the histochemical staining procedure insofar as it measures the optimal attainable activity under most favorable conditions, whereas the histochemical staining procedure used for evaluation of myocardial damage may often reflect the depletion of labeled substrates and cofactors from the infarcted muscle (Nachlas and Shnitka, 1963).

The functional significance of the enzyme profile is further complicated by the oscillatory performance of metabolic pathways, where activities vary over a large range, indirectly demonstrating control features which are imposed upon the pattern at multiple sites along the pathway.

Despite all these difficulties, recent studies have indicated that the myocardial enzyme profile may change significantly in response to pathologic situations.

Assay of Enzyme Activity

The activity of an enzyme is defined by the rate of the reaction catalyzed by the enzyme. The rate of the chemical reaction is defined by the rate of change in optical density (OD) indicating a decrease of the reacting compound with time or an increase of the reaction product. Substrate transformations involving NAD- and NADP-linked dehydrogenase reactions are measured in this way.

The rate of an enzyme reaction means the initial rate, v_0. This rate is obtained from the slope of the tangent to the reaction curve at zero time. An approximate value can be obtained by plotting several measurements made just after the start of the reaction and then extrapolating to $t = 0$. With nonlinear reaction curves the intervals at which measurements are made should be small. It is incorrect to take only a few measurements after a relatively long incubation time.

Like all chemical reactions, reactions catalyzed by enzymes are sensitive to changes in temperature. The temperature coefficient of the reaction rate is 10 percent per degree or more. Consequently, a 10°C rise in temperature may cause 100 percent increase in the reaction rate. Constant temperature is therefore essential in the assay of enzyme activity.

All enzymes have an optimum pH range for their activity, and often this range is very narrow. With increasing concentration of substrate the rate of the enzyme-catalyzed reactions finally reaches a maximum value. According to the equation of Michaelis and Menten, further increase in concentration should no longer change the rate. Many enzymes are, however, inhibited by a large excess of substrate. The optimum substrate concentration may also depend on the pH and the temperature.

The measurement of enzyme activity is always carried out with the optimum substrate concentrations, and if necessary the enzyme sample is diluted. The substrate must be pure, since contamination with substrate or other enzymes leads to errors. The reaction is started by addition of the substrate. Since the sample cannot be deproteinized, all the enzymes contained in it are active; they can react with their substrates if those are present in the sample and can cause considerable interference with the measurements. It may therefore be necessary to let the endogenous substrates react first, and after the initial reaction has stopped the actual measurements are started by addition of the substrate.

Coupled reactions can be used for the measurements of reaction rates in a manner similar to their use in the determination of substrates. The indicator enzyme is usually an NAD- or NADP-linked dehydrogenase. The role of the indicator reaction in determination of enzyme activity is to indicate the amount of reaction product formed with time. For this type of assay it is important to know how much more rapid the indicator reaction must be than the reaction to be measured, and frequently a hundredfold to a thousandfold excess of indicator enzyme is required. By "excess" is understood not the amount of enzyme, but rather the product of the amount of the specific activity or turnover number of the enzyme. With an unfavorable ratio for the turnover numbers (specific activities) the amount of indicator enzyme that is required may be very large.

Three component assays are relatively rare, because it is more difficult to obtain a sufficiently rapid rate for the auxiliary reaction in comparison to the primary reaction and for the indicator reaction in comparison to the auxiliary reaction. Only if the ratios of the specific activities of the participating enzymes are favorable can this type of assay be carried out.

It must be emphasized that the procedures outlined in this chapter represent guidelines, and they must be reexamined with respect to optimum assay conditions. The optimum substrate and cofactor concentrations may differ depending upon the species or the organ. It is therefore recommended that the optimum assay conditions should be established for the organ and species that will be studied.

Enzyme Units

One unit of an enzyme is the amount that will catalyze the transformation of one micromole of substrate per minute under defined conditions. The conditions of measurements of enzyme units should be standardized. The suggested temperature is 25°C. The suggested standard pH and substrate concentrations are those that give optimal activity.

The concentration of an enzyme solution is normally given in units per milliliter (or in moles per liter).

The specific activity of an enzyme is the number of units per milligram of protein.

The molecular activity of an enzyme is the number of units per micromole of enzyme. Thus, the molecular activity gives the number of molecules of substrate transformed per minute per molecule of enzyme.

The catalytic center activity of an enzyme is the number of units per micromole of catalytic centers. The molecular activity and the catalytic center activity will be identical if the enzyme contains only one active center per molecule.

Tissue Extraction for Enzyme Determinations

MATERIAL

Turn on refrigerated ultracentrifuge so it will be cool when needed. Place in a 4°C room all equipment needed for homogenizing the tissue samples:

- 1 size C Potter-Elvehjem glass tissue grinder with Teflon pestle for each tissue sample
- 1 50-ml beaker for each tissue sample
- 1 40-ml glass tube for each tissue sample
- 1 20-ml heavy-walled tube for the extract
- 1 test tube rack for holding tubes
- 1 10-ml graduated pipette
- 1 small glass rod for each tissue sample
- 1 scissors
- Polymer centrifuge tubes and caps for proper centrifuge rotor
- Rotor for centrifuge.

EXTRACTION

Prepare small labeled glass containers and place in an ice bath, one container for each tissue sample to be extracted, and give to experimenter. It is important that the tissue be kept cool at all times.

Remove the endocardium and epicardium from the heart muscle and weigh a 1-gram sample. Place each weighed tissue sample into a respectively labeled piece of aluminum foil. Process immediately if possible, or freeze with liquid nitrogen and place in freezer overnight.

Remove tissue samples from freezer and place in respective 50-ml beakers in the 4°C room.

Pipette into fresh or frozen samples eight volumes of the homogenization buffer.

Example: 1.05 g of heart or liver
× 8
8.40 ml buffer

When the tissue thaws, cut it into small pieces with scissors. Pour the suspension into the thick-walled tube of the tissue grinder. The pestle is inserted in a stirrer motor which will rotate the pestle rapidly. The tube is pushed up and down on the rotating pestle by hand. The tube is cooled to prevent overheating by submersing it in a beaker of ice water while homogenizing. Pour the homogenate into a polymer tube, cap, and place in the rotor. Centrifuge at 100,000 × *g* (about 38,000 rpm) for 15 minutes. Decant the supernatant into the labeled 40-ml tube.

Pipette four volumes of homogenization buffer onto the pellet remaining in the polymer tube. Suspend the pellet with a glass rod and pour the suspension into the tube of the tissue grinder. Homogenize, remembering to keep the tube cool. Pour the homogenate into the same polymer tube, cap, and place in the rotor. Centrifuge at 100,000 × *g* (about 38,000 rpm) for 15 minutes. Add the supernatant to the supernatant already in the 40-ml tube.

Again pipette four volumes of homogenization buffer onto the pellet in the polymer tube. Suspend with the glass rod and pour the suspension into tube of the tissue grinder. Homogenize, keeping the tube cool. Pour homogenate into the polymer tube, cap, and place in the rotor. Centrifuge at 100,000 × *g* (about 38,000 rpm) for 15 minutes. Add the supernatant to the 40-ml tube and mix all the supernatants together.

Divide the combined supernatants (the extract): one half is placed in a thick-walled tube for freezing and the other half is used for the enzyme determinations that day.

REAGENTS:

1. 0.1 M potassium phosphate buffer, pH 7.2. (a) Weigh 13.6 g KH_2PO_4 and dissolve in a liter of distilled water. (b) Weigh 17.4 g K_2HPO_4 and dissolve in a liter of distilled water.

   Using a glass electrode to check the pH, mix "a" and "b" together in a beaker until the pH of 7.2 is reached. Make about a liter of buffer at pH 7.2.
2. 0.1 M potassium phosphate buffer with 0.002 M ethylenedinitrilotetraacetic acid (EDTA). Weigh 744 mg EDTA (m.w. 372.25) and place in a liter volumetric flask. Pour into flask about 750 ml 0.1 M potassium phosphate buffer (reagent 1). Checking pH with glass electrode, adjust pH by using reagent 1a or 1b to pH 7.2, making sure not to go over mark but up to the mark. Refrigerate.
3. Homogenization buffer. Weigh 184.2 mg glutathione (GSH), 0.01 M. Weigh 33.0 mg adenosine diphosphate (ADP), 0.001 M. Dissolve both in 60 ml of 0.1 M potassium phosphate buffer with EDTA (reagent 2).

The GSH and ADP must be added to the buffer only on the day the extraction is to be done. The 60-ml volume is enough for only three tissue samples. Place in 4°C room with other equipment.

*Biuret Protein Determination on Enzyme Extracts**

REAGENTS:

1. Biuret solution
   a. Make a liter of 0.2 N NaOH (carbonate-free) from a stock saturated solution; 11.6 ml stock, diluted to 1 liter with distilled water.
   b. Weigh 9.0 g potassium sodium tartrate, 4 H_2O (Rochelle salt), m.w. 282.2. Place in a large beaker with a magnetic stirrer and add 400 ml (approx.) of 0.2 N NaOH. Allow to stir until completely dissolved.

*From Henry et al. 1957. *Anal. Chem.*, 29:1491.

c. Weigh 3.0 g cupric sulfate, 5 H_2O (m.w. 249.68). Add to the solution in the beaker and allow to dissolve completely.
d. Weigh 5.0 g potassium iodide (m.w. 166). Add to the solution in the beaker and allow to dissolve completely.
e. Pour the solution into a liter volumetric flask and rinse the beaker with 0.2 N NaOH and add to the flask. Bring up to the liter mark with 0.2 N NaOH and mix by inversion.

2. 50 percent trichloroacetic acid (TCA).
   Weigh 50 g TCA and add distilled water; fill up to 100 ml.

PROCEDURE:

Measure 1-ml aliquots of the extract samples and add 0.1 ml 50 percent TCA and mix. Centrifuge and discard the supernatant. Invert the tubes and allow the precipitate to drain dry. The precipitates may be frozen and run at a later time. Add 2.5 ml biuret solution to the tubes with the precipitate, mix thoroughly, and place on a shaker for 30 minutes. The time period begins upon addition of the biuret to the tubes.

After the 30 minutes are up, add 2.5 ml distilled water and mix. Read the optical density on a spectrophotometer at 546 mμ against a biuret blank and a standard.

Assay of Enzyme Activity

Phosphofructokinase (Fructose-6-Phosphate Kinase)*

REACTIONS:

1. Fructose-6-phosphate + ATP $\longrightarrow$ Fructose-1,6-diphosphate + ADP
2. Fructose-1,6-diphosphate $\xleftrightarrow{\text{Aldolase}}$ glyceraldehyde-3-phosphate (GAP) + dihydroxyacetone phosphate (DHAP)
3. GAP $\xrightarrow{\text{Triosephosphate-isomerase}}$ DHAP
4. 2 DHAP + 2 NADH + 2 H $\xleftrightarrow{\alpha\text{-GPDH}}$ 2 α-glycerophosphate + NAD

REAGENTS:

1. 0.05 M TRA buffer with 0.005 M EDTA, pH 7.5.
2. 0.02 M fructose-6-phosphate (F-6-P) barium salt.
3. 0.06 M adenosine triphosphate (ATP).
4. 0.01 M reduced nicotinamide adenine dinucleotide (NADH) in 1 percent $NaHCO_3$.
5. 0.01 M magnesium chloride ($MgCl_2 \cdot 6H_2O$).
6. 0.20 M cysteine, pH 7.0.
7. Aldolase, 10/ml ammonium sulfate.

*From Bucher et al. 1964. Hoppe-Seyler/Thierfelder, Handbuch der Physiologisch und Pathologisch-Chemischen Analyse, 6A:292.

8. α-glycerophosphate dehydrogenase/triosephosphate isomerase (α-GPDH/TIM), 2 mg/ml ammonium sulfate (C.P.).

PROCEDURE:

Into a clean cuvette, pipette (wiping pipette before measuring):

2.10 ml TRA buffer with EDTA
0.10 ml F-6-P
0.10 ml ATP
0.05 ml NADH
0.30 ml $MgCl_2$
0.10 ml cysteine HCl
0.10 ml aldolase
0.05 ml α-GPDH/TIM

Mix and record optical density until constant.

Add: 0.10 ml extract sample diluted 1:10 with distilled water
3.00 ml total volume in cuvette

Mix and record optical density.

CALCULATIONS:

$$\frac{\Delta OD/\text{minute}}{6.22} \times \frac{\text{total vol. in cuvette}}{\text{sample vol. in cuvette}} \times \text{sample dilution} = \text{units/ml extract}$$

$$\Delta OD/\text{minute} \times 48.2 = \text{units/ml extract}$$

$$\text{specific activity} = \frac{\text{units/ml}}{\text{mg protein/ml}} = \text{units/mg protein}$$

*Aldolase**

REACTIONS:

1. Fructose-1,6-diphosphate $\xrightleftharpoons{\text{Ald}}$ dihydroxyacetone phosphate (DHAP) + glyceraldehyde-3-phosphate (GAP)
2. DHAP $\xrightleftharpoons{\text{TIM}}$ GAP
3. DHAP + NADH + H $\xrightarrow{\alpha\text{-GPDH}}$ α-GP + NAD^+

REAGENTS:

1. 0.05 M TRA buffer with 0.005 EDTA, pH 7.5.
2. 0.1 N NaOH.
3. 0.012 M reduced nicotinamide adenine dinucleotide (NADH).
4. 1 percent $NaHCO_3$.
5. 0.147 M fructose-1,6-diphosphate (F-1,6-DP).

*From Bruns and Bergmeyer. 1963. *In* Methods of Enzymatic Analysis, Academic Press, Inc., p. 736.

6. α-glycerophosphate dehydrogenase/triosephosphate isomerase, from rabbit muscle (α-GPDH/TIM).

PROCEDURE:

Into a clean cuvette, pipette:

2.73 ml TRA buffer with EDTA
0.05 ml NADH
0.04 ml α-GPDH/TIM (pipetting onto a mixing spoon then adding)
0.10 ml extract, sample diluted 1:10 with distilled water

Mix and record optical density, should equilibrate in 5 to 10 minutes.

Add: 0.08 ml F-1,6-DP
3.00 ml total volume in cuvette

Mix and record optical density. Optical change is usually linear with time.

CALCULATIONS:

$$\frac{\Delta OD/\text{minute}}{6.22} \times \frac{\text{total vol. in cuvette}}{\text{vol. of sample in cuvette}} \times \frac{\text{sample dilution}}{2} = \text{units/ml extract}$$

The correction factor of 2 takes into consideration the formation of two moles of triosephosphates per mole of fructose-1,6-diphosphate.

$$\Delta OD/\text{minute} \times 24.1 = \text{units/ml extract}$$

$$\text{specific activity} = \frac{\text{units/ml}}{\text{mg protein/ml}} = \text{units/mg protein} = \mu\text{moles/minute} \times \text{mg}$$

*Glyceraldehyde-3-Phosphate Dehydrogenase**

REACTIONS:

1. D-3-phosphoglycerate + ATP $\xrightleftharpoons{PGK}$ D-1,3-diphosphoglycerate + ADP
2. D-1,3-diphosphoglycerate + NADH + H^+ $\rightleftharpoons$ D-glyceraldehyde-3-phosphate + NAD + Pi

REAGENTS:

1. 0.05 M TRA Buffer with EDTA, pH 7.5.
2. 0.009 M reduced nicotinamide dinucleotide (NADH) in 1 percent $NaHCO_3$.
3. 0.21 M adenosine triphosphate (ATP)
4. 0.198 M magnesium sulfate ($MgSO_4 \cdot 7H_2O$).
5. 0.072 M glutathione (GSH).

*From Delbruck et al. 1959. *Biochem. Z.*, 331:273.

6. 3-phosphoglyceratekinase (3-PGK), 2 mg/ml ammonium sulfate (C.P.).
7. 1.5 M 3-phosphoglycerate-Na_3 (3-PG).

PROCEDURE:

Into a clean cuvette, pipette:

2.55 ml TRA buffer with EDTA
0.05 ml NADH
0.05 ml ATP
0.05 ml $MgSO_4$
0.05 ml GSH
0.05 ml 3-PGK
0.10 ml extract sample diluted 1:100 with distilled water.

Mix and record optical density until constant.

Add: 0.10 ml 3-PG
3.00 ml total volume in cuvette

Mix and record optical density: $OD_0 - OD_{10} = \Delta$ OD/10 minutes.

CALCULATIONS:

$$\frac{\Delta\text{OD/minute}}{6.22} \times \frac{\text{total vol. in cuvette}}{\text{sample vol. in cuvette}} \times \text{sample dilution} = \text{units/ml extract}$$

$$\Delta\text{OD/minute} \times 482 = \text{units/ml extract}$$

$$\text{specific activity} = \frac{\text{units/ml}}{\text{mg protein/ml}} = \text{units/mg protein}$$

*α-Glycerophosphate Dehydrogenase**

REACTION:

dihydroxyacetone phosphate + NADH + H^+ $\xrightleftharpoons{\alpha\text{-GPDH}}$ α-glycerophosphate + NAD^+

REAGENTS:

1. 0.05 M TRA buffer with 0.005 M EDTA, pH 7.5.
2. 0.012 M reduced nicotinamide adenine dinucleotide (NADH).
3. Glycerophosphate dehydrogenase (α-GPDH), 2 mg/ml ammonium sulfate (C.P.).
4. Dihydroxyacetone phosphate (DHAP):
   a. Dissolve 25 mg DHAP (dicyclohexylamine salt, dimethylketal) $\cdot H_2O$ (m.w. 432.5) in 2.0 ml distilled water.
   b. Add 500 mg Dowex 50W H^+ ion exchange resin (stock #50X4-200) and swirl for 30 seconds.

*From Delbruck et al. 1959. *Biochem. Z.*, 331:273.

c. Filter into a tube suitable for freezing and wash the resin with 1.0 ml distilled water. Incubate filtrate at 38° to 40°C for 4 hours to hydrolyze ketal.
d. Adjust to pH 4.5 with 1 percent $NaHCO_3$ and run an assay on yield of DHAP.
DHAP Assay:
Into a clean cuvette, pipette:

2.97 ml TRA buffer (reagent 1)
0.05 ml NADH (reagent 3)
0.02 ml DHAP (above preparation onto a spoon)

Mix and read optical density (OD_1) until constant.

Add: 0.05 ml α-GPDH
3.09 ml total volume in cuvette

Mix and read final optical density (OD_2) until constant.

$$\frac{OD_1 - OD_2}{6.22} \times \frac{3.09}{0.02} = \mu\text{moles/ml DHAP}$$

Assay is usually 8 to 11 μmoles/ml. For the α-GPDH test, 0.6 to 0.7 μmoles/ml are needed:

$$\frac{0.6\,\mu\text{moles}}{x\text{ ml}} = \frac{8\text{ to }11\,\mu\text{moles}}{1\text{ ml}}$$

where x ml = 0.075 to 0.055 ml prepared DHAP to be used in α-GPDH test. Store frozen.

PROCEDURE:

Into a clean cuvette, pipette:

2.83 ml TRA buffer with EDTA
0.05 ml NADH
0.05 ml undiluted extract sample

Mix and record optical density until constant or a constant rate of change.
Add: 0.06 ml or necessary amount for 0.6 to 0.7 μmoles DHAP, altering buffer volume to keep total total volume in cuvette equal to 3.00 ml.
Mix and record optical density. Optical density change is usually linear with time.
$OD_0 - OD_{10} = \Delta$ OD/10 minutes.

CALCULATIONS:

$$\frac{\Delta\text{OD/minute}}{6.22} \times \frac{\text{total vol. in cuvette}}{\text{vol. of sample in cuvette}} \times \text{sample dilution} = \text{units/ml extract}$$

$$\Delta\text{OD/minute} \times 9.65 = \text{units/ml extract}$$

$$\text{specific activity} = \frac{\text{units/ml}}{\text{mg protein/ml}} = \text{units/mg}$$

*Lactic Dehydrogenase**

REACTION:

$$\text{pyruvate} + \text{NADH} + H^+ \rightleftharpoons \text{lactate} + \text{NAD}^+$$

REAGENTS:

1. 0.05 M potassium phosphate buffer, pH 7.5. (a) Weigh 6.8 grams KH_2PO_4 and dissolve in a liter of distilled water. (b) Weigh 8.7 grams K_2HPO_4 and dissolve in a liter of distilled water. Using a glass electrode to check pH, mix "a" and "b" together in a beaker until pH is 7.5.
2. 0.012 M reduced nicotinamide adenine dinucleotide (NADH) in 1 percent $NaHCO_3$.
3. 0.008 M sodium pyruvate.

PROCEDURE:

Into a clean cuvette, pipette:

2.87 ml 0.05 M potassium phosphate buffer, pH 7.5
0.05 ml NADH
0.05 ml extract sample diluted 1:100 with distilled water

Mix and record optical density until constant.

Add: 0.03 ml pyruvate (onto mixing spoon then adding)
3.00 ml total volume in cuvette

Mix and record optical density OD_0: $OD_0 - OD_{10} = \Delta\ OD/10$ minutes.

CALCULATIONS:

$$\frac{\Delta OD/\text{minute}}{6.22} \times \frac{\text{total vol. in cuvette}}{\text{sample vol. in cuvette}} \times \text{sample dilution} = \text{units/ml extract}$$

$$\text{specific activity} = \frac{\text{units/ml}}{\text{mg protein/ml}} = \text{units/mg} = \frac{\mu\ \text{moles}}{\text{minute} \times \text{mg}}$$

Glucose-6-Phosphate Dehydrogenase†

REACTION:

$$\text{glucose-6-phosphate} + \text{NADP}^+ \rightleftharpoons \text{6-phosphogluconate} + \text{NADPH} + H^+$$

REAGENTS:

1. 0.05 M TRA buffer with 0.005 M EDTA, pH 7.5.
2. 0.03 M nicotinamide adenine dinucleotide phosphate (NADP).
3. 0.1 M glucose-6-phosphate (G-6-P) in 1 percent $NaHCO_3$.

*From Bergmeyer et al. 1963. *In* Methods of Enzymatic Analysis, Academic Press, Inc., p. 736.

†From Lohr and Waller. 1963. *In* Methods of Enzymatic Analysis, Academic Press, Inc., p. 744.

PROCEDURE:

Into a clean cuvette, pipette:

2.36 ml TRA buffer with EDTA
0.05 ml NADP
0.50 ml undiluted extract sample

Mix and record optical density until constant.

Add: 0.09 ml G-6-P
3.00 ml total volume in cuvette

Mix and record optical density: $OD_0 - OD_{10} = \Delta OD/10$ minutes.

CALCULATIONS:

$$\frac{\Delta OD/\text{minute}}{6.22} \times \frac{\text{total vol. in cuvette}}{\text{sample vol. in cuvette}} \times \text{sample dilution} = \text{units/ml extract}$$

$$\Delta OD/\text{minute} \times 0.965 = \text{units/ml extract}$$

$$\text{specific activity} = \frac{\text{units/ml}}{\text{mg protein/ml}} = \frac{\text{units}}{\text{mg protein}}$$

*6-Phosphogluconate Dehydrogenase**

REACTION:

6-phosphogluconate + $NADP^+$ $\rightleftharpoons$ D-ribulose-5-phosphate + CO_2 + NADPH + H^+

REAGENTS:

1. 0.05 M TRA buffer with 0.005 M EDTA, pH 7.5.
2. 0.10 M magnesium chloride ($MgCl_2 \cdot 6H_2O$).
3. 0.03 M nicotinamide adenine dinucleotide phosphate (NADP).
4. 0.021 M 6-phosphogluconate (G-6-P).

PROCEDURE:

Into a clean cuvette, pipette:

2.05 ml TRA buffer with EDTA
0.03 ml $MgCl_2$
0.05 ml NADP
0.05 ml undiluted extract sample

Mix and record optical density.

CALCULATIONS:

$$\frac{\Delta OD/\text{minute}}{6.22} \times \frac{\text{total vol. in cuvette}}{\text{sample vol. in cuvette}} \times \text{sample dilution} = \text{units/ml extract}$$

*From Glock. 1964. Hoppe-Seyler/Thierfelder, Handbuch der Physiologisch and Pathologisch Chemischen Analyse. 6A:414.

$$\Delta OD/\text{minute} \times 0.965 = \text{units/ml extract}$$

$$\text{specific activity} = \frac{\text{units/ml}}{\text{mg protein/ml}} = \text{units/mg protein}$$

*NAD-Specific Isocitrate Dehydrogenase**

REACTION:

$$\text{D-isocitrate} + NAD^+ \longrightarrow \alpha\text{-ketoglutarate} + CO_2 + NADH + H^+$$

REAGENTS:

1. 0.1 M potassium phosphate buffer, pH 7.6.
2. 0.24 M magnesium chloride ($MgCl_2 \cdot 6H_2O$).
3. 0.05 M nicotinamide adenine dinucleotide (NAD).
4. 0.12 M isocitrate sodium salt.
5. 0.06 M adenosine diphosphate (ADP).

PROCEDURE:

Into a clean cuvette, pipette:

2.55 ml potassium phosphate buffer, pH 7.6
0.10 ml $MgCl_2$
0.10 ml NAD
0.10 ml ADP
0.05 ml undiluted extract sample

Mix and record optical density until constant.

Add: 0.10 ml isocitrate-Na_3
3.00 ml total volume in cuvette

Mix and record optical density. Optical density change is usually linear with time. $OD_0 - OD_{10} = \Delta\ OD/10$ minutes.

CALCULATIONS:

$$\frac{\Delta OD/\text{minute}}{6.22} \times \frac{\text{total vol. in cuvette}}{\text{sample vol. in cuvette}} \times \text{sample dilution} = \text{units/ml extract}$$

$$\text{specific activity} = \frac{\text{units/ml}}{\text{mg protein/ml}} = \text{units/mg protein}$$

NADP-Specific Isocitrate Dehydrogenase†

REACTION:

$$\text{D-isocitrate} + NADP \longrightarrow \alpha\text{-ketoglutarate} + CO_2 + NADPH + H^+$$

*From Goebell and Klingenberg. 1964. *Biochem. Z.*, 340:441.

†From Delbruck et al. 1959. *Biochem. Z.*, 331:273; and Bucher et al. 1964. Hoppe-Seyler/Thierfelder, Handbuch der Physiologisch und Pathologisch Chemischen Analyse. 6A:292

REAGENTS:

1. 0.05 M TRA buffer with 0.005 M EDTA, pH 7.5.
2. 0.718 M magnesium sulfate ($MgSO_4 \cdot 7H_2O$).
3. 0.03 M nicotinamide adenine dinucleotide phosphate (NADP).
4. 0.15 M isocitrate sodium salt.

PROCEDURE:

Into a clean cuvette, pipette:

2.65 ml TRA buffer with EDTA
0.05 ml $MgSO_4$
0.05 ml NADP
0.10 ml extract sample diluted 1:10 with distilled water

Mix and record optical density until constant.

Add: 0.15 ml isocitrate-Na_3
3.00 ml total volume in cuvette

Mix and record optical density. $OD - OD_{10} = \Delta\ OD/10$ minutes.

CALCULATIONS:

$$\frac{\Delta OD/\text{minute}}{6.22} \times \frac{\text{total vol. in cuvette}}{\text{sample vol. in cuvette}} \times \text{sample dilution} = \text{units/ml extract}$$

$$\text{specific activity} = \frac{\text{units/ml}}{\text{mg protein/ml}} = \text{units/mg protein} = \frac{\mu\ \text{moles}}{\text{minute} \times \text{mg}}$$

*Malic Dehydrogenase**

REACTION:

$$\text{L-malate} + NAD^+ \underset{}{\overset{\text{MDH}}{\rightleftharpoons}} \text{oxaloacetate} + NADH + H^+$$

REAGENTS:

1. 0.05 M TRA buffer with 0.005 M EDTA, pH 7.5.
2. 0.009 M reduced nicotinamide adenine dinucleotide (NADH) in 1 percent $NaHCO_3$.
3. 0.015 M oxalacetic acid (OAA).

PROCEDURE:

Into a clean cuvette, pipette:

2.80 ml TRA buffer with EDTA
0.05 ml NADH
0.05 ml extract sample diluted 1:100 with distilled water

*From Bergmeyer and Bernt. 1963a. *In* Methods of Enzymatic Analysis, Academic Press, Inc., p. 757; and Bucher et al. 1964. Hoppe-Seyler/Thierfelder, Handbuch der Physiologisch und Pathologisch Chemischen Analyse, 6A:292.

Mix and record optical density until constant.

Add: $\frac{0.10 \text{ ml OAA}}{3.00 \text{ ml total vol. in cuvette}}$

Mix and record optical density.

CALCULATIONS:

$$\frac{\Delta\text{OD/minute}}{6.22} \times \frac{\text{total vol. in cuvette}}{\text{sample vol. in cuvette}} \times \text{sample dilution} = \text{units/ml extract}$$

$$\Delta\text{OD/minute} \times 965 = \text{units/ml extract}$$

$$\text{specific activity} = \frac{\text{units/ml}}{\text{mg protein/ml}} = \frac{\text{units}}{\text{mg}} = \frac{\mu\text{ moles}}{\text{minute} \times \text{mg}}$$

*Glutamate Oxaloacetate Transaminase**

REACTIONS:

$$\text{L-glutamate} + \text{oxaloacetate} \xrightleftharpoons{\text{GOT}} \text{L-aspartate} + \alpha\text{-ketoglutarate}$$

$$\text{oxaloacetate} + \text{NADH} + H^+ \xrightleftharpoons{\text{MDH}} \text{malate} + \text{NAD}^+$$

REAGENTS:

1. 0.1 M potassium phosphate buffer with 0.24 M aspartate, pH 7.6.
2. 0.009 M reduced nicotinamide adenine dinucleotide (NADH) in 1 percent $NaHCO_3$.
3. Malic dehydrogenase (MDH), 0.5 mg/ml ammonium sulfate.
4. 0.3 M α-ketoglutaric acid, sodium salt, pH 7.6 (α-KG).

PROCEDURE:

Into a clean cuvette, pipette:

2.66 ml 0.1 M phosphate buffer with aspartate
0.05 ml NADH
0.05 ml MDH
0.01 ml extract sample diluted 1:100 with distilled water

Mix and record optical density until constant.

Add: $\frac{0.14 \text{ ml } \alpha\text{-KG}}{3.00 \text{ ml total volume in cuvette}}$

Mix and record optical density.

CALCULATIONS:

$$\frac{\Delta\text{OD/minute}}{6.22} \times \frac{\text{total vol. in cuvette}}{\text{sample vol. in cuvette}} \times \text{sample dilution} = \text{units/ml extract}$$

*From Delbruck et al. 1959. *Biochem. Z.*, 331:273; and Bergmeyer and Bernt. 1963b. *In* Methods of Enzymatic Analysis, Academic Press, Inc., p. 837.

$$\text{specific activity} = \frac{\text{units/ml}}{\text{mg protein/ml}} = \text{units/mg} = \frac{\mu\text{ moles}}{\text{minute} \times \text{mg}}$$

*Creatine Phosphokinase**

REACTIONS:

$$\text{creatine} + \text{ATP} \xrightleftharpoons{\text{CPK}} \text{creatine phosphate} + \text{ADP}$$

$$\text{ADP} + \text{phosphoenolpyruvate} \xrightarrow{\text{PK}} \text{ATP} + \text{pyruvate}$$

$$\text{pyruvate} + \text{NADH} + H^+ \xrightarrow{\text{LDH}} \text{lactate} + \text{NAD}^+$$

REAGENTS:

1. 0.1 M creatine-0.1 M glycine buffer, pH 9.0.
2. 0.10 M magnesium chloride ($MgCl_2 \cdot 6H_2O$).
3. 0.07 M adenosine triphosphate (ATP).
4. 0.05 M phosphoenolpyruvate (PEP).
5. 0.012 M reduced nicotinamide adenine dinucleotide (NADH) in 1 percent $NaHCO_3$.
6. Lactate dehydrogenase (LDH), 5 mg/ml ammonium sulfate.
7. Pyruvate kinase (PK), mg/ml ammonium sulfate.

PROCEDURE:

Into a clean cuvette, pipette:

2.41 ml creatine-glycine buffer
0.10 ml $MgCl_2$
0.20 ml ATP
0.10 ml PEP
0.10 ml NADH
0.02 ml LDH (pipette onto mixing spoon)
0.02 ml PK (pipette onto mixing spoon)

Allow to stand about 30 minutes to equilibrate. There will be a substrate reaction occurring due to the ATP.
Mix and record the optical density until constant.

Add: $\frac{\text{0.05 ml extracted sample diluted 1:10 with distilled water}}{\text{3.00 ml total volume in cuvette}}$

Mix and record optical density.

CALCULATIONS:

$$\frac{\Delta\text{OD/minute}}{6.22} \times \frac{\text{total vol. in cuvette}}{\text{sample vol. in cuvette}} \times \text{sample dilution} = \text{units/ml extract}$$

*From Bernt and Bergmeyer. 1963. *In* Methods in Enzymatic Analysis, Academic Press, Inc., p. 859.

$$\Delta OD/\text{minute} \times 96.5 = \text{units/ml extract}$$

$$\text{specific activity} = \frac{\text{units/ml}}{\text{mg protein/ml}} = \text{units/mg protein} = \frac{\mu\ \text{moles}}{\text{minute} \times \text{mg}}$$

See Table 1, page 58.

ANALYSIS OF MYOCARDIAL LIPIDS

Introduction

Lipid metabolism of cardiac muscle has been studied in vivo and in vitro, in whole homogenates, cell-free systems, isolated mitochondria, etc. Numerous methods have been employed for these studies, and the best of these require considerable investment (e.g., gas-liquid chromatography). In this chapter we will describe the use of relatively inexpensive methods to separate complex lipids into the main lipid classes. These methods may suffice for many studies that are directed toward examination of the main lipid classes.

An attempt will not be made to describe any of the many procedures for in vitro experiment, since those depend upon the system used and upon the question that is being asked.

The in vivo studies have consisted of analysis of lipid extraction and utilization by the heart (i.e., analysis of arterial and coronary sinus blood) and of analysis of lipid synthesis by the heart (i.e., by incorporation of a tracer such as acetate-1-^{14}C into myocardial lipids).

Lipid Extraction from Blood and Tissue

BLOOD –Allow the blood sample to clot at room temperature for about 30 minutes. Centrifuge the samples at 2,500 rpm for 30 minutes. If the serum is clotted, rim the top of the sample with a wooden stick and centrifuge again. Remove the serum and store in a small, labeled, screw-cap tube. Refrigerate until needed.

EXTRACTION. Using 50-ml tubes or graduate cylinders with ground-glass stoppers, extract the samples. Pipette 20 ml chloroform:methanol (2:1, v/v) into the cylinder and add 1.0 ml serum sample (Folch et al., 1957). Measure the sample using volumetric pipettes. Allow the shaken sample to stand at room temperature for 30 minutes. The samples may be stored at 4°C and completed the next day. If refrigerated, allow the samples to return to room temperature before continuing.

Set up a separatory funnel (250 ml) and a funnel with Whatman #1 filter paper with a 250-ml evaporation flask under the separatory funnel. Check all glassware for cracks. Do not place the separatory funnels in the refrigerator because the Teflon stopcock and glass contract at different rates and the samples will be lost.

TABLE 1

*Specific Activities (μmoles substrate/min × mg) of Heart Muscle Enzymes from Normal, Uninfarcted Heart (Normal) and from the Center (Ic) and Periphery (Ip) of Infarcted Heart Muscle**

Enzymes	× f	normal N = 12	5 hr N = 4		24 hr N = 6		48 hr N = 4		10 days N = 4		10 weeks N = 8	
			Ic	*Ip*	*Ic*	*Ip*	*Ic*	*Ip*	*Ic*	*Ip*	*Ic*	*Ip*
Aldolase	$\times 10^{-1}$	1.76 ±0.12	1.41 ±0.12	1.16 ±0.24	0.34 ±0.09	0.90 ±0.15	0.34 ±0.09	0.63 ±0.22	0.22 ±0.03	0.66 ±0.10	0.59 ±0.16	1.29 ±0.21
GAPDH	× 1	2.85 ±0.56	1.89 ±0.06	2.19 ±0.24	1.21 ±0.34	1.22 ±0.25	0.71 ±0.21	1.29 ±0.16	0.92 ±0.17	1.41 ±0.27	1.51 ±0.22	2.20 ±0.22
LDH	× 1	3.84 ±0.34	3.53 ±0.21	3.20 ±0.38	1.84 ±0.34	1.94 ±0.28	0.97 ±0.23	1.81 ±0.73	0.84 ±0.05	1.97 ±0.37	0.87 ±0.27	2.15 ±0.35
α-GPDH	$\times 10^{-2}$	10.5 ±0.54	10.1 ±1.3	9.1 ±1.3	3.3 ±0.6	5.6 ±1.1	2.0 ±1.0	3.6 ±1.0	0.65 ±0.16	2.98 ±0.81	11.21 ±4.47	8.69 ±2.06
NAD-IDH	$\times 10^{-2}$	8.66 ±0.46	4.83 ±0.71	4.73 ±0.63	1.98 ±0.51	4.06 ±1.00	0.79 ±0.45	2.21 ±1.13	0.69 ±0.88	2.70 ±0.61	1.51 ±0.27	4.16 ±0.65
NADP-IDH	$\times 10^{-1}$	3.54 ±0.52	3.37 ±0.33	2.85 ±0.17	1.30 ±0.35	1.39 ±0.25	0.58 ±0.18	1.19 ±0.40	0.44 ±0.05	1.22 ±0.18	0.81 ±0.09	2.51 ±0.46
MDH	× 1	13.20 ±1.31	14.60 ±1.73	11.20 ±1.91	7.56 ±1.05	9.33 ±1.96	4.68 ±0.23	6.45 ±0.95	1.86 ±0.41	5.15 ±0.99	5.35 ±1.92	10.27 ±1.68
GOT	× 1	2.86 ±0.22	2.28 ±0.18	2.23 ±0.18	1.68 ±0.49	1.59 ±0.23	1.35 ±0.30	1.66 ±0.31	0.29 ±0.11	0.69 ±0.18	0.74 ±0.15	1.84 ±0.31
G-6-PDH	$\times 10^{-3}$	1.03 ±0.04	3.81 ±0.51	4.82 ±0.84	8.76 ±1.60	7.91 ±1.67	9.66 ±1.57	7.54 ±1.37	35.03 ±5.80	23.97 ±3.80	6.58 ±1.51	1.93 ±0.33
6-PGDH	$\times 10^{-3}$	0.83 ±0.08	4.13 ±0.29	6.23 ±1.76	4.74 ±0.56	4.37 ±0.66	6.30 ±1.55	5.43 ±1.37	25.37 ±1.65	21.33 ±0.01	4.89 ±0.76	2.00 ±0.22
Extractable protein	mg / g tissue	84.0 ±1.2	68.0 ±3.6	70.7 ±3.2	75.4 ±3.1	78.5 ±4.0	72.4 ±6.0	72.1 ±5.5	63.0 ±6.3	66.8 ±3.9	38.6 ±3.4	64.3 ±8.2

*From Gudbjarnason et al. 1968. *Cardiologia*, 51:148.

± Standard error of the mean.

The specific activity, in μmoles of substrate converted to product per minute and per mg of protein, is obtained by multiplying the numbers with the respective factor in the second column.

The specific activities were determined at different times after infarction, from 5 hr to 10 weeks.

Pour the 20 ml of 2:1 chloroform:methanol plus the 1.0 ml serum sample onto the filter paper. Rinse the mouth of the cylinder with 5.0 ml 2:1 chloroform:methanol (C:M) and add to the funnel. Rinse the cylinder three times with 5.0 ml 2:1 C:M and add to the funnel. Rinse the filter paper three times with 5.0 ml 2:1 C:M, allowing the filter to drain between each rinse. The separatory funnel now contains 55 ml total volume of 2:1 C:M. Add 11 ml 0.73 percent saline to the separatory funnel (1 ml per 5 ml of 2:1 C:M). Stopper and shake, being careful to release the pressure. Shake vigorously. Replace in the rack and release the pressure. Allow to stand overnight.

Continue with the procedure the next morning. The bottom chloroform layer contains the lipids. Remove the bottom layer into the evaporation flask. Rinse the funnel with two 5-ml volumes of lower-phase solvent. Rinse the neck of the funnel and its sides, and add each volume to the evaporation flask. Rinse the stem of the separatory funnel and the neck of the evaporation flask with 2:1 C:M.

If some of the upper phase is allowed to get into the evaporation flask, add 5 ml upper-phase solvent to the evaporation flask, and aspirate off. Repeat three or four times, then add 5 ml methanol and mix into one phase.

Evaporate the flasks to dryness at 40° to 50°C. Add 2:1 C:M and acetone to the flask and take to dryness. Add only acetone and take to dryness again.

Add a small amount of 2:1 C:M to the dried sample and rotate to redissolve. Transfer the sample to a small screw-cap vial. Add another volume of 2:1 C:M and transfer to the vial. Repeat washing of the evaporation flask four more times. Evaporate the solvents in the small vial to dryness under a stream of nitrogen gas. The vial is placed in the refrigerator for thin-layer chromatography.

REAGENTS:

1. Chloroform:methanol (2:1 v/v).*
2. 0.73 percent saline (NaCl).
3. Lower-phase solvent (84:16:1):

chloroform	84 ml
methanol	16 ml
0.73 percent saline	1 ml

4. Upper-phase solvent (3:47:48):*

chloroform	3 ml
methanol	47 ml
0.73 percent saline	48 ml

*Mix chloroform and methanol very carefully.

TISSUE (HEART MUSCLE).—Remove the endocardium and epicardium from the muscle. Weigh one gram sample and place in a size C glass tissue grinder. Add 10 ml chloroform:methanol (2:1, v/v). Use the same reagents as in the above procedure.

Using an adaptor to hold the pestle in the stirring motor, homogenize the tissue by pushing the tube up and down on the rotating pestle. Have the tissue grinder in an ice bath to prevent overheating. Transfer the homogenate to a 50-ml beaker, rinse the tissue grinder twice with 5 ml each of C:M, and add to the beaker. Allow the beaker to stand at room temperature for 30 minutes. (Remember to extract with at least 20 ml chloroform:methanol (2:1) per gram of tissue.)

Set up 250-ml separatory funnels (Teflon stopcocks) with a Whatman #1 filter paper in a funnel. Pour the 20 ml of 2:1 C:M and the tissue in the beaker onto the filter. Rinse the beaker three times with 5-ml volumes of 2:1 C:M and add to the filter. Rinse the filter three times with 5-ml volumes of 2:1 C:M, allowing the filter to drain between each rinse (total volume of 2:1 C:M is 50 ml). Add 10 ml 0.73 percent saline to the separatory funnel (1 ml per 5 ml of 2:1 C:M). Stopper and shake, being careful to release the pressure. Shake vigorously. Place in the rack and release the pressure. Allow to stand overnight.

Continue with the procedure the next morning. Remove the bottom layer containing the lipids into the evaporation flask. Rinse the funnel with two 5-ml volumes of lower-phase solvent. Rinse the neck of the funnel and its sides, and add each volume to the evaporation flask. Rinse the stem of the separatory funnel and the neck of the evaporation flask with 2:1 C:M.

If some of the upper phase is allowed to get into the evaporation flask, add 5 ml upper-phase solvent to the evaporation flask and aspirate off. Repeat three or four times, then add 5 ml methanol and mix into one phase.

Evaporate to dryness at 40° to 50°C. Add to the flask a small amount of 2:1 C:M and acetone, and dry again. Then add only acetone, and dry.

Add a small amount of 2:1 C:M to the dried sample and rotate to redissolve. Transfer the sample into a 25-ml volumetric flask. Add another volume of 2:1 C:M and transfer to the flask. Repeat washing the evaporation flask four more times. Bring to 25 ml in the volumetric flask with 2:1 C:M and mix by inversion. Pipette aliquots for TLC and for column chromatography. Evaporate each to dryness under a stream of nitrogen and store in the refrigerator.

Thin-Layer Chromatography

A TLC coating is prepared by spreading a slurry, consisting of a specific sorbent powder and a suitable liquid (usually water), on a glass plate. After the thin layer is dried and activated in an oven, the sample mixture is applied to one end of the plate, either in the form of a spot or as a line. The plate is then mounted vertically in a developing tank with the sample just above the solvent level near the bottom of the plate.

Ascending development, where the solvent is drawn through the layer by capillary action, is the most common procedure. Because the migration rates of different compounds vary, the original sample mixture is resolved into individual spots. The invisible spots are identified by staining with iodine vapors. For quantification of radioactivity, the spots are scraped into a scintillator and placed in a scintillation counter.

PREPARATION OF TLC PLATES FOR LIPID SEPARATION.—On the standard mounting board, place two 20- by 40-cm plates, one 20- by 20-cm plate, and two 20- by 5-cm plates (one at each end of the board). Check the plates for any scratches or nicks; if any, place on the bottom side of the plate, being careful to handle only edges of the plates. Under each plate place a few drops of water to hold the plates in place, again being careful not to touch the top surface of the plates. Push the plates against the white plastic guide rail on the mounting board. Using distilled water and gauze, clean the top surface of the plates.

In a hood, weigh 60.0 g of Silica Gel H (without $CaSO_4$ binder) into a 400-ml beaker. Add 135 to 140 ml distilled water and mix thoroughly, tapping the beaker to wet all particles. Complete mixing is a must for smooth plates. The slurry is now ready for use.

The Model S-11 Applicator (Brinkman Instruments), with an internal rotating reservoir chamber, is used to spread the slurry. The applicator is set to spread a 0.5-mm-thick plate and is placed on the 20- by 5-cm plate on the end of the mounting board without a guide rail. Open the chamber on the applicator to the plates and make a few practice pulls across the plates. (Have your feet placed so that the pull is continuous across all plates.)

Pour the mixed slurry into the chamber closed to the plates. Open the chamber to the plates and pull the applicator across the plates and rest it on the 20- by 5-cm plate at the end; close the chamber. Wash the applicator with tap water and dry immediately. The two 20- by 5-cm end plates are discarded. The layer on the other plates should be smooth and without any change in thickness.

Allow the plates to air-dry and then place on a drying rack, wiping the water from the bottom of the plate. Place plates and rack in a desiccator until needed.

PROCEDURE FOR LIPID SEPARATION ON TLC PLATES.—Place 20- by 40-cm plates on a drying rack in a 120°C oven for *one hour* to activate.

While the plates are activating, prepare developing tanks. The tanks must be prepared the day they are needed. Line the two tanks with Whatman #3 chromatography paper and place a trough on the bottom of each tank.

Make the two solvent systems in 500-ml volumetric flasks (Freeman and West, 1966):

POLAR SOLVENT SYSTEM I

Benzene	271.2 ml
Diethyl ether	216.9 ml
Ethyl alcohol	10.8 ml
Acetic acid	1.1 ml

NONPOLAR SOLVENT SYSTEM II

Hexane	470 ml
Diethyl ether	30 ml

One solvent system is to be used for each tank. Add 200 ml of the solvent system to the trough and pour another 200 ml down the sides of the tank, wetting the chromatography paper in the process. This portion of the solvent should be in the bottom of the tank with the paper dipping into it. Seal the glass plate cover to the jar with stopcock grease. Allow at least one hour to equilibrate before using.

After activating the plates for one hour in the oven, remove the plates and allow them to cool in a desiccator. On the cooled plates, make a mark 2 cm from the bottom of the plate on the outer edge. Place marks 25 cm and 33 cm above the 2-cm mark, also on the outer edge. The 2-cm level will be the level of the origin of the samples. Place a plastic template over the TLC plate with the bottom of the template at the 2-cm mark.

Now that the plate has been marked and the template is in place, remove the dried lipid extract samples from the refrigerator (see p. 59). Just before spotting, add 0.1 ml chloroform to the sample vial, cap, and rotate to redissolve sample into the chloroform. Using a mechanical microsyringe with a pushbutton dispenser, remove a 10-microliter fraction from the sample vial and recap the vial tightly. At the 2-cm level on the plate, spot the 10-microliter fraction, applying a small amount of the fraction, allowing it to dry (one may use a blower to help drying), and then spotting another small amount, and so on until the entire 10-microliter fraction is spotted onto the plate. Repeat the procedure for the next sample spot. Do not spot any more than six samples per plate plus one standard spot (see below), a total of seven spots per plate.

The lipid standard spot is a 20-microliter sample of a 1 percent solution of a representative of each lipid class. Weigh 100 mg of each and dissolve them altogether in 10 ml of chloroform:

Palmitic acid
Tripalmitin
Cholesterol palmitate
Monopalmitin
Cholesterol
D,L-α-lecithin
Dipalmitin

After all the samples and the standard have been spotted and dried, the plate is placed vertically in the prepared tank with polar solvent system I. The solvent is allowed to move by capillary action to the 25-cm mark on the plate (about 60 minutes). When the mark is reached, the plate is removed from the tank and air-dried to remove all residue from the first solvent system. The plate is then placed in the other tank with nonpolar solvent system II. This solvent is allowed to move to the 33-cm mark on the plate (about 100 to 120 minutes); then the plate is removed and air-dried.

After completion of this double-development procedure, the lipid classes are visualized by a brief development in iodine vapor. The plate is placed in a closed container with iodine crystals. After a brief exposure to the iodine vapor, the separated lipids and standard samples become visible as yellow spots. The phospholipids remain at the origin, and the other lipids are recovered in the following order of increasing mobility: monoglyceride (MG), free fatty acids (FA), free cholesterol (FC), diglycerides (DG), triglycerides (TG), and cholesterol esters (CE).

Remove the plate from the iodine container and encircle the lipid spots which have been separated so that when the iodine vapor coloration disappears you will be able to locate the lipids.

If the lipid samples are radioactive, it may be advantageous to remove the phospholipids from the plate before the development with iodine vapor. The phospholipids tend to stain deeply, and the staining may cause a reduction in counting efficiency.

In order to count the radioactivity of the individual lipid samples, the silicic acid containing the lipid spot is scraped off the plate with a razor blade onto glycine paper and transferred to a prelabeled counting vial containing 15 ml of scintillator (see below). Cap the vial tightly and shake well. Scrape a portion of the silicic acid from thc top of thc platc and placc in a vial to be used as a blank.

The results can be expressed in a number of ways—for example, as incorporation of the tracer into a lipid per gram of tissue or as fractional distribution, i.e., incorporation of the tracer into a specific lipid class relative to total incorporation.

TOLUENE SCINTILLATOR: Weigh 100 mg POPOP (1,4-bis-2-[5-phenyloxazolyl]-benzene) and 4 g PPO (2,5-diphenyloxazole) and dissolve in one liter of toluene. Allow to stand overnight before using.

Silicic Acid Column Chromatography

The following is a shortened and simplified modification of the method of Hirsch and Ahrens (1958):

1. Preparation of silicic acid columns:
   a. Use Mallinckrodt silicic acid, CC-4, 100-200 mesh.
   b. Heat silicic acid in oven at 110° to 120°C for 12 to 16 hours in 400-ml beaker filled to 100-ml mark.
   c. After activation, remove from oven and carefully slurry *immediately* with anhydrous ether.
   d. Decant and wash several times with hexane until the ether has been *completely* removed.
   e. Pour silicic acid slurry into hexane moistened columns, using a funnel to prevent spillage.
   f. Stir columns to remove air bubbles and apply N_2 pressure to settle: *never permit columns to run dry.*

Transfer samples prepared according to the above-mentioned procedure to the columns by dissolving the dried sample in a small amount of hexane and carefully adding the solutions to the top of each column. Wash sample containers twice with hexane and add washings to the columns.

2. A three-step elution is done as follows:
   a. Eluant No. 1:100 ml of 15 percent benzene in hexane to elute esterified cholesterol.
      (1) Add the eluant to the columns in two separate 50-ml washings. Add first washing carefully to avoid unsettling lipids.
      (2) Collect eluate in 250-ml evaporation flask: wash stem of column with hexane after eluant has run through to remove remaining CE's.
      (3) Take samples to dryness; add 50 ml ethanol:anhydrous ether (3:1 v/v) and mark completely around the flask with dotted line at 50-ml level. Add 0.5 ml 10 N KOH and cover with watch glass.
      (4) Saponify on steam bath at 100°C for 2 to 4 hours. Add small amounts of ethanol if necessary to prevent flasks from becoming dry.
      (5) Remove from bath and cool to room temperature. Add 25 ml distilled H_2O; then adjust to 50-ml mark with absolute ethanol. (A 50 percent alcoholic solution is optimal for complete cholesterol recovery.)
      (6) Add 60 ml petroleum ether, stopper, shake and allow to stand for at least 4 hours or overnight.
      (7) The following day, transfer the top (petroleum ether) layer containing nonsaponifiable lipids to separatory funnel, using minimal vacuum to avoid splashing. Surface wash flask five times to insure complete recovery.
      (8) Wash sample in separatory funnel with 50 ml distilled water to remove ionic contaminants. Remove and discard bottom (H_2O) layer and wash funnel stem with methanol.
      (9) Drain petroleum ether into evaporating flasks; wash funnel several times with petroleum ether, then methanol.
      (10) Take samples to dryness. Add acetone to remove water and take to dryness again.
      (11) When samples are dry, add 50 ml petroleum ether to all flasks. Transfer by suction into 100-ml volumetric flasks, using additional washings with petroleum ether to insure complete transfer. (For tissue samples, use 10-ml volumetric flasks.)
      (12) Fill flasks to mark and take aliquots for colorimetric determination.
      (13) Transfer remaining sample or appropriate aliquots to evaporating flasks, take to dryness, and transfer to counting vials with methanol: chloroform (1:2).
      (14) To saponification flasks containing potassium salts of CEFA, add 1 ml concentrated HCl (or 10 ml 1.5N HCl) and 60 ml petroleum ether. Stopper and shake. Allow to stand for a minimum of 4 hours or overnight.
      (15) The following day, remove the top (petroleum ether) fraction containing the saponifiable lipids and transfer to separatory funnels, using minimal vacuum. Surface wash flask five times with additional petroleum ether.
      (16) Wash sample in separatory funnel with 50 ml distilled water to remove ionic contaminants. Remove and discard bottom (H_2O) layer and wash funnel stem with methanol.

(17) Drain remaining petroleum ether into evaporating flasks; wash funnel several times with petroleum ether, then with methanol.
(18) Take samples to dryness, adding acetone to remove water.
(19) Transfer CEFA to a volumetric flask and fill to volume with chloroform.
(20) Take aliquots for counting vials and for colorimetric determination of fatty acids.

b. Eluant No. 2: 20 ml chloroform and 130 ml anhydrous ether to elute free cholesterol, glycerides, and free fatty acids.
   (1) Add 20 ml chloroform to columns and allow to run through (do not allow to run dry); this conditions the column and renders it less likely to fissure from the ether. Add first amount of chloroform to columns very carefully with a Pasteur pipette to prevent unsettling the lipids.
   (2) The chloroform will move the lipid front down the columns about one inch; addition of ether, with its greater polarity, will bring the lipids down with the solvent front. Add the ether in three separate washings of 30 ml, 50 ml, and 50 ml.
   (3) Collect eluate in 250-ml evaporating flasks; wash stem of column with hexane after eluant has run through to remove any adhering lipids.
   (4) Take samples to dryness and add 25 ml petroleum ether to flasks. Aspirate into separatory funnels, using additional petroleum ether washings to remove all lipids.
   (5) Shake each sample three times with 20-ml volumes of alcoholic NaOH (0.05 N in 50 percent ethanol) to extract the FFA's. Collect NaOH washings in evaporation flasks; wash stem of funnels with ethanol after final extraction and set flasks aside. (50 ml 1 N NaOH diluted to 500 ml distilled water plus 500 ml ethanol.)
   (6) To petroleum ether fraction remaining in separatory funnels (containing free cholesterol and glycerides), add 25 ml 50 percent ethanol and shake.
   (7) Remove and discard bottom (water) layer. Wash petroleum ether fraction into extraction flasks, using additional washings of petroleum ether and methanol to insure recovery of all lipids.
   (8) Take flasks to dryness, adding acetone to remove water. Transfer to 25-ml volumetric flasks with hexane. Dilute to volume and transfer 25 ml (or appropriate aliquot) to evaporation flasks for saponification.
   (9) Take flasks to dryness and add 50 ml ethanol:ether (3:1, v/v). Mark completely around flask at 50-ml level with dotted lines.
   (10) Add 0.5 ml 10 N KOH and cover with watch glass.
   (11) Saponify on steam bath at 100°C for 2 to 4 hours; add small amounts of ethanol if necessary, to prevent from becoming dry.
   (12) Remove from steam bath and cool to room temperature.
   (13) Add 25 ml distilled water, then adjust to 50-ml mark with absolute ethanol (a 50 percent alcoholic solution is optimal for complete cholesterol recovery.)
   (14) Add 60 ml petroleum ether, stopper, shake, and allow to stand for at least 4 hours or overnight.

(15) *Free fatty acid fraction:* Acidify each FFA sample (extracted with alcoholic NaOH, see step 5) with 5 ml HCl:H_2O (1:1, v/v); add 60 ml petroleum ether, stopper, shake, and allow to stand for several hours. Following equilibration, aspirate top (petroleum ether) layer containing FFA's into separatory funnels, surface-wash five times with additional petroleum ether to insure complete recovery. Wash samples in separatory funnels once each with 50 ml distilled water. Remove and discard bottom (H_2O) layer and wash funnel stem with methanol. Drain petroleum ether fraction into evaporating flasks, washing funnels with additional petroleum ether and methanol. Take flasks to dryness, adding acetone to remove water. Set aside for FFA colorimetric test. Bring FFA up to 10 ml with chloroform in a volumetric flask. Use 5 ml for colorimetric test, 4 ml for counting.

(16) *Glyceride/free cholesterol extract* (5/25 remaining in volumetric flask): Since the glyceride colorimetric test is a test involving the glycerol moiety, this test must be run on an unsaponified sample. Hence, aliquots are taken from the remaining extract (see step 8) for this analysis. (For glyceride colorimetric test: use 1 ml of serum samples; 0.2 ml of tissue samples.) Additional portions are taken for cholesterol analysis (as a check for cholesterol recovery following saponification) and for counting (1 ml for counting from the 5/25 ml remaining).

(17) *Saponification flasks:* After equilibration (step 14), top (petroleum ether) layer containing free cholesterol is aspirated into separatory funnels, using minimal vacuum to avoid splattering. Surface wash all flasks five times each to insure complete recovery of FC.

(18) Wash samples in separatory funnels with 50 ml distilled water to remove ionic contaminants. Remove and discard bottom (H_2O) layer and rinse funnel stem with methanol.

(19) Drain petroleum ether fraction containing free cholesterol into evaporating flasks, using additional washings of petroleum ether and methanol.

(20) Take samples to dryness, using acetone to remove water.

(21) When completely dry, add 50 ml petroleum ether to all flasks.

(22) Aspirate into 100-ml volumetric flasks using additional washings of petroleum ether to insure complete recovery.

(23) Dilute to volume and take appropriate aliquots for cholesterol colorimetric test.

(24) Take remaining sample or appropriate aliquot to dryness in evaporating flask and transfer to counting vial with methanol:chloroform (1:2, v/v).

(25) To saponification flasks (see step 17), which contain potassium salts of glyceride fatty acids, add 1 ml concentrated HCl; add 60 ml petroleum ether, stopper, shake, and allow to equilibrate for at least 4 hours or overnight.

(26) The next day, aspirate top (petroleum ether) fraction into separatory funnels using additional surface washes, as indicated previously.

(27) Wash samples in separatory funnels with 50 ml distilled water; remove and discard bottom (H_2O) layer.

(28) Drain petroleum ether fraction containing glyceride fatty acids into evaporating flasks, washing funnels with petroleum ether and methanol.
(29) Take flasks to dryness and transfer to counting vials with methanol: chloroform (1:2, v/v).

c. Eluant No. 3: 150 ml methanol to elute phospholipids.
(1) Add the eluant to the column in two separate washings: first 50 ml, then 100 ml. As indicated previously, add the first amount carefully with a Pasteur pipette to avoid unsettling the lipids.
(2) Collect eluate in a 200-ml volumetric flask; wash stem of column with additional methanol after eluant has run through to recover adhering phospholipids.
(3) Dilute to volume and remove appropriate aliquots for colorimetric test (1 ml from 200 ml total)
(4) Transfer remaining sample or appropriate aliquot to evaporation flask, take to dryness, and transfer to radioactive counting vials with methanol: chloroform (1:2, v/v).

Determination of radioactivity:
The aliquots are evaporated to dryness in the counting vial and redissolved in 0.5 ml of petroleum ether or methanol (phospholipids). Add 15 ml of toluene scintillator and place the counting vial in a liquid scintillation spectrometer.

Colorimetric Determinations

*Phospholipids**

REAGENTS:†

1. Nitric acid, 1 mg calcium nitrate per ml. Stock: 2.5 Ca $(NO_3)_2 \cdot 4H_2O$ in 425 ml HNO_3. Store in brown bottle. Working: Dilute 1 ml stock to 50 ml with HNO_3.
2. 10 percent trichloroacetic acid (TCA).
3. 10 percent ascorbic acid (fresh).
4. 1 percent ammonium molybdate.
5. Arsenite-citrate: Place 20 g sodium arsenite and 20 g sodium citrate in a 1-liter volumetric flask. Add approximately 800 ml of water and dissolve completely. Then add 20 ml acetic acid and fill flask to mark with distilled water.
6. Standard. Stock: Dissolve 438.1 mg of potassium dihydrogen phosphate in distilled water in a 100-ml volumetric flask and dilute to volume. Working: Dilute 0.25 ml of the stock solution to 100 ml with distilled water (0.0025 mg inorganic phosphorus/ml).

PROCEDURE:

1. Evaporate appropriate aliquot to dryness in sand bath. Place three glass beads into each tube.
2. Add 2 ml nitric acid-calcium nitrate. Mix.

*From Baginski and Zak. 1960. *Clin. Chim. Acta,* 5:834.

†All glassware is not acid-washed.

3. Evaporate to dryness using Meker burner. All nitric acid fumes must be expelled.
4. Cool.
5. Add 2 ml TCA and shake.
6. Add 0.5 ml ascorbic acid and shake.
7. Add 1 ml ammonium molybdate and shake.
8. Add 2 ml arsenite-citrate. Must be added within 4 minutes of the ammonium molybdate.
9. Mix and wait 15 minutes.
10. Read OD at 700 m against reagent blank.

CALCULATIONS:

$$\frac{0.0025 \times DF \times CF \times OD_{sample}}{OD_{standard}} \times 25 = \text{mg phospholipid/g of tissue or serum}$$

0.0025 = mg inorganic phosphorus in standard

DF = dilution factor (usually 200/1 because 1 ml sample represents a total of 200 ml)

CF = correction factor (usually the results are expressed per gram sample)

25 = factor to convert mg phosphorous to mg phospholipid

*Glycerides**

REAGENTS:

1. Alcoholic KOH, 1 ml of 7 N KOH/100 ml absolute alcohol.
2. 0.2 N H_2SO_4.
3. Sodium periodate, 0.025 M or 0.5 percent (5.347 g/liter).
4. Chromotropic acid (4,5-dihydroxy-2,7-naphthalenedisulfonic acid disodium salt), 0.2 percent in 60 percent H_2SO_4. Add 200 ml distilled water to 600 ml H_2SO_4. Dissolve 2 g salt in 200 ml water. Allow to cool and mix together. Store in brown bottle.
5. Standard: 0.05 mg tripalmitin/ml hexane. Use 1.0 ml.
6. 0.5 M sodium arsenite.

PROCEDURE

1. Take the sample containing glycerides to dryness.
2. Add 0.5 ml alcoholic KOH.
3. Saponify at 60° to 70° C for 15 to 20 minutes.
4. Remove from the water bath and add 0.5 ml H_2SO_4. Shake.
5. Place in boiling water bath. (Water level should be less than ½ height of tubes.) Boil 10 to 12 minutes until there is no alcohol smell. There should be about 0.3 ml in tube. Adjust with distilled water.

*From Van Handel et al. 1957. *J. Lab. Clin. Med.*, 50:152.

6. Cool to room temperature.
7. Add 0.05 ml sodium periodate (or one drop) and shake each tube.
8. Wait 10 minutes.
9. Add 0.05 ml or one drop sodium arsenite. Shake and wait 10 minutes.
10. Add 5 ml chromotropic acid and *mix thoroughly.*
11. Place in boiling water bath for 30 minutes. (Water level should be above the contents of the tube.)
12. Cool and read OD at 570 m against a reagent blank.

CALCULATIONS:

$$\frac{0.05 \times DF \times CF \times OD_{sample}}{OD_{standard}} = \text{mg glyceride/g of tissue or serum}$$

0.05 = mg glyceride in standard

DF = dilution factor (usually 25/0.2 for tissue, 25/1 for serum)

CF = correction factor to one gram

*Cholesterol**

REAGENTS:

1. Concentrated sulfuric acid, reagent grade.
2. Ethyl acetate, reagent grade.
3. Ferric chloride, $FeCl_3 \cdot 6\ H_2O$.
4. Color reagent: 1 g ferric chloride/liter ethyl acetate.
5. Standard: 0.05 mg cholesterol/ml. Use 1 ml.

PROCEDURE:

1. Take appropriate aliquot of cholesterol sample to dryness on a water bath.
2. Add 3 ml color reagent and shake.
3. Add 2 ml concentrated sulfuric acid and mix immediately.
4. Cool to room temperature (10 minutes).
5. Read OD at 550 mμ against a reagent blank.

CALCULATIONS:

$$\frac{0.05 \times DF \times CF \times OD_{sample}}{OD_{standard}} = \text{mg cholesterol/g of tissue or serum}$$

0.05 = mg cholesterol in standard
DF = dilution factor (usually 10/3 because a 3 ml sample from a total of 10 ml was tested)
CF = correction factor to one gram

*From Babson et al. 1962. *Clin. Chim. Acta,* 7:800.

*Free Fatty Acids**

REAGENTS:

1. Sodium diethyldithiocarbamate (Na-DEDTC), 0.1 percent in *n*-butanol (stable for a week).
2. 1 M triethanolamine (13.55 ml/100 ml distilled water).
3. 6.45 percent cupric nitrate (16.13 g/250 ml distilled water).
4. 1 M acetic acid.
5. Reaction mixture: 10 $Cu(NO_3)_2$:9 triethanol amine:1 acetic acid.
6. Standard: 1 mg palmitic acid/ml chloroform. Use 0.1 ml.

PROCEDURE:

1. Take appropriate aliquot of fatty acid sample and place in wide ignition tube.
2. Bring up to 10 ml total volume with chloroform.
3. Add 5 ml reaction mixture and shake on vortex mixer until well mixed. Bottom layer should be clear.
4. Remove top layer with suction.
5. Pour chloroform layer in Sorvall tubes and centrifuge for 5 minutes.
6. Pour supernatant into fresh tubes and transfer a 3-ml aliquot into small tubes.
7. Add 0.5 ml Na-DEDTC and mix.
8. Read OD at 440 m against a reagent blank.

CALCULATIONS:

$$\frac{0.1 \times DF \times CF \times OD_{sample}}{OD_{standard}} = \text{mg free fatty acid/g of tissue or serum}$$

0.1 = mg free fatty acid in standard

DF = dilution factor (usually 10/5 since 5 ml sample is from 10 ml total)

CF = correction factor to one gram

MYOCARDIAL BLOOD FLOW DETERMINATION WITH RUBIDIUM-84

Introduction

The determination of coronary blood flow is valuable for the correlation of myocardial metabolic studies with oxygen consumption by the heart. The development of coincidence counting and injections of Rubidium-84 chloride (^{84}RbCl) allows the clinical determination of myocardial blood flow (MBF) without

*From Anstall and Trujillo. 1965. *Clin. Chem.*, 11:741.

cardiac catheterization (Nolting et al., 1958; Bing et al., 1964). This method determines clearance of $^{84}RbCl$ by the myocardial nutritional blood flow to the heart (MBF), rather than the total coronary perfusion flow.

Rubidium, a member of the same atomic family as potassium, is actively transported across the cell membrane. Rubidium-84 decays by the emission of positrons (β^+). Positrons travel a few millimeters from their origin before annihilation with a negative electron and emission of two gamma photons of 0.51 million electron volts each which travel in opposite directions. Counts are registered when a gamma photon pair strikes an opposing (180°) pair of radiation detectors within the same 0.05 second (i.e., "coincidence"). Rubidium-84 has a 33-day half-life which is convenient for clinical use. The double-coincidence counting system* consists of two pairs of sodium iodide scintillation detection crystals, each pair arranged anteriorly and posteriorly to the chest 180° apart. One pair of scintillation detectors, 4 inches in diameter, is aligned over the fluoroscopically outlined border of the heart. A second pair of scintillation detectors, 2 inches in diameter, is aligned over the right side of the chest in a position free of the larger thoracic vessels. Background activity detected from the right side of the chest is electronically subtracted from the combined heart and chest activity, resulting in an expression of myocardial activity alone.

Major advantages of the double-coincidence counting technique are the ability to detect activity in the cylindrical space between the detectors without elaborate collimation and the separation of the activity of the heart from that of the surrounding structures. When the method was first developed in this laboratory, the $^{84}RbCl$ was injected intravenously at a constant rate by a pump. The slopes of activity from the coincidence pairs and arterial blood were recorded on a strip chart as average counts per seven seconds. The test procedure was divided into three 7-minute steady-state periods. The main advantage of the constant infusion method was that the rate of isotopic uptake by the heart was recorded. The main disadvantages of the constant infusion method are that changes of MBF during short periods cannot be detected, no convenient reference for comparison is possible, and calculations are cumbersome. The more recent development of rapid bolus injections by Donato et al. (1964) and the application of this technique to coincidence counting of $^{84}RbCl$ bolus injections by McHenry and Knoebel (1967) allow the simple and reproducible measurement of MBF during short periods of time. Bolus injections can be easily compared with simultaneous direct Fick principle measurements.

Experimental Procedure

ELECTRONIC STANDARDIZATION.—Calibration of the electronic apparatus requires adjustment of the high voltage source so that the most sensitive detector, the well counter, which measures activity in arterial blood, has a constant response to a known standard radioactivity source. The response of each detector

*Co-Insitron. American Science and Engineering, Inc., Cambridge, Mass.

to a known standard source at various voltage window openings is plotted. The detector is then set at the portion of the voltage response curve which gives the widest range of constant response to this source.

PREPARATION OF RUBIDIUM SOURCE.—Each shipment of $^{84}RbCl$ is accompanied by radiation activity data expressed in terms of microcuries per milliliter of sterile solution at pH 7.4. A decay curve is plotted, and about 10 microcuries (determined by weight) is diluted to 25 ml. The 4-inch diameter source dish is filled with this solution and the volume determined by weighing. The dish is sealed with waterproof tape and sprayed with quick-drying adhesive. From the remainder of the 25-ml dilution, 1 ml is diluted to 100 ml, and a Radicoil is filled with a measured volume of this solution and the ends sealed with clamps. These sources are used for routine daily calibrations.

TEST PROCEDURE.—The details of the test are explained to each patient; informed consent is obtained. The heart borders are drawn on the chest with a crayon during fluoroscopy. A polyethylene cannula (large Intracath*) is introduced percutaneously into an antecubital vein. The opposite antecubital fossa is scrubbed and infiltrated with Xylocaine (1 percent). A needle is introduced into the brachial artery and 100 mg of heparin is injected into the artery. The arterial needle is then connected to a 10-ml Radicoil in the arterial well counter. The distal Radicoil tubing is connected to a withdrawal pump calibrated to withdraw 40 ml/min. While arterial blood is being withdrawn through the Radicoil, $^{84}RbCl$ (0.2 microcuries/lb body weight) is injected intravenously as a bolus at the head of a 10-ml normal saline flush. The sums of activity per 3 seconds of the well counter and the myocardial activity are continuously recorded by a rapid recorder as a printout. Arterial activity is recorded during the first circulation (about 30 to 40 seconds). Precordial activity is recorded for 3 minutes, beginning 90 seconds after initial appearance. At the end of the test the needles are withdrawn and pressure is applied for 5 minutes to the arterial puncture site.

CALCULATION OF DATA.—Myocardial blood flow (MBF) in terms of the clearance of rubidium by the heart is calculated by the equation:

$$MBF = K_x \frac{U_H(t)}{A_1(t)dt}$$

$U_H(t)$ represents average myocardial uptake (counts/minute) for 3 minutes (from 90 seconds after precordial appearance of activity). $A_1(t)dt$ is the primary curve area of arterial activity redrawn on semilogarithmic paper. K represents a factor calculated for each study to convert injectate activity to values comparable to

*Manufactured by C. R. Bard, Inc., Murray Hill, N.J.

arterial counts from the well counter and to correct for transmission factors, distances between crystal pairs, chest density, and the geometry of the chest.

$$K = 0.86 \times \frac{\text{CHO} \times \text{AWO}}{\text{CHL} \times \text{COHO}}$$

The factor 0.86 is a constant number representing the transmission, the volume and dilution factors for the dish and Radicoil, the mass of the heart, and the geometry of the heart. CHO is the coincidence counting rate of the rubidium-84 source without the patient on the table. CHL is the coincidence counting rate of the rubidium-84 source placed over the precordial area. AWO is the counting rate of the source solution. COHO is the counting rate with rubidium-84 source between the upper and lower precordial crystals at the level of the heart, but without the patient on the table. COHO is recorded when the patient leaves the table after the test. The two precordial crystal pairs are made equisensitive to the rubidium-84 source by introducing a factor (F) into the scaler:

$$F = \frac{\text{CHL}}{\text{CBR}} \div 2$$

CBR is the coincidence counting rate of the rubidium-84 source over the right side of the chest.

SAMPLE CALCULATION:

Patient #700. The activity of the bolus is calculated:

0.2 microcuries/lb × weight (188 lb) = 37.6 microcuries

The activity of the rubidium-84 for the test day is obtained from the decay curve, and the desired bolus activity is divided by this to determine the volume of rubidium-84 solution:

37.6 microcuries ÷ 133 microcuries/ml (5/3/68) = 0.28 ml ^{84}RbCl

The accuracy of the bolus activity is checked by determining the weight of the syringe before and after injection of the rubidium-84 solution:

3.34 g (syringe and rubidium) – 3.06 g (syringe) = 0.28 ml

The primary arterial activity is counted over a period of about 20 seconds. Precordial activity level is 44 counts/3 seconds, K equals 535, and A_1 is 3,733 counts/3 seconds, 20 equals conversion of seconds to a minute. Therefore:

$$\text{MBF} = \frac{44 \times 20}{3{,}733} \times 535 = 126 \text{ ml/minute}$$

The method outlined permits, in a relatively simple fashion, the calculation of total and nutritional (effective) blood flow in man and in the anesthetized animal. Its advantages over other isotope methods used in the determination of coronary blood flow are the application of coincidence counting and the rapidity with which the test can be performed.

REFERENCES

Anstall, H. B., and Trujillo, J. M. 1965. Determination of free fatty acids in plasma by a colorimetric procedure: An appraisal of the method and comparison with other technics. Clin. Chem., 11:741.

Babson, A. L., Shapiro, P. O., and Phillips, G. E. 1962. A new assay for cholesterol and cholesterol esters in serum which is not affected by bilirubin. Clin. Chim. Acta, 7:800.

Baginski, E., and Zak, B. 1960. Micro-determination of serum phosphate and phospholipids. Clin. Chim. Acta, 5:834.

Bergmeyer, H. U., ed. 1963. Methods of Enzymatic Analysis. New York, Academic Press, Inc., and Verlag Chemie.

---- and Bernt, E. 1963a. Malic dehydrogenase. *In* Methods of Enzymatic Analysis. Bergmeyer, H. U., ed. New York, Academic Press, Inc., and Verlag Chemie, p. 757.

— and Bernt, E. 1963b. Glutamate-oxaloacetate transaminase. *In* Methods of Enzymatic Analysis. Bergmeyer, H. U., ed. New York, Academic Press, Inc., and Verlag Chemie, p. 837.

— Bernt, E., and Hess, B. 1963. Lactic dehydrogenase. *In* Methods of Enzymatic Analysis. Bergmeyer, H. U., ed. New York, Academic Press, Inc., and Verlag Chemie, p. 736.

Bernt, E., and Bergmeyer, H. U. 1963. Creatine phosphokinase. *In* Methods of Enzymatic Analysis. Bergmeyer, H. U., ed. New York, Academic Press, Inc., and Verlag Chemie, p. 859.

Bing, R. J., Bennish, A., Bluemchen, G., Cohen, A., Gallagher, J. P., and Zaleski, E. J. 1964. The determination of coronary flow equivalent with coincidence counting technique. Circulation, 24:833.

Bruns, F. H., and Bergmeyer, H. U. 1963. Fructose-1,6-diphosphate aldolase. *In* Methods of Enzymatic Analysis. Bergmeyer, H. U., ed. New York, Academic Press, Inc., and Verlag Chemie, p. 724.

Bücher, T., Luh, W., and Pette, D. 1964. Einfache und zusammengesetzte optische Tests mit Pyridinnucleotiden. Hoppe-Seyler/Thierfelder Handbuch der Physiologisch und Pathologisch Chemischen Analyse, 6A:292.

Delbruck, A., Zebe, E., and Bücher, T. 1959. Über Verteilungsmuster von Enzymen des Energieliefernden Stoffwechsels im Flugmuskel, Sprungmuskel und Fettkorper von Locusta Migratoria und ihre Cytologische Zuordnung. Biochem. Z., 331:273.

Donato, L., Bartolomei, G., and Giordani, R. 1964. Evaluation of myocardial blood perfusion in man with potassium or rubidium and precordial counting. Circulation, 29:195.

Folch, J., Lees, M., and Sloane Stanley, G. H. 1957. A simple method for the isolation and purification of total lipids from animal tissues. J. Biol. Chem., 226:497.

Fox, A. C., and Reed, G. E. 1969. Changes in lactate dehydrogenase composition of heart with right ventricular hypertrophy. Amer. J. Physiol., 216:1026.

Glock, G. E. 1964. Glucose-6-phosphate dehydrogenase and 6-phosphogluconate dehydrogenase. Hoppe-Seyler/Thierfelder Handbuch der Physiologisch and Pathologisch Chemischen Analyse. 6A:414.

Goebell, H., and Klingenberg, M. 1964. DPN-Spezifische Isocitrate-Dehydrogenase der

Mitochondrien. 1. Kinetische Eigenschaften, Vorkommen und Funktion der DPN-Spezifischen Isocitrate-Dehydrogenase. Biochem. Z., 340:441.
Gudbjarnason, S., and Priver, D. 1968. LDH-Isoenzymes in infarcted heart muscle. Life Sci., 7:623.
— Cowan, C., Braasch, W., and Bing, R. J. 1968. Changes in enzyme pattern of heart muscle in response to myocardial infarction. Cardiologia, 41:148.
— DeSchryver, D., Hunn, G., and Bing, R. J. 1964. Changes in myocardial enzyme pattern in human heart disease. J. Lab. Clin. Med., 64:796.
Henry, R. J., Sobel, C., and Berkman, S. 1957. Interferences with biuret methods for serum proteins. Anal. Chem., 29:1491.
Hirsch, J., and Ahrens, E. H. 1958. The separation of complex lipid mixtures by the use of silicic acid chromatography. J. Biol. Chem., 233:311.
Lohr, G. W., and Waller, H. D. 1963. Glucose-6-phosphate dehydrogenase (Zwischenferment). *In* Methods of Enzymatic Analysis. Bergmeyer, H. U., ed. New York, Academic Press, Inc., and Verlag Chemie, p. 744.
McHenry, P. L., and Knoebel, S. B. 1967. Measurement of coronary blood flow by coincidence counting and a bolus of ^{84}RbCl. J. Appl. Physiol., 22:495.
Nachlas, M. M., and Shnitka, T. K. 1963. Macroscopic identification of early myocardial infarcts by alterations in dehydrogenase activity. Amer. J. Path., 42:379.
Nolting, D., Mack, R., Luthy, E., Kirsch, M., and Hogancamp, C. 1958. Measurement of coronary blood flow and myocardial rubidium uptake with Rubidium^{86}. J. Clin. Invest., 37:921.
Van Handel, E., Silversmit, B. B., and Bowman, K. 1957. Micromethod for the direct determination of serum triglycerides. J. Lab. Clin. Med., 50:152.

CHAPTER 3

Isolated Atrial Preparations

Joseph V. Levy
Research Laboratories, Presbyterian Hospital, Pacific Medical Center
San Francisco, California

INTRODUCTION

This chapter deals with methods, techniques, and procedures that can be used for studying drug effects on the contractile properties of atrial myocardium in vitro. Particular emphasis will be given to the description of methods involving rabbit atrial tissue, although in most instances the techniques can also be applied to atria from other species.

Rabbit atrial muscle offers distinct advantages for the in vitro study of myocardial function and the action of drugs. Among these features are (1) thinness of tissue permits good oxygen diffusion in vitro; (2) extensive tissue trimming or slicing is not necessary; (3) uniformity of tissue size eliminates need for tissue selection; (4) tissue size permits easy recording of contractile tension without high electronic recording amplification; (5) easy separation of right and left atria for experiments using spontaneously beating or stimulated preparations; (6) tissue size

This chapter was prepared by the author during tenure of a Research Career Program Award from the National Heart Institute, NIH.
Original work by the author cited in this survey was supported in part by grants from the American Heart Association, NIH, San Francisco and San Mateo Heart Association, American Medical Association, and various private donors and contributors.

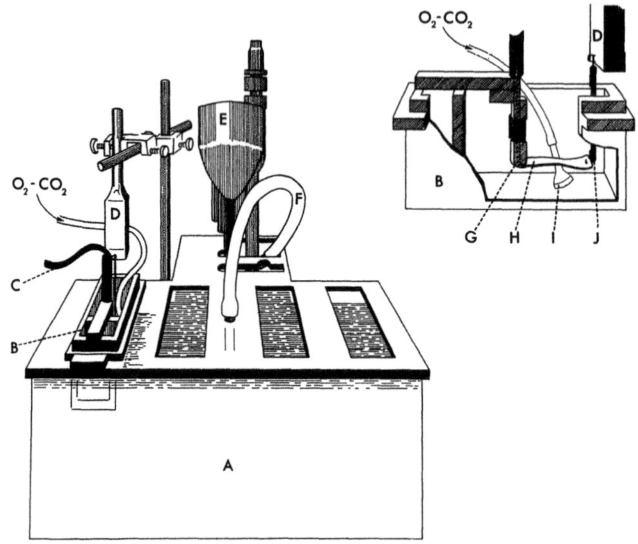

FIG. 1. Multi-chamber apparatus for studying cardiac muscle. (A) Constant temperature tank with one muscle chamber (B) in position. (B: Insert) Detail of muscle chamber. (C) Electrode connections to electronic stimulator. (D) Force-displacement transducer. (E) Constant temperature heater-circulator. (F) Hose connection from pump circulator to tank. (G) Platinum electrode (shielded)-muscle clamp device. (H) Muscle strip. (I) gas delivery (dispersion) disc. (J) Muscle hook attached to cantilever arm of transducer. (Levy, unpublished).

and shape permits direct coupling of tissue with holding clamp and electrodes to recording transducer without the use of ties or ligatures; (7) preparations show good contractile tension and stability over many hours under usual experimental conditions; (8) tissue size and mass permit most chemical and biochemical analyses without the necessity of pooling atria of different experiments. Other specific advantages of using atrial tissue for in vitro cardiac muscle experiments will be presented under specific sections to follow.

PHYSICAL APPARATUS

Muscle Chambers

A variety of muscle chambers or myographs have been developed for holding isolated atrial tissue. These variations reflect special requirements depending on the general type of experiment being conducted. These variations usually involve general access of muscle, mounting and placement procedures, changing perfusate solutions, placement of electronic accessories, temperature regulation, tissue oxygenation, and other manipulations that are required for any given experimental protocol.

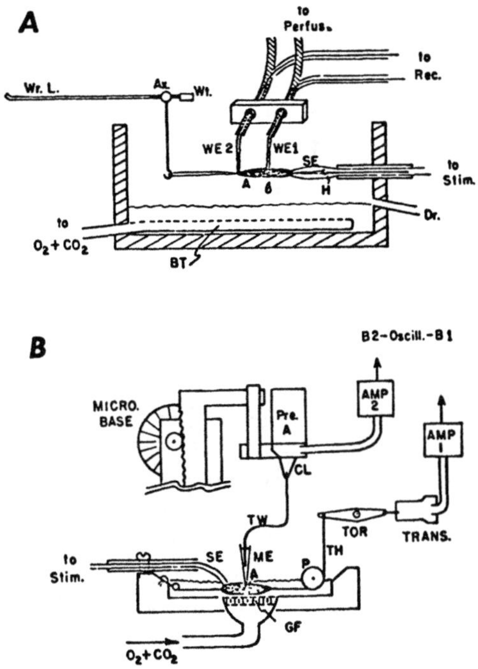

FIG. 2. Example of horizontal muscle chamber. (A) Schematic diagram showing electrode, tissue, and recording system arrangement. (B) Arrangement for experiments using microelectrode (ME) recording. (From Furchgott et al., 1960.)

The author has found over many years of working with a variety of muscle chambers that most, if not all, of the important requirements for in vitro experiments are conveniently met using a horizontal muscle chamber arrangement. Figure 1B shows a typical configuration of a muscle chamber which has a functional volume of 50 ml. Other examples of muscle chambers which have been used for studying atria in a horizontal position are illustrated in Figures 2, 3A, and 4.

The chamber illustrated in Figure 1B is constructed of Plexiglas brand of acrylic plastic (Rohm and Hass). Joints are secured and sealed with an ethylene dichloride solvent. The inside dimensions of the chamber are 7.0 L by 2.9 W by 4.0 D cm. The bottom may be canted to facilitate muscle chamber drainage during wash procedures. Whatever materials are chosen for construction of the basic muscle chamber, it is important to remember that they must be (1) nontoxic to the muscle, (2) chemically nonreactive with solvents, drugs, salt solutions, or other materials added to the muscle perfusate, (3) glues, adhesives, or solvents must afford secure joint seals to avoid leakage of chamber contents.

Ease of fabrication of Plexiglas chambers makes for low unit cost, thus permitting discarding of units when excessive surface pitting or defects appear with repeated detergent washings. The chamber must be of sufficient strength and

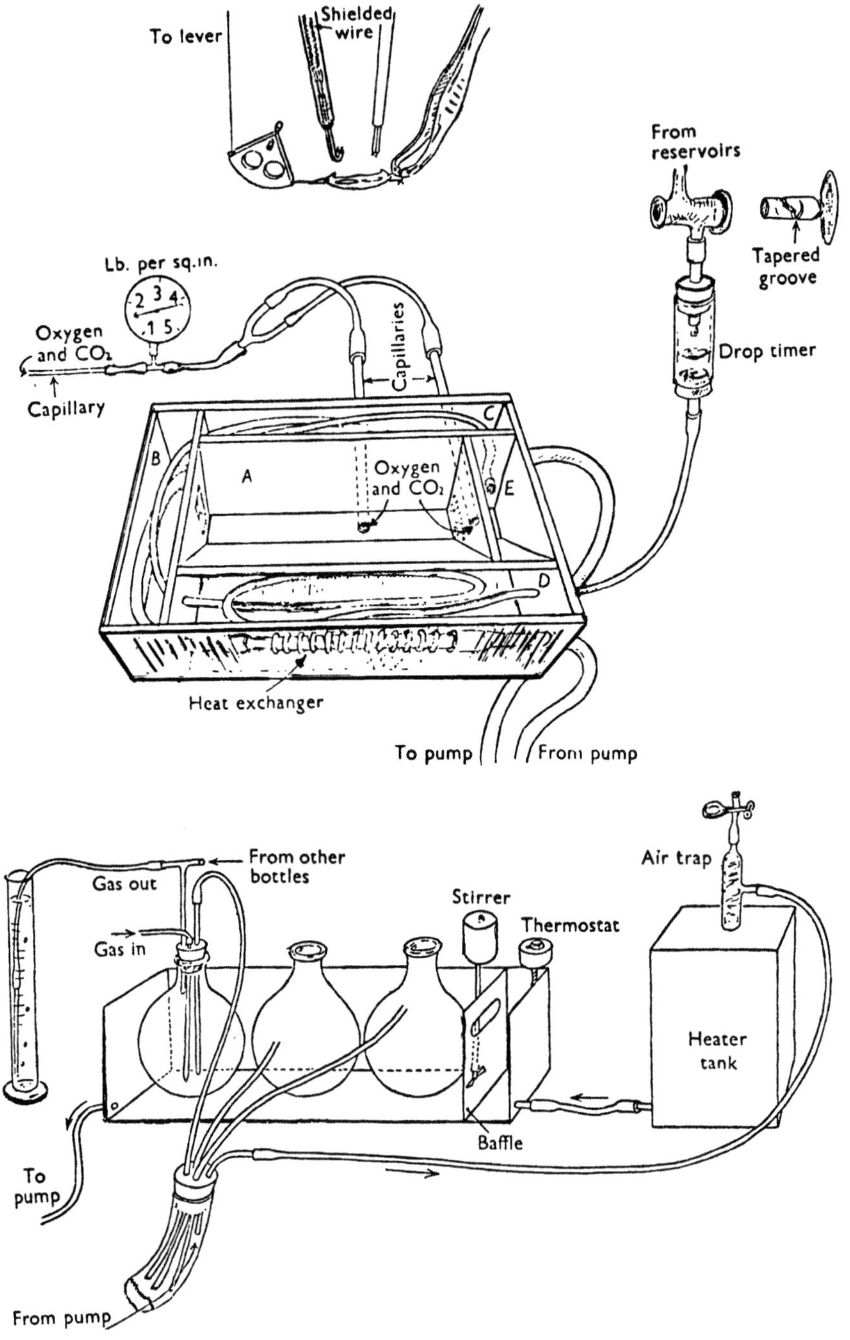

FIG. 3. (Top) Muscle chamber for studying the electrical and contractile properties of isolated atrial myocardium. Insert shows arrangement of muscle stimulating and recording electrodes, and transducer pulley. (Bottom) Arrangement for external perfusion of muscle chamber using perfusate reservoirs. (From Vaughan Williams, 1955.)

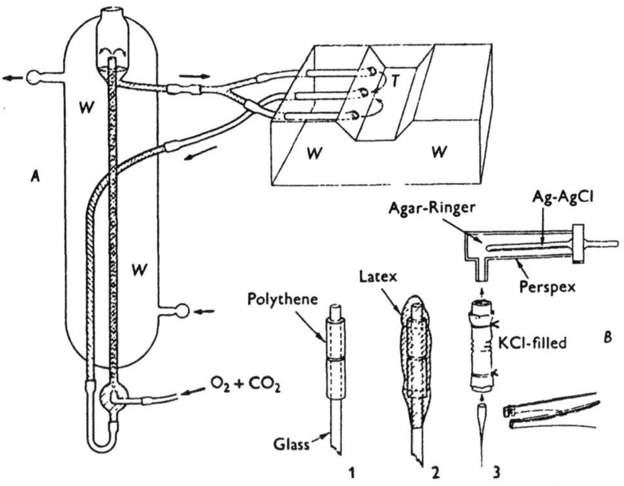

FIG. 4. Modified perfusion circulation system for isolated muscle chamber. (B) Microelectrode mount and assembly details. (From Szekeres and Vaughan Williams, 1962.)

rigidity to permit mounting of brackets, electrodes, and other chamber attachments. The thickness of the Plexiglas must be such as to minimize the temperature gradient from inside to outside when the chamber is placed in a constant temperature tank. Figure 1A shows a simple suggested multichamber configuration permitting the study of one to four preparations.

For intracellular recordings using microelectrode techniques, the horizontal tissue arrangement affords ample room for placement of the electrode, electrode probe, and associated manipulators. Thus, simultaneous recording of transmembrane electrical events and mechanical functions of the muscle can be made (Figs. 2A, 2B, 3A, 4).

When it is deemed desirable to use an atrial preparation in a vertical muscle chamber configuration, a variety of methods and techniques are available. Figures 5, 6, 7, 8, and 9 illustrate typical examples of chambers, clamps, electrodes, and associated equipment for studying isolated cardiac muscle in a vertical position. It will be noted, however, that the methods shown require that one or both ends of the muscle be secured via ties or threads connected to the appropriate holding block and/or recording transducer. Also note that in the vertical configuration, access to the tissue is difficult or impossible insofar as recording from the surface of the muscle with electrodes. However, vertical configurations offer the advantage of ease of bath perfusate exchange and minimum loss of bath contents through evaporative loss because of a smaller bath cross-sectional area compared to most horizontal chamber arrangements.

Stimulating Electrodes

In experiments where it is required that the atrial tissue be excited with external electrical stimuli, it is important to recognize the advantages and

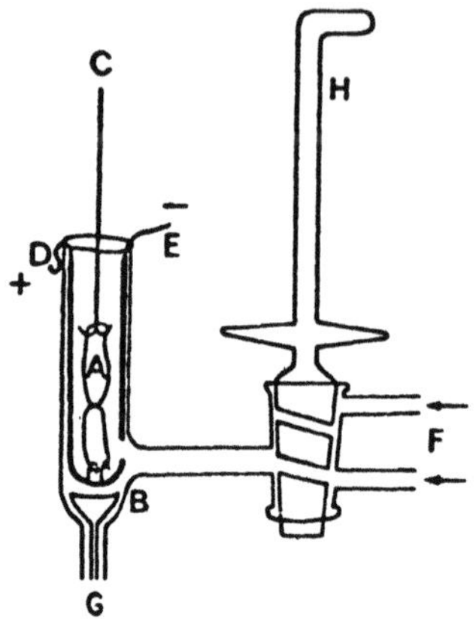

FIG. 5. Small volume (5–7.5 ml) muscle chamber for studying contractile functions of isolated atrial muscle. (A) Atrial appendage. (B) Glass muscle chamber. (C) Connection from muscle to recording transducer. (D, E) Stimulating electrodes (field). (F) Perfusate delivery through stopcock assembly H. (From Thorp and Cobbin, 1967.)

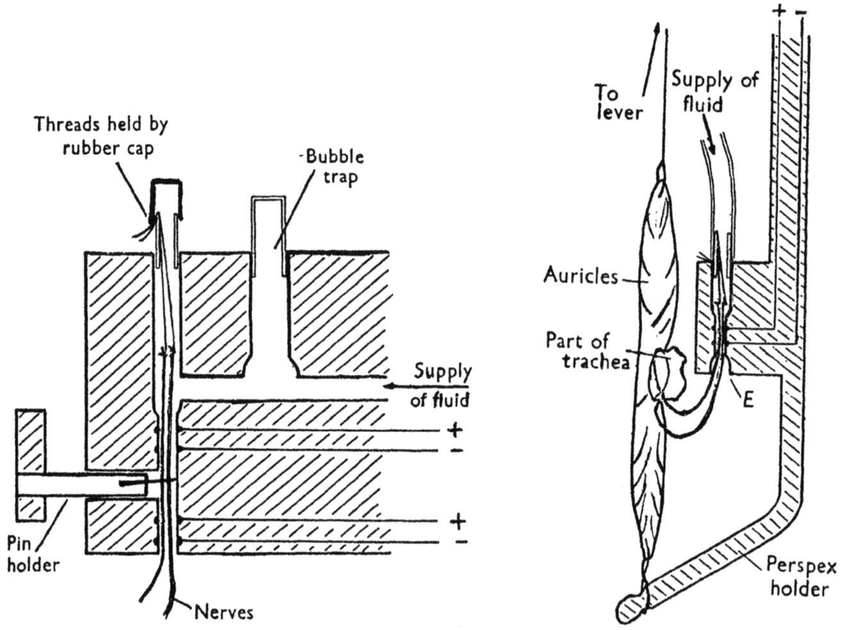

FIG. 6. Nerve-auricle (atria) preparation. Insert on left shows arrangement for stimulation of vagus nerves supplying atrial muscle. Figure on right shows vertical arrangement of muscle for recording of contractile functions. Perspex holder is immersed in constant temperature chamber. (From McEwen, 1956.)

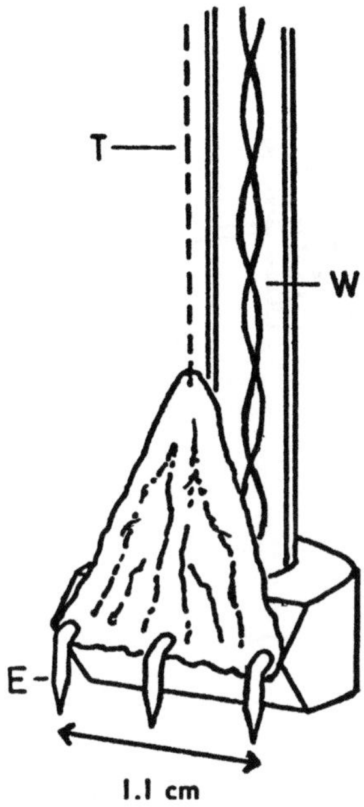

FIG. 7. Isolated atrial appendage. Atrium is mounted vertically by anchoring base on three pins that also serve as stimulating electrodes (E). Other end of muscle is held with a tie that is led to a transducer for recording of contraction (T). (From Lock, 1963.)

disadvantages of the type of electrodes used for this purpose.

Three basic types of electrodes have been described. Two involve direct contact of the electrode with the muscle; the other involves excitation of the muscle through use of "field stimulation." Figures 1B, 2, 7, and 8A illustrate examples of stimulating electrodes in contact with the tissue; Figures 8B, 8C, and 9 (inset) show examples of the use of "field stimulation" electrodes.

The use of the latter type of electrode is generally advocated when it is desirable to provide simultaneous excitation of the muscle by applying a transverse or longitudinal current flow along the whole length of the muscle. Stimulation of the muscle by this technique is recognized to cause excessive release of neurotransmitter substances (e.g., norepinephrine and acetylcholine) from the myocardium, since intramural nerve endings are also excited along with the muscle fibers. This effect may be reduced by using stimulating currents only slightly above the threshold needed to excite the muscle. This procedure is self-defeating, however, since synchronous excitation of the tissue (for which "massive" or "field electrodes" are designed) cannot be assumed because the stimuli probably depolarize the tissue at limited sites.

Some advantages of using "massive stimulation" techniques are (1) minimizing contractile or electrical variability due to conduction along the muscle fibers, (2) synchrony of contraction in multifiber preparations is nearly optimum, and (3)

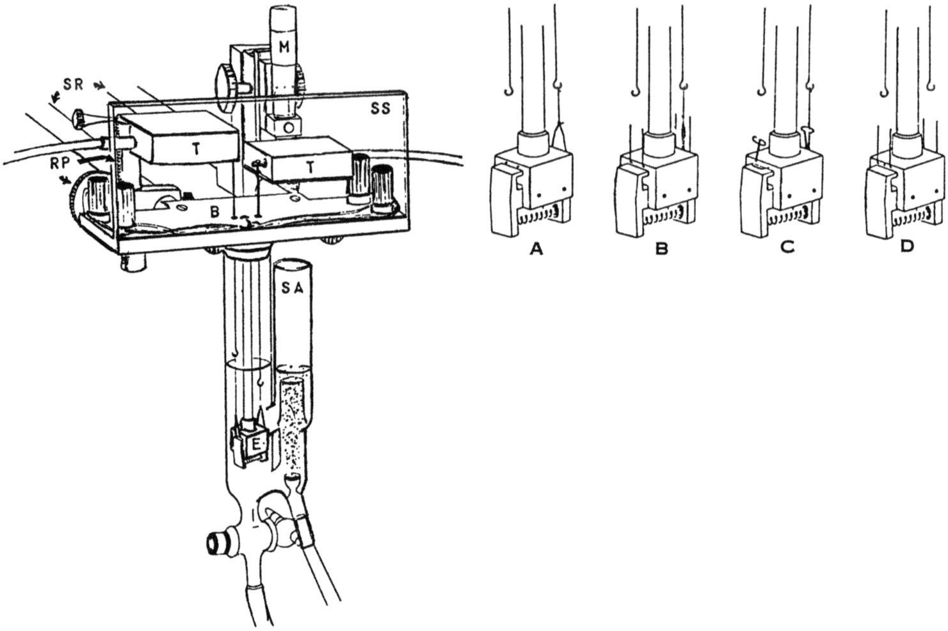

FIG. 8. Apparatus for recording contraction of isolated heart muscle. (E) Electrode-clamp assembly. (A) Enlargement of (E) showing one atrial appendage in position. Stimulating electrodes are of punctate type. (B) Baseplate for attaching recording and electrical accessories. (T) Force-displacement transducers. (M) Micrometer head. (SR) Support rods. (RP) Rack and pinion. (SS) Spray shield. (SA) Side arm of glass vessel for physiologic salt solution. The glass vessel is immersed in a constant-temperature tank after mounting the muscle on the electrode block. (From Blinks, 1965.)

changes in electrode-tissue resistance are absent due to avoiding contact with the tissue.

To achieve effective "field" or "massive stimulation" of isolated muscle, the following problems must be recognized and overcome: (1) low resistance of the physiologic salt solution through which the electrical stimulus traverses, (2) requirement of high current values from the stimulator in order that short pulse durations can be used, (3) no current should flow during intervals between application of the square wave stimuli.

Punctate and bar electrodes in direct contact with the muscle offer advantages in that they excite only a small portion of the tissue. Propagation of the impulse producing depolarization and contraction is more "physiologic" since fiber-conducting mechanisms are involved. Even then, if high-intensity (suprathreshold) stimuli are used, such small electrodes still can release neurotransmitter substances through excitation of nerve fibers in the muscle. In addition to this, it has been noted that the effects on atrial muscle produced by high-voltage high-frequency stimulation varied with the position of the electrode.

Thus, the advantages and disadvantages of punctate or contact electrodes versus plate or mass electrodes must be individually determined. Moreover, when

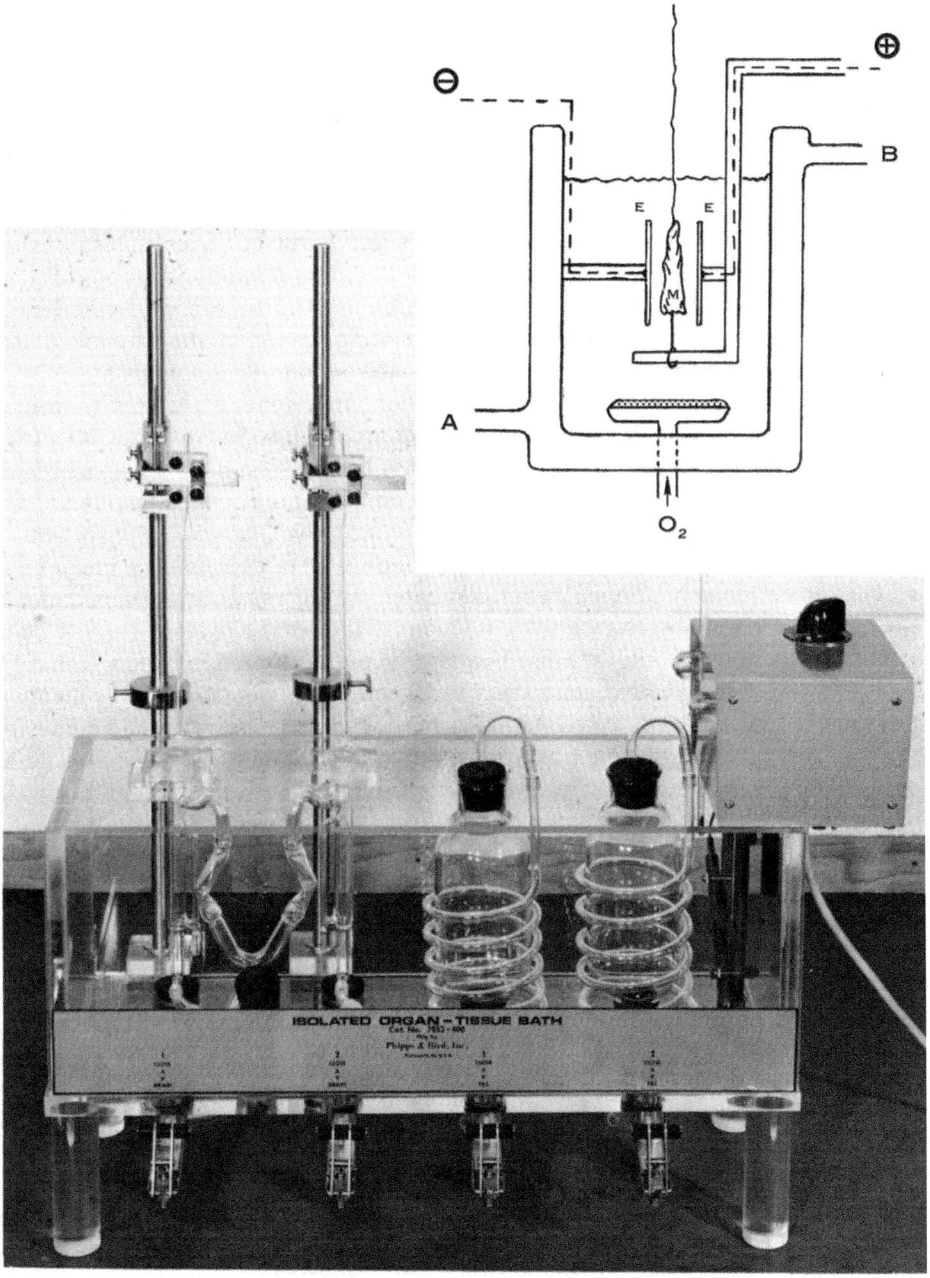

FIG. 9. Isolated organ-tissue bath assembly with constant temperature regulating units (Phipps and Bird, Inc., Model 7053-400). Inset shows diagram of muscle chamber assembly for studying contractions of isolated cardiac muscle. Water inlet (A) and outlet (B) for water jacket to maintain desired bath temperature. Electrodes (E) on either side of muscle (M) are of the "massive" or "field" type.

drug studies are involved, the differential effect of a drug on the threshold for nerve excitation and that of muscle must not be overlooked.

Stimulating electrodes are made most commonly of platinum, silver, silver-silver chloride, or platinum-iridium. While cost may be a factor in using such metals, the advantages far outweigh this initial investment. Of particular importance is the fact that nonstainless ferrous or copper-containing metals should be avoided if they are in an oxygenated saline environment. Thus, metal corrosion with release of Fe or Cu ions into the bath perfusate may introduce difficulties, especially when studies with catecholamines are involved. Such substances are vulnerable to trace-metal oxidation, and the degree and duration of their pharmacologic effects may be greatly altered by the presence of trace-metal contamination. In such instances, use of chelating agents in the physiologic salt solution may circumvent this problem. (See later section on solutions.)

The action of electrochemical polarization on electrode surfaces in contact with the muscle must be appreciated. Apparent changes in tissue electrical excitability or threshold for excitation may be the result of electrochemical polarization. This may be particularly so for commonly used stainless steel electrodes. For the noble metals such as platinum, silver, or gold, electrochemical polarization is avoided. Moreover, use of nonnoble metals results in a greater part of the current density applied being dissipated in the polarization impedance of the electrodes, and therefore only a fraction of the total delivered current being applied to the muscle. Another disadvantage of use of nonnoble metals is that the threshold for electrolytic gas generation and electrode discoloration of the anode of bipolar electrode pairs is often within range of current output used in in vitro studies. This problem does not arise with noble-metal electrodes. Thus, electrodes made from such metals can pass sufficient electric current without normally changing the chemical environment in the vicinity of the electrode-tissue junction.

Transducer Frame and Holder

An integral part of any in vitro muscle chamber arrangement is the unit used to hold and manipulate the force-displacement transducer used for recording muscle contractile activity.

The general requirements for such a transducer holder are (1) stability and freedom from external vibration, (2) compact size to permit close approximation to muscle chamber, (3) coarse and fine rack and pinion movement for adjustment of transducer position, (4) corrosion-resistant construction or shielding.

The relationship of the holder and transducer to the muscle chamber will vary with the configuration of the muscle chamber. Figure 1A illustrates a simple holder with a semimicromanipulator clamp allowing horizontal and vertical movement of a vertical transducer arrangement using a horizontal muscle chamber. Figure 10 shows the use of a modified isometric tension clamp* as a transducer holder and

*Harvard Instrument Co., Dover, Massachusetts.

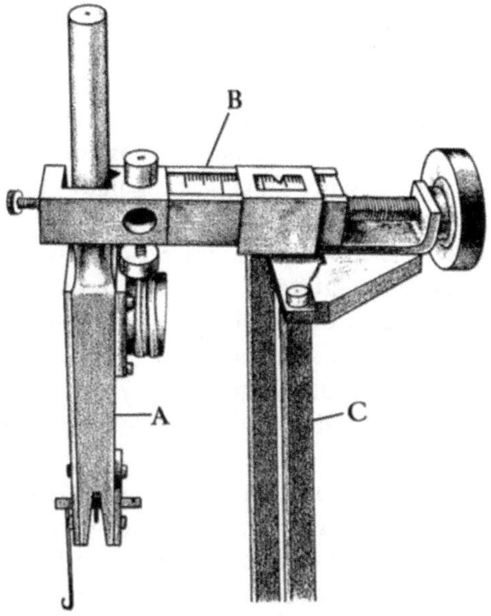

FIG. 10. Modified isometric tension clamp (B) (Harvard Instrument Co.) used for holding transducer (A) and serving as macro-manipulator. This unit is compatible with the apparatus shown in Figure 1. (C) Mounting rods for attaching unit to constant temperature tank.

manipulator for a horizontal muscle bath which is also applicable to the configuration shown in Figure 1.

More elaborate rack and pinion holders and manipulators may be used, as illustrated in Figures 2B and 8. The individual must determine the requirements for his own system depending on the force-displacement transducer used and the need for gross or fine adjustment capability.

Muscle Chamber Oxygenation

Adequate oxygenation of the buffer solution in which the tissue preparation is immersed is one of the critical requirements for in vitro studies of cardiac muscle. Assuming that the tissue meets the other requirements such as appropriate thickness (see later section), its functional state is critically dependent on the delivery to, and uptake of oxygen from, the physiologic salt solution.

The general requirements of a muscle chamber oxygenator include (1) ability to deliver gasses close to the muscle, (2) avoiding excessive movement of muscle or muscle chamber contents by mechanical disturbance caused by gas stream or bubbles, (3) minimum disturbance of muscle chamber temperature regulation, (4) avoidance of evaporative effect caused by dry gas bubbling through solution, and (5) ease of cleaning or replacement of gas delivery or dispersing unit.

Figures 1B and 2B illustrate one of the simplest oxygenator devices. These consist of a Pyrex disc (No. 39535) connected to an oxygen-delivery line. The disc in Figure 1B has a diameter of 12 mm and fits easily under the tissue in the horizontal configuration shown. The sintered glass system yields a fine stream of gas bubbles which not only adequately diffuse past the tissue, but also serve to stir and mix the chamber perfusate. The flow of gas through such a disc is adjusted and maintained by use of any two-stage gas regulator at the gas source in addition to adjustable tubing clamps. The gas is "scrubbed" before being delivered to the bath by passing it through a wash or gas scrub bottle (Pyrex No. 29142). This assures that the gas is water-saturated and thus minimizes evaporative loss from the muscle chamber caused by dry gas bubbling through the perfusate.

A single orifice oxygenator such as a hypodermic needle or polyethylene tube is to be avoided because of inadequate delivery of a stream of bubbles past the tissue without causing objectionable vibration of the muscle or tissue-transducer coupling system.

For vertical muscle chamber configurations, adequate oxygenation can be achieved by delivering the stream of gas bubbles vertically past the muscle via a sintered disc at the bottom of the bath, as in Figures 5 and 9A. Another technique is to use a side arm in communication with the main muscle chamber (Fig. 8). The side arm chamber containing the salt solution can be vigorously gassed; and then the solution can be directed toward the muscle in the main chamber.

Temperature Regulation

Unless experiments are to be done at ambient room temperature, it is usually desirable to control the temperature of the perfusate bathing the isolated muscle. Such temperature regulation may be achieved by several methods.

One technique involves perfusing the muscle chamber continuously with oxygenated physiologic salt solution brought to desired temperature by gassing through a heat-exchange system external to the muscle chamber (e.g., Figs. 3A, 3B, 4). Sufficient heat-exchange area must be provided so that, if rates of flow are increased, the solution has been temperature-equilibrated to be at the desired temperature when it is delivered to the muscle chamber.

A more commonly used temperature-regulating system involves the placement of the muscle chamber in a constant temperature tank, or delivering a flow of water around the muscle chamber via a water jacket arrangement (e.g., Figs. 3A and 9).

In the example shown in Figure 1A, it is often necessary to regulate the tank temperature slightly higher than the temperature desired in the muscle chamber. This is necessary because of evaporative loss and heat dissipation caused by oxygenation and by the limitation of heat exchange through the walls of the muscle chamber immersed in the tank. The smaller the chamber area exposed to the air and the deeper it can be immersed in the temperature-regulated water tank, the less difference there will be in the tank and muscle chamber temperatures.

In those instances where the bath design utilizes a water jacket technique for maintaining constant temperature of the muscle chamber contents, it is necessary that a satisfactory circulating water pump be employed. Depending on the volume of circulating water required, several commercially available pumps are available for such applications. In general, it is desirable to have the temperature-regulating device, whether pump or stirrer, separate from the main muscle chamber assembly to avoid artifacts caused by mechanical vibration of the units.

ELECTRONIC APPARATUS

Stimulators

In those experiments where it is required that the muscle be excited by external electrical stimuli, a suitable electronic stimulator is required. Electronic stimulators to be used in delivering electrical current to a muscle immersed in a salt solution should have the following general characteristics and functions:

1. Stimulator should have sufficient output capacity (power) to deliver necessary current to tissue independent of load.
2. Individual pulses delivered should be rectangular in wave form and unaffected by load impedance variations.
3. Stimulus intensity, duration, and frequency parameters must be easily read, changed, and reset, using continuously adjustable operating controls.
4. Output should be completely isolated from power and ground.
5. A variety of modes of operation should be possible without use of external synchronization or control systems. These modes should include (a) single shocks, (b) repetitive (continuous) stimulation, (c) single pairs of stimuli, (d) single trains of stimuli, (e) repetitive pairs of stimuli. (See Figures 11 and 12 for examples of commonly used commercially available stimulators of this class.)
6. Design features should provide either a nearly constant voltage or constant current output.

The latter type of stimulator is being increasingly used (e.g., Fig. 13B). This is because it can deliver a stimulus through the stimulating electrodes independent of the resistance of the muscle, electrodes, and saline environment. Thus, the voltage between two stimulating electrodes will vary directly with resistance changes for any given stimulating current setting.

In a constant-voltage stimulator, a stimulus of any given voltage is delivered independent of the resistance on the electrodes. However, this constant output will only be delivered down to a lower limit of electrode-tissue-saline resistance. This constancy is set by the current delivering capacity of the stimulator.

Most constant-voltage stimulators may be converted to constant-current types through the use of constant-current regulators (Fig. 13A). These regulators are designed for use with any sine or square wave generator. The regulators provide

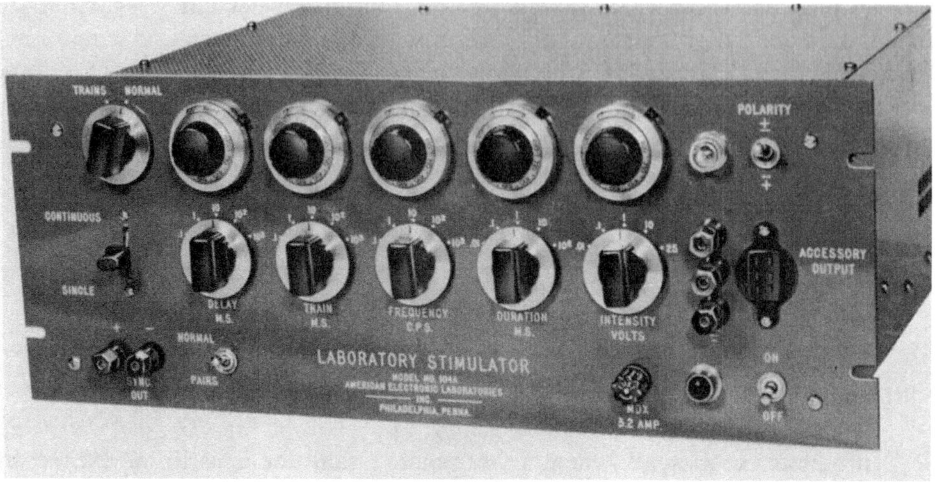

FIG. 11. Electronic stimulator (American Electronics Labs, Inc., Model 104A).

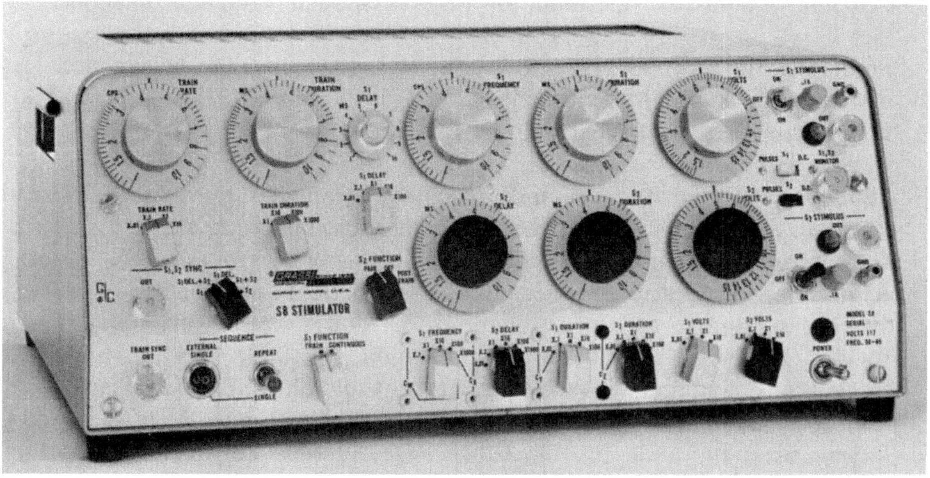

FIG. 12. Electronic stimulator (Grass Instrument Co., Model S8).

controls which allow adjustment of constant-current pulses, although frequency and pulse duration modes are controlled from the wave form generator. Figure 14 illustrates the schematic layout for a typical stimulator constant-current regulator arrangement.

Another major advantage of some constant-current stimulators is that they do not require separate stimulation isolation units when used in conjunction with most wave form generators. Also, such units eliminate polarization effects common to stimulating electrodes because they maintain constant-output current while voltage varies with load resistance changes due to electrode-tissue polarization. This

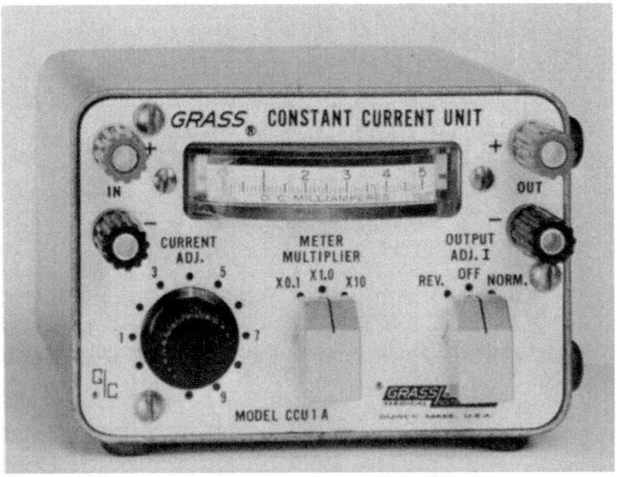

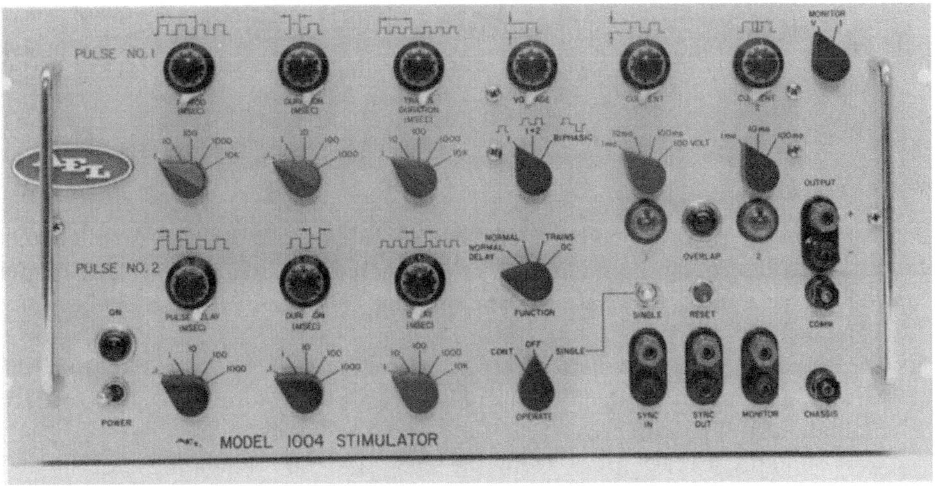

FIG. 13. A and B. Example of constant current stimulators. (A, Top) Grass Instrument Co.; (B, Bottom) AEL Model 1004.

assures that true rectangular current pulses are delivered to the muscle. Single, repetitive, pairs, trains, repetitive trains, repetitive pairs, etc., are capable of triggering most constant-current regulators.

A possible major limitation or disadvantage in using constant-current stimulators is the rise in voltage that can occur at a stimulating electrode if electrode-muscle resistance rises. The voltage will increase to compensate for the added current X resistance drop at the electrode. This can cause excessive power dissipation at the electrode-muscle junction, with the result that the tissue may be

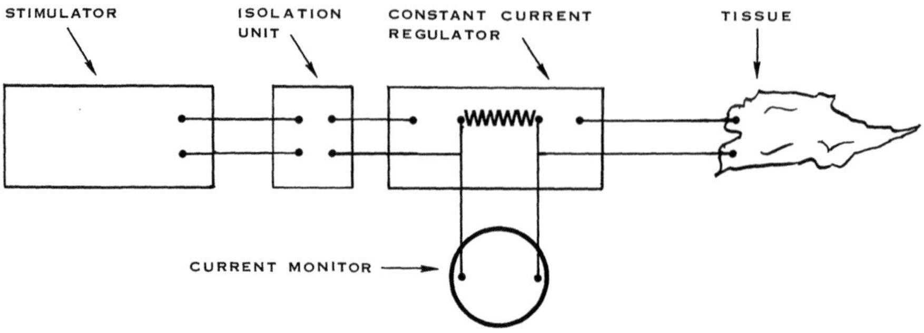

FIG. 14. Schematic circuit for typical stimulator-constant current regulator arrangement used for in vitro studies.

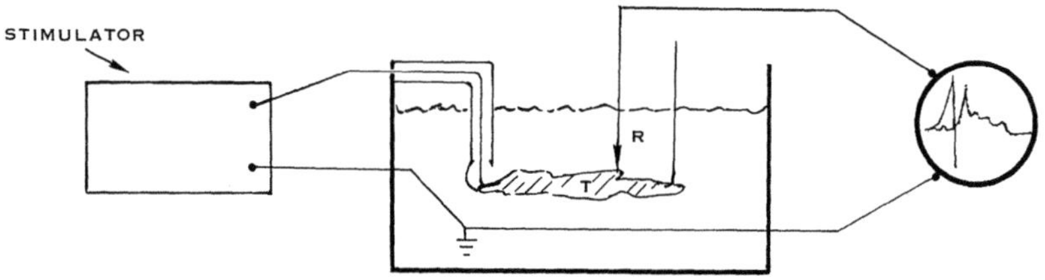

FIG. 15. Diagram illustrating improper arrangement of stimulating and recording electrodes for isolated muscle preparation.

burned or damaged, especially where the stimulator can deliver high enough voltage. This danger can be minimized or eliminated by having the voltage output controllable or limited to a safe maximum value. For most in vitro applications, this value will be as low as a few volts.

In those experiments where electrical recordings are to be made from the muscle that is being stimulated, it is usually necessary to utilize a device to reduce or eliminate stimulus artifacts.

The stimulus artifact arises from the fact that the stimulating current and voltage are usually many hundreds or thousands of times greater than the bioelectric potential being recorded. Thus, as the stimulating current passes to the tissue to the recording electrode, it will obscure the recorded signal. This occurs during the time the stimulus current is flowing and also after. This will usually cause the recording pen or oscilloscope trace to go off scale. The degree and magnitude of this artifact is related to the recording amplifier. It is most apparent with AC coupled amplifiers. Direct coupled amplifiers eliminate this problem, although they tend to be less stable than AC coupled amplifiers.

Figure 15 illustrates schematically the way stimulating and recording electrodes are *improperly* arranged. With this configuration, large stimulus artifacts will appear between ground electrode and the recording electrode (R).

However, by using a stimulus isolator device (e.g., Fig. 16) this artifact may be eliminated. Such a stimulus isolator unit is usually a shielded transformer. The

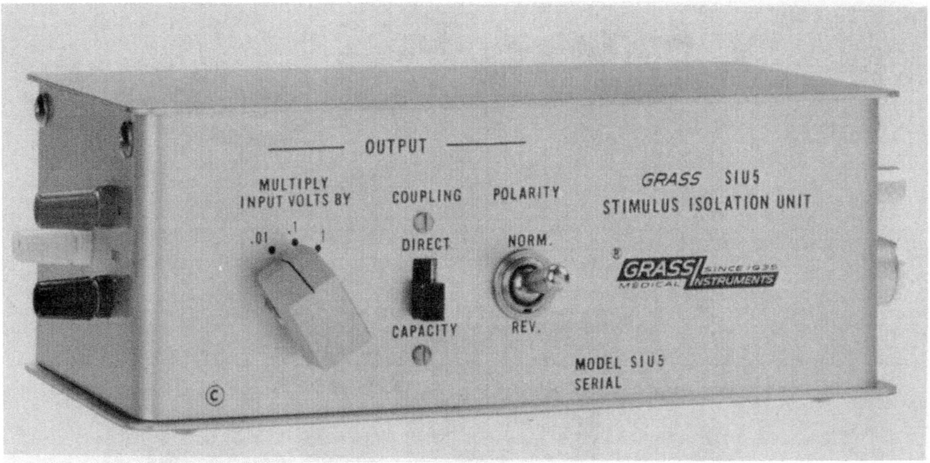

FIG. 16. Stimulus isolation unit (Grass Instrument Co., Model SIU5).

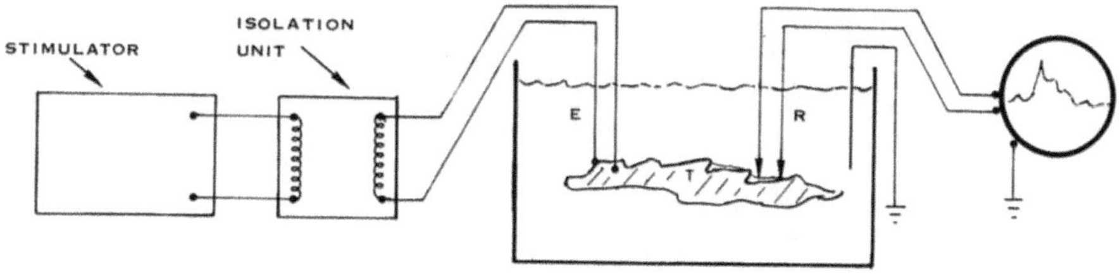

FIG. 17. Diagram illustrating proper arrangement of stimulating electrodes, tissue, ground connection, stimulus isolator unit, and recording electrodes.

effect of the stimulus isolator unit is to isolate the two stimulating electrodes from ground. The unit converts the stimulus to a radio frequency (RF) at the primary coil and back to the original stimulus wave form at the secondary. Figure 17 illustrates the *correct* placement of stimulating electrodes, tissue, ground, stimulus isolator unit, and recording electrodes (bipolar). It is important that the two recording electrodes be placed as close together as possible. This applies to the stimulating electrodes also. The preparation should be grounded by a separate electrode.

Force-Displacement Transducers

Modern techniques for recording contraction of isolated cardiac tissue invariably depend on electronic force-displacement transducers. These transducers fall into seven main operating categories: (1) Wheatstone (strain-gage) bridge type, (2) variable inductive, (3) variable capacitance, (4) mechanoelectronic triode, (5) differential transformer, (6) photoelectric, (7) piezoelectric.

Table 1 summarizes some of the electronic properties and requirements of these transducer types. By far the most commonly used type is the strain gage

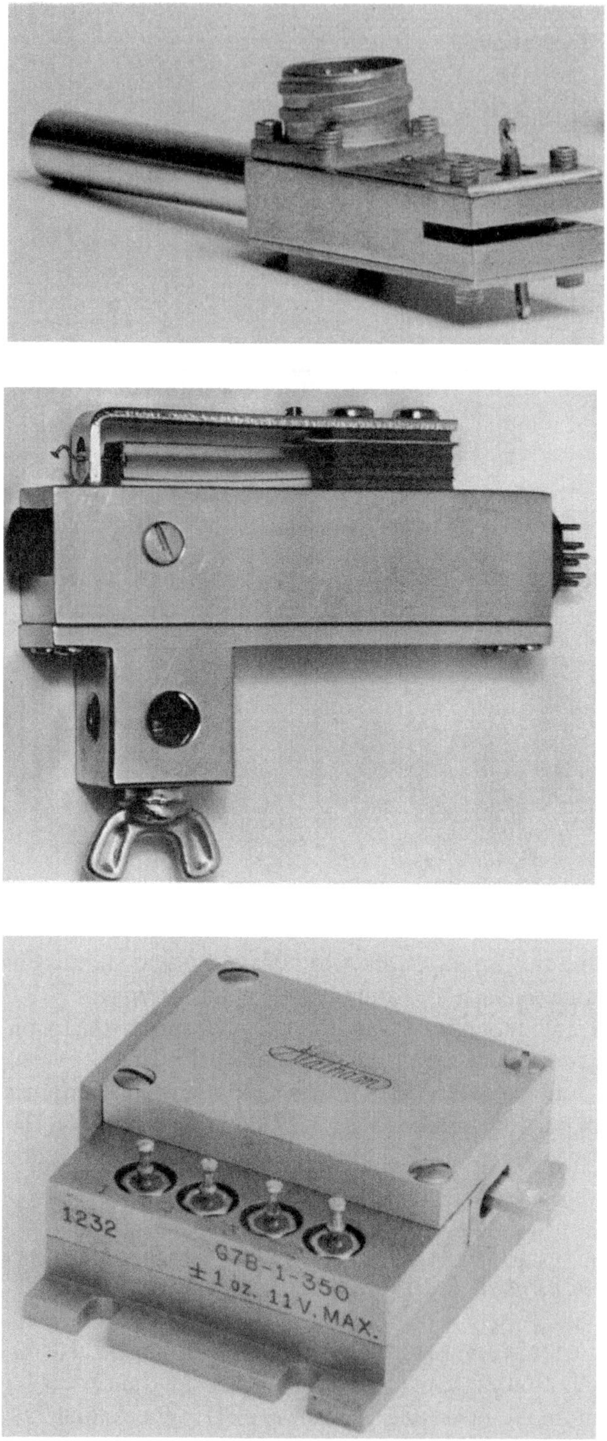

FIG. 18. Examples of commercially available force-displacement transducers. (A, Top) Grass Instrument Co., Model FT. 03. (B, Center) E and M Instrument Co., Myograph and Myograph Tension Adjuster. This is an isotonic, photoelectric transducer. (C, Bottom) Statham Instruments, Model G7B.

utilizing resistive elements in a Wheatstone bridge configuration. Transducers of the types listed in Table 1 are commercially available. Various descriptions for specialized gages and associated circuits may also be referred to when commercial gages are not satisfactory for any given recording requirement (see references).

The selection of any given transducer type will depend on (1) anticipated contractile force range, (2) isometric versus isotonic recording, (3) availability of appropriate amplifiers or recording device, (4) physical size and mechanical (external) coupling requirements, (5) natural frequency of device, (6) ambient temperature changes, (7) ease of calibration and balancing.

The transducer illustrated in Figure 18A is a model FT 0.03 force-displacement transducer manufactured by Grass Instrument Co., Quincy, Massachusetts. By use of springs in the cantilever beam housing, the FT 0.03 is capable of recording tensions from single fibers to that from whole muscles developing up to 2 kg force. Figure 18 illustrates several other types of commonly used, commercially available transducers.

PHYSIOLOGIC SALT SOLUTIONS

There are nearly as many variations in the composition of physiologic salt solutions used for in vitro cardiac muscle studies as there are investigators using them. To recommend one solution over another arbitrarily is irrational without knowing the specific requirements of the experiment. However, there are several basic solutions which have been found to be most useful for mammalian tissues, and which have found wide use for isolated atrial muscle.

Table 2 summarizes the composition of these basic solutions and their requirements insofar as gas phase is concerned.

The following comments and principles are applicable to all these solutions and their modifications:

1. The NaCl concentration used is required for isotonicity. When NaCl must be decreased, yet isotonicity maintained, an osmotically active material must be added in appropriate concentration. A 97.9 g per liter sucrose solution, for example, is nearly isotonic with a 9.0 g per liter NaCl solution.

2. If $NaHCO_3$ is used as a buffering salt, the final pH of the solution will depend on both the CO_2 in the gas phase and the concentration of buffer as well as the temperature.

For example, a solution at 30°C passed with 1 percent CO_2 - 99 percent O_2, with a bicarbonate concentration of 5.8 mM, would have a pH of 7.4. By changing only the bicarbonate to 2.9 or 11.6 mM, pH's of 7.1 and 7.7 could be obtained, respectively. Alternatively, by keeping the bicarbonate constant, and altering the percent CO_2 in the gas phase, changes in pH can be obtained. These are best checked with a pH meter directly, even though equations are available for estimating the changes in pH depending on the $[HCO_3]/[CO_2]$ ratio used.

3. The use of glucose as an energy substrate for cardiac muscle in vitro is well founded. The amount used, however, depends on the particular need of the experiment. Generally, for long experiments, a 0.1 to 0.2 percent glucose

TABLE 1

Force Transducer Characteristics

Strain Gage Type	Advantages	Disadvantages
Resistive	Simple construction; versatile; ease of calibration; rugged; low mass (inertia); high stiffness (dF/dx)	Relative low gage factor
Variable inductance	Large voltage output/deflection; measure displacement without affecting system being measured; medium mass; low stiffness	Usually two separate balance adjustments
Differential transformer	Balance by centering transducer armature; medium mass; low stiffness	Electronic zeroing circuit complex
Variable capacitance	Inherent frequency response better than resistance gages; medium mass; low stiffness	Temperature unstable
Photoelectric	Good frequency response; low coupling inertia; very low mass and stiffness; good for isotonic contractions	Mechanical instability; linearity depends on correct alignment of light source and phototube
RCA 5734 (Triode Tube)	Large voltage output/deflection (40 v/degree deflection); direct coupling of output to high input impedance recorders	Mechanical and temperature unstable; heat sink required; maximum allowable deflection ±0.5.
Piezoelectric	High frequency response; simplicity; ease of balance	Cannot measure sustained force (no DC response)

TABLE 2

Commonly Used Physiologic Salt Solutions for In Vitro Muscle Studies

	Common Name							
			Krebs-Henseleit			Tyrode		
Component*	Mammalian Ringers	Krebs	*I*	*II*	Locke	*I*	*II*	Modified Ringer-Locke
NaCl	9.0	6.90	6.90	6.92	9.2	8.0	8.0	9.0
KCl	0.42	0.35	0.35	0.35	0.42	0.20	0.2	0.42
$CaCl_2$	0.24	0.28	0.28	0.28	0.17	0.10	0.2	0.24
$NaHCO_3$	0.30	2.10	1.00	2.1	0.15	1.0	1.0	0.50
$MgCl_2 \cdot 6H_2O$	–	0.11	–	–	–	0.1	0.05 AH†	0.005
$NaH_2PO_4 \cdot H_2O$	–	0.14	–	–	–	0.05	0.04 AH†	–
Glucose	–	2.00	1.0	2.0	1.0	1.0	1.0	0.50
$MgSO_4 \cdot 7H_2O$	–	–	0.293	–	–	–	–	–
KH_2PO_4	–	–	0.162	0.16	–	–	–	–
pH @ 37.5°C	–	–	7.4	–	7.5	8.0	6.8-7.2	7.4
H_2O-dist. (ml)	1,000	1,000	1,000	1,000	1,000	1,000	1,000	1,000
Gas phase	95% O_2 5% CO_2	95% O_2 5% CO_2	95% O_2 5% CO_2	95% O_2 5% CO_2	95% O_2 5% CO_2	95% O_2 5% CO_2	95% O_2 5% CO_2	95% O_2 5% CO_2

*Amount of each component given in grams.

†AH = Anhydrous salt.

concentration is adequate to maintain contractile function. Insulin (5 units/L) has been used to facilitate uptake and utilization of glucose by the myocardium.

4. For the solutions listed in Table 2, the order of mixing is often critical to assure complete solubility of each salt and the avoidance of precipitates. The NaCl, KCl, and $NaHCO_3$, for example, should be dissolved in a little water and brought into solution by thorough mixing. The $CaCl_2$ should be added after the other salts, and the entire solution gassed with 95 percent O_2 - 5 percent CO_2. If KH_2PO_4 and $MgSO_4$ are used, they should be added last. Glucose can be added shortly before using the solution.

An excellent review by Lockwood (1961) lists about 100 different physiologic salt solutions for a variety of species and tissues. This should be consulted for further information. It should be kept in mind that an artificial salt solution with nutrients, hormones, and physically dissolved gasses is a physiologic compromise, at best. Often, selection of a given solution will be based on the practicality of being able to compare one's own results with previously published experiments utilizing the same solution. However, the constant modification and "customizing" of physiologic salt solutions to suit one's own needs is not to be discouraged if the modification is based on sound physiologic principle or fact, or is desired as an experimental intervention in itself.

TISSUE TECHNIQUES

Animal Selection

Rabbits weighing between 2 and 3 kg have been found to yield atrial preparations of uniform size and contractile function. White New Zealand rabbits of either sex are popularly used. In my own work, the animal supplier is able to provide the desired rabbits in a very narrow weight range, usually varying by less than 0.2 to 0.5 kg. This uniformity of body size minimizes variations in contractile function resulting from large differences in heart size. This weight range is also associated with minimum fat deposits in and around the heart.

Before they are used, all animals are maintained on standard Rabbit Purina Chow and water *ad lib.*

Tissue Preparation

SACRIFICE OF ANIMAL AND REMOVAL OF HEART.—For rabbits of the size just described, it has been found that the most satisfactory way of sacrificing the animal for removal of the heart is by administering a sharp blow to the animal's head. This procedure, if properly done, immediately renders the animal unconscious and insensible to pain. Its main advantage is that it does not introduce the undesirable variable of anesthetic agents.

The animal is kept as quiet and calm as possible during preparative procedures. It is then placed on a flat surface or table near a faucet with running cold water. An assistant places the animal on the bench or table, holding the animal quiet with one hand on the back, one near the head. The animal should be handled carefully to avoid excitement and unnecessary movement which might cause excessive sympathoadrenal discharge.

A second assistant then administers a sharp blow to the occipital region of the animal's head using a club or mallet of sufficient size and weight to assure that the animal is rendered unconscious without repeated application of blows.

The animal's head is quickly placed under a stream of running water. The body is held vertically while it is exsanguinated by rapidly cutting the carotid and jugular blood vessels with a scalpel. The animal is held in this position for 20 to 30 seconds. The animal is then placed on its back and a thoracotomy performed by rapidly cutting into the rib cage above the xiphoid process. With appropriate bone-cutting scissors, the heart can be completely exposed within 5 to 10 seconds. The pericardium is usually cut open at this point. A rat-tooth forceps is used to grasp the apex of the ventricles, and the heart is elevated so that a pair of curved scissors may be placed nearly parallel to the exposed spinal cord. Usually with one or two cuts, the heart is freed from its vascular and connective tissue attachments. It is immediately placed into a beaker containing oxygenated physiologic salt solution at room temperature (20° to 22°C).

The elapsed time from applying a blow to the animal's head to placing the heart in the beaker should be of the order of 60 seconds.

If properly performed, the removal of the heart leaves both atria undamaged. The heart should be beating vigorously during the entire procedure. By exsanguinating the animal prior to opening the chest, a relatively bloodless field is obtained. Moreover, undesirable intracardiac blood clots are avoided. Rarely is it necessary to remove clots from the atrial chambers if proper sacrifice, exsanguination, and dissection procedures are followed.

REMOVING ATRIA AND FINE DISSECTION.—Figure 19A-C shows the position of the atria relative to the ventricles. The heart, having been beating in a beaker with physiologic salt solution for approximately 15 to 20 seconds, is then transferred to a dissecting dish (e.g., a petri dish) containing physiologic salt solution which is continuously oxygenated via a sintered disc placed in the solution. The right and left atria are separated, intact, from the ventricles by cutting along the atrioventricular groove (dotted line, Fig. 19B,C). Care should be taken to keep the atria immersed in the salt solution. The resulting atrial preparation should be beating vigorously. The amputated ventricles may be discarded.

The intact atrial preparation is then transferred to another petri dish containing oxygenated physiologic salt solution for final trimming and dissection. This involves first trimming off excess fat and vascular tissue which is easily identifiable from the atrial myocardium. If the spontaneously beating right atrium is to be studied, care should be used not to damage or cut into the SA node area.

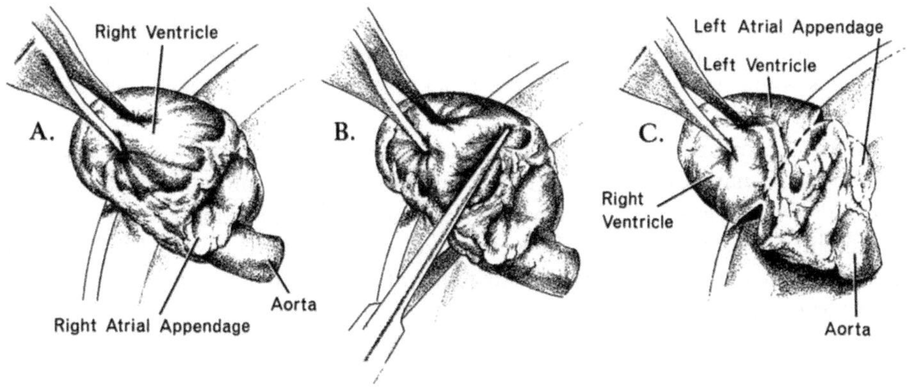

FIG. 19. Dissection of atria from ventricles of isolated rabbit heart. (A) Heart is held over ridge of petri dish immersing atria, as scissors are used to cut atria from ventricles along the atrioventricular groove (B,C).

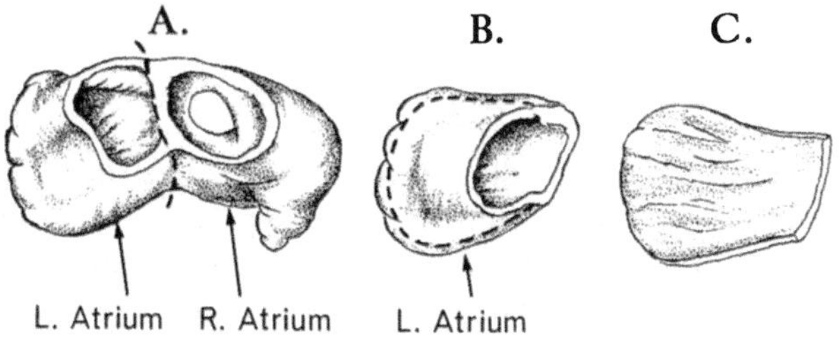

FIG. 20. Separation of right and left atria of rabbit heart. Atria are separated by cutting at the interatrial septum. Right atrium is identified by the irregularly shaped appendage ("auricle"). Left atrium is further cut (B) to yield a fan-shaped preparation as in (C).

This is an area roughly bounded by the junction of the superior and inferior vena cavae and right atrium.

If the left atrium is to be studied, it is cut off from the right, midway between the two appendages (Fig. 20A). If properly placed, this cut will result in a quiescent left atrium and spontaneously beating right atrium.

The right atrial appendage may be further identified anatomically by the irregularly shaped appendage (Fig. 20A) as compared to the more symmetrical left atrium.

To assure adequate oxygen diffusion through the tissue in the muscle bath, an additional trimming procedure is recommended. This involves cutting open the left atrial appendage, yielding two halves, as shown in Figure 20B,C.

The larger of the fan-shaped pieces is used. For muscle bath arrangements requiring ties, appropriate thread, wire, or suture material is attached to one or both ends of the muscle as desired. In the muscle bath arrangement shown in Figure 1B, the fan-shaped atrial muscle can be placed directly into the muscle clamp by placing the widest portion against the electrode-clamp assembly (G). The opposite end of the muscle is then secured to the transducer hook (J) directly.

The only time the tissue is not being vigorously oxygenated in physiologic salt solution is when it is being transferred quickly from beaker to dissection dish, and then to the muscle chamber.

With appropriate experience, the entire procedure from sacrifice to mounting in the chamber should not take longer than three or four minutes. Experience has indicated that the longer this period, the less viable a preparation is obtained, even though the preparation is well oxygenated in the dissecting dish. This is particularly evident for the quiescent left atrium, but less critical for the spontaneously beating right atrium.

EXPERIMENTAL PROCEDURES

After the atrium has been placed in the chamber containing oxygenated physiologic buffer solution, several procedures are generally required.

Electrically Driven Tissue

If the left atrium is being studied, it must be driven with an external electrical stimulus. Initially, a stimulus of sufficient intensity is delivered to demonstrate a contractile response. A fixed pulse duration and frequency are set. Once the muscle is beating, the intensity of stimulus is lowered to that value where no response is observed. It is then increased again in fine steps until a contractile response is produced. This is the threshold stimulus intensity. It is noted and, depending on the specific protocol followed, retained at this value or changed to some value higher than threshold (e.g., 20, 50, 100, 300 percent, etc., greater than threshold).

It is now well known that the stimulus parameters used for in vitro studies with myocardial tissue can greatly influence the contractile responses observed, as well as influence the effects of drugs on the tissue. Thus, when threshold intensity stimulation is used with pulse durations of 2 to 5 msec, release of catecholamines from intracardiac nerve endings is minimized (see earlier section on electrodes). Use of stimulus intensities 20 to 50 percent greater than threshold may produce detectable catecholamine release, although this is minimized with punctate electrodes. Suprathreshold stimulation of the order of two or three times threshold intensity may produce detectable release of catecholamines as revealed by increases in contractile force when switching from threshold to suprathreshold stimulation (see Fig. 21). This is more apparent at higher stimulus frequencies (e.g., 100 to 200 beats per minute).

For any given stimulus intensity, increasing pulse duration also tends to excite intracardiac nerve fibers with subsequent release of autonomic transmitter substances. For cardiac tissue, square wave pulse durations of 2 to 5 msec are employed in experiments where this parameter is not altered. Threshold intensity is determined at the pulse duration selected.

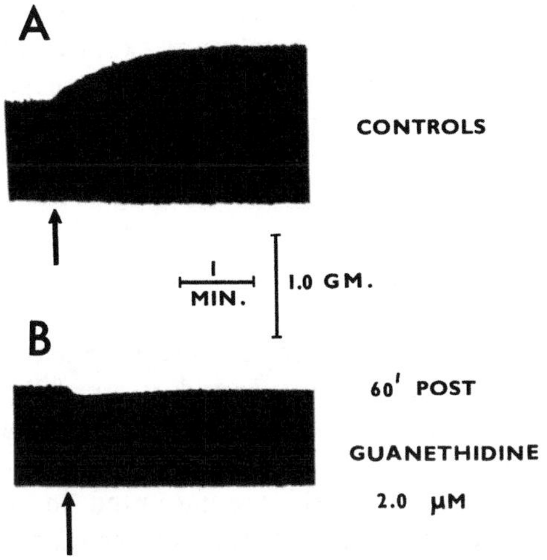

FIG. 21. Recordings of contractile response of isolated, electrically driven rabbit left atrium. (A) At first arrow, stimulus intensity was raised from threshold to three times threshold value. Note increase in contractile tension. (B) Same muscle as in A. Response to suprathreshold stimulation after 60 minutes treatment with guanethidine-SO_4 (2.0 μM). Note the complete abolishment of the positive inotropic response to an increase in stimulus intensity. Stimulus frequency: 120 beats/min. Pulse duration: 5.0 msec. (From Levy, 1967.)

While it is appreciated and recognized that stimulus intensities greater than threshold may cause some release of autonomic transmitter substances from the tissue, this must be balanced against the desirability of a steady-state contractile pattern or anticipation of elevation of threshold value by experimental manipulations. Thus, selecting a stimulus intensity 1.5 to 3.0 times threshold for a short pulse duration allows study when a wide variety of experimental inverventions which might affect tissue excitability are involved and when it is undesirable to change stimulus intensity during the course of the experiment.

Whatever stimulation conditions are selected, they should be stated completely, particularly in relation to the type of electrodes used.

Length-Tension Relation

Once the tissue has been beating for several minutes, it is usually desirable to adjust diastolic tension. The Frank-Starling mechanism for heart muscle predicts the effect of changes in diastolic tension or rest length. Some authors prefer to affix an arbitrary rest tension on the isolated muscle. This may typically be of the order of 0.5 to 1.5 g. More frequently, however, it is desirable to adjust diastolic tension systematically by changing muscle length with an appropriate micrometer arrangement (e.g., Fig. 10) until contractile force is maximal (i.e., at the peak of the length-tension curve). This length is individually determined for each muscle. Once the curve has been determined, rest length can be adjusted so that the tissue is functioning at some known point on this curve. Some authors prefer to do experiments at the peak of the length-tension curve. Others may select a rest length somewhat below this point. Rarely are experiments performed on the descending portion of the length-tension curve unless an experimental intervention is being evaluated particularly for its effect on depressed contractility associated with greater than optimum resting lengths.

Equilibration-Stabilization Period

Experience with most isolated cardiac muscle preparations indicates that a suitable equilibration or stabilization period is needed before commencing experimental interventions. This is particularly so with rabbit left atrial preparations, in the author's view.

Typically, when rabbit left atria are mounted in the muscle chamber, stimulated, stretched, and threshold intensity determined, a predictable period must elapse before a steady-state contractile tension is observed. The following protocol has been found to yield a consistent pattern of response.

Within five minutes after mounting, threshold is determined, and preliminary adjustment of rest length is made. Approximately 20 to 30 minutes later, stimulus threshold is redetermined, and final adjustment of resting length is made to assure the muscle is functioning near the peak of its length-tension curve. At 40 minutes after placing the tissue in the muscle chamber, contractile tension has usually reached a steady state. An accurately measured, known quantity of fresh physiologic buffer solution is added to the muscle chamber at this time. Stimulus threshold is again redetermined and the final appropriate stimulus intensity delivered as a multiple of this threshold value. At exactly 60 minutes after mounting the tissue in the muscle chamber, experimental procedures are begun. This is taken as "0" time or "postequilibration time."

With these techniques, good contractile tension is maintained for long periods of time. At 60 minutes (stimulated at 120 beats per minute at 3 times threshold intensity), untreated control preparations show 98 ± 4.7 percent (mean ± standard error) of the postequilibration contractile force. At 120 minutes, contractile force is still 74 ± 5.6 percent of the control (postequilibration) value. These values are typical for experiments done at 37.5°C. Using a lower temperature may frequently prolong the viability of the muscles with still smaller decreases in contractile properties.

IN VITRO DRUG ADDITIONS

This section outlines some of the basic principles of drug studies with isolated cardiac muscle. Among these principles, one may list the following:

1. Drugs to be added to the muscle chamber should be made up in the same physiologic salt solution used to bathe the muscle. If unstable in such buffers,

they should be made up in simple isotonic solutions. If this is not possible, distilled water may be used, using a high enough drug concentration so that small volumes can be administered to the muscle chamber to minimize dilution effects.

2. When organic solvents are used to dissolve drugs, appropriate solvent control experiments must be made for all dosing volumes used. Appropriate correction of drug effects must be made by adding or subtracting the effects seen with the solvent alone.
3. Drug solutions should be made just prior to the experiment, if possible. If made hours or days ahead, the solution should be frozen or refrigerated at low temperatures.
4. Light-sensitive drug solutions should be stored in dark containers.
5. Catecholamine solutions (norepinephrine, epinephrine, phenylephrine, etc.) are extremely vulnerable to oxidation from light and heat. Adjustment of pH to an acid range by addition of ascorbic acid or HCl helps to protect from these oxidative changes. Trace-metal ion contamination also facilitates oxidation of such solutions. The activity of norepinephrine in distilled water or isotonic sodium chloride solution is diminished by as much as 40 to 60 percent when stored for 48 hours at 18°C. Alkaline pH accelerates this degradation. For shorter periods (4 hours), norepinephrine made up in 0.9 percent sodium chloride or a 1.4 percent bicarbonate buffer retains 96 to 100 percent of its initial concentration. Both epinephrine and norepinephrine are destroyed in a few minutes when in a Krebs bicarbonate buffer at 37°C at pH 7.4 and gassed with a carbogen gas mixture. In a Krebs-Henseleit bicarbonate buffer gassed with 95 percent O_2-5 percent CO_2, epinephrine shows only 50 percent of its initial activity after only 5 minutes.

   Biologic effects of stable catecholamine solutions may be prolonged in vitro by the presence of disodium EDTA (20 to 40μM) in the physiologic buffer.

REFERENCES

Blinks, J. R. 1965. Convenient apparatus for recording contractions of isolated heart muscle. J. Appl. Physiol., 20:755-757.

Dean, M., and Douglas, R. D., eds. 1962. Semiconductor and Conventional Strain Gages. New York, Academic Press, Inc.

Furchgott, R. F., Sleator, W., and DeGubareff, T. 1960. Effects of acetylcholine and epinephrine on the contractile strength and action potential of electrically driven guinea pig atria. J. Pharmacol., 129:405-416.

Haggendal, J., and Johnsson, G. 1967. The stability of noradrenaline infusion solutions. Acta Pharmacol., 25:461-464.

— and Svedmyr, N. 1967. Studies on the destruction of adrenaline in nutrient solution. Acta Pharmacol., 25:364-368.

Levy, J. V. 1967. Catecholamine stores and the negative inotropic effect of beta-adrenergic blocking drugs on the isolated rabbit heart. Arch. Int. Physiol. Biochem., 75:381-404.

Lock, J. A. 1963. Observations on the use of the hen and rabbit isolated auricles for the determination of inotropic potency. Brit. J. Pharmacol., 21:393-401.

Lockwood, A. P. 1961. Ringer solutions and some notes on the physiological basis of their ionic composition. Comp. Biochem. Physiol., 2:241-289.

McEwen, L. M. 1956. The effect on the isolated rabbit heart of vagal stimulation and its modification by cocaine, hexamethonium and ouabain. J. Physiol., 131:678-689.
Szekeres, L., and Vaughan Williams, E. M. 1962. Antifibrillatory action. J. Physiol., 160:470-482.
Thorp, R. H., and Cobbin, L. B. 1967. Cardiac stimulant substances. *In* Medicinal Chemistry Series, Vol. 7. New York, Academic Press, Inc.
Turner, R. A. 1965. Screening Methods in Pharmacology. New York, Academic Press, Inc.
Vaughan Williams, E. M. 1955. The individual effects of CO_2, bicarbonate and pH on the electrical and mechanical activity of isolated rabbit auricles. J. Physiol., 129:90-110.

CHAPTER **4**

Cardiac Muscle Function Studies

William W. Parmley and
Edmund H. Sonnenblick
Cardiovascular Unit, Peter Bent Brigham Hospital and Harvard Medical School, Boston, Massachusetts

INTRODUCTION

The purpose of this chapter is to discuss certain principles of cardiac muscle physiology as they are influenced by pharmacologic interventions, in order to outline a specific approach for testing the effects of drugs on the heart. It should be emphasized that the administration of a drug to the intact circulation may induce complex reflex changes as well as vascular, neuronal, hormonal, or metabolic effects which may not reflect the direct action of the drug on the heart. Thus, in order to separate the central cardiac effects of a drug from its peripheral effects, it is desirable to study the actions of any drug on rigorously controlled in vivo preparations and in vitro heart muscle preparations. Such studies provide a basic knowledge of the action of a drug on heart muscle so that the more complex effects in the presence of an intact circulation can be more clearly interpreted. After

Supported in part by U.S. Public Health Service Grant No. HE-11306-02 and American Heart Association Grant No. 67 782.

outlining some basic principles of cardiac muscle physiology, certain in vitro tests of cardiac muscle function will be described and then extended to the study of the intact heart. This chapter will be concerned only with ventricular muscle since Chapter 3 deals specifically with atrial muscle.

BASIC PRINCIPLES OF MUSCLE PHYSIOLOGY

When heart muscle is activated it can develop tension and shorten. Unlike skeletal muscle, it cannot be tetanized so that these activities occur during a limited time. The properties of the activated muscle can be described in terms of a three-component mechanical model as first proposed by Hill and associates (Hill, 1938; Wilkie, 1956) (Fig. 1). In this model, a contractile element (CE), which is assumed to be freely extensible at rest, is arranged in series with an elastic element (SE), which behaves like a passive spring. Resting tension is supported by another elastic element in parallel with the CE, i.e., the PE. With activation the CE can develop tension and shorten. During an isometric contraction where the ends of the muscle are fixed, the CE shortens and stretches the SE, which results in the development of tension. The rate of tension development (dP/dt) is thus dependent on velocity of shortening of the CE, (dl/dt), and the stress strain relations of the SE, (dP/dl): $dP/dt = (dl/dt)_{CE} \times (dP/dl)_{SE}$ (Sonnenblick, 1964; Parmley and Sonnenblick, 1967).

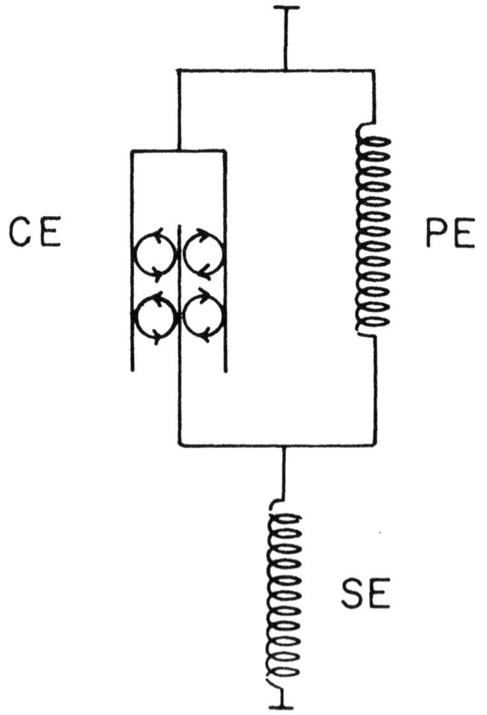

FIG. 1. A three-component mechanical model analogue of heart muscle, consisting of a contractile element (CE), a series elastic element (SE), and a parallel elastic element (PE).

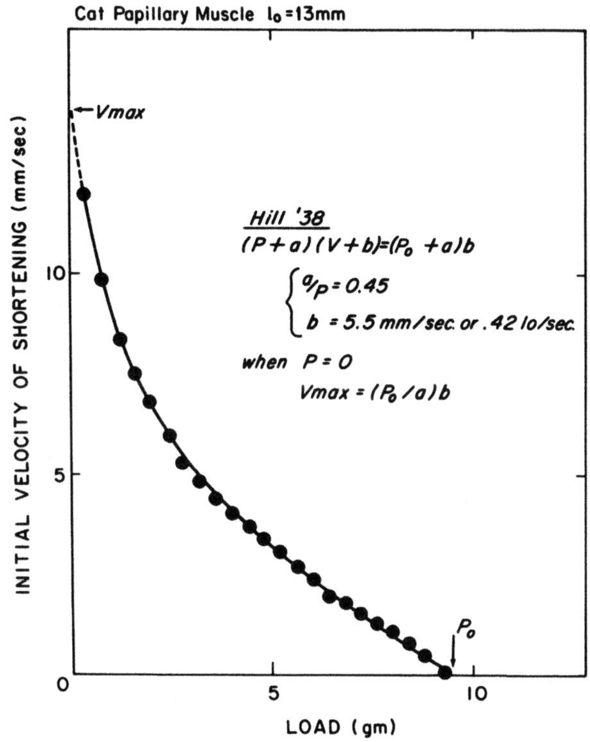

FIG. 2. Force-velocity relation obtained from a cat papillary muscle, with its accompanying Hill equation (1).

During isotonic contraction, the CE velocity of shortening (dl/dt) is inversely related to the tension developed, and the resultant hyperbolic curve is termed the *force-velocity relation* (Abbott and Mommaerts, 1959; Sonnenblick, 1962a, 1962b) (Fig. 2). The force-velocity relation has been termed the most fundamental property of muscle, since it is also directly related to the energetics of heat measurements (Hill, 1938). When this curve is extrapolated to zero tension, velocity is maximal (V_{max}), while the other end of the curve defines the isometric tension (P_0). Force-velocity relations have usually been obtained in vitro, by sequentially increasing afterload and measuring the peak velocity of shortening (Abbott and Mommaerts, 1959; Sonnenblick, 1962a, 1962b). Although the force-velocity relation thus obtained is different from the course of CE velocity during isometric contraction (Parmley and Sonnenblick, 1967), or from instantaneous force-velocity curves obtained by quick-release methods (Sonnenblick, 1965; Brady, 1965; Jewell and Blink, 1968), it is a reliable, simple, and reproducible method which can be easily compared with similar curves obtained after pharmacologic interventions.

There are two general ways in which the force of contraction of heart muscle can be altered, and these are readily distinguishable through the study of force-velocity relations. The *first* mechanism, which does not involve a change in contractility (or, synonymously, contractile state or inotropic state), is the change in force of contraction brought about by a change in initial muscle length. With

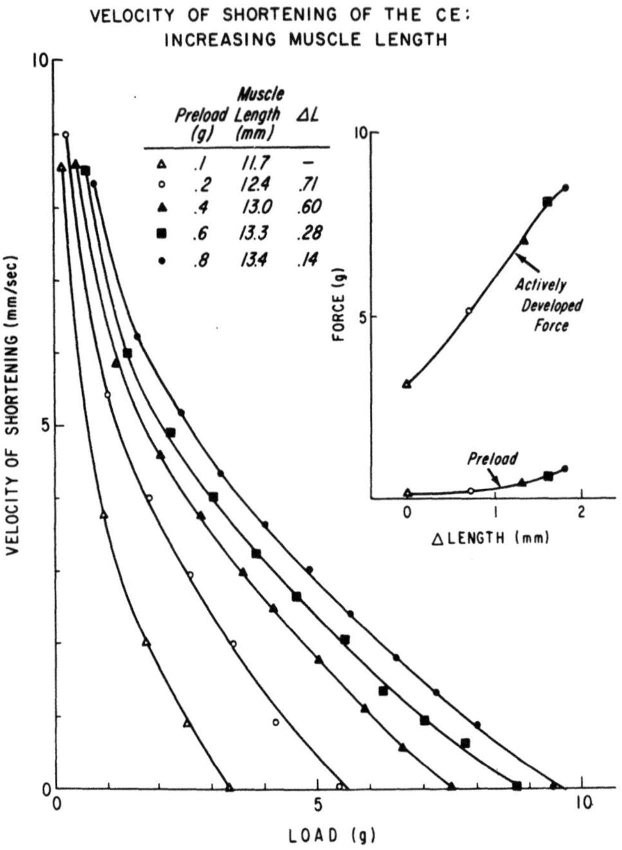

FIG. 3. Force-velocity relations (cat papillary muscle) obtained at different initial muscle lengths (preloads). Although P_0 is increased, V_{max} is constant. The inset illustrates the corresponding resting and active length-tension curves.

sequential increases in resting tension (or preload), the force-velocity curve is shifted to the right with a progressive increase in isometric tension (P_0) but, significantly, without a change in V_{max} (Sonnenblick, 1962a, 1962b) (Fig. 3).

The *second* mechanism, changing contractility, which is brought about by an inotropic influence such as norepinephrine or digitalis, is characterized by a shift in the force-velocity relation upward and to the right with an increase in maximum velocity of shortening (V_{max}), and usually, but not necessarily, an increase in P_0 (Fig. 4). Thus V_{max} is a sensitive index of the contractile state of heart muscle since it is changed only by inotropic interventions and not by changes in preload (Sonnenblick, 1962a, 1962b). The manner in which the force-velocity relation is altered, therefore, provides an easily reproducible method for determining the magnitude of positive or negative inotropic effects of any intervention. Further, it is apparent that an evaluation of contraction involves delineation of *speed, force,* and *time,* as well as *muscle length* (Sonnenblick, 1965; Brady, 1968).

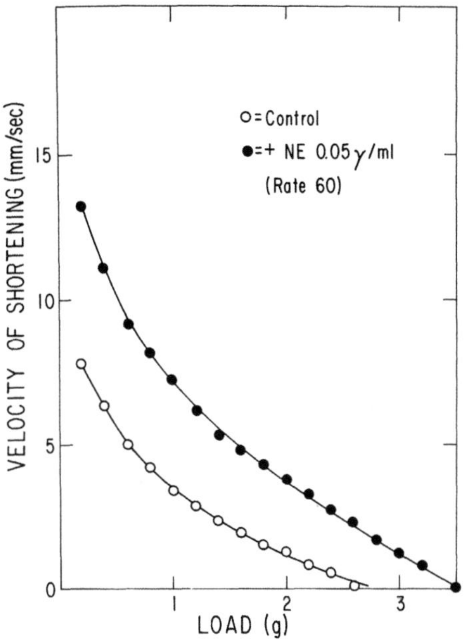

FIG. 4. Effect of norepinephrine (NE) on the force-velocity relation, with an increase in both P_0 and V_{max}.

The SE has the properties of an exponential spring (Fig. 5) with a modulus of elasticity (dP/dl) which is linearly related to the tension (P): $dP/dl = KP + C$, where K and C are constants (Sonnenblick, 1964; Parmley and Sonnenblick, 1967; Parmley et al., 1968). The properties of the SE or the PE are not altered by changes in contractility, so that any changes in the force-velocity or length-tension relations are directly related to changes in the contractile state of the CE (Sonnenblick, 1964; Parmley and Sonnenblick, 1967; Parmley et al., 1968).

IN VITRO PREPARATION

The most commonly used preparation for in vitro studies of myocardial function is the cat papillary muscle. The linear arrangement of muscle fibers and the cylindrical shape of the muscle simplifies the measurements of shortening and tension development. In the intact heart, by contrast, the irregular geometry of ventricular shape and activation and the changing direction of muscle bundles make similar measurements of shortening and tension development much more complex and difficult to interpret.

The following brief description outlines the principal steps involved in preparing a cat papillary muscle for in vitro studies of cardiac contractility. The cat is anesthetized with an intraperitoneal injection of sodium pentobarbital, 40 mg

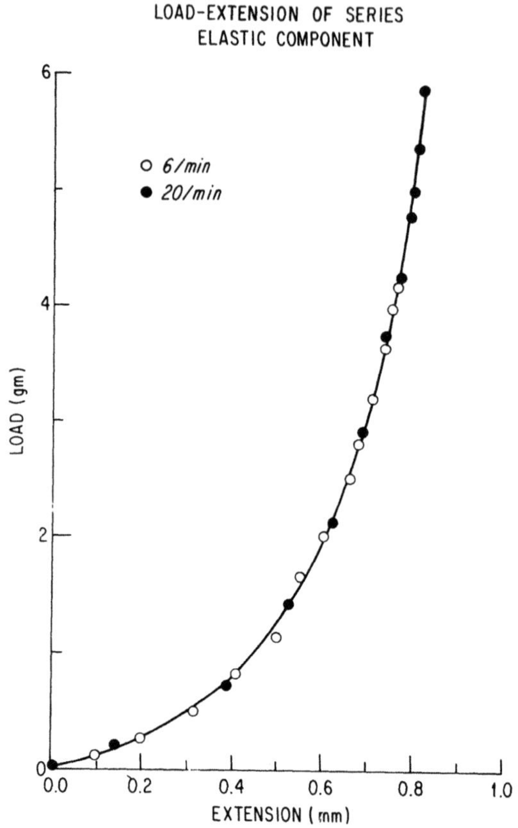

FIG. 5. Representative load extension curve of series elastic element (cat papillary muscle). Although contractility is increased by changing the stimulation rate from 6 to 20 per min, the series elastic curve is unchanged.

per kg, which produces satisfactory anesthesia in 5 to 10 minutes. The heart is removed rapidly from the chest and the free wall of the right ventricle opened. The first large anterior papillary muscle encountered is generally too thick to be a satisfactory preparation and should rarely be used. The ideal papillary muscle is long and thin with a cross-sectional area of 1.0 mm^2 or less. A 0000 silk tie is placed around the muscle tendon junction and the distal tendon severed. The muscle can then be severed at its base from the ventricle and placed in the muscle bath with special care to avoid trauma. The cut muscular end of the muscle is attached to a tension transducer while the tendinous end is attached to the tip of an isotonic lever system by wire or fine chain (Fig. 6A). Care should be taken with the connections to avoid excessive stray compliance. Specially designed spring-loaded clips are very satisfactory for this purpose. One can thus record changes in length (L) and tension (P) (Fig. 6B), and, by electronically differentiating these two measurements, velocity of shortening (dl/dt) and the rate of tension development (dP/dt) are obtained. A suitable Krebs bicarbonate solution for the muscle bath

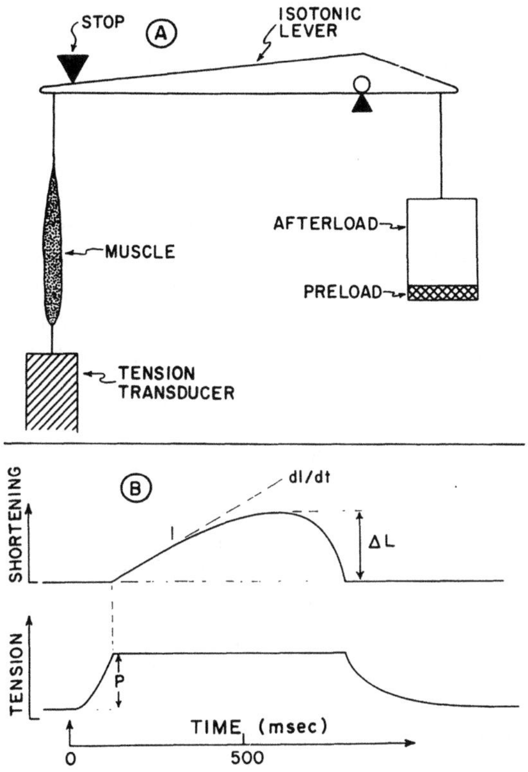

FIG. 6. (A) Schematic arrangement of isotonic lever system for the study of isolated heart muscle. The preload determines the initial length of the muscle. After the stop is placed on top of the lever to prevent further stretching of the muscle, any additional load is termed afterload. (B) Representative length and tension traces obtained during a single afterloaded isotonic contraction.

(Na^+ 148, K^+ 4.0, Ca^{++} 5.0, Mg^{++} 2.5, Cl^- 128, and HCO_3^- 125 mEq/liter; phosphate 1.2 and glucose 5.6 mM at pH 7.4) is bubbled with 95 percent O_2 and 5 percent CO_2.

Stimulation can be accomplished by either contact electrodes or electrodes placed parallel to the muscle. Although point stimulation has some theoretical advantages (Jewell and Blinks. 1968), these are minor, and satisfactory results can be obtained with mass stimulation through the bathing medium from platinum electrodes placed parallel to the muscle (Abbott and Mommaerts, 1959; Sonnenblick, 1962a). Pulses of short duration (5 msec or less), stimulus voltages just above threshold (10 percent)and low rates of stimulation are desirable to avoid the release of stored catecholamines in the muscle (Jewell and Blinks. 1968). Temperature should be maintained constant with a temperature bath which circulates either the bathing solution or water in a surrounding water jacket. Muscle function may be unstable below 20°C or near 37°C, so that most studies can be satisfactorily performed in a midrange such as 29° to 30°C with Q_{10}

measurements from 24° to 34°C. A stimulation rate of 6 to 24 per minute is satisfactory for most studies, while the preparation may deteriorate at prolonged stimulation rates above 30 per minute. Muscles studied within these ranges have been shown to be metabolically intact in terms of high-energy phosphate stores—viz., creatine phosphate and adenosine triphosphate (ATP) (Pool et al., 1967). After one or two hours of equilibration in the bath the muscle will remain stable for several hours. After studying the effects of a given drug, the bath solution may be replaced with fresh Krebs solution, and after an equilibration of 30 to 60 minutes the muscle may be restudied (if the drug is not irreversibly bound to muscle). Repeated washing, however, may lead to deterioration of muscle function and should be avoided. Special equipment for quick stretch or quick release experiments are valuable in studying the course of active state, but are not necessary for routine studies (Brady, 1968; Sonnenblick, 1967).

IN VITRO STUDIES

The positive or negative inotropic effects of any drug are best described in terms of its effects on (1) *isometric tension development* and (2) the *force-velocity relations*. The following general protocol describes how these two aspects of muscle physiology can be satisfactorily studied.

In the study of the isometric contraction, initial muscle length is generally fixed at the apex of the length-active-tension curve. The isometric trace, recorded at rapid paper speeds, provides a useful measure of the course of muscle activity. The rate of tension development (dP/dt), peak developed tension (P), and the time to peak tension (TTP) can be studied (Sonnenblick, 1967) (Fig. 7). Since the maximum rate of tension development (dP/dt) is linearly related to the average rate of tension development (P/TTP), measurement of any two of these parameters will define the third (Buccino et al., 1967).

The isometric contraction has been demonstrated to be directly related to the course of active state as measured by either quick stretch or quick release methods (Brady, 1965; Sonnenblick, 1967). Active state has been defined as a measure of those processes at contractile sites that generate force and shortening. With each contraction these processes are turned on, become maximal, and then are turned off. It has been shown that maximum dP/dt is linearly related to the maximum intensity of active state, while time to peak tension is linearly related to the time to reach maximum active state (Sonnenblick and Parmley, 1967). Thus simple measurements of the isometric contraction also characterize the course of active state without the necessity of repeating the laborious quick stretch or quick release measurements.

Different positive inotropic interventions affect isometric tension development in different ways. For example, catecholamines tend to shorten time to peak tension (Fig. 7) more than calcium or digitalis (Sonnenblick, 1962a, 1962b), while glucagon does not affect TTP in spite of a substantial increase in P and dP/dt (Glick et al., 1968). It is probable that such differences are related to the specific mechanism of action of the different interventions, although the precise meaning of such differences has yet to be defined.

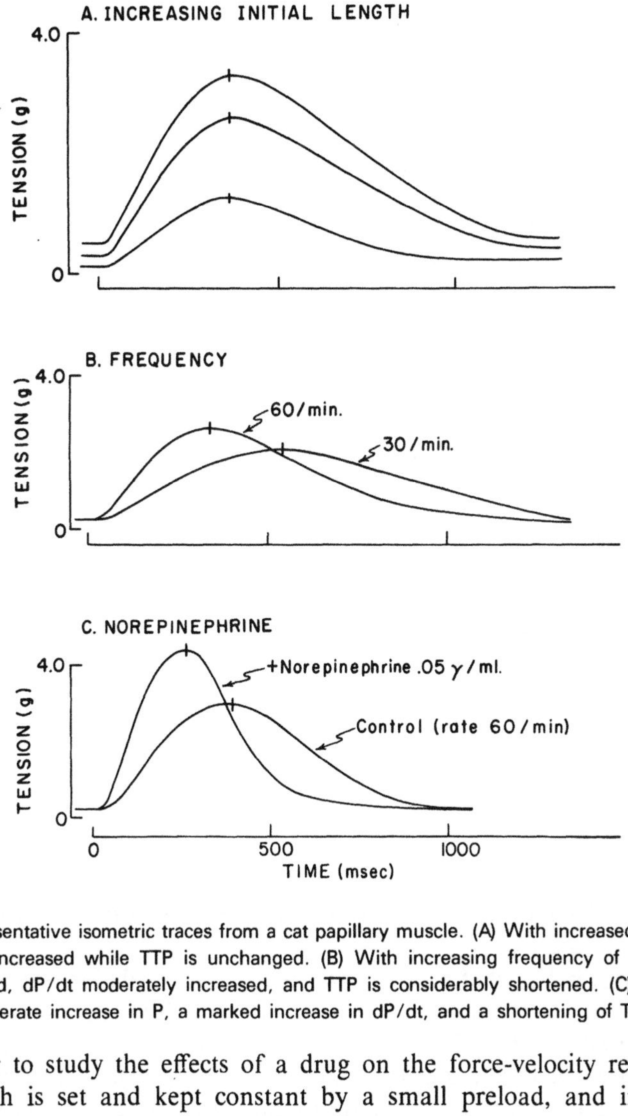

FIG. 7. Representative isometric traces from a cat papillary muscle. (A) With increased initial length, P and dP/dt are increased while TTP is unchanged. (B) With increasing frequency of stimulation, P is slightly increased, dP/dt moderately increased, and TTP is considerably shortened. (C) Norepinephrine results in a moderate increase in P, a marked increase in dP/dt, and a shortening of TTP.

In order to study the effects of a drug on the force-velocity relation, initial muscle length is set and kept constant by a small preload, and increments of afterload are sequentially added. The velocity of shortening is measured at each increase in afterload until the contraction is isometric (Sonnenblick, 1962a). The plot of velocity of shortening relative to afterload is the force-velocity curve. Resting tension is then increased to bring the muscle to the top of its length-active-tension curve, at which point control measurements of the tension (P), dP/dt, and TTP are obtained. Sequential logarithmic doses of the drug to be studied are then added to the bath to define the cumulative dose response curve. The higher concentration of drug is added only when the effects of the previous lower concentration has reached a steady state. The effect of the drug on the force-velocity relation is then determined by reducing the resting tension (or preload) to the level of the control and repeating the measurements of the force-velocity

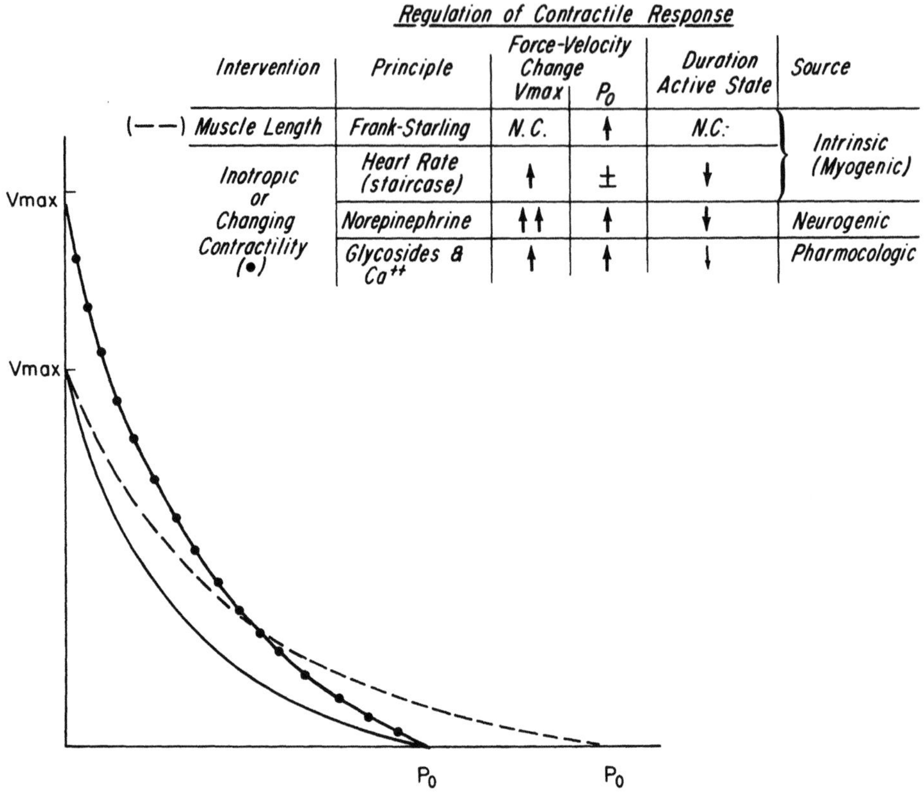

FIG. 8. Diagrammatic representation of the effects of common interventions on the force-velocity relation.

relation. The effects of common interventions on the force-velocity relation are summarized in Figure 8.

The change in V_{max} that occurs in the force-velocity relation is a sensitive index of a change in contractility (Sonnenblick, 1962b). Similarly, the change in P, maximum dP/dt, and TTP are indices of alterations in the active state as previously described (Sonnenblick and Parmley, 1967). The cumulative dose response curve is necessary to establish meaningful relationships with other cardioactive drugs.

When it has been determined that a drug has a positive inotropic effect, it is important to determine the relationship of this effect to both intrinsic catecholamine stores and beta adrenergic receptors. By reserpine pretreatment or denervation, intrinsic catecholamine stores can be depleted (Spann et al., 1966a), as confirmed by the addition of tyramine (10^{-5} to 10^{-4} M) to the bath or subsequent tissue analysis for catecholamines. If the positive inotropic action of a drug persists in tissues depleted of catecholamines [e.g., digitalis (Spann et al., 1966b)], it is clear that the drug does not act by releasing local stores of cathecholamines. To determine if the drug acts by stimulating beta adrenergic receptors, satisfactory beta adrenergic blockade can be obtained with 10^{-5} to 10^{-4} M *dl*-propanolol (Blinks, 1967). If the drug action persists [e.g., glucagon (Glick et al., 1968).], then it does not act by stimulation of beta adrenergic receptors. If the dose concentration-response curve is shifted in a parallel manner following beta adrenergic blockade [e.g., Isoproterenol (Blinks, 1967)], then it is apparent that the drug and propanolol are in competition for beta receptor sites.

When studying the action of drugs on the isolated cat papillary muscle it is valid to use either the muscle as its own control or a different group of normal control muscles if the former method is not possible. Since the cat papillary muscle is such a reproducible preparation, the results from groups of muscles fall in a very narrow normalized range (Spann et al., 1966a, 1966b), thus validating either horizontal or longitudinal studies.

SPECIAL MUSCLE PREPARATIONS

In addition to the normal preparations already described, papillary muscles have been removed from cats following particular interventions for special studies. A few of these preparations follow as examples.

Catecholamine depletion can be produced by pretreatment of cats with intraperitoneal reserpine, 3 mg/kg, on each of two days prior to study, which will reduce myocardial catecholamine content to negligible amounts (Spann et al., 1966a). Surgical denervation will also deplete catecholamines (Spann et al., 1966a), but is a much more difficult procedure and is thus unsuitable for routine use.

Hyperthyroidism can be induced by the intraperitoneal administration of thyroxin, 1 mg/kg/day, for 10 to 14 days with substantial changes in cardiac muscle function as measured in vitro or in vivo (Buccino et al., 1967). Conversely, hypothyroidism can be produced by the intraperitoneal administration of ^{131}I (1 mcg/kg), with subsequent study of the animals three months later (Buccino et al., 1967).

Right ventricular hypertrophy can be produced in a few days by placing a clip of diameter 2.8 or 3.5 mm around the pulmonary artery of cats, which will produce 90 and 80 percent constriction respectively (Spann et al., 1967a). The right ventricular papillary muscles from such a preparation have been used as a model for mechanical and pharmacologic studies of hypertrophied and failing cardiac muscle (Spann et al., 1967b).

IN VIVO PREPARATION

The open-chested dog is the most commonly used animal preparation for in vivo studies of the effects of drugs on myocardial contractility. However, the cat may be used quite adequately for the same purpose and indeed more economically. In general the same approaches utilized in isolated muscle can be extended to the intact heart. These can be discussed under three general headings: (1) *strain-gage measurement,* (Boniface et al., 1953), (2) *ventricular function curves* (Sarnoff and Mitchell, 1962), and (3) *muscle mechanics* applied to the *intact heart*(Ross et al., 1966; Taylor et al., 1967).

An index of ventricular wall tension can be recorded directly by suturing a Walton-Brodie strain-gage arch to the right (or left) ventricle (Boniface et al., 1953). For more complex evaluations of function, left ventricular pressure is recorded by a pressure transducer attached to a cannula which is inserted into the left ventricular cavity through the apical dimple or through the left atrial appendage and mitral valve. The left ventricular pressure at high gain permits the measurement of end-diastolic left ventricular pressure which serves as an index of ventricular volume prior to systole (Sarnoff and Mitchell, 1962). The measurement of mean atrial pressures as an index of ventricular filling pressure is much less reliable, especially at rapid heart rates. Arterial pressure is recorded from a femoral or carotid artery catheter attached directly to a pressure transducer, and intravenous injections are made through a catheter inserted into the femoral or jugular vein. Cardiac output can be determined by dye dilution techniques or by the use of an electromagnetic flowmeter placed about the root of the aorta.

Additional modifications of this basic preparation, to be listed, may be of further value in interpreting the observed hemodynamic effects. For example, coronary flow can be measured with the right heart bypass preparation, by tying off the pulmonary artery and pumping blood from the venae cavae directly to the pulmonary artery. Blood collected from the right atrium and right ventricle constitutes all of the coronary blood flow, less the minor flow that returns to the left ventricle by thebesian veins. Further, cardiac output in this right heart bypass preparation can be controlled with a roller pump. The influence of the vagus nerve can be abolished by vagotomy. Norepinephrine depletion in the ventricle may be produced by pretreating the dog with reserpine, 0.5 mg/kg intravenously, in divided doses on each of the two days preceding the study. However, satisfactory beta adrenergic blockade can be produced at the time of study by the intravenous administration of *dl*-propanolol (0.5 mg/kg). Since heart rate changes can directly alter contractility (Covell et al., 1967), heart rate is controlled by crushing the sinoatrial node or blocking the A-V node with an intramyocardial injection of formaldehyde (Steiner and Kovalick, 1968) and electrically pacing the heart. Changes in arterial pressure may also influence interpretation. Accordingly, it is desirable to maintain a constant mean aortic pressure, which can be done by adjusting the height of a volume reservoir of blood connected to the femoral artery (Downing and Sonnenblick, 1964).

IN VIVO STUDIES

Strain-Gage Measurements

The attachment of a strain gage (Boniface et al., 1953) to either the right or left ventricle permits measurement of the isometric contractile force beneath the gage. Once the gage is attached, the fibers beneath it are stretched so that they move relatively little and are less affected by changes in overall ventricular size. The resultant measurements provide a gross but useful index of the force of contraction of the wall of the heart. The recordings have little meaning in absolute terms, but relative changes following the administration of a drug can provide useful directional information. As is found in the isolated muscle under isometric conditions (discussed previously), the peak tension developed (T), rate of tension development (dT/dt), and the time to peak tension (TTP) provide useful information. A positive inotropic response to an agent which increases contractility is characterized by an increase in dT/dt and T, with a shortening [e.g., norepinephrine (Sonnenblick, 1962a)], little change [e.g., calcium or glycosides (Sonnenblick, 1962a)], or essentially no change [e.g., glucagon (Glick et al., 1968)] in TTP. It is also clear that were TTP to shorten adequately to offset an increase in dT/dt, no change in T might occur (Buccino et al., 1967), e.g., increased heart rate within certain limits (Sonnenblick, 1962a). This too would indicate an increase in contractility. Thus the measurement of T alone may not be satisfactory. Strain-gage measurements are of greatest value in studying the direct effect of drugs on the intact heart using the animal as his own control. One limitation to the use of force gages is the necessity to open the animal's chest, while imposing deep anesthesia. Further, strain-gage measurements may be altered by large alterations in either aortic pressure or ventricular volume, and these may require control.

Ventricular Function Curves

The analysis of the function of the intact heart as a pump has focused on the Frank-Starling mechanism–viz., the ability of the heart to increase its output as venous filling pressure of the heart is augmented. Sarnoff and Mitchell (1962) expanded this concept by describing ventricular function curves as a measure of the contractile state of the heart (Fig. 9). The relation between stroke work (stroke volume times left ventricular pressure) and left ventricular end-diastolic pressure (LVEDP) is shifted upward when the contractile state of the heart is increased and is likewise depressed when contractility is decreased (Fig. 9).

This type of analysis, however, may be inadequate when there are changes in arterial pressure and reflex changes in the resistance vessels of the peripheral circulation. Stroke work (approximated by stroke volume times arterial pressure) is by definition dependent on aortic pressure. Thus, unless pressure is held constant, the stroke work may be altered independently of any changes in contractility (Downing and Sonnenblick, 1964). Also it is often difficult to obtain complete ventricular function curves, since large shifts in blood volume are required to obtain these curves. This in itself may alter the contractility of the heart. Further, very extensive surgical manipulation of the heart is required prior to study, which may alter the physiologic setting substantially.

Implicit in the ventricular function curve is the relation between stroke volume (SV) and end-diastolic volume (EDV)–i.e., the ejection fraction (SV/EDV). The ejection fraction may be measured in a variety of ways. It may be obtained directly from the step functions of dye or temperature washout curves (Hugenholtz et al., 1968).

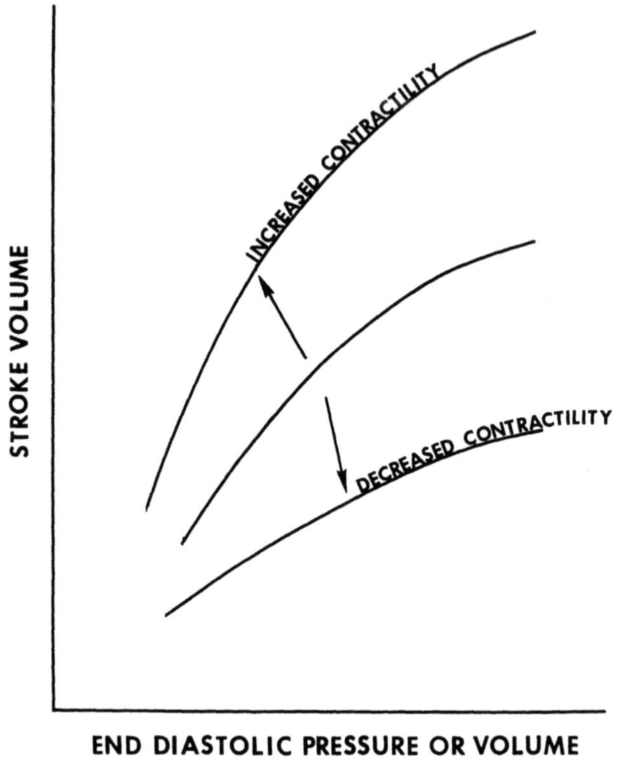

FIG. 9. Diagrammatic representation of the effect of changes in contractility on the ventricular function curve.

EDV may be measured from angiocardiograms and the SV calculated from the dye cardiac outputs or, in the dog, from flowmeter measurements. The ejection fraction as a measure of contractility is based on the fact that the SV/EDV is relatively independent of EDV, and with increased contractility, the same SV can be ejected from a smaller EDV–i.e. SV/EDV increases. However, the extent of muscle shortening, and hence the SV, is dependent on resistance to shortening. Thus increases in aortic pressure may decrease the ejection fraction, while lowering impedance to ejection [e.g., arteriovenous shunt or mitral regurgitation (Urschell et al., 1967)] will increase the SV/EDV, despite the absence of a change in contractility. Hence, the ejection fraction has a confined use, especially in a pathologic setting.

Muscle Mechanics in the Intact Heart

In the analysis of tension records from a strain gage sutured directly to the ventricle, an increase in contractility is present if the rate of development of wall tension is increased, as long as heart rate is held constant and LVED does not rise. Similarly, a rise in LV dP/dt at a constant heart rate with no increase or a decrease in LVED also indicates an increase in the contractile state of the myocardium. Since an increase in wall tension or LV dP/dt can occur with a rise in left ventricular end-diastolic pressure (LVEDP) and volume, without a change in the contractile state of the myocardium, interpretation of any results associated with a rise in LVEDP is difficult. Further, since most inotropic agents increase heart rate, which of itself augments contractility, it is most important to test the effect of any drug both before and after heart rate is held constant by electrical pacing.

A more recent approach to defining the contractile state of the heart has been the application of the force-velocity relation, as defined by in vitro papillary muscle studies, to the intact heart (Ross et al., 1966; Sonnenblick et al., 1968). This relation is most conveniently obtained by using an isovolumic beat technique (Ross et al., 1966; Taylor et al., 1967). An essentially isovolumic contraction is obtained by suddenly distending a balloon in the root of the aorta during diastole so as to prevent ejection of blood during the next systole. Utilizing the records of LV pressure and dP/dt from this one beat and assuming a hollow thin- or thick-walled spherical shape for the heart, a force-velocity curve for the ventricular muscle can be calculated (Fig. 10) (Taylor et al., 1967; Sonnenblick et al., 1968). Such calculations have confirmed the value of V_{max} as an index of myocardial contractility as first demonstrated for the isolated cat papillary muscle. With positive inotropic interventions, V_{max} is increased, while negative inotropic interventions decrease V_{max}. Thus, the principles of muscle physiology derived from in vitro papillary studies are fully applicable to the intact heart and provide a more sensitive index of contractility than pressure or flow measurements alone, which under certain circumstances can even be misleading (Covell et al., 1966). For example, in normal man, digitalis glycosides always induce an increase in cardiac contractility when measured directly. Nevertheless, cardiac output is unchanged or even decreased under these conditions (Sonnenblick et al., 1966).

When a particular agent has a demonstrated positive inotropic effect, it is then necessary to determine whether or not this effect is mediated by stimulation of beta adrenergic receptors. This is done by again testing the effects of the drug after satisfactory beta adrenergic blockade has been obtained with 0.5 mg/kg propanolol IV intravenously. Similarly, to determine whether or not an agent is acting by release of catecholamines, one can deplete such stores by pretreatment of the dog with 1.5 mg/kg/day reserpine on two days preceding the study. The degree of catecholamine depletion can be verified by a lack of response to 0.05 mg/kg tyramine intravenously or subsequent tissue analysis.

It should be emphasized at this juncture that merely because an agent has a demonstrated positive inotropic effect on the heart, it may not necessarily have a beneficial effect on the circulation. For example, the arrhythmogenic properties of an inotropic agent may be too dangerous to use for a slight increase in inotropy. Similarly, the increased oxygen requirements associated with an increase in myocardial contractility (Graham et al., 1968) may have a deleterious effect if the oxygen supply to the heart is limited by coronary vessel disease. Conversely the fact that an agent has a negative inotropic action on the heart does not necessarily

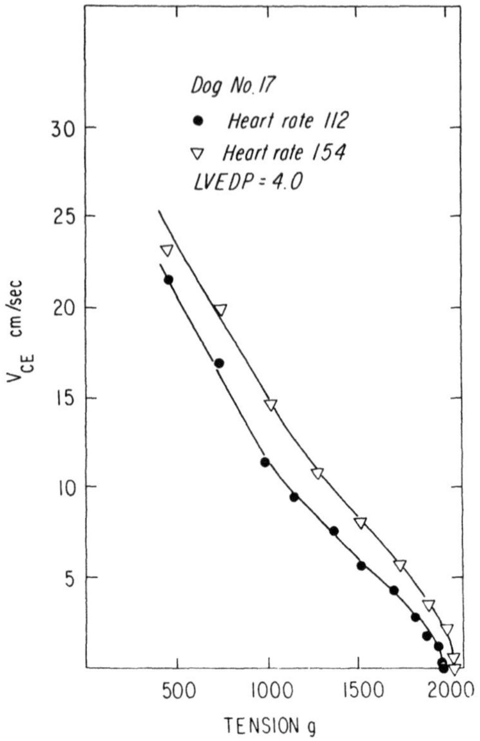

FIG. 10. Example of force-velocity relations in the intact dog calculated from single isovolumic contractions. Increasing contractility by increasing the heart rate shifts the force-velocity relations upwards and to the right.

imply that this is a deleterious effect. For example, *dl*-propanolol is of value in patients with angina pectoris primarily because it reduces the oxygen requirements of the heart by reducing both heart rate and cardiac contractility. Similarly, all antiarrhythmic agents have a negative inotropic effect on the ventricle (Parmley and Braunwald, 1967). Thus the clinical value of a drug may not be related to its inotropic effects per se but to its specific clinical application and particularly its degree of arrhythmogenic potential.

In summary, the effects of any agent on the heart are best characterized by a combination of both in vitro studies on isolated heart muscle and studies in the intact animal. The combined information obtained from both preparations allow one to interpret and quantitate drug action more clearly and more easily define its interrelated effects.

Recent studies (Pollack, 1970) have emphasized the importance of analyzing the force-velocity relations of the contractile element (CE) in terms of different three-component models. In particular, when resting tension becomes appreciable, the force-velocity relations of the *contractile element,* will differ depending on which three-component model of muscle is chosen. When one is measuring the force-velocity relations of the *muscle,* however, using isotonic afterloaded contractions as described in this chapter, the extrapolated maximum velocity of shortening, V_{max}, is indeed unchanged by changes in muscle length. It should be emphasized, however, that the force-velocity relations of the *muscle* obtained in this manner are not the same as the force-velocity relations of the *contractile element* which have to be calculated according to the specific three-component model being employed. Thus the measurement of force-veolocity relations of isolated heart muscle and extrapolated V_{max} as described in this chapter remain useful measurements of the effects of a given drug on contractile state in vitro.

When the attempt is made to calculate force-velocity relations in the intact heart, the situation is more complex. Since one cannot measure isotonic muscle shortening in this situation, one must calculate the velocity of the contractile element. Previous studies in the intact heart have been performed at relatively low end-diastolic pressures and volumes, and have thus employed a simple two-component model consisting of a contractile element in series with an elastic element. At these low end-diastolic pressures, the extrapolated maximum velocity of shortening, V_{max}, has been shown to be relatively independent of initial muscle length. Recent unpublished studies (Urschel and Sonnenblick), however, have demonstrated that a simple two-component model is no longer appropriate at higher end-diastolic pressures. These latter studies suggest that a more appropriate model to use in the intact heart is a three-component model wherein the parallel elastic (PE) is in parallel with both the contractile element and the series elastic. This is easily accomplished by employing developed pressure, rather than total pressure, in the equations for the calculation of contractile element velocity (Sonnenblick, 1968).

REFERENCES

Abbott, B. C., and Mommaerts, W.F.H.M. 1959. Study of inotropic mechanisms in papillary muscle preparation. J. Gen. Physiol., 42:533-551.

Blinks, J. R. 1967. Evaluation of the cardiac effects of several beta adrenergic blocking agents. Ann. N.Y. Acad. Sci., 139:673-685.

Boniface, K. J., Brodie, O. J., and Walton, R. P. 1953. Resistance strain gauge arches for direct measurement of heart contractile force in animals. Proc. Soc. Exp. Biol. Med., 84:263.

Brady, A. J. 1965. Time and displacement dependence of cardiac contractility: problems in defining active state and force velocity relations. Fed. Proc., 24:1410-1420.

—1968. Active state in cardiac muscle. Pharmacol. Rev., 48:570-600.

Buccino, R. A., Pool, P. E., Spann, J. F., Jr., Sonnenblick, E. H., and Braunwald, E. 1967. Influence of the thyroid state on the intrinsic contractile properties, and energy stores of the myocardium. J. Clin. Invest., 46:1669-1682.

—Sonnenblick, E. H., Spann, J. F., Jr., Friedman, W. F., and Braunwald, E. 1967. Interactions between changes in the intensity and duration of the active state in the characterization of inotropic stimuli on heart muscle. Circ. Res., 21:857-867.

Covell, J. W., Ross, J., Jr., Taylor, R., Sonnenblick, E. H., and Braunwald, E. 1967. Effects of increasing frequency of contraction on the force-velocity relation of the left ventricle. Cardiovasc. Res., 1:2-8.

—Ross, J., Jr., Sonnenblick, E. H., and Braunwald, E., 1966. Comparison of the force-velocity relation and the ventricular function curve as measures of the contractile state of the intact heart. Circ. Res., 19:364-372.

Downing, S. E., and Sonnenblick, E. H. 1964. Cardiac muscle mechanics and ventricular performance: force and time parameters. Amer. J. Physiol., 207:705-715.

Glick, G., Parmley, W. W., Wechsler, A. S., and Sonnenblick, E. H. 1968. Glucagon: its enhancement of cardiac performance on the cat and dog and persistence of its inotropic action despite beta-receptor blockade with propanolol. Circ. Res., 22:789-799.

Graham, T. P., Jr., Covell, J. W., Sonnenblick, E. H., Ross, J., Jr., and Braunwald, E. 1968. Control of myocardial oxygen consumption: relative influence of contractile state and tension development. J. Clin. Invest., 47:375-385.

Hill, A. V. 1938. Heat of shortening and dynamic constants of muscle. Proc. Roy. Soc. (Biol.)., 126:136-195.

Hugenholtz, P. G., Wagner, H. R., and Sandler, H. 1968. The in vivo determination of left ventricular volume: Comparison of the fiber optic-indicator dilution and the angiocardiographic methods. Circulation,37:489-508.

Jewell, B. R., and Blinks, J. R. 1968. Drugs and the mechanical properties of heart muscle. Ann. Rev. Pharmacol., 8:113-130.

Parmley, W. W., and Braunwald, E., 1967. Comparative myocardial depressant and antiarrhythmic properties of d-propanolol, dl-propanolol and quinidine. J. Pharmacol. Exp. Ther., 158:11-21.

—and Sonnenblick, E. H. 1967. Series elasticity in heart muscle: its relation to contractile element velocity and proposed muscle models. Circ. Res., 20:112-123.

—Spann, J. F., Taylor, R. R., and Sonnenblick, E. H. 1968. The series elasticity of cardiac muscle in hyperthyroidism, ventricular hypertrophy, and heart failure. Proc. Soc. Exp. Biol. Med., 127:606-609.

Pollack, G. H. 1970. Maximum velocity as an index of contractility in cardiac muscle: a critical evaluation. Circ. Res., 26:111-127.

Pool, P. E., Chandler, B., Sonnenblick, E. H., and Braunwald, E. 1967. Integrity of energy stores in cat papillary muscle in vitro. The Pharmacologist, 9:222.

Ross, J., Jr., Covell, J. W., Sonnenblick, E. H., and Braunwald, E. 1966. Contractile state of the heart characterized by force-velocity relations in variably afterloaded and isovolumic beats. Circ. Res., 18:149-163.

Sarnoff, S. J., and Mitchell, J. H. 1962. Control of function of the heart. *In* Handbook of Physiology. Hamilton, W. F., and Dow, P., eds. Washington, D.C., American Physiological Society, Vol. 1, Sec. 2, p. 758.

Sonnenblick, E. H. 1962a. Force velocity relations in mammalian heart muscle. Amer. J. Physiol., 202:931-939.

—1962b. Implications of muscle mechanics in heart. Fed. Proc., 21:975-990.

—1964. Series elastic and contractile elements in heart muscle: changes in muscle length. Amer. J. Physiol., 207:1330-1338.

—1965. Determinants of active state in heart muscle: force, velocity, instantaneous muscle length, time. Fed. Proc., 24:1396-1409.

—1967. Active state in heart muscle. Its delayed onset and modification by inotropic agents. J. Gen. Physiol., 50:661-676

—and Parmley, W. W. 1967. Active state in heart muscle: force-velocity-length relations and the variable onset and duration of maximum active state in factors influencing myocardial contractility. New York, Academic Press, Inc., pp. 65-83.

—Parmley, W. W., and Urschell, C. W. 1968. The contractile state of the heart as expressed by force-velocity relations. Amer. J. Cardiol. (In press.)

—Williams, J. F., Jr., Glick, G., Mason, D. T., and Braunwald, E. 1966. Studies on digitalis XV. Effects of cardiac glycosides on myocardial force-velocity relations in the non-failing human heart. Circulation, 34:532-539.

Spann, J. F., Jr., Buccino, R. A., and Sonnenblick, E. H. 1967a. Production of right ventricular hypertrophy with and without congestive heart failure in the cat. Proc. Soc. Exp. Biol. Med, 125:522-524.

—Buccino, R. A., Sonnenblick, E. H., and Braunwald, E. 1967b. Contractile state of cardiac muscle obtained from cats with experimentally produced ventricular hypertrophy and heart failure. Circ. Res., 21:341-354.

—Sonnenblick, E. H., Cooper, T., Chidsey, C. A., Willman, V. L., and Braunwald, E. 1966a. Cardiac norepinephrine stores and the contractile state of heart muscle. Circ. Res., 19:317-325.

—Sonnenblick, E. H., Cooper, T., Chidsey, C. A., Willman, V. L., and Braunwald, E. 1966b. Studies on digitalis XIV. Influence of cardiac norepinephrine stores on the response of heart muscle to digitalis. Circ. Res., 19:326-331.

Steiner, C., and Kovalik, T. W. 1968. A simple technique for production of chronic complete heart block in dogs. J. Appl. Physiol., 25:631-632.

Taylor, R. R., Ross, J., Jr., Covell, J. W., and Sonnenblick, E. H. 1967. A quantitative analysis of left ventricular myocardial function in the intact, sedated, dog. Circ. Res., 21:99-115.

Urschell, C. W., Covell, J. W., Sonnenblick, E. H., Ross, J., Jr., and Braunwald, E. 1967. Myocardial mechanics in aortic and valvular regurgitation: the concept of instantaneous impedance as a determinant of performance of the intact heart. J. Clin. Invest., 47:867.

Wilkie, D. R. 1956. Mechanical properties of muscle. Brit. Med. Bull., 12:177-182.

CHAPTER 5

Experimental Hypertension

Hubert C. Stanton*

Department of Pharmacology, Baylor College of Medicine
Houston, Texas

INTRODUCTION

Although experimental hypertension may be induced in rats by many methods, it is not known if any model closely approximates primary hypertension in man. The merits of these models are not discussed in this chapter, but instead we have described certain methods used to record blood pressure and to induce experimental hypertensive cardiovascular disease in the rat. Since space was not available to describe all methods, only references are given in many cases.

The descriptions of techniques in this chapter are, in most instances, limited and only intended to aid the investigator in choosing a procedure for his individual needs. The methods for fabricating and implanting direct blood pressure catheters in rats, however, are described in detail. This seems justified in view of the uniqueness of the procedures, their technical difficulty, and our experience in this area.

The final portion of the chapter describes some of our studies on the effects of commonly employed antihypertensive agents on normotensive, metacorticoid hypertensive, and adrenal regeneration hypertensive rats.

*Present address: Biological Sciences Research Center, Shell Development Company, Modesto, California.

BLOOD PRESSURE RECORDING

Arterial blood pressure has been recorded in hypertensive rats under three conditions: directly from anesthetized animals, directly from unanesthetized rats using implanted arterial catheters, or indirectly in unanesthetized animals by sensing the systolic pulse in an extremity such as the leg or tail. We will not consider anesthetized animals, since the effects of anesthesia on hemodynamics are many and varied and may seriously influence blood pressure responses. Although the unanesthetized rat is preferred for blood pressure studies, there may be a choice between direct and indirect recording methods. In most instances, this choice depends upon a balance between two major considerations–the reliability of the measurement and the convenience with which it can be performed.

Small differences in recording technique may have less effect on the reliability of arterial blood pressures measured directly compared to indirectly. Furthermore, a continuous recording for a specified period of time may be obtained by direct methods, and blood pressure fluctuations associated with movement or environmental stress may be more easily recognized. Systolic and diastolic pressures can both be approximated directly, and heart rate may be obtained from the blood pressure record. Warming the rat before or during indirect blood recording significantly influences hemodynamics and, unless the conditions of warming are rigidly controlled, may affect the reproducibility of repeated measurements. Similarly, the position of the occluding cuff on the extremity may determine the blood pressure obtained (Weeks and Jones, 1960; Fregly, 1963).

In order to improve the reliability of repeated, indirect, blood pressure measurements in the rat, Sturtevant (1957) employed a "blind" procedure where the individual recording the blood pressure was not aware of the drug treatment. Coded antihypertensive agents of known activity were also included with unknown drugs. A similar procedure may be desirable if unknown drugs are routinely evaluated using indirect blood pressure recording techniques.

Direct methods for chronically recording blood pressure in unanesthetized rats require surgical skills and techniques that are moderately difficult to master and time-consuming. Implanted catheters may remain functional for two or more weeks if frequent recordings are taken, although following the progress of experimental hypertension over long periods of time is generally difficult. Indirect recording methods do not require special surgical skills and are particularly useful for studying large numbers of hypertensive animals or following the course of the disease over long periods of time. It is paramount that the conditions under which these indirect determinations are made be standardized if repeated measurements are to be compared.

Direct Measurements

Several methods have been described for chronically measuring blood pressure directly from anesthetized rats. In our laboratory, the Weeks and Jones

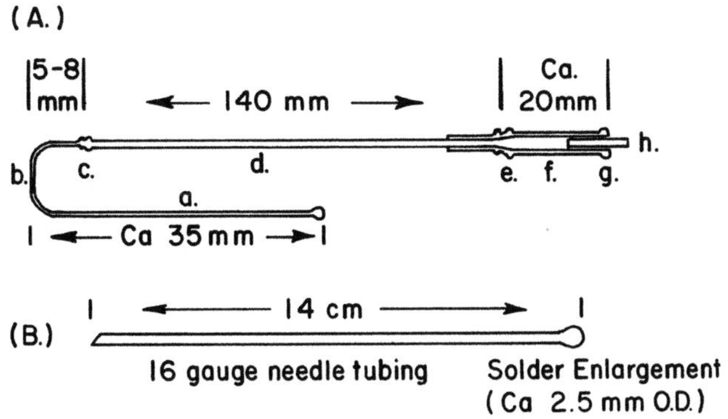

FIG. 1. (A) Aortic blood pressure catheter. (B) Trocar used to pass the aortic catheter through the body to the back of the neck of the rat.

(1960) modification of the method of Still and Whitcomb (1956) has been found to be satisfactory for moderate-sized animals (> 150 g). This procedure will be described in detail. The catheter, with the dimensions for each segment, is illustrated in Figure 1A and is fabricated as follows:

1. Standard polyethylene tubing of the following sizes is cut to the following approximate lengths: PE 10 = 50 mm, PE 50 = 170 mm, PE 160 = 50 mm.
2. A 6- to 8-inch length of 21-gauge needle stylet with a 3- to 4-mm tapered tip is passed through the PE 50 tubing and firmly inserted into the lumen of the PE 10 segment. The PE 50 tubing is then slipped as far as possible over the PE 10. If this cannot be accomplished, the tip of the stylet must be tapered more.
3. The PE 50 and PE 10 junction is sealed together by rapidly rotating the stylet and tubing against the tip of a warm soldering iron (Ungar 23½ watt with a No. 332 tiplet, Allied Radio Corp.). The ridge, (c) in Figure 1A, is raised by gently pushing the two segments of tubing together while they are rotated against the iron. Proper soldering iron temperature can be controlled with a conventional rheostat set at about 70. The tubes will mold to the shape of the stylet if the soft, polyethylene joint is rotated between the fingers while it cools and hardens.
4. With the 21-gauge needle stylet in the PE 50 tubing, slip a 30-mm segment of PE 160 tubing over the PE 50 until the ends are flush. The PE 50 and 160 are sealed together 20 to 25 mm from the end of the catheter, as shown in (e) in Figure 1A.
5. The ends of the tubing are sealed to form the flange, (g) in Figure 1A.
6. The tip of the PE 10 tubing is sealed against the soldering iron.
7. The J shape, (b) in Figure 1A, is obtained by loosely forming the PE 10 tubing around an L-shaped glass rod and momentarily immersing in boiling water.
8. The catheter is tested underwater by attempting to inject 1 ml of air into the catheter from a 2-ml syringe equipped with a 21-gauge blunt needle. Air bubbles appear at faulty seals, and these catheters are discarded or repaired.
9. The 7-mm metal plug, (h) in Figure 1A, is fashioned from an 18-gauge needle

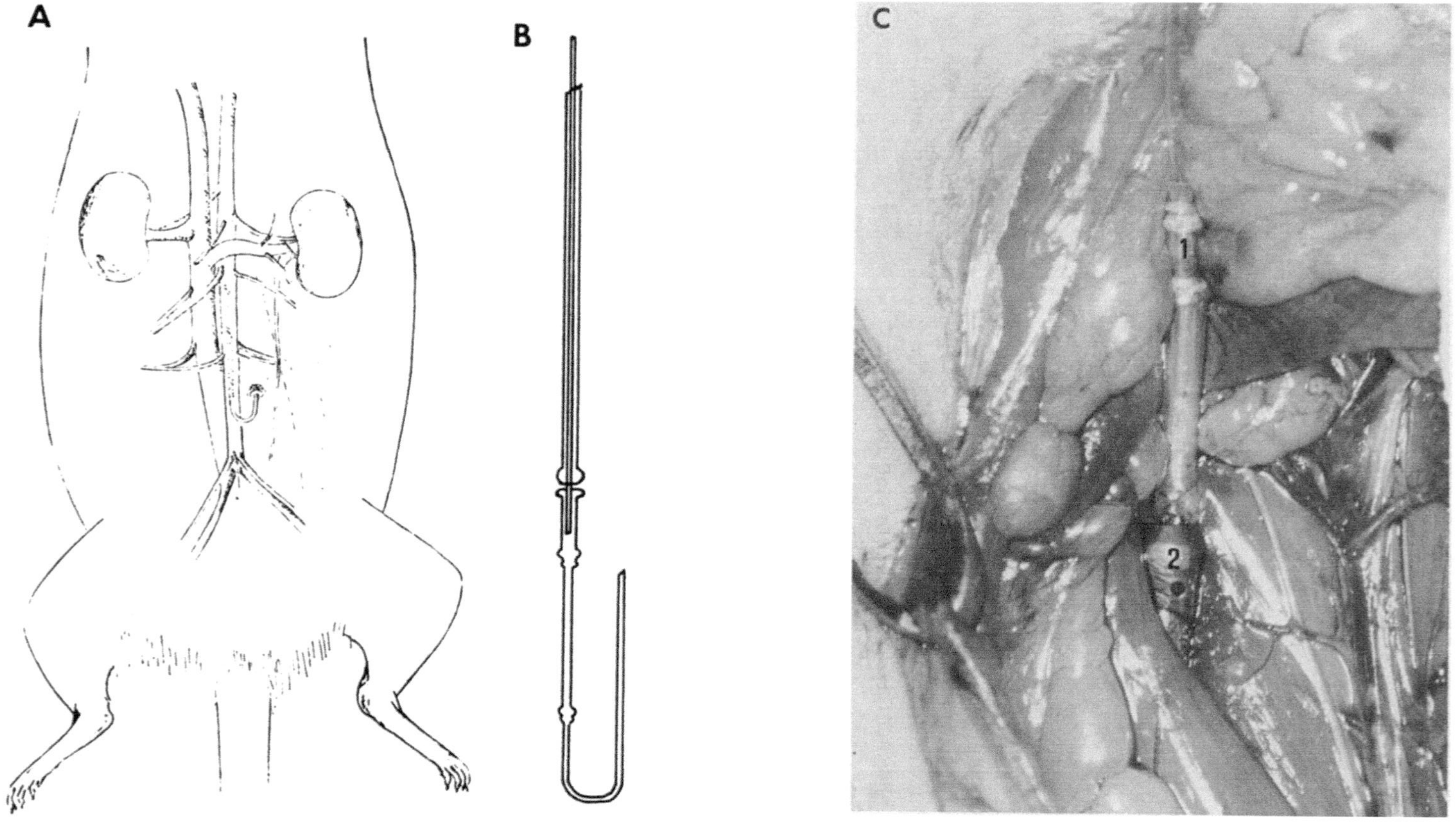

FIG. 2. (A) Diagram showing the catheter in the aorta. (After McIlreath et al., 1965. *Arch. Int. Pharmacodyn.*, 157:330–338.) (B) Aortic catheter attached to the trocar by means of needle tubing. (C) Catheter, 1, and trocar, 2, in place in the living animal. The catheter follows as the trocar is drawn through the tissues.

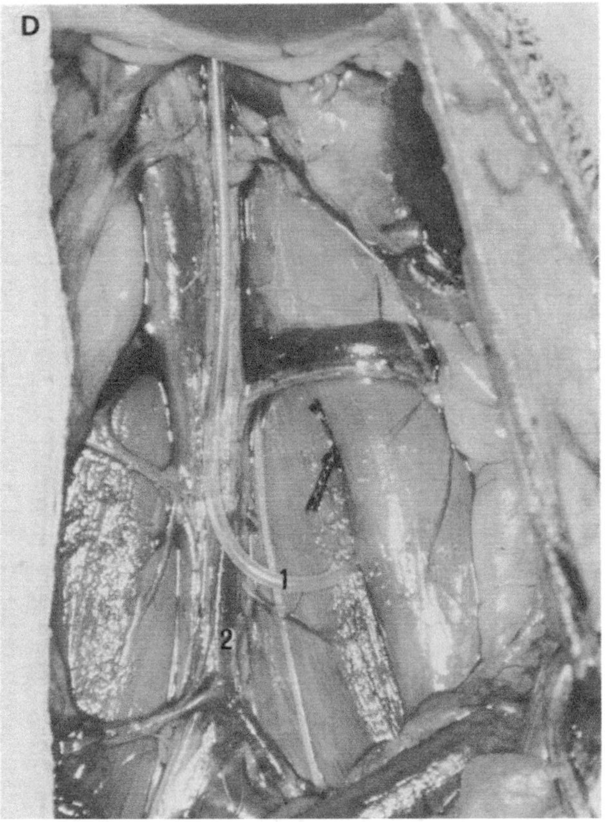

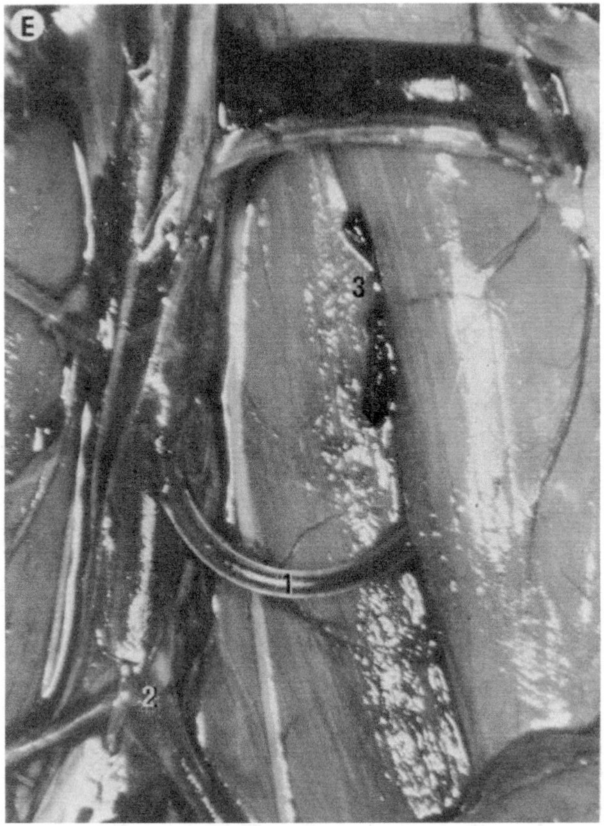

FIG. 2. (*cont.*) (D) The position of the PE 10 segment, 1, of the catheter inserted into the aorta above the bifurcation of the iliac arteries, 2. The catheter has been secured to the psoas muscles with silk suture, 3.

stylet by cutting and polishing the metal with a dental separating disc attached to a Moto tool (Dremel Manufacturing Co., Racine, Wisconsin). This disc, which is also used to taper the 21-gauge needle stylet, is moistened with a stream of water during the grinding process.

10. Silk suture, size 0000, is tied at position (c) (Fig. 1A) and is used to secure the catheter to the tissue.

These catheters fit rats weighing 250 to 350 g, but the dimensions can be altered to fit smaller animals. When catheters are to be implanted for several weeks, allowances should be made for growth. Heatley and Weeks (1964) have described, in detail, other methods for fashioning polyethylene tubing for use in animal experimentation.

The rat is anesthetized with ether and the neck and abdominal area clipped and cleansed with 70 percent ethanol. The rat is placed on its back on an animal board with the legs extended and fastened with rubber bands. Anesthesia is maintained by placing a small, Gooch crucible containing ether-saturated cotton over the animal's nose when needed. Sterile conditions are not necessary, although it is desirable to immerse the surgical instruments and sutures in 70 percent ethanol or other antiseptic before use. A small incision is made at the back of neck, approximately 15 mm behind the ears. A midline, abdominal incision is extended 4 to 5 cm from the junction of the pelvis, and the viscera are gently removed and covered with sterile, moist gauze. A segment of abdominal aorta just above the bifurcation of the iliac arteries is gently wiped with a cotton-tipped applicator stick. If this area is rubbed too vigorously, the inferior vena cava may be torn.

A trocar, illustrated in Figure 1B, is passed through the psoas muscles adjacent to the cleared segment of aorta (lateral to the genitofemoral nerve and medial to the left ureter), through the muscles of the back and under the skin until it emerges from the incision at the back of the neck. A 20-cm segment of 22-gauge needle tubing is inserted through the trocar and tightly attached to the catheter, as shown diagrammatically in Figure 2B. A photograph of the trocar and catheter in the animal is seen in Figure 2C. The trocar and needle tubing with the catheter attached are simultaneously pulled through the tissues until the end of the catheter protrudes from the neck incision. The catheter is positioned so that the J portion faces, and the segment of PE 10 tubing lies parallel to, the aorta (Fig. 2D). This PE 10 segment is cut on a bevel to a length that reaches slightly below the renal arteries. The catheter is loosely anchored to the psoas muscles with the silk suture attached at point (c) (Fig. 1A). The catheter is filled with saline and connected to a Statham P23Dc pressure transducer with PE 50 tubing.

The aorta, occluded with the tip of the first finger, is punctured in the cleared area above the bifurcation with a bent 27-gauge hypodermic needle attached to a 0.5-ml glass syringe. The tip of the PE 10 catheter is inserted into the needle hole using fine forceps and is advanced up the aorta. The catheter remains inserted in the artery, and blood pressure is recorded if the J segment is properly situated. The position of the catheter in the animal is shown diagrammatically in Figure 2A and in the living rat in Figure 2E. Occasionally the PE 10 tubing enters the fascia surrounding the aorta and blood pressure can not be recorded. If this happens, it will be necessary to puncture the aorta again and reinsert the catheter. The catheter will also occasionally pass through the aorta if the angle at which the vessel is entered is too steep.

The viscera are replaced if the catheter is functional and the abdominal cavity closed with 0000 chromic gut suture followed by 0000 silk suture. A loose silk suture is placed in the neck incision and the catheter loosely anchored to the skin at point (e) (Fig. 1A). Antibiotic treatment is not generally needed after the surgery if cleanliness is observed during the procedure. Weeks and Jones (1960) do not recommend heparin, although we fill our catheters with dilute (0.2 mg/ml) heparin sodium in 0.9 percent sodium chloride solution before they are closed. The catheters are flushed by gently occluding the polyethylene portion protruding through the skin (Fig. 3A) with a hemostat with rubber tubing on the jaws, removing the metal plug with another hemostat and then inserting a blunt 22-gauge needle attached to a 2-ml syringe into the catheter (Fig. 3B).

The first blood pressures are recorded three days after surgery from animals lightly wrapped in a towel (Fig. 3C). The towel is light cotton, measures 14 by 16 inches, and has a buttonhole sewn in the corner for the catheter end to protrude. Most animals struggle during the first recording but adapt after two or three trials and are quiet enough for consistent blood pressure measurements (Fig. 3D). McIlreath et al. (1965) recorded direct blood pressures from rats which were free to move about in small cages (Fig. 4). This is preferable to restraining the animals, but the free animals may chew the extension tube which passes from the catheter to the transducer. A catheter saddle and swivel (Weeks, 1964) is commercially available (Lehigh Valley Electronics, Fogelsville, Pennsylvania) and may be utilized to record direct arterial blood pressures from a few unanesthetized, relatively unrestrained animals.

It is sometimes possible to open a blocked catheter with gentle flushing, while in other instances the catheter may be opened by gently massaging the aorta through the abdominal wall. Certain animals develop hind limb paralysis two to three days following catheter implantation and must be sacrificed. Occasionally, the catheter will be occluded in such a manner that it is possible to inject fluid but not to record pressure or withdraw blood. Rats prepared in our laboratory are generally useful for at least one or two weeks, even though blood pressures are frequently taken. Weeks and Jones (1960), on the other hand, use animals much longer than this (6 to 12 months). There is some suggestion that frequent catheter flushing increases the likelihood of failure or hind limb paralysis.

We have also employed rats with indwelling aortic catheters to determine glucose tolerance curves since small, serial blood samples are easily obtained from unanesthetized animals (Kvam and Stanton, 1964).

Indirect Methods

Systolic arterial blood pressure has been estimated in the unanesthetized rat by a variety of indirect methods. The commonly employed procedures correlate the pressure in a pneumatic, occluding cuff placed on an extremity with the appear-

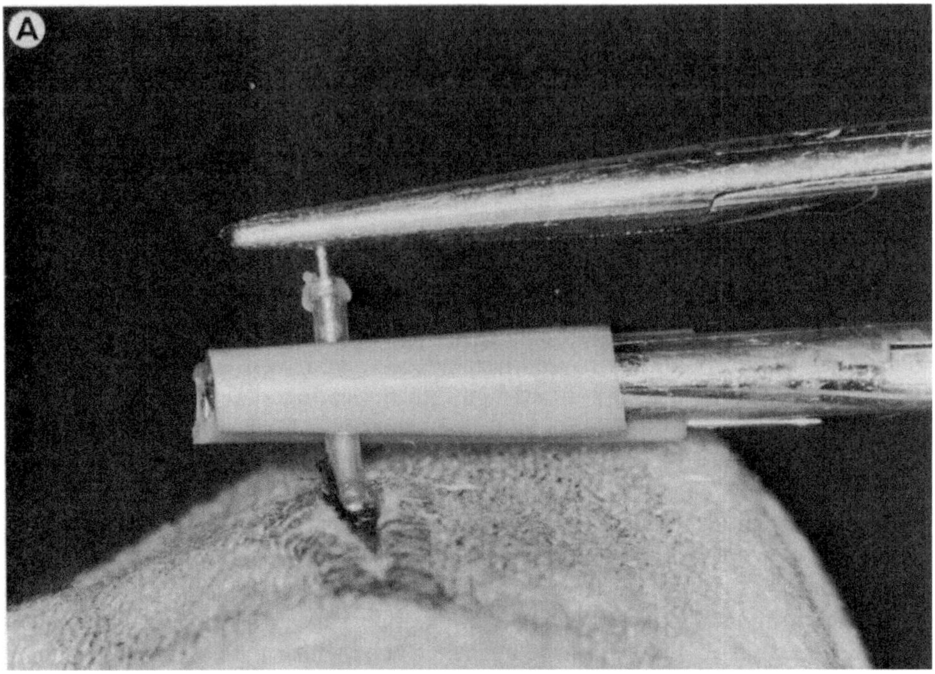
A

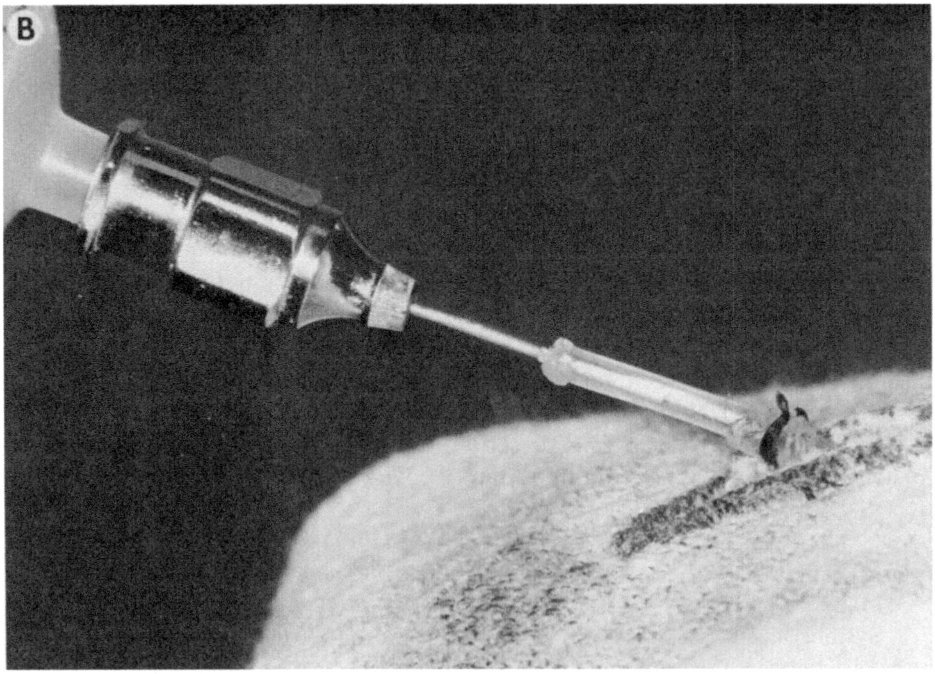
B

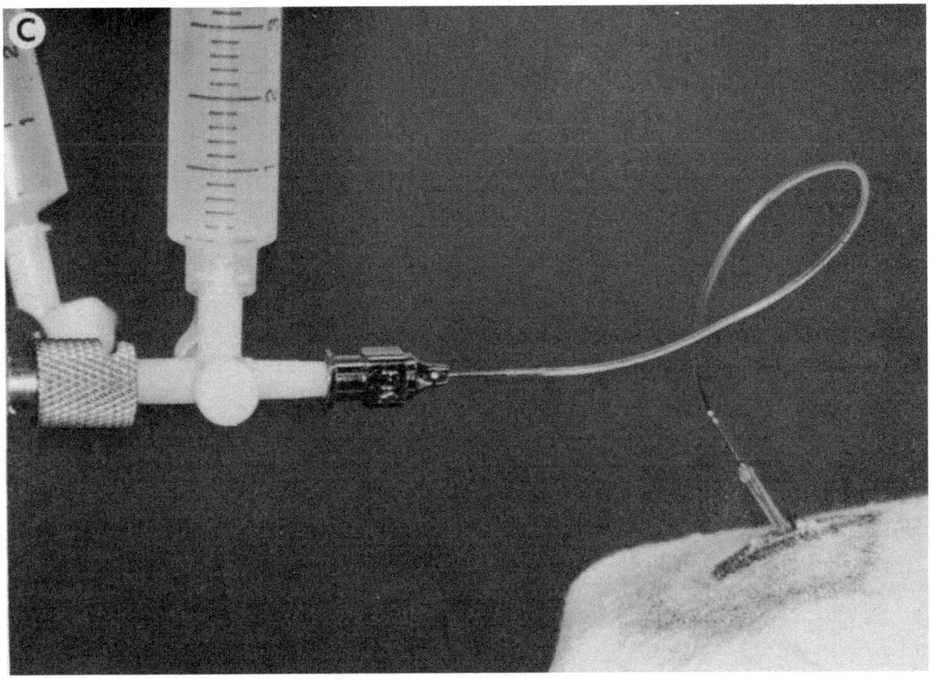

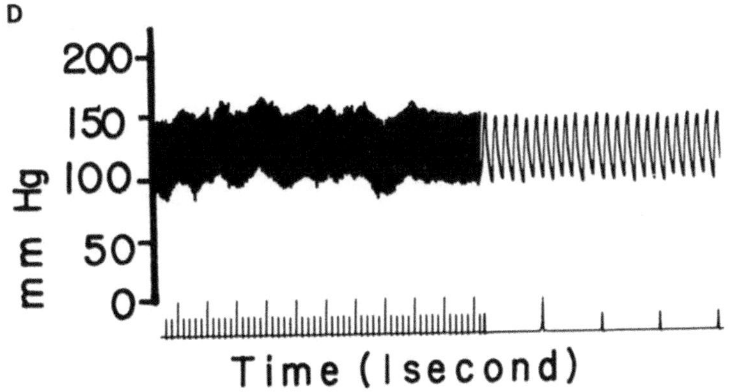

FIG. 3. (A) Occluding the catheter and removing the metal plug. The catheter end at the back of the rat's neck protrudes through a buttonhole in the restraining towel. (B) Flushing the catheter. (C) Recording aortic blood pressure from a restrained rat with an indwelling aortic catheter. PE 50 tubing connects the catheter to the transducer. (D) Blood pressure recording taken from an unanesthetized, normotensive rat with an indwelling aortic catheter. (From Stanton and Cooper, 1966. *Cardiovasc. News Bull.*, 5:16-28.)

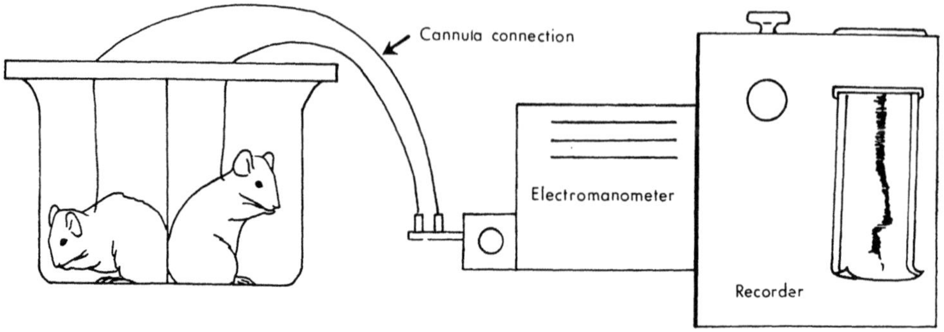

FIG. 4. Diagram illustrating the recording of direct, aortic blood pressure from unrestrained rats. (From McIlreath et al., 1965. *Arch. Int. Pharmacodyn.*, 157:330-338.)

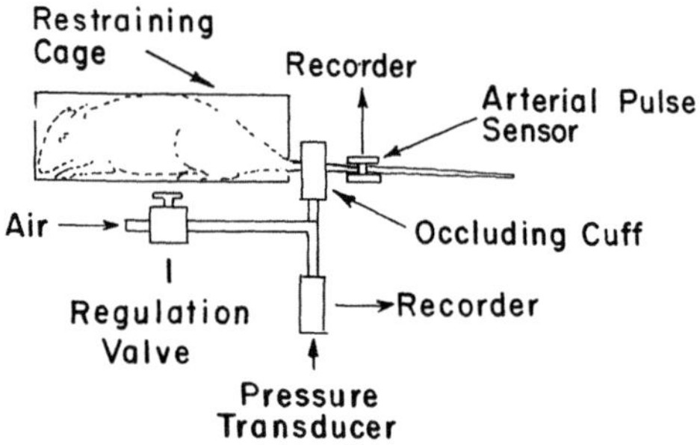

FIG. 5. Diagram showing the principles involved when indirectly recording systolic blood pressure from the tail of a rat.

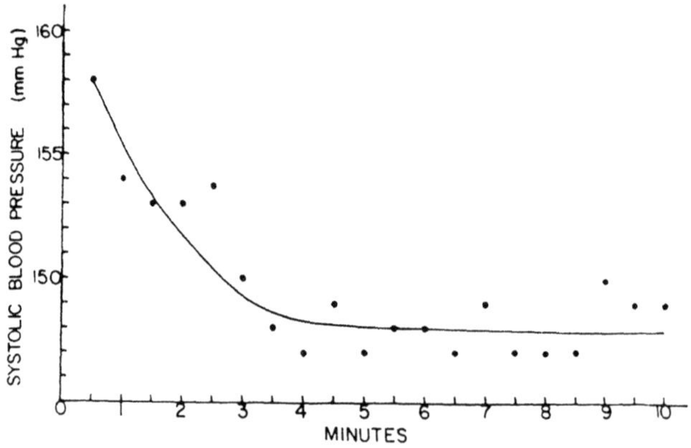

FIG. 6. The effect of repeated (30 second) measurements of systolic blood pressure of rats beginning immediately after the cessation of warming. Blood pressure reached a stable level in 4 minutes, suggesting an initial period of stress with elevated blood pressure. (From Fregly, 1963. *J. Lab. Clin. Med.*, 62:223-230. Courtesy of The C. V. Mosby Company.)

ance of the first systolic pulse. The methods used to detect this pulse include a microphone, a sensitive plethysmograph, a photoelectric cell, or an unbonded strain gage.

TAIL.—The general position of the rat, the occluding cuff, and the pulse sensing device, regardless of type, are illustrated diagrammatically in Figure 5. Since the rat is restrained and this is stressful, training is necessary before meaningful pressures are obtained. Fregly (1963) observed that the systolic blood pressure, measured indirectly from the tail after heating, was highest during the first four minutes the animals were restrained but then stabilized at a lower level (Fig. 6).

The rat is generally warmed before indirectly measuring blood pressure from the tail in order to dilate small arteries that are normally constricted and allow better detection of blood flow through the extremity. However, the hemodynamics of the animal are also influenced by this treatment, which undoubtedly affects the validity of blood pressure measurements. Utmost care must therefore be taken to standardize the duration and degree of warming. Proskauer et al. (1945) observed, using anesthetized as well as unanesthetized rats, that fluctuations in cutaneous temperature could be correlated in magnitude and time with changes in blood pressure. Olmsted et al. (1951) studied the affects of various methods of heating on the blood pressure of rats and observed a steady increase in blood pressure with warming. Stable blood pressures were obtained by initially heating the rats for 3 minutes at 45°C and then maintaining the temperature at 40°C. Similar blood pressure levels were obtained if only the tails were heated at 45°C for 15 minutes. Many investigators warm the animals in a box before and/or during the blood pressure measurement, while others warm the restraining cage. The exact procedure is probably not as critical as the careful standardization of the conditions under which the rats are warmed and the blood pressures are recorded.

The width of the occluding cuff and its position on the tail are important if reproducible, blood pressure measurements are to be obtained when the cuff is frequently removed and replaced. Fregly (1963) reported that blood pressures were lower when the occluding cuff width was increased (Fig. 7A) and chose a cuff width of 37.5 mm. He suggested, however, that each investigator prepare a cuff width-blood pressure curve and determine the optimum cuff width under his experimental conditions.

Fregly (1963) also noted that the position of the cuff on the tail was important, and found that blood pressure decreased as the cuff was moved from the base of the tail (Fig. 7B). The investigator should therefore mark the position of the cuff on the tail and duplicate this position each time he uses the animal.

A diagram of the tail occluding cuff used by Fregly (1963) is shown in Figure 8. Occluding cuffs are commercially available (E & M Instrument Co., Inc., Houston, Texas), but the custom model may provide more flexibility for adjusting the width to the investigator's needs.

The systolic arterial pulse sound is commonly detected with a small carbon microphone attached over the caudal artery. A thin metal trough is often soldered to the diaphragm of the microphone to better fit the tail. Fregly (1963) used a

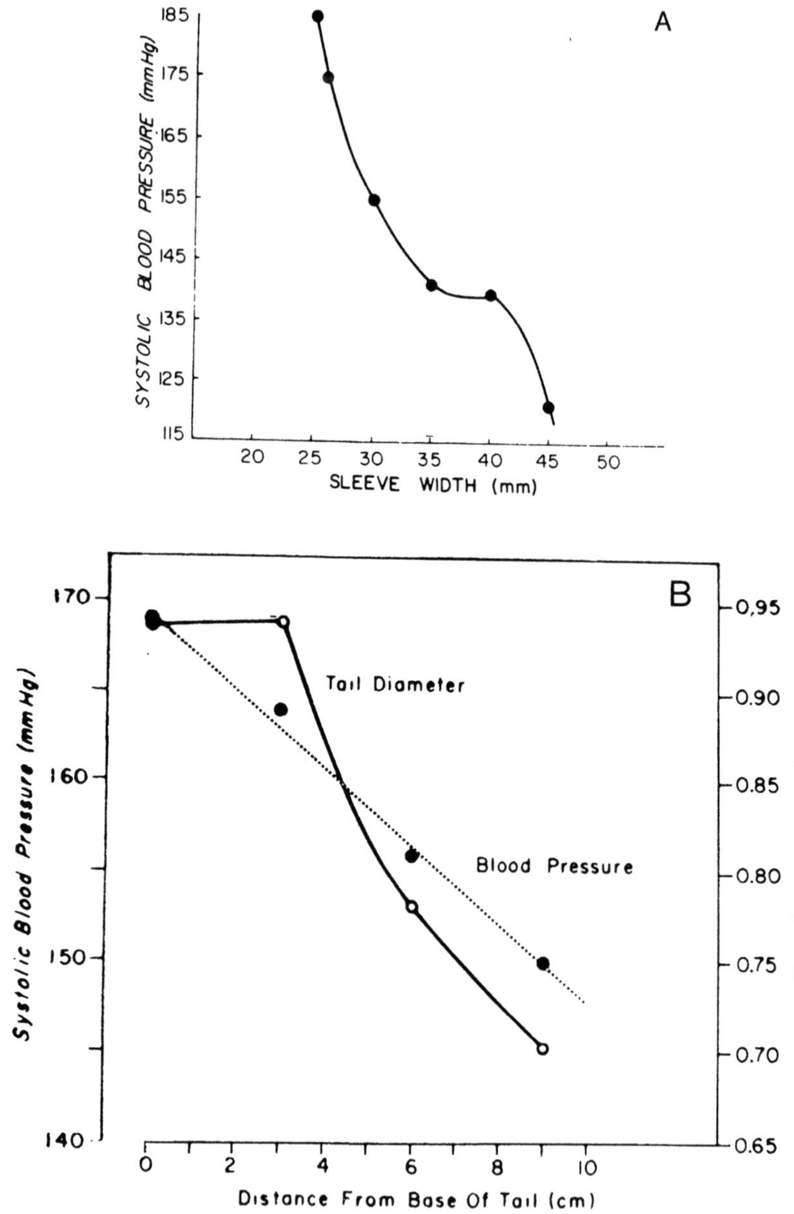

FIG. 7. The effect of changing the width of the rubber sleeve of the occluding cuff on the measurement of systolic blood pressure in the rat. (From Fregly, 1963.) (B) The effect of the placement of the occluding cuff at various distances from the base of the tail on the measurement of blood pressure. The black dots represent mean blood pressures taken from five rats. The open circles represent mean tail diameters of the same five rats taken at various distances from the base of the tail. (From Fregly, 1963. *J. Lab. Clin. Med.*, 62:223-230. Courtesy of The C. V. Mosby Company.)

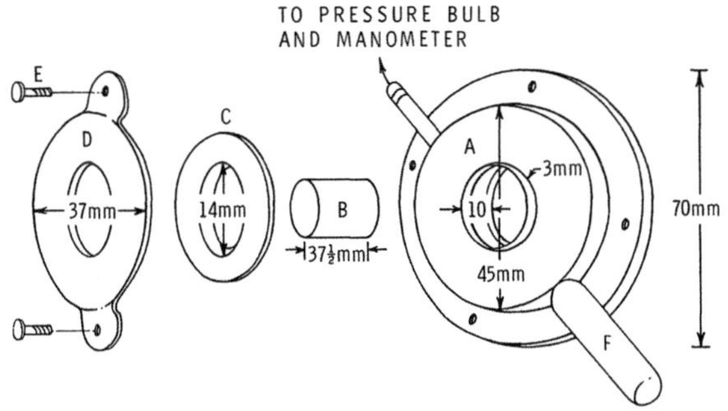

FIG. 8. An exploded view of the metal occluding cuff used for the indirect measurement of systolic blood pressure of the rat. Only one side of the cuff is shown. The air chamber (A) in the body of the cuff is 45 mm in diameter. A 3-mm lip protrudes beyond the surface of the air chamber on both sides of the cuff. A rubber sleeve (B) fits into the chamber and the ends of the tubing (Penrose drainage tubing 1/2 inch in diameter) fit over each lip. The brass insert (C) (one on each side) fits inside the lip of the air chamber and makes that portion of the rubber tubing over the lip of the air chamber a gasket to seal the chamber. The brass plate (D) (one on each side) then goes over the brass insert screws to the cuff (E). The metal bar (F) clamps the cuff to a ring stand. (From Fregly, 1963. *J. Lab. Clin. Med.,* 62:223-230. Courtesy of The C. V. Mosby Company.)

model T-30-R microphone (Aircraft Radio Industries, New Haven, Connecticut), but similar microphones are also available from many other sources, including the Spinco Division of Beckman Instrument Co. The microphone is firmly fastened to the ventral surface of the tail with tape or elastic cloth. The pressure in the occluding cuff pressure is raised above the arterial systolic pressure and then slowly released. When this pressure falls below systolic pressure, there is an audible pulse from the caudal artery which, when detected, can be amplified and heard with earphones or recorded oscillographically. A schematic diagram for a low-frequency sound amplifier used with a capacitor microphone was described by Friedman and Freed (1952). Further information on the amplifier systems and coupling to a specific recorder can usually be obtained from the manufacturer of the microphone or recorder. Movements of the tail may cause noise and obscure the pulse sounds, thus making the end point difficult to detect.

The caudal arterial pulse may also be detected plethysmographically using an inexpensive device similar to that described by Williams et al. (1939) or a more sophisticated electronic transducer system with appropriate amplifiers coupled to a recorder. A system using a rubber, pneumatic sensor connected to a sensitive pressure transducer is commercially available from E & M Instrument Co., Inc., Houston, Texas. This system includes a pneumatic sensor, occluding cuff, transducer, a sphygmomanometer-preamplifier combination, and a rat holder-warmer with control unit. A photograph of this unit with attachments is illustrated in Figure 9. Preamplifiers for recording EKG and respiration are also available and may be added if desired. A custom occluding cuff and air pressure regulator valve may be preferable to the bulb and cuff shown with the system. If the Physiograph TM recorder is not available and another type of recorder is used, a transducer monitor-coupler (Fig. 9) must be used to match the preamplifiers to the recorder.

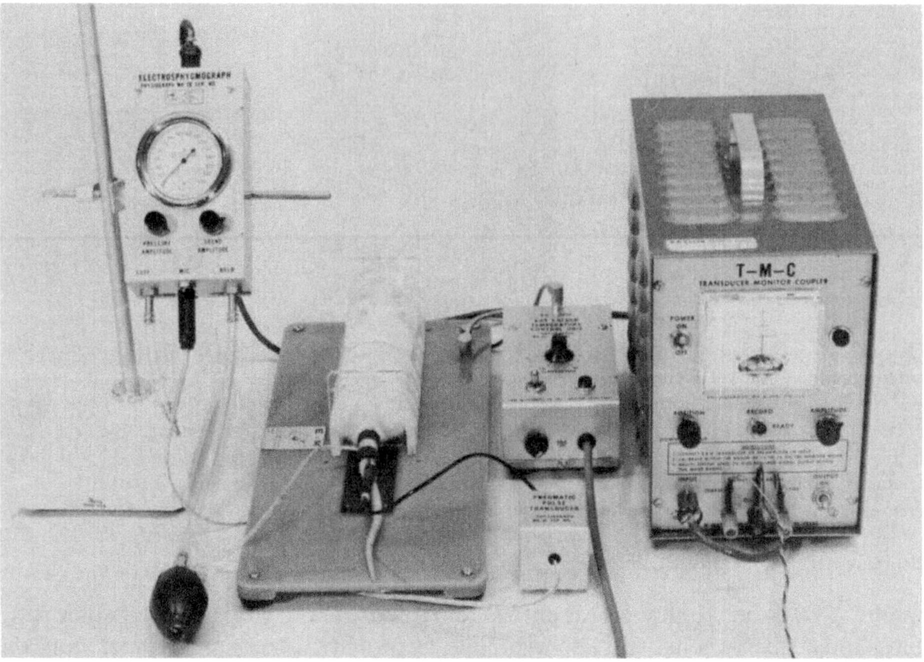

FIG. 9. Small-animal blood-pressure measurement unit manufactured by E & M Instrument Co., Houston, Texas. The occluding cuff and the pneumatic sensor are attached to the rat's tail. The transducer-monitor-coupler is needed if a recorder other than the Physiograph is used.

This significantly increases the cost of the system. Similar systems can, of course, be built by the investigator using common, commercially available pressure transducers.

FOOT.—Blood pressure has been measured indirectly in the rat without warming using a photoelectric cell to rapidly detect volume changes in the foot (Kersten et al., 1947). The animal is restrained in a special chamber which allows access to the hind leg and foot, and the paw is placed in a special holder over an aperture so that light passes from a source below, through the foot, and onto a photoelectric cell situated on the dorsal surface (Fig. 10). If blood flow through the foot is normal, the light sensed by the photocell is constant; but when the leg is occluded, the foot swells and the amount of light striking the photocell is reduced. In the original Kersten et al. (1947) method, blood flow to the leg was occluded by applying pressure (250 mm Hg) to a latex cuff and the ammeter, used to detect the amplified photocell response, was adjusted to 150 ma. The pressure in the cuff was slowly released, and arterial blood flow was restored when systolic pressure was reached. The resulting increase in foot volume reduced the amount of light transversing the paw, and the ammeter needle fell rapidly. When venous pressure was reached, venous return was reestablished, foot volume was reduced, and the needle rose. This procedure has been modified so that the photocell response is

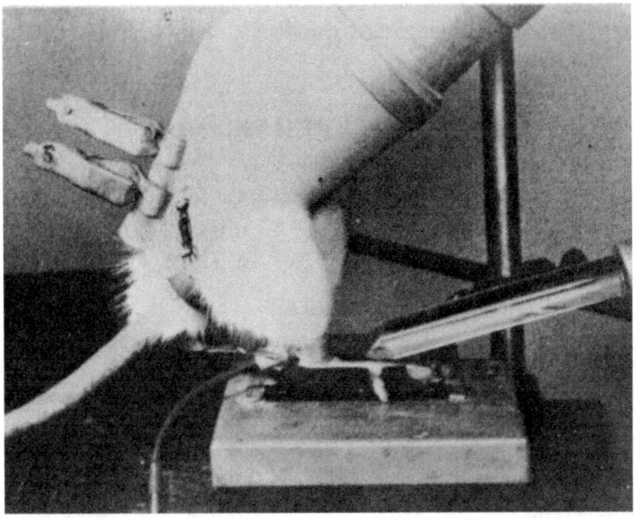

FIG. 10. Restraining chamber, foot holder, and photoelectric cell used to detect blood flow in the foot of an unanesthetized rat. (From Kersten et al., 1947. *J. Lab. Clin. Med.*, 32:1090-1098. Courtesy of The C. V. Mosby Company.)

amplified and recorded simultaneously with the occluding cuff pressure on a suitable recorder. The details for fabricating or assembling the various components of the system are clearly provided in the original description of the method. Easily modified, commercially available leg cuffs were described by Rosett and Handler (1957). In studies by Weeks and Jones (1960), repeated direct blood pressures, measured in the same animals from aortic catheters, agreed closely with indirect pressures measured from the foot with a photoelectric tensometer if the leg cuff remained in one place. However, variations as great as ± 70 mm Hg were encountered if the cuff was removed and replaced. Since cuff pressure must be reduced at an optimal, uniform rate, an easily controlled air valve, similar to that described by Olmsted et al. (1951), seems indicated for more reproducible results.

Olmsted et al. (1951) described an indirect method for recording blood pressure in the rat using a procedure similar to Kersten et al. (1947) but detecting the systolic pulse in the foot with a sensitive, unbonded, strain gage.

Summary

Direct blood pressure recording methods in unanesthetized rats are technically difficult and, in many instances, inconvenient. However, the measurements are probably more reliable and reproducible when results from independent laboratories are compared. Methods for indirectly recording blood pressure in the rats using the tail or the foot are relatively easy to master. However, in order to obtain meaningful and reproducible results, experimental detail must be standardized, with particular emphasis on the width of the occluding cuff, the placement of the cuff on the extremity, the training of the animal and, if necessary, the warming of the rat. It may be desirable to use a "blind" system for drug evaluations where coded reference agents are submitted randomly with unknown compounds.

EXPERIMENTAL HYPERTENSION

We have limited our descriptions of methods to induce hypertension in rats to two forms of endocrine and two forms of renal. Many other procedures are described in the literature and are tabulated in Table 1.

TABLE 1

*Methods for the Induction of Experimental Hypertension in Rats**

Types of Hypertension	References
Steroid	
Acute DOCA + NaCl	Selye et al. (1943)
Post-DOCA + NaCl	Friedman et al. (1951)
Aldosterone + NaCl	Gross et al. (1957), Kumar et al. (1957)
Cortisone acetate	Knowlton et al. (1952)
Adrenal regeneration	Skelton (1956)
Renal	
Renal artery constriction	Wilson & Byron (1941)
Perinephritic (silk, cellophane, latex, figure 8 ligature	Abrams & Sobin (1947), Page (1939) Grollman (1944)
Macromolecules (polyvinyl alcohol or methyl cellulose)	Hall & Hall (1961), (1962)
Choline or K^+ deficiency	Hartroft & Best (1949), Grollman & White (1958)
Renoprival	Grollman et al. (1942), Braun-Menendez & von Euler (1947)
Experimental pyelonephritis	Heptinstall (1962)
Heterologous and homologous renin administration	Masson et al. (1966), (1964)
High NaCl intake	Sapirstein et al. (1950)
Teratogenic	Smirk & Hall (1958) Grollman & Grollman (1962)
Neurogenic	
Buffer nerve denervation	Krieger (1964)
Psychogenic (stress)	Farris et al. (1945), Hudak & Buckley (1961), Clay & Kaufman (1958)

*From Stanton and Cooper, 1966. *Baylor College of Medicine Cardiovasc. Res. Bull.*, 5:16-28.

"Active" DOCA and "Metacorticoid" Hypertension

Deoxycorticosterone acetate (DOCA) administration to rats, coupled with increased sodium intake, results, within one week, in a significant elevation of arterial blood pressure. If DOCA treatment is discontinued within one to two weeks, blood pressure may slowly return to control, and the animals are said to have "active" DOCA hypertension. If the DOCA is continued for four to six weeks, the animals develop a self-sustaining disease known as metacorticoid hypertension (Friedman et al., 1951). Rats are considered to have metacorticoid hypertension if the arterial blood pressure remains elevated or continues to rise even though DOCA treatment is discontinued and sodium intake returned to normal. Pathologic changes observed at this stage of the disease include lesions in small arteries (particularly of the kidneys and mesentery) accompanied by cardiac and renal hypertrophy (Sturtevant, 1958). The severity of hypertension is enhanced if one kidney is removed before treatment. The disease is most consistently induced in young (50 to 100 g) animals.

Similar results are obtained if DOCA is administered by a variety of methods. Sturtevant (1958) induced metacorticoid hypertension in 75-g male rats by subcutaneously implanting an extruded, 40-mg, 1.6- by 11-mm pellet consisting of a 2:1:1 mixture of DOCA, Carbowax 4000 (Carbide and Carbon Chemical Co., New York, New York), and Flexowax C light (Glyco Chemicals, Inc., New York, New York). (The press used to extrude the pellet is described by U.S. patent #2,413,419.) The drinking fluid in these studies contained 0.86 percent sodium chloride. Pellet fluid in these studies contained 0.86 percent sodium chloride. Pellet remnants, taken from the animal after three months, contained 0.2 to 0.3 percent of the original quantity of DOCA. Other types of DOCA pellets (Schering Corporation) have also been employed to induce "active" DOCA and metacorticoid hypertension in rats (Hall and Hall, 1965; Rubin et al., 1962). When DOCA pellets are used to induce metacorticoid hypertension, the investigator should be certain that little or no hormone remains at the site of implantation in order to correctly classify the condition as metacorticoid-induced.

The following procedure has been used in our laboratory to induce metacorticoid hypertension:

1. Female Wistar rats weighing 70 to 90 grams are unilaterally nephrectomized under ether anesthesia.
2. A microsuspension containing DOCA, 20 mg/ml, is prepared in a mortar and pestle with Tween 80 (0.25 percent), carboxymethyl cellulose (0.125 percent), and sodium chloride solution (0.9 percent). This suspension (0.1 ml/100 g body weight) is injected subcutaneously, once daily, five days per week for four weeks. The rats are given 1 percent sodium chloride solution to drink during DOCA treatment, but tap water is substituted for saline when the DOCA injections are stopped. The animals are maintained on water for at least one week before blood pressures are measured.
3. Indwelling, aortic, blood pressure catheters are implanted, as described in the previous section, and direct arterial blood pressures measured.
4. Rats exhibiting mean arterial blood pressures of more than 140 mm Hg are considered to have metacorticoid hypertension. This represents a blood pressure of at least three standard deviations above our normotensive control. Systolic, diastolic, and mean aortic blood pressures obtained from normotensive rats and rats with metacorticoid hypertension are shown in Table 2.

Sixty to 70 percent of DOCA-treated animals survive, while 75 to 80 percent of these survivors develop metacorticoid hypertension using our criteria of mean

TABLE 2

*Arterial Blood Pressure of Normotensive and Hypertensive Rats**

	Blood Pressure (mm Hg ± SD)†		
Parameter	*NORMOTENSIVE*	*"METACORTICOID" HYPERTENSION*	*ADRENAL REGENERATION HYPERTENSION*
Systolic	134.4 ± 12.3	197.6 ± 20.7	203.3 ± 25.4
Diastolic	86.9 ± 9.1	132.7 ± 16.4	141.5 ± 17.2
Mean	108.0 ± 10.7	167.8 ± 15.9	172.8 ± 20.7
No. of rats	100	100	62

*From Stanton and Cooper, 1966. *Baylor College of Medicine Cardiovasc. Res. Bull.*, 5:16-28.

†SD = standard deviation.

arterial blood pressure of over 140 mm Hg. The mortality rate is much higher in rats with respiratory infections than in healthy animals.

Adrenal Regeneration Hypertension

Many aspects of adrenal regeneration hypertension in rats were reviewed by Skelton (1959). The procedures used in our laboratory for the induction of this disease are as follows:

Immature female Wistar rats (50 to 70 g) are unilaterally nephrectomized under ether anesthesia. The right adrenal gland is removed and the left enucleated, by incising the capsule and gently extruding the glandular tissue with forceps (Ingle and Higgins, 1938). This removes the medullary tissue and most of the cortex, leaving a few cells of the zona glomerulosa attached to the capsule. Sodium is supplied as 1 percent sodium chloride in the drinking water. Indwelling aortic catheters are implanted after at least five postoperative weeks and direct aortic blood pressures are recorded. Diastolic, systolic, and mean arterial blood pressures, obtained from 63 rats with adrenal-regeneration hypertension, are shown in Table 2. Eighty to 85 percent of the animals surgically prepared for adrenal regeneration hypertension survive for five weeks, while 75 to 80 percent of these have blood pressures in excess of 140 mm Hg. Rats with adrenal regeneration hypertension do not seem to tolerate the indwelling aortic catheters as well as normotensive or metacorticoid hypertensive rats.

Adrenal regeneration, like metacorticoid hypertension, becomes more severe when started in young animals. Furthermore, the disease may develop faster in young female than in male rats (Brownie et al., 1966).

Adrenal regeneration hypertension, like metacorticoid hypertension, may become self-sustaining, although this facet has not been adequately studied. The removal of the regenerating adrenal gland or substitution of tap water for saline resulted in only a modest decline in the systolic blood pressure of rats with established adrenal regeneration hypertension (Skeleton, 1957).

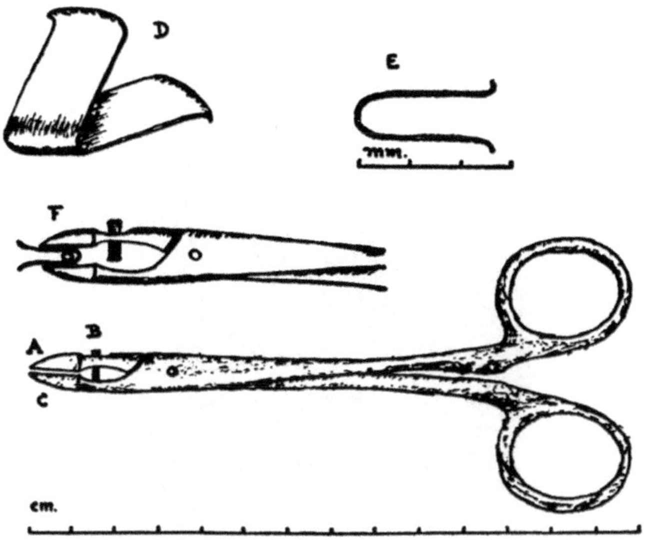

FIG. 11. The instrument, the silver clips, and the method for applying the clips to the renal artery of rats. The distance between the jaws A and C of the surgical needle holder is adjusted with the set screw B. The serrations have been removed from the jaws of the instrument. The form and dimensions of the silver clip (which can be prepared from annealed, rolled, silver ribbon 2 mm wide and 0.127 mm thick) is shown in D and E. The position of the clip in the jaws of the instrument is shown in F. (From Shaffenburg, 1959. *Proc. Soc. Exp. Biol. Med.,* 101:676-677.)

Renal Hypertension

Renal hypertension may be induced in mature rats by two methods: (1) partial occlusion of the renal artery ("Goldblatt"-type), (2) compression of the kidney with ligatures, silk, cellophane, or rubber capsules (perinephritic-type). There have been no definitive studies to determine if animals with different types of renal hypertension respond differently to antihypertensive drugs; hence, no model can be favored over another as a pharmacologic test system. Sustained renal hypertension ("metarenal") may occur in some animals if the affected kidney is removed from animals with renal hypertension of long duration (Green, 1953).

"GOLDBLATT"–TYPE RENAL HYPERTENSION.–Silver clips can be applied to the renal artery of rats using a modified needle holder where the distance between the jaws can be adjusted with a screw (Schaffenburg, 1959). This instrument (Codman and Shurtleff, Inc., Boston, Massachusetts) and the clips are illustrated in Figure 11. Silver clips may be prepared from "fine" silver, 0.0005 inch thick and 2 inches wide (Handy and Harmon, Inc., Chicago, Illinois). This material must be heated over a flame in order to render it pliable enough for use. The kidney is exposed through a costo lumbar incision; the renal artery, near its

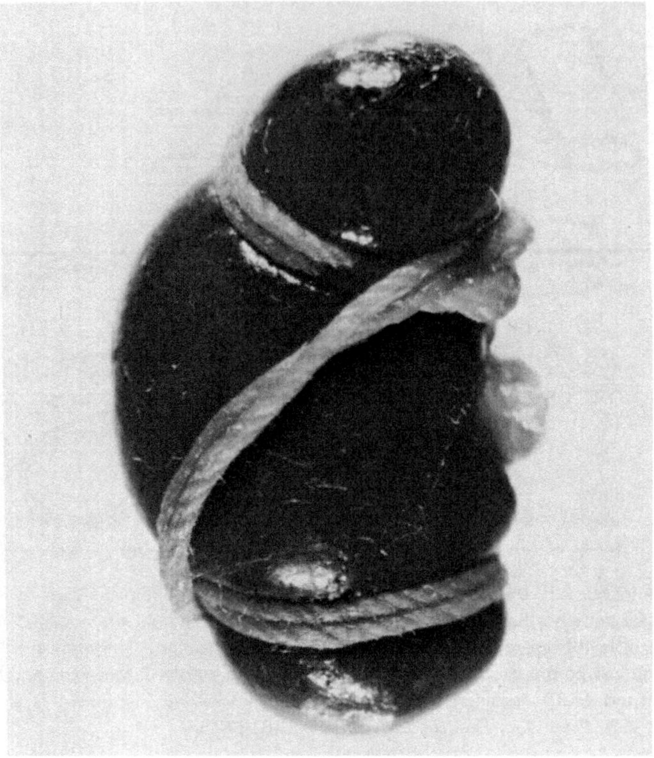

FIG. 12. Figure-8 ligature applied to the kidney of a rat.

origin from the abdominal aorta, is gently cleaned with a cotton-tipped applicator stick; and the clip is applied with the special forceps. The degree of renal artery constriction is critical, and the investigator may determine the optimal for his animals. Inadequate constriction does not induce hypertension, whereas constriction that is too tight leads to renal necrosis. The following free spaces within the clips were recommended by Schaffenburg (1959) for female rats: (1) 150-g animals = 0.014 inch, (2) 200-g animals = 0.015 inch, (3) 250-g animals = 0.016 inch. In rapidly growing male rats the constriction used for female rats may become tight as the animal grows and may cause renal necrosis.

The severity of "Goldblatt" hypertension is enhanced if the normal kidney is removed five to seven days after the clip is applied.

PERINEPHRITIC TECHNIQUES.

Figure-8 Ligature: Grollman (1944) utilized the method of Chanutin and Ferris (1932) to compress the poles of the kidney of laboratory animals (mouse, dog, rabbit, rat) with a figure-8 ligature. In the rat, the kidney is exposed through a lumbar incision, the renal capsule is removed by gentle traction, and a figure-8

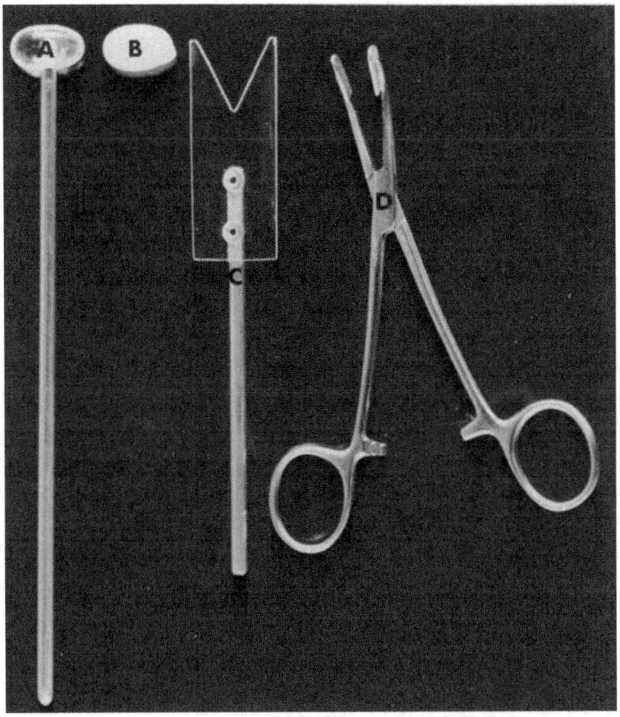

FIG. 13. Equipment needed to encapsulate the kidneys. The latex rubber capsules (B) are formed by dipping the molds (A) into liquid latex. The exposed kidney is supported with the platform (C) which is coated with latex, and the capsule is applied with the wide-jawed Kelley forceps (D).

ligature applied as illustrated in Figure 12. This ligature should be tight enough to deform the kidney but not tight enough to cut the tissue. Hard silk suture seems to have more tendency to cut than softer materials such as heavy cotton thread. Care should be exercised to avoid damaging or constricting the blood vessels or ureters emerging from the hilus of the kidney. Grollman (1944) reported that 10 to 20 percent of his animals developed hypertension within three to six months when one kidney was constricted. A larger number of rats will become severely hypertensive within three to four weeks if both kidneys are compressed or one kidney is removed and the other compressed.

Renal Encapsulation With Latex Rubber: Renal hypertension may be induced in the rat by encapsulating both kidneys with latex rubber capsules (Abrams and Sobin, 1947). The items needed for the preparation of the animals and the application of the capsule are shown in Figure 13A-D. The molds (A) used to fabricate the capsules may be formed from glass or plastic using a kidney, taken from a rat of appropriate size, as a model. The clear plastic molds used in our laboratory were formed in a lathe and threaded for a steel handle. Several molds of each size are needed to economically prepare a large number of latex capsules. These capsules (B) are prepared by dipping the molds in liquid latex (Fisher Chemical Co.) and allowing them to dry in the air. Three applications of latex are generally applied before the capsules are toughened by placing them under running warm tap water (45° to 50°C) for two to three hours. The capsules are coated with starch, removed from the mold and stored dry or in 75 percent ethanol. The starch must be removed, the capsules sterilized in ethanol, and this rinsed away in sterile saline before use. The kidney, exposed by a lumbar incision, is placed on a-V-shaped platform (C) to stabilize it during the application of the capsule. This platform is prepared from one-sixteenth-inch Lucite plastic and coated with latex to protect the kidney and to prevent slippage. The renal capsule is gently removed by traction or forceps before encapsulation. The latex capsule is then inverted over the special, widened points of the Kelly hemostat (D) and applied to the kidney. The applicator is held firmly against the platform and the lower edge of the capsule drawn down and over the lower pole of the kidney with forceps. The upper end of the capsule is then guided over the upper pole of the kidney. Extreme care must be exercised to prevent constricting the renal blood vessels or ureter. The kidney is returned to its original anatomical position, and the incision is closed. Persistent hypertension (165 to 240 mm Hg) was obtained within two to three weeks in 75 percent of the animals following renal encapsulation of male 190- to 200-g rats (Abrams and Sobin, 1947).

ANTIHYPERTENSIVE DRUGS

Drugs with potential antihypertensive activity are frequently evaluated in rats with experimental hypertension. Unfortunately, there have been few studies reported where currently used, clinically effective agents were compared in hypertensive animals. This is particularly true with renal hypertension, a model frequently employed for the evaluation of drugs.

The effects of several antihypertensive drugs on normotensive rats and rats with metacorticoid or adrenal regeneration hypertension have been studied in our laboratory (Stanton and White, 1965; Stanton and Cooper, 1967). These agents were administered subcutaneously and the blood pressures recorded from unanesthetized animals prepared with chronically indwelling, aortic catheters. The activities of single doses of a drug were assessed by recording blood pressures at 0, 0.5, 1, 3, 6, 24, and, in some instances, 48 hour intervals. The linear portion of a curve relating maximal mm Hg blood pressure reduction to log dose was analyzed by linear regression analysis. The dose inducing a 25 mm Hg fall in mean arterial blood pressure (ED25) was calculated from the regression equation, and the values are tabulated in Table 3. Most active agents lowered the blood pressure of normotensive as well as hypertensive rats, although the changes (mm Hg) were greater in hypertensive than normotensive animals, and the drug effects were easier to detect. Many drugs (chlorisondamine, hydralazine, reserpine, protoveratrine A and B, methyl dopa) were more active in rats with adrenal regeneration hypertension compared to animals with metacorticoid hypertension. Guanethidine

TABLE 3

*Potency of Antihypertensive Drugs in Normotensive and Hypertensive Rats**

Drug (Trade Name)	Drug Dose Units/kg, Sc	ED_{25}† With Standard Errors NORMOTENSIVE	"METACORTICOID" HYPERTENSIVE	ADRENAL REGENERATION HYPERTENSIVE
Chlorisondamine (Ecolid)	μg	109.6 (89.1-134.9)	51.3 (38.9-67.6)	18.2 (10.7-30.9)
Hydralazine (Apresoline)	μg	575.5 (426.6-776.2)	380.2 (316.2-457.1)	186.2 (144.5-239.9)
Reserpine	μg	128.8 (123.0-134.9)	40.7 (30.2-55.0)	12.0 (6.8-21.4)
Protoveratrine A & B (Veralba)	μg	134.9 (107.2-169.8)	67.6 (51.3-89.1)	41.7 (33.1-52.5)
Methyl dopa (Aldomet)	mg	213.8 (154.0-295.1)	43.7 (34.7-55.0)	26.9 (17.8-40.7)
Diazoxide	mg	30.2 (26.3-34.7)	7.1 (6.0-8.3)	7.6 (6.3-9.1)
Guanethidine	μg	—	—	269.2 (123.0-588.8)

*From Stanton and Cooper, 1966. *Baylor College of Medicine Cardiovasc. Res. Bull.*, 5:16-28.
†ED_{25} dose including a 25 mm Hg reduction in MABP.

induced an acute, dose-related fall in the blood pressure of rats with adrenal regeneration hypertension. This acute action was also noted with animals with metacorticoid hypertension although not dose-related. Guanethidine, administered once daily, did not induce a consistent, sustained blood-pressure-lowering action in any of these studies. The time required for maximal hypotensive activity and the durations of action of the acutely active drugs are shown in Table 4 .

TABLE 4

*Time of Maximal Hypotension and Duration of Effect**

Drug	Time of Peak Hypotension (Hours Post-Drug) N†	M†	AR†	Duration of Response (Range in Hours Post-Drug) N†	M†	AR†
Chlorisondamine	0.5-1	0.5-1	0.5	3-6	6-24	6-24
Hydralazine	0.5-1	0.5-1	0.5	6-24	6-24	6-24
Protoveratrine A & B	0.5-1	0.5-1	0.5	3-6	3-6	6-24
Reserpine	3-6	3-6	6	24-30	24-30	30-48
Alpha methyl dopa	3	3	3	6-24	6-24	6-24
Diazoxide	0.5-1	0.5-1	0.5	3-24	3-24	3-6
Guanethidine	–	0.5-1	0.5	–	3-24	6-24

*From Stanton and Cooper, 1966. *Baylor College of Medicine Cardiovasc. Res. Bull.*, 5:16-28.
†N = Normotensive, M = Metacorticoid, AR = Adrenal regeneration.

Hydrochlorothiazide (2.5 or 10 mg/kg, subcutaneous route), administered once daily for five to six days, significantly lowered the blood pressure of metacorticoid hypertensive rats but was not active in normotensive or adrenal regeneration hypertensive animals.

An injection of saline often induced a transient, hypotensive response of varying degrees in normotensive, adrenal regeneration or metacorticoid hypertensive rats. This is probably a response to handling and should be considered when evaluating the antihypertensive actions of unknown drugs. Furthermore, this emphasizes the need for establishing dose-effect relationship when using hypertensive animals to evaluate new chemical compounds.

REFERENCES

Abrams, M., and Sobin, S. 1947. Latex rubber capsule for producing hypertension in rats by perinephritis. Proc. Soc. Exp. Biol. Med., 64:412-416.
Braun-Menendez, E., and von Euler, U. S. 1947. Hypertension after bilateral nephrectomy in the rat. Nature (London), 160:905.
Brownie, A. C., Bernardis, L. L., Niwa, T., Kamura, S., and Skelton, F. R. 1966. The influence of age and sex on the development of adrenal regeneration hypertension. Lab. Invest., 15:1342-1356.
Chanutin, A. and Ferris, E. B. 1932. Experimental renal insufficiency produced by partial nephrectomy. Arch. Intern Med., 49:767-787.
Clay, M. M., and Kaufman, L. 1958. Effect of chronic stress upon systolic blood pressure of albino rats. J. Geron, (Abstract), 13:435.
Farris, E. J., Yeakel, E. H. and Medoff, H. S. 1945. Development of hypertension in emotional gray Norway rats after air blasting. Amer. J. Physiol., 144:331-333.
Fregly, M. J. 1963. Factors affecting indirect determination of systolic blood pressure of rats. J. Lab. Clin. Med., 62:223-230.
Friedman, M., and Freed, S. C. 1949. Microphonic manometer for indirect determination of systolic blood pressure in the rat. Proc. Soc. Exp. Biol. Med., 70:670-672.
Friedman, S. M., Friedman, C. L., and Nakashima, M. 1951. Sustained hypertension following the administration of deoxycorticosterone acetate. J. Exp. Med., 93:361-371.
Green, D. M. 1953. Hypertension. *In* Selye, H. and Horava, A., Third Annual Report on Stress. Montreal, Acta Inc., pp 277-297.
Grollman, A. 1944. A simplified procedure for inducing chronic renal hypertension in the mammal. Proc. Soc. Exp. Biol. Med., 57:102-104.
— and White, F. N. 1958. Induction of renal hypertension in rats and dogs by potassium and choline deficiency. Amer. J. Physiol., 193:144-146.
— and Grollman, E. F. 1962. The teratogenic induction of hypertension. J. Clin. Invest., 41:710-714.
— Harrison, T. R., and Williams, J. R., Jr. 1942. The mechanism of experimental renal hypertension in the rat. Amer. J. Physiol., 139:293-298.
Gross, F., Loustalot, P., and Meier, R. 1957. Production of experimental hypertension by aldosterone. Acta Endocr. 26:417-423.
Hall, C. E. and Hall, O. 1965. Hypertension and Hypersalimentation. II. Deoxycorticosterone hypertension. Lab. Invest., 14:1727-1735.
— and Hall, O. 1961. Experimental hypertension elicited by injections of methyl cellulose. Experientia, 17:544-545.
— and Hall, O. 1962. Macromolecular hypertension: hypertensive cardiovascular disease from subcutaneously administered polyvinyl alcohol. Experientia, 18:38-40.
Hartroft, S. W., and Best, C. H. 1949. Hypertension of renal origin in rats following less than one week of choline deficiency in early life. Brit. Med. J., 1:423-426.
Heatley, N. G., and Weeks, J. R. 1964. Fashioning polyethylene tubing for use in physiological experiments. J. Appl. Physiol., 19:542-545.
Heptinstall, R. H. 1962. Experimental pyelonephritis. The effect of chronic infection on the blood pressure in the rat. Brit. J. Exp. Path., 43:333-339.

Hudak, W. J., and Buckley, J. P. 1961. Production of hypertensive rats by experimental stress. J. Pharm. Sci., 50:263-264.

Ingle, D. J., and Higgins, G. M. 1938. Regeneration of the adrenal gland following enucleation. Amer. J. Med. Sci., 196:232-239.

Kersten, H., Brosene, Jr., W. G., Ablondi, F., and Subba Row, Y. 1947. A new method for the indirect measurement of blood pressure in the rat. J. Lab. Clin. Med., 32:1090-1098.

Knowlton, A. I., Loeb, E. N., Stoerk, H. C., White, J. P., and Hefferman, J. F. 1952. Induction of arterial hypertension in normal and adrenalectomized rats given cortisone acetate. J. Exp. Med., 96:187-205.

Krieger, E. M. 1964. Neurogenic hypertension in the rat. Circ. Res., 15:511-521.

Kumar, D., Hall, A. E. D., Nakashima, R., and Gornall, A. G. 1957. Studies on aldosterone. II. Hypertension as a cumulative effect of aldosterone administration. Canad. J. Biochem., 35:113-118.

Kvam, D.C., and Stanton, H. C. 1964. Studies on diazoxide hyperglycemia. Diabetes, 13:639-644.

Masson, G. M., Kashii, C., Matsunaga, M., and Page, I. H. 1966. Hypertensive vascular disease induced by heterologous renin. Circ. Res., 18:219-227.

— Kashii, C., Matsunaga, M., and Page, I. H. 1964. Hypertensive vascular disease produced by homologous renin. Science, 145:178-180.

McIlreath, F. J., DeGraw, W., and Kadar, V. 1965. A method for evaluating drug action on the cardiovascular system. Arch. Int. Pharmacodyn., 157:330-338.

Olmsted, F., Corcoran, A. C., Page, I. H. 1951a. Blood pressure in the unanesthetized rat. Circulation, 3:722-726.

— Corcoran. A. C., and Page, I. H. 1951b. Blood pressure in the unanesthetized rat. II. Spontaneous variations and effect of heat. Circulation, 3:727-729.

Proskauer, G. G., Neumann, C., and Graef, I. 1945. The measurement of the blood pressure in rats with special reference to the effect of changes in temperature. Amer. J. Physiol., 143:290-296.

Rosett, T., and Handler, P. 1957. Cuff for use with end point devices for estimation of arterial blood pressure of the rat. Proc. Soc. Exp. Biol. Med., 96:391-392.

Rubin, A. A., Roth, F. E., Taylor, R. M., and Rosenpilde, H. 1962. Pharmacology of diazoxide, an antihypertensive, nondiuretic benzothiadiazine. J. Pharmacol. Exp. Ther., 136:344-352.

Sapirstein, L. A., Brandt, W. L., and Drury, D. R. 1950. Production of hypertension in the rat by substituting hypertonic sodium chloride for drinking water. Proc. Soc. Exp. Biol. Med., 73:82-85.

Schaffenburg, C. A. 1959. Device to control constriction of main renal artery for production of hypertension in small animals. Proc. Soc. Exp. Biol. Med., 101:676-677.

Selye, H., Hall, C. E., and Rowley, E. M. 1943. Malignant hypertension produced by treatment with desoxycorticosterone acetate and sodium chloride. Canad. Med. Assoc. J., 49:88-92.

Skelton, F. R. 1959. Adrenal regeneration and adrenal regeneration hypertension. Physiol. Rev., 39:162-182.

— 1956. Adrenal-regeneration hypertension and factors influencing its development. Arch. Int. Med., 98:449-462.

— 1957. Studies on the natural history of adrenal regeneration hypertension. Circulation, 16:938-939.

Smirk, F. H., and Hall, W. H. 1958. Inherited hypertension in rats. Nature (London), 182:727.

Stanton, H. C., and White, J. B., Jr. 1965. Hypotensive actions of drugs on unanesthetized normotensive and metacorticoid hypertensive rats determined by a direct recording technique. Arch. Int. Pharmacodyn., 154:351-363.

— and Cooper, C. M. 1966. Comparison of effects of antihypertensive agents on normotensive rats and rats with metacorticoid and adrenal regeneration hypertension. Baylor University Cardiovasc. Res. Bull., 5:16-28.

— and Cooper, C. M. 1967. Antihypertensive effects of drugs measured in unanesthetized rats with established adrenal regeneration hypertension. Arch. Int. Pharmacodyn., 168:1-13.

Sturtevant, F. M. 1957. Pharmacology of a new hypotensive steroid. 17 α propyl-4.5 β-dihydro-19-nortestosterone. J. Pharmacol. Exp. Ther., 121:369-377.

— 1958. The biology of metacorticoid hypertension. Ann. Intern. Med., 49:1281-1293.

Still, J. W., and Whitcomb, E. R. 1956. Technique for permanent long-term intubation of rat aorta. J. Lab. Clin. Med., 48:152-154.

Weeks, J. R. 1964. Experimental narcotic addiction. Sci. Amer., 210:46-52.

— and Jones, J. A. 1960. Routine measurement of arterial pressure in unanesthetized rats. Proc. Soc. Exp. Biol. Med., 194:646-648.

Williams, J. R., Jr., Harrison, T. R., and Grollman, A. 1939. A simple method for determining the systolic blood pressure of the unanesthetized rat. J. Clin. Invest., 18:373-376.

Wilson, C., and Byrom, F. B. 1941. The vicious circle in chronic Bright's disease. Experimental evidence from the hypertensive rat. Quart. J. Med., 10:65-93.

CHAPTER 6

Methods for Evaluating Antiarrhythmic Agents

Laszlo Szekeres

Institute of Pharmacology, University Medical School of Szeged
Dóm tér 12, Szeged, Hungary

INTRODUCTION

The search for new drugs able to prevent or to correct heart rhythm disturbances is rendered difficult by the fact that so far there is no generally accepted procedure for the quantitative assay of these substances. This is partly due to the fact that investigation of clinically useful antiarrhythmic agents would require the induction in experimental animals of model arrhythmias corresponding to the pathologic phenomena observed in patients. The overwhelming majority of the various experimental arrhythmias introduced up to now seem not to be able to answer fully the foregoing requirement. This is not surprising if we bear in mind that, insofar as existing theories and views concerning the pathomechanism of arrhythmias and fibrillation are concerned, bases for every rational therapy are rather contradictory.

A systematic investigation of new antiarrhythmic substances is hindered by the lack of uniform criteria for evaluating antiarrhythmic activity of drugs. Though in the literature there are some older and also some more recent attempts to review the techniques for measuring antiarrhythmic action in animals (Dawes, 1952;

The author wishes to express his thanks to Dr. J. Gy. Papp for his valuable help.

Winbury, 1956; Turner, 1965; Moe and Mendez 1964; Katzung, 1968) and in men (Dreifus et al., 1964, 1965), in view of the aforementioned and of the ever increasing number of new procedures for testing antiarrhythmic drugs, a critical survey of the assay methods used so far, as well as of those recently recommended, seems justified.

In this chapter the general principles of antiarrhythmic assay, the different techniques for production of experimental arrhythmias, as well as the various procedures for evaluating antiarrhythmic activity, with concluding remarks on a rational screening program, will be discussed.

BASIC PRINCIPLES UNDERLYING THE APPLICATION OF ANTIARRHYTHMIC ASSAY METHODS

The ultimate object of the search for new antiarrhythmic agents is to produce clinically useful drugs. Accordingly the program for screening effective compounds should involve, besides evaluating antiarrhythmic activity, the detection of possible undesirable side effects. Since experimental arrhythmias are different from those occurring in patients, it is extremely difficult to predict clinical usefulness from the results of pharmacologic analysis (Terry, 1956). In view of this, the first condition to be considered in selecting antiarrhythmic substances is a satisfactory agreement between results of pharmacologic and clinical evaluation, including side effects. Furthermore the method used should be reproducible, simple, and inexpensive.

Antiarrhythmic assay methods may be classified according to the type of preparation or according to the species used. Antiarrhythmic action may be studied on isolated parts of the heart (on isolated atria, or on isolated papillary muscle preparation), on the isolated heart (on the Langendorff heart preparation or on the heart-lung preparation), and finally in the more or less intact animal, anesthetized or unanesthetized. Moreover in some selected cases, patients suffering from arrhythmia may also be suitable media for testing antiarrhythmic agents.

As regards species, arrhythmias induced in cold-blooded animals are so different in nature from those produced in higher organisms that, with exception of the toad heart occasionally employed for investigation of certain theoretical problems (Brooks et al., 1955), they are not used for evaluation of antiarrhythmic drugs. Mammals, for this purpose, may be divided into two groups according to the size of heart. The first group includes animals possessing a relatively small heart and therefore capable of spontaneously restoring ventricular fibrillation to normal rhythm. These include the rat, guinea pig, rabbit, and cat. Animals belonging to the second group are those with relatively larger hearts such as the dog or the monkey and are not inclined to spontaneous defibrillation.

The rat is particularly suitable for assays where a large number of experimental animals are required for purposes of statistical evaluation. The guinea pig and rabbit heart represent good media for isolated preparations (e.g., the papillary muscle or auricular preparation, or the Langendorff heart), and the intact animal is also suitable for assay. The rabbit, being rather quiet by nature and with easily accessible ear veins for injection, is especially useful for evaluation of antiarrhythmic activity in the unanesthetized animal. The cat is among the largest species capable of spontaneous defibrillation. Its heart is highly resistant to injuries but at the same time sufficiently sensitive to cardioactive drugs. It lends itself well to surgical operations such as thoracotomy and fixation of electrodes on the heart. Therefore, the cat represents one of the most useful species for the assay of antiarrhythmic drugs. In contrast to the cat, the dog is highly inclined to develop lasting ventricular fibrillation upon external stimuli. Its susceptibility exceeds even that of man, and due to its relatively large heart size, spontaneous defibrillation is very rare. Accordingly, it seems to be less suitable for screening of antiarrhythmic compounds than the aforementioned smaller and cheaper animals, except for a detailed analysis of selected substances with marked antiarrhythmic activity, where it is advisable to study their action on the highly sensitive dog before passing over to the clinical trial. The probability of good agreement between pharmacologic results and successful application in therapy may be enhanced by employing monkeys for assay, but unfortunately the use of this species is limited due to relatively high costs. Pharmacologic testing in humans suffering from arrhythmia seems to be the most satisfactory procedure, but in view of the multiplicity of different disturbances of rhythm that occur in man, it is important to apply it in very carefully selected cases; otherwise misleading results may be obtained.

As already mentioned, there are numerous procedures for evaluation of antiarrhythmic activity, employed mainly on an empirical basis without appropriate theoretical foundation. Nevertheless all antiarrhythmic assay methods used so far are based on the following three fundamental principles (Szekeres, 1964):

1. Some type of experimental arrhythmia is produced, and the dose of the antiarrhythmic drug determined, which is able to
   a. abolish persisting arrhythmia (suspending dose) or
   b. prevent the production of arrhythmia (preventive dose).
2. Increase due to the antiarrhythmic agent in the intensity of the threshold stimulus just eliciting arrhythmia is determined.
3. Changes induced by antiarrhythmic drugs in the fundamental properties of the heart, as conductivity, excitability, refractoriness, and automaticity, assumed to play a role in the development or perpetuation of arrhythmias, are compared.

TECHNIQUES USED FOR PRODUCTION OF EXPERIMENTAL ARRHYTHMIAS

In the foregoing we have already alluded to the importance of the production of adequate experimental arrhythmias as a basis for evaluation of antiarrhythmic drugs. In addition, they may yield valuable data on the pathomechanism of the arrhythmia involved.

Sometimes the factors eliciting and those maintaining arrhythmia can be distinguished. Burn et al. (1955) precipitated auricular fibrillation in the dog by electrical stimulation of the auricles when acetylcholine was infused simultaneously. In this case, electrical stimulation acts only as an eliciting factor, since arrhythmia persists even after its cessation as long as acetylcholine, the factor responsible for perpetuation of the arrhythmia, is present.

In the method for production of experimental arrhythmia by the combined use of epinephrine and chloroform, cyclopropane, or halothane, epinephrine acts as the factor precipitating the heart rhythm disturbance, whereas chloroform, cyclopropane, or halothane sensitizes the myocardium to the arrhythmogenic action of epinephrine.

Arrhythmia and fibrillation may be elicited by such external factors as mechanical, thermal, chemical, osmotic, or electrical stimuli, which have to reach a certain intensity to induce arrhythmia. Changes in the cardiac muscle itself, such as depressed conduction, shortening of the refractory period, increased excitability and ectopic activity, development of local blocks, uneven propagation of impulses, and nonuniform recovery of excitability in the heart, may also precipitate heart rhythm disturbances and may under certain circumstances enhance the arrhythmogenic action of external stimuli. Myocardial changes favoring the development of arrhythmias may be produced by hypoxia or ischemia of the heart, by local circulatory disturbances (cardiac infarction) or cooling of the myocardium, by changes in the autonomic nervous regulation of the heart, by increase of the catecholamine level in the blood, and by other means.

The techniques used for production of experimental arrhythmias may be classified as follows:

1. Electrical stimulation of the heart.
2. Drugs or other chemical agents–applied locally to the heart or administered through the bloodstream.
3. Mechanically or thermically produced local blocks and ectopic foci in the heart.
4. Direct excitation of the central nervous system.

Production of Arrhythmias by Electrical Stimulation of the Heart

Electrical stimulation of the heart represents the oldest and most widespread technique for producing experimental arrhythmias. It has several advantages over all other stimuli: it is not harmful to the myocardium; its effect is, except for extremely strong stimuli, fully reversible; the analogy with the natural impulse is more evident than with all other methods; and the strength and duration of the stimulating current may be very accurately measured and controlled.

Production of arrhythmia or fibrillation by electrical stimulation of the heart may be performed by (1) a single electrical shock, (2) serial shocks, (3) progressively increasing rate of stimulation, or (4) prolonged application of galvanic current.

First attempts to produce ventricular (Vulpian, 1847) and auricular fibrillation (Rothberger and Winterberg, 1914) were performed by faradic stimulation. Later Lewis et al. (1921) produced auricular flutter and fibrillation by increasing the rate of suprathreshold stimuli up to 350 to 500 a minute. Moreover De Boer (1921) succeeded in precipitating a fibrillation-like disturbance in the frog heart by a single electrical shock, applied near the end of systole, after the refractory period. Validity of this observation for the mammalian heart was demonstrated by Andrus and Carter (1930), finding that a single shock applied under vagal stimulation at the end of the refractory period often elicits auricular fibrillation in the dog heart in situ. Wiggers and Wégria (1940) presented an extensive analysis of the problem and showed that, from the point of view of fibrillation, the heart is most vulnerable to a single DC or AC stimulus at the end of systole. This so-called vulnerable period, demonstrable in all hearts, coincides more or less with the relative refractory period, when part of the heart muscle fibers are still refractory to stimuli, whereas other fibers have already recovered their excitability. They could also show that weak stimuli applied to the vulnerable period evoked only extrasystoles; but when they increased the intensity of electrical shocks to a certain critical value (to the so-called fibrillation threshold), fibrillation appeared. Nevertheless, if applied during diastole, even strong stimuli never precipitated fibrillation, only extra beats. The vulnerable period coincides with the dip in excitability curve as shown by Brooks et al. (1951).

In order to understand the mechanism by which electrical stimulation affects the myocardium and evokes arrhythmias, it is advisable to start from the analysis of action of the single shock, since effects of all other types of electrical stimuli can be derived from this model. The electrical stimulus, like that originating from the pacemaker cells, depolarizes the membrane at the site of its action and under appropriate circumstances gives rise to a propagating wave of depolarization. Weak stimuli may only temporarily reduce the membrane potential. The latter returns to its initial value after cessation of the stimulus. This can be explained on the basis of the present ionic theory of excitation by the assumption that the depolarizing action of sodium entry to the cell is counterbalanced by potassium efflux. If the electrical stimulus is strong enough to reduce the membrane potential to the critical value (called "threshold potential"), the depolarizing factor, namely the sodium entry, will prevail over the repolarizing potassium outflux, and the membrane will become fully depolarized, leading to a propagating action potential. The minimal strength of current required for originating a propagated action potential–i.e., that able to depolarize the membrane to the threshold potential–is the so-called diastolic threshold (a measure of excitability of the heart).

There are certain differences even among adjacent cardiac fibers with respect to conductivity, refractoriness, and excitability. Accordingly, the boundary between the refractory zone of the advancing excitation wave and the areas recovering their excitability is an irregular line, which means that some of the fibers may be excitable again, whereas adjacent fibers may still be refractory to excitation. If a weak stimulus (yet strong enough to evoke a propagated action potential) is applied at the vulnerable period, the wave of excitation spreads over the myocardium in the wake of, but outside of, the retreating border of the absolute refractory zone of the preceding natural excitation wave of pacemaker origin. In the ECG it will appear in the form of an extrasystole.

If the stimulus applied at the vulnerable period is strong enough, the depolarization will extend to a larger area and may at places reach the irregular borderline of the absolute refractory zone of the preceding wave of excitation. At these sites the second wave of depolarization is extinguished, whereas at other sites recovery of excitability in the wake of the wave of excitation is so much advanced that the second wave may stimulate adjacent fibers and propagate in an unhindered manner. Thus, a difference in phase in the spreading of excitation among closely located sections of the myocardium will arise, leading to a gradually increasing disorganization of the cardiac action and ending in fibrillation.

On the basis of the foregoing considerations, it is not difficult to understand the mechanism of the fibrillation-inducing action of serial impulses. If the myocardium is stimulated by serial shocks of high frequency (10 to 20 cycles/sec) and the strength of the stimulus is gradually increased, first extrasystoles, later tachycardia, flutter, and finally fibrillation will appear, irrespective of the form of stimulation (rectangular pulses, faradic current, or simple alternating current) (Fig. 1). Thus, with the aid of serial electrical stimulation it is possible to reproduce some of the main types of arrhythmias of clinical importance. Possible explanation of these findings may be the following: If at first weak stimuli of increasing strength are applied, the diastolic threshold is soon reached and extra beats are elicited. Weak stimuli, however, are not sufficient to break through the subsequent refractory phase. By further increasing the current even during the relative refractory period of the extrasystoles, a propagated wave of excitation can be elicited. Thus, the cycle length and the refractory period become shorter and shorter, and the serial shocks will evoke exstrasystoles progressively earlier within the cardiac cycle. The heart rate increases as long as the heart is able to follow the stimulation. The maximal frequency still followed is determined by the so-called effective refractory period—i.e., the shortest interval between two stimuli to which the heart responds with contraction. The tachycardia smoothly changes into flutter. Since some of the very frequent stimuli will hit the heart within the vulnerable period, if strength of the stimulating current is further increased, fibrillation may be evoked just as in the case of a single stimulus.

A very similar mechanism is present in arrhythmias and fibrillation produced by gradually increasing the rate of suprathreshold stimuli (Lewis et al., 1921). With progressively shorter cycle length the refractory period also becomes shorter, thus enabling the heart to follow the steadily increasing rate of stimulation until tachycardia and then flutter appears. If the rate of stimulation exceeds the maximal frequency the heart is able to follow, soon one or more stimuli will fall within the vulnerable period and, if sufficiently strong, evoke fibrillation.

Prolonged application of galvanic current may also depolarize the myocardium to the extent of eliciting arrhythmia. Depolarizing current accelerates the slow diastolic depolarization characteristic of the action potential of the pacemaker cells and thus increases their firing rate. As ventricular conductive tissue possessing latent automaticity (Purkinje fibers) is also affected, increase of heterotopic impulse generation results, and thus conditions for an irregular cardiac activity are established. However, the technique of prolonged application of galvanic current has not become popular for production of experimental arrhythmias.

For a better understanding of the factors promoting or inhibiting the appearance of flutter or fibrillation, it is necessary to define the concept of

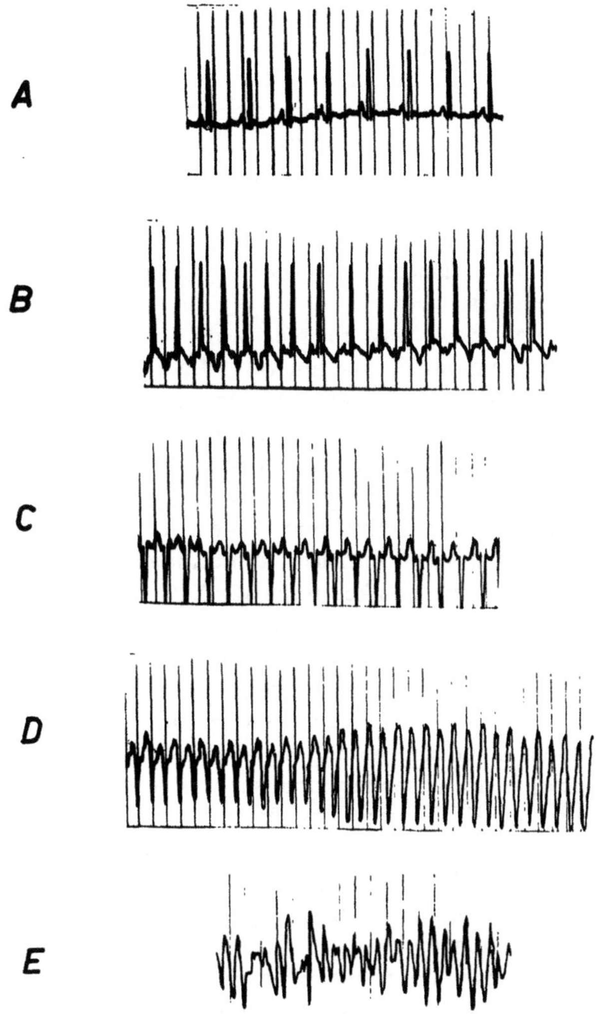

FIG. 1. ECG changes due to serial electrical shocks of gradually increasing intensity applied to the right ventricle of the cat heart. (Rectangular impulses of 20 c/sec frequency and 1 msec duration were used. ECG was recorded in the II lead. Time signal: 100 msec.)
(A) Control—Heart rate: 240 beats/min.
(B) Strength of stimulus: 0.28 mA—Heart rate: 350 beats/min.
(C) Strength of stimulus: 0.30 mA—Heart rate: 400 beats/min.
(D) Strength of stimulus: 0.70 mA—Ventricularfibrillo-flutter, heart rate: 600 beats/min.
(E) Strength of stimulus: 0.90 mA—Ventricular fibrillation.

susceptibility or tendency to flutter and fibrillation. This concept covers two, partly separable phenomena: (1) the possibility of an easier or of a more difficult production of fibrillation or flutter and (2) the tendency of the elicited fibrillation or flutter to persist or to cease spontaneously. These two phenomena are not necessarily parallel. Sometimes it is difficult to evoke fibrillation, but once established, it may prove very resistant to antifibrillatory measures. Fibrillation is occasionally easily produced and nevertheless may end spontaneously.

Since precipitation of flutter or fibrillation is more difficult after the use of antiarrhythmic agents, it is of great importance to know how easily these heart rhythm disturbances may be elicited by external stimuli. This can be accomplished very accurately with the determination of the electrical fibrillation threshold–i.e., the minimum current intensity just able to precipitate auricular or ventricular fibrillation. The higher the tendency or susceptibility to fibrillation, the lower current intensity will be sufficient to elicit this phenomenon (lower fibrillation threshold), and vice versa.

In practice, there are two ways for measuring fibrillation thresholds. The first possibility is to increase gradually the intensity of a single electrical shock applied in the vulnerable period until fibrillation appears. This method, though its theoretical basis has been very carefully elaborated by Wiggers and Wégria (1940) and Brooks et al. (1955), has never become popular for routine assay of antiarrhythmic drugs. This is mainly due to the great technical requirements associated with the use of the method and to other factors limiting the application of this procedure. Thus, in order to place the precipitating shock in the vulnerable period, first the natural pacemaker impulses have to be excluded, either by crushing the sinoatrial node or by locally applying chemical agents depressing automaticity. Furthermore the heart has to be driven artificially and a second stimulus applied at different intervals from the driving stimulus in order to determine the exact position of the vulnerable period. If the heart rate is constant and the extra stimulus sufficiently long to fall easily into the vulnerable period, driving of the heart is not absolutely necessary. Here the extra stimulus may be controlled by one of the ECG waves, usually the R wave, and timed in the suitable interval from this latter. Both procedures require elaborate equipment. In addition, artificial driving affects the fundamental properties of the myocardium, e.g., conductivity, refractoriness, etc. A further disadvantage of the method is that precipitation of fibrillation by a single shock requires the use of a rather high current strength which may injure the myocardial tissue, especially if the shock is applied in each cycle to get a smooth gradual increase of stimulus intensity. Therefore, it is advisable to apply the second stimulus only after 5 to 10 cycles. Of course, this type of determination of fibrillation threshold becomes a very time-consuming and elaborate procedure, and rapidly changing processes may escape the investigator. Determination may be retarded by the use, if necessary, of electrical defibrillation, which, due to the powerful shocks applied, necessitates a delay of 10 to 15 minutes between two measurements to allow complete recovery of the myocardium, the latter being a preliminary condition of reproducible thresholds. On the basis of the aforementioned,Wegria and Nickerson (1943) concluded that the single-shock procedure for determination of the fibrillation threshold is rather difficult and little suited for assay of antiarrhythmic drugs.

The advantage of using serial shocks for this purpose may be summarized as follows: (1) There is no need for an artificial pacemaker, as well as for determination of the vulnerable period. This enables one to measure the electrical threshold from minute to minute and thus to follow closely rapidly changing processes. (2) Serial shocks require a much lower current intensity than a single shock to produce fibrillation, probably as a consequence of summation of stimuli falling in the vulnerable period. (3) The effective refractory period, i.e., the maximum frequency followed, can be established from the ECG. Thus changes in refractoriness can be estimated approximately. (4) The use of serial shocks enables one to introduce the concept of "flutter threshold." This latter is of practical value, since production of flutter requires a lower current intensity compared to fibrillation. Flutter or fibrilloflutter thus induced stops immediately in the relatively small cat heart after cessation of the electrical stimulation. This is particularly important if changes in ventricular susceptibility to fibrillation or flutter have to be determined. Under circumstances where strong serial stimuli are applied, even in cats, persistent ventricular fibrillation may sometimes arise, requiring the use of cardiac massage or of defibrillatory shocks.

There is no such problem in connection with atrial flutter and fibrillation, since the tendency of the auricles to spontaneous defibrillation is greater than that of the ventricles. Also the hemodynamic consequences of auricular fibrillation are by far not so potentially fatal as those of ventricular fibrillation.

The immediate recovery from ventricular flutter may be at least partly due to the aforementioned fact–that the stimulus strength required to produce flutter or fibrilloflutter is much lower, by about one-third or one-fourth, than that needed to elicit fibrillation. In spite of this, the hemodynamic consequences of ventricular flutter so produced, correspond to those of ventricular fibrillation; i.e., the blood pressure falls abruptly and the circulation is minimal or stops completely.

The usefulness of the method for determination of flutter threshold is enhanced by the fact that flutter appears with a very sharply defined margin, the values are reproducible, they can be frequently repeated under the same circumstances, and they tend to return to the original value even after different interventions. In addition there is good correlation between flutter threshold and fibrillation threshold on the same heart (Szekeres and Papp, 1970). Thus, it seems justifiable to infer, from flutter threshold data, the susceptibility of the heart to fibrillation.

The appearance of flutter may be established by direct inspection of the heart in the open-chest animal, by the abrupt fall of blood pressure, and by ECG. Appearance of fibrillation can be verified only from the ECG, as fibrilloflutter of high frequency is hardly separable from fibrillation by direct inspection of the heart, and the blood pressure fall is present in both types of arrhythmia.

In dogs, which are highly susceptible to external fibrillating stimuli, even determination of the flutter threshold with serial shocks involves the risk of precipitating a self-sustaining and prolonged ventricular fibrillation. Here, determination of the ventricular multiple response threshold is the method of choice–i.e., measurement of the lowest current intensity of a single shock applied in the vulnerable period that is just able to elicit multiple ventricular response. This latter usually manifests itself in the form of a few ventricular extrasystoles, but sometimes fibrillation potentials may appear for a very short time. Nevertheless, the danger of producing lasting ventricular fibrillation in the dog heart when using

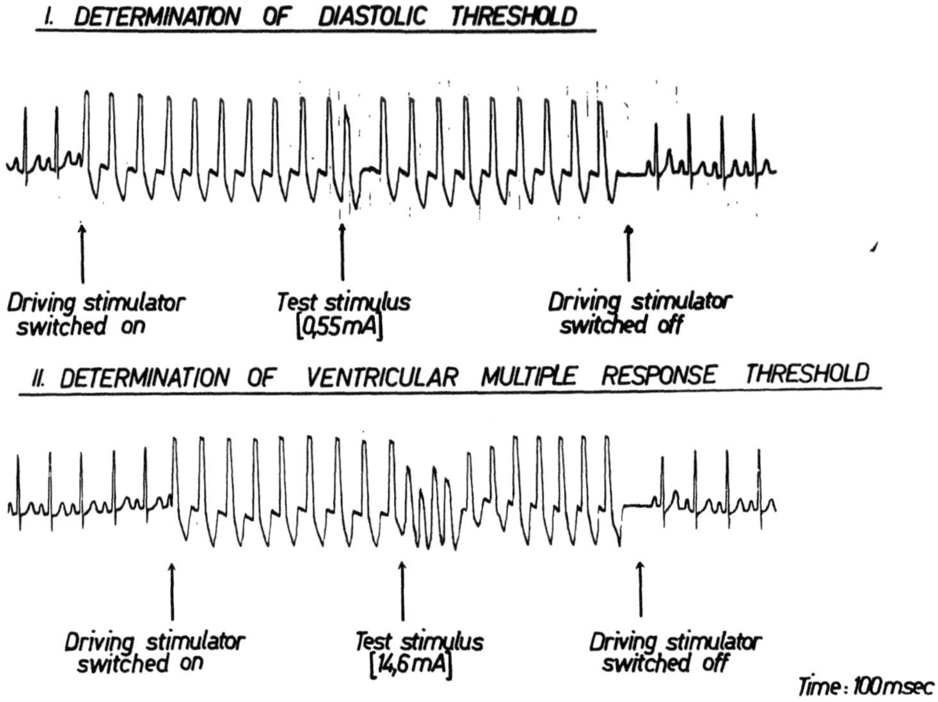

FIG. 2 Determination of the electrical diastolic threshold, as well as of the ventricular multiple response threshold, in the anesthetized dog. Recording: II lead ECG; driving and test electrodes on the right anterior ventricular wall.

this method is less than with all other techniques previously discussed. As the minimal current strength for production of ventricular multiple response is only slightly lower than that required for production of fibrillation (Hoffman et al., 1955), the multiple response threshold seems to be just as useful for estimation of the susceptibility of the heart to external arrhythmogenic stimuli as the "true" electrical fibrillation threshold (Han et al., 1964; Papp and Szekeres, 1968). It also has a great advantage over the latter method in that it enables nearly continuous determination of cardiac susceptibility to arrhythmogenic stimuli. Measurement of the multiple response threhold may be carried out in artifically driven hearts, where a second stimulus of adjustable intensity applied at the desired time within the cardiac cycle serves to detect the vulnerable period. It is advisable to use stimuli of increasing intensity in intervals of 10 msec starting from the border of the absolute and relative refractory periods and approaching the end of the cycle until multiple ventricular responses appear. An example for determination of the ventricular diastolic threshold and of the ventricular multiple response threshold in the dog is given in Figure 2, which also demonstrates the great difference between intensity of threshold stimuli needed to elicit a single extrasystole and multiple extrasystoles, respectively.

Production of Arrhythmias by Drugs or Other Chemical Agents

Various substances with different chemical structure and biologic action have been employed for producing experimental arrhythmias. Their arrhythmogenic effect is due to their influence on one or several fundamental properties of the myocardium. Since the site of action is different with various kinds of agents, it is not justified to assume that these substances exert their arrhythmogenic effect by the same mechanism. Consequently, it is not satisfactory to determine antiarrhythmic activity on the basis of a test arrhythmia produced by a single arrhythmogenic agent.

Arrhythmogenic agents are either applied locally, i.e., directly to the myocardium, or injected into the bloodstream.

1. *Local application* of chemical substances is theoretically based on the assumption that they act as a permanent stimulus at the site of application giving rise to ectopic activity.

Scherf et al. (1948) introduced the method of applying *aconitine* on the atrial surface of the dog heart, either by using a cotton pledget immersed into aconitine solution, by applying aconitine crystals, or by subepicardial injection of the drug. As a consequence, auricular tachycardia, flutter, and eventually fibrillation appeared, depending upon the concentration used. Local cooling abolished the arrhythmia which reappeared on rewarming, a fact serving as an argument in favor of the ectopic focus theory of fibrillation. Accordingly, drugs preventing or abolishing arrhythmias produced by local application of aconitine may themselves act by primarily influencing the ectopic activity. Electrophysiologic support of this assumption is given by the observation that slow diastolic depolarization, which is characteristic of cells possessing automaticity, is accelerated by aconitine (Schmidt, 1958).

Delphinine crystals applied to the auricle of the dog heart evoke supraventricular tachycardia which changes into auricular flutter lasting sometimes as long as 40 minutes (Scherf et al., 1963). It is noteworthy that neither auricular flutter nor ventricular tachycardia induced by application of the drug to the auricles and ventricles, respectively, will change into auricular or ventricular fibrillation. Both arrhythmias may be abolished by cooling the site of application.

Acetylcholine, if applied locally on the auricle, may induce auricular flutter and fibrillation, as shown by Nahum and Hoff (1940), in the dog and rat heart. This is mainly due to the acceleration of repolarization and shortening of the refractory period (Burgen and Terroux, 1953; Trautwein and Dudel, 1956). The acetylcholine-induced arrhythmia may be effectively antagonized by atropine even if this is applied locally (Hoff and Nahum, 1934). A certain minimal mass of myocardial tissue is necessary for the production of cholinergic arrhythmia, as stated by West and Landa (1962), showing that it is not possible to evoke or to maintain acetylcholine-induced arrhythmia if the atrial mass is less than 30 mg, thereby furnishing evidence for the "circus movement mechanism" operating in cholinergic arrhythmia.

Veratrum alkaloids, if applied directly to the myocardium, may also produce heart rhythm disturbances similar to those induced by aconitine (Scherf and Chick, 1951).

Cardiac glycosides, known to precipitate arrhythmias if given in sufficiently high doses, may also elicit extrasystoles by local application—e.g., by subepicardiac injection into the auricular myocardium (Scherf, 1944).

2. Arrhythmogenic action of the aforementioned substances also occurs if administered *through the bloodstream by intravenous injection.* However, the mechanism of precipitating arrhythmia by this method may not necessarily be due to an increase of ectopic firing, which probably is caused by the effect of local application. Other basic properties of the heart are also affected.

The principles of the mechanism responsible for the local arrhythmogenic effect of acetylcholine and aconitine are also valid for the general action of these substances.

Veratrum alkaloids reduce in low concentrations, but increase in large concentrations, the susceptibility of the heart to fibrillation (Brooks et al., 1951). They may precipitate arrhythmia or even tachycardia and ventricular fibrillation (Krayer and Acheson, 1946). This is mainly due to the marked slowing of conduction, especially in the atrioventricular bundle, not compensated for by the prolongation of the absolute and relative refractory period in the auricular and ventricular tissue or by the decrease of the myocardial excitability (Brooks et al., 1951). The repolarization phase of the action potential is extremely prolonged; irregular oscillations appear, which are indicative of spontaneously firing ectopic foci.

Cardiac glycosides were among the first substances known to produce arrhythmia. Therefore their mode of arrhythmogenic action has been extensively studied. According to Vassalle et al. (1963), two types of arrhythmias may appear after infusion of 0.10 to 0.15 mg/kg/min strophanthin in dogs. At the beginning, ventricular automaticity is depressed, but later it is more and more pronounced. All this may be concealed by the dominance of the sinoatrial pacemaker, which can be eliminated by vagus stimulation. Sometimes the ventricular automaticity may be permanently inhibited. If in addition atrioventricular block is induced, as occurs frequently with digitalis, cardiac activity may cease. If, on the contrary, automaticity of the Purkinje fibers increases beyond a certain limit, its own frequency will be higher then the sinoatrial rate.

The second type of arrhythmia appears in the form of extrasystoles which may, in prolonged digitalis intoxication, develop into paroxysmal tachycardia of shorter or longer duration, frequently precipitating ventricular fibrillation. Dudel and Trautwein (1958) have shown in the isolated cat papillary muscle and on the dog Purkinje fiber that, in the phase of accelerated spontaneous activity, membrane resistance increases, whereas in the phase of toxic depression, resistance and excitability diminish. According to West (1964), cardiac glycosides shorten the absolute refractory period if the vagus innervation is intact, and they prolong its duration in the denervated heart. The underlying ionic changes are reduced permeability to potassium (mainly the inward flux is inhibited), consequent loss of potassium from the myocardium, prolonged repolarization and the rate of the sodium outflow is reduced, while the inflow of sodium increases.

The digitalislike action of $BaCl_2$ on the frog heart, first increasing contractility, then evoking arrhythmia, and finally cardiac standstill, was described by Boehm in 1875. Later it has been shown that, in the mammalian heart, injection of $BaCl_2$ may induce ventricular extrasystoles, tachycardia, and fibrillation (Rothberger and Winterberg, 1911; Levy, 1914), which is mainly due to its action enhancing rhythmicity of the myocardium (Kruta, 1934; Greiner and Garb, 1950). It prolongs the action potential by reducing the efflux of potassium (Kleinfeld et al., 1954). In the nerve it enhances depolarization and increases the afterpotential (Lorente de Nó and Feng, 1946).

Ventricular fibrillation produced after a large dose of $CaCl_2$ was observed by Gross as long ago as 1903 in the isolated Langendorff heart. Intravenous injection of $CaCl_2$ to the intact animal induced ventricular arrhythmia and eventually fibrillation, which was attributed by Rothberger and Winterberg (1911) to the direct action of Ca^{++} on the myocardium. Malinow et al. (1953), on the other hand, assumed that $CaCl_2$ exerts its arrhythmogenic action mainly through the central nervous system, notably through the sympathetic branch. Although $CaCl_2$ in physiologic concentrations reduces excitability of the heart (Greiner and Garb, 1950), it also enhances spontaneous ectopic activity in the myocardium by direct and reflex stimulation of the peripheral adrenergic structures (Grumbach et al., 1954). Diminution of excitability under the influence of high Ca^{++} concentrations is not uniform in various parts of the myocardium; thus, asynchronous propagation of impulses and arrhythmia result (Brooks et al., 1955). Low Ca^{++} concentration may also precipitate arrhythmia, since excitability and spontaneous impulse generation are enhanced throughout the heart (Brooks et al., 1955).

Levy's classical experiments (1914) first showed that intravenous administration of epinephrine to dogs under moderately deep chloroform anesthesia may precipitate ventricular fibrillation. Han and Moe (1964) have shown that chloroform is capable of increasing the temporal dispersion of recovery of excitability in the ventricle of the dog. Also, other agents "sensitizing" epinephrine were described, such as benzol (Nahum and Hoff, 1934), cyclopropane (Meek et al., 1937), amarine (Brooks et al., 1955), and halothane (Raventos, 1956; Andersen and Johansen, 1963; Takaori and Loehning, 1965). According to Hauswirth (1969), halothane facilitates the development of arrhythmias mainly for the following reasons: a) decreased conduction velocity due to increased internal resistance, b) shortening of the refractory period, and c) pronounced disparity of the refractory period between Purkinje and ventricular fibers. Norepinephrine may also act as a precipitating agent (Garb and Chenoweth, 1948). Isoproterenol (Dresel et al., 1963) and direct or reflex stimulation of the sympathetic nervous system may produce a similar effect to that of epinephrine and norepinephrine. Chloroform may sensitize the heart to the action of endogenous catecholamines (Levy, 1914), which explains the mechanism of arrhythmias induced by chloroform alone. The "sensitizing" effect of the preceding depressants is present only with low concentrations of the drug. In deep anesthesia, sensitization does not appear to occur (Levy, 1914). As shown by Brooks et al. (1955), low concentrations of chloroform and benzol shorten the refractory period but do not affect or moderately increase the excitability of the heart. Higher concentrations definitely prolong the refractory period and depress excitability without significantly affecting the fibrillation thresholds.

Thus, the simultaneous stimulating and depressing action of chloroform may be at least partly responsible for the sensitization to the arrhythmogenic action of epinephrine. In addition, excitation of the cardiac sympathetic and vagus nerve may also contribute to this action, since administration of sympatholytic, parasympatholytic, or ganglion-blocking agents may inhibit the development of arrhythmias produced by the foregoing depressants.

On the other hand, the fibrillation-precipitating action of instantaneous intravenous injection of epinephrine lasts only for a very short time, the effective period being not longer than 30 seconds after administration of the drug (Nickerson and Nomaguchi, 1949). This observation is in good agreement with our findings (Szekeres, 1964b) in which epinephrine infused in doses higher than 3 μg/kg/min, after a short temporary increase, markedly reduced susceptibility to fibrillation.

Succinyldicholine may also produce arrhythmia on repeated administration to animals under halothane or cyclopropane (Williams et al., 1961) but not under thiopenthal anesthesia.

Some hormones may also exert arrhythmogenic action, such as insulin alone (Strouse et al., 1932) or in combination with glucose and acetylcholine (Levêque, 1964, 1965); possibly the insulin-induced hypokalemia sensitizes the heart to the arrhythmogenic action of acetylcholine or epinephrine. Leveque used this test arrhythmia for assay of antiarrhythmic drugs. He also recommends the precipitation of arrhythmia by acetylcholine in animals pretreated with thyroid extract, but owing to the short duration (10 to 30 sec) of the fibrillation thus elicited, it does not seem suitable for assay. Walker (1952) described ventricular tachycardia, sometimes flutter, or even fibrillation in pregnant rats on the inhalation of ether.

It has already been mentioned in the introduction that electrical stimulation as a precipitating measure may, in the presence of various drugs acting as "sensitizing" agents or as agents perpetuating arrhythmia, produce lasting heart rhythm disturbances. This has been shown for acetylcholine which induces auricular fibrillation in the dog heart-lung preparation (Burn et al., 1955), for epinephrine which elicits ventricular arrhythmias in the dog (Gilbert et al., 1959), or even for hypertonic solutions (NaCl, mannite), all of which prolong the duration of auricular fibrillation in the dog induced by electrical stimulation (Swain and Curtis, 1966).

Induction of Arrhythmias by Mechanically or Thermically Produced Local Blocks and Ectopic Foci

The interventions discussed in this section have a certain analogy with the local application of such drugs as aconitine or veratrine insofar as they alter fundamental properties of the heart within a circumscribed area of the myocardium, giving rise to local blocks and to spontaneously firing ectopic foci. These in turn may cause asynchronous propagation of impulses leading to irregular cardiac activity.

Local ischemia of the heart brought about by ligation of the coronary arteries is one of the most adequate and popular forms of application of the foregoing principle. Arrhythmias so produced are etiologically similar to the arrhythmias occurring in man in association with local ischemia brought about by heart infarction.

After coronary ligation, myocardial excitability increases in the ischemic area as a consequence of hypoxic instability of the membrane (Brooks et al., 1961). Moreover the action potential is shortened. All these factors favor the appearance of extrasystoles. In prolonged ischemia the resting membrane potential is reduced. Ligation of the left descending coronary artery in dogs produces ventricular fibrillation in 30 percent of the cases, according to Varma et al. (1963). Harris (1950) introduced the two-stage ligation technique to avoid ventricular fibrillation. For this purpose, at least a 30-minute interval between partial and total ligation of the artery is needed. The chest is then closed under aseptic conditions, and spontaneous respiration restored. Arrhythmia in the form of a lasting ventricular tachycardia appears five to seven hours following complete occlusion, but maximal ectopic activity suitable for assay of drugs appears only on the second day after operation (Winbury and Hemmer, 1955). On the other hand, Varma et al. (1963), aiming at the elaboration of a test arrhythmia suitable for evaluation of the preventive action of drugs, succeeded in increasing the incidence of ventricular fibrillation following left anterior coronary ligation in dogs from 30 to 100 percent if coronary ligation was associated with hypothermia. The latter alone caused a 40 percent incidence of ventricular fibrillation.

The two-stage ligation method may serve as a sensitizing intervention which prolongs and increases the severity of the arrhythmias produced by epinephrine or norepinephrine in dogs (Moran et al., 1962) and in pigs (Winbury et al., 1962). The catecholamines are administered on the fourth or fifth day after ligation, when cardiac rhythm is normal again, but the latent ectopic foci still present may be reactivated by the above mentioned drugs.

Although both local heating and cooling of the myocardium may induce under certain circumstances severe heart rhythm disturbances, these methods are not used for assay of antiarrhythmic drugs, since reproducibility of the arrhythmia so induced seems not to be satisfactory for this purpose. Additional effort is required for standardization of the technique. The mechanism is probably based on the fact that in the heated area the refractory period becomes shorter and at the same time conduction velocity increases. In addition, ectopic firing may appear. Nevertheless, local temperature differences sufficient to elicit complete disorganization of the cardiac activity may be brought about only by heating the area to a temperature already impairing the myocardium (Brooks et al., 1955).

Local cooling is not so harmful in this respect, as local temperature differences sufficient to precipitate arrhythmias are more easily established, as shown by Scherf and Schott (1953). An injury current appears between the cooled and normal myocardium (Hoff and Stansfield, 1949). The slowing of conduction provides a preliminary condition for a circus movement of excitation.

The method introduced by Rosenblueth and Garcia-Ramos (1947), producing atrial flutter by crushing the intervena caval portion of the atrial myocardium and by simultaneous electrical stimulation of the heart, represents an argument in favor of the circus movement theory and a technique suitable for testing drugs against atrial flutter.

Induction of Arrhythmias by Direct Stimulation of the Central Nervous System

Direct stimulation of the central nervous system by electrical, chemical, or mechanical stimuli may also induce heart rhythm disturbances. These are not accepted as routine methods for assay due to the difficulties in standardization and reproducibility. Nevertheless, they seem to be valuable for predicting the usefulness of a given drug in arrhythmias of central origin appearing in certain clinical conditions (e.g., acute increase of intracranial pressure).

METHODS FOR SELECTING EFFECTIVE ANTIARRHYTHMIC DRUGS

Methods Based on the Principles of Preventing the Appearance of Arrhythmia or Abolishing Persisting Arrhythmia

The methods based on the preceding principles most nearly meet the requirements for an ideal antiarrhythmic agent–i.e., the ability to prevent a latent, or to suspend an existing, heart rhythm disturbance. A great advantage of an assay of this kind is that it may also supply information regarding the duration of the antiarrhythmic action, since after cessation of the drug's action, arrhythmia may reappear. However, production of a fairly long-lasting experimental arrhythmia is needed for this purpose; otherwise it is very difficult to interpret not only the duration of the antiarrhythmic action but also whether the arrhythmia was abolished by the antiarrhythmic drug itself or whether it ceased spontaneously in consequence of the elimination of the arrhythmogenic drug.

Another important requirement is that the arrhythmia should be standardizable and reproducible; i.e., identical intervention should produce heart rhythm disturbance of identical severity. This is particularly important in arrhythmias produced by chemical substances. A further problem arises in connection with assay of drugs effective against ventricular fibrillation. Since prolonged ventricular fibrillation may develop, provision should be made to maintain circulation by some sort of heart-oxygenator. Up to this time, only electrical defibrillation has proved effective in abolishing ventricular fibrillation, and so far no known drug is able to terminate it with absolute certainty.

In the light of the foregoing facts, theoretically nearly all types of experimental arrhythmias reviewed would be suitable for the assay of antiarrhythmic drugs. Their practical value depends mainly on how closely they represent the model arrhythmia, considering also the conditions needed for its production, and how far they are comparable to that occurring in clinical practice.

If the selection of the methods is made from the preceding point of view, the technique used by Holland (1957)–inducing lasting fibrillation in the isolated rabbit atria by diminishing the potassium content of the medium and by applying at the same time high concentrations of acetylcholine and simultaneous electrical stimulation–can hardly be considered appropriate for testing antiarrhythmic drugs. This is obvious if we take into account that changes in the ionic composition of the medium are of an extent that is never present in the intact organism, except in extreme conditions. Also, the concentration of acetylcholine is much higher than that usually applied in the intact animal. All of this represents a rather rough intervention into processes related to cell permeability and metabolism.

Evaluation of antiarrhythmic action with the aid of combined methods for producing experimental arrhythmias–as the use of acetylcholine along with electrical stimulation (Burn et al., 1955) or the widely used combinations of epinephrine and chloroform, epinephrine and benzol, or epinephrine and cyclopropane–is rendered difficult by the fact that instead of a single arrhythmogenic factor, we have to take into account two, each of them acting directly on the heart and also indirectly through reflexes influencing heart and vessels. The interaction of these two factors–different concentration and different activity and duration of action–will determine not only the type of the arrhythmia so produced, but also the nature of the antiarrhythmic action to be measured. Thus, if one of the arrhythmogenic factors is an autonomic transmitter, such as epinephrine or acetylcholine, we cannot tell whether the antiarrhythmic action observed is due to the specific blockade of the mediator by sympatholytic or cholinolytic action of the drug in question, or to a nonspecific quinidinelike antiarrhythmic effect appearing directly on the myocardium, or to both.

The combination of acetylcholine and electrical stimulation has yielded poor correlation with other methods for assay of antiarrhythmic drugs (Rand and Walker, 1958). The minimum dose of catecholamines (adrenaline, isoprenaline) required to produce ectopic beats during vagal stimulation is determined before and after administration of antiarrhythmic agents in the vagus-amine test (Roberts and Baer, 1960). The method provides a relatively simple means of examining antiarrhythmic action in vivo, but it is rather time-consuming and, because of the frequent deterioration of the stimulated nerve, the results are not always reproducible in the same animal.

Combinations of epinephrine with depressants are more current. It has been shown (Wégria and Nickerson, 1943) that among the sensitizing agents, benzol gives the most reliable combination with epinephrine for producing arrhythmia and ventricular fibrillation. A further step forward was the introduction of electrical defibrillation. All this increased applicability of the method, since formerly, on one hand, arrhythmia could not be reliably produced and, on the other, if the antiarrhythmic drug tested proved to be ineffective, the animal was lost in consequence of ventricular fibrillation. A very detailed critical review on this type of combined assay is given by Dawes (1952).

Better results can be expected with methods using a single substance only for production of arrhythmia, with well-known modes of action or conditions similar to those observable in human pathology.

Thus the method of Scherf and Terranova (1949), inducing auricular flutter and fibrillation by local application of aconitine, as well that of Rosenblueth and Garcia-Ramos (1947), producing auricular flutter by atrial crushing and electrical stimulation, proved to be equally useful for testing drugs, acting mainly on atrial flutter and fibrillation, respectively. Winbury (1956) found that antiarrhythmic potencies determined by these methods appear to be highly consistent, despite the fact that arrhythmias produced by the Rosenblueth and Garcia-Ramos method are probably evoked by circus movement, while local application of aconitine precipitates arrhythmia mainly by increasing ectopic activity.

The drawback of both methods is that they require thoracotomy. Consequently deep anesthesia and artificial respiration are needed. This deficiency can be eliminated by closing the chest and restoring spontaneous respiration. Whereas the Rosenblueth-Garcia-Ramos flutter is usually long-lasting, duration of the aconitine flutter is limited by the absorption of the drug. Constant drip of aconitine solution (0.04 percent) on the filter paper applied to the auricle may solve the problem.

Auricular fibrillation was produced in anesthetized closed-chest dogs by applying suprathreshold electrical stimuli through a catheterlike monopolar electrode introduced through the femoral vein into the auricle (Ellis, 1956). But the auricular fibrillation thus produced is very unstable. It may last from 15 seconds to 2 hours and therefore seems to be less suitable for assay of antiarrhythmic compounds.

In the following paragraphs, techniques for evaluating drugs acting mainly against heart rhythm disturbances of ventricular origin will be discussed. A widely adopted method for assaying antiarrhythmic drugs is the use of toxic doses of cardiac glycosides alone or in combination with other drugs. Besides its being a valuable tool for screening, the method has a great importance also from a purely clinical-toxicologic standpoint, in view of the frequent occurrence of arrhythmias due to digitalis overdosage. According to Van Dongen (1936), ventricular fibrillation induced by intravenous injection in the cat of half the lethal dose of strophanthin, followed by 20 mg/kg ephedrine, is suitable for assay of antiarrhythmic agents. But toxic doses of ouabain (110 μg/kg) alone may produce ventricular tachycardia in the dog responding well to antiarrhythmic agents, whereas subsequent ventricular fibrillation causing the death of more than two-thirds of the animals can only be prevented with quinidine (Clark and Cummings, 1956). Since intoxication with cardiac glycosides is a progressive process, it does not lend itself to standardization. Nevertheless the early phase of intoxication is suitable for estimating the lowest dose of antiarrhythmic drug still able to suspend ventricular tachycardia. This is shown in Figure 3, demonstrating that even lower doses (70 μg/kg) of strophanthin-G may produce prolonged ventricular tachycardia in the dog, and are suitable for measuring not only suspension of arrhythmia by the antiarrhythmic agent but also duration of antiarrhythmic action. After elimination of the antiarrhythmic drug, ventricular tachycardia appears again (Papp, 1967).

As mentioned earlier, rapid intravenous injection in rats of $CaCl_2$ in doses ranging from 120 mg/kg (Fekete and Borsy, 1964) to 200 mg/kg (Malinow et al., 1953; Nieschulz et al., 1955) may precipitate arrhythmias of ventricular origin, enabling the assay of antiarrhythmic agents. The differences in doses cited by various authors to elicit ventricular tachycardia and fibrillation, respectively, are mainly due to the different speed of injection (Nieschultz et al., 1955) and also to the widely differing sensitivity of the strains of rat used. In a critical evaluation of the method, Papp (1967) showed that rapid intravenous injection of 140 mg/kg $CaCl_2$ (in 2.5 percent solution) in rats precipitated, in 80 percent of the cases, lasting ventricular fibrillation leading to death of the animals (Fig. 4, Part I); whereas in the remaining 20 percent, transient atrioventricular block and ventricular extrasystole with scattered fibrillation potentials appeared, but the animals survived (Fig. 4, Part II). In rare instances, a single $CaCl_2$ injection

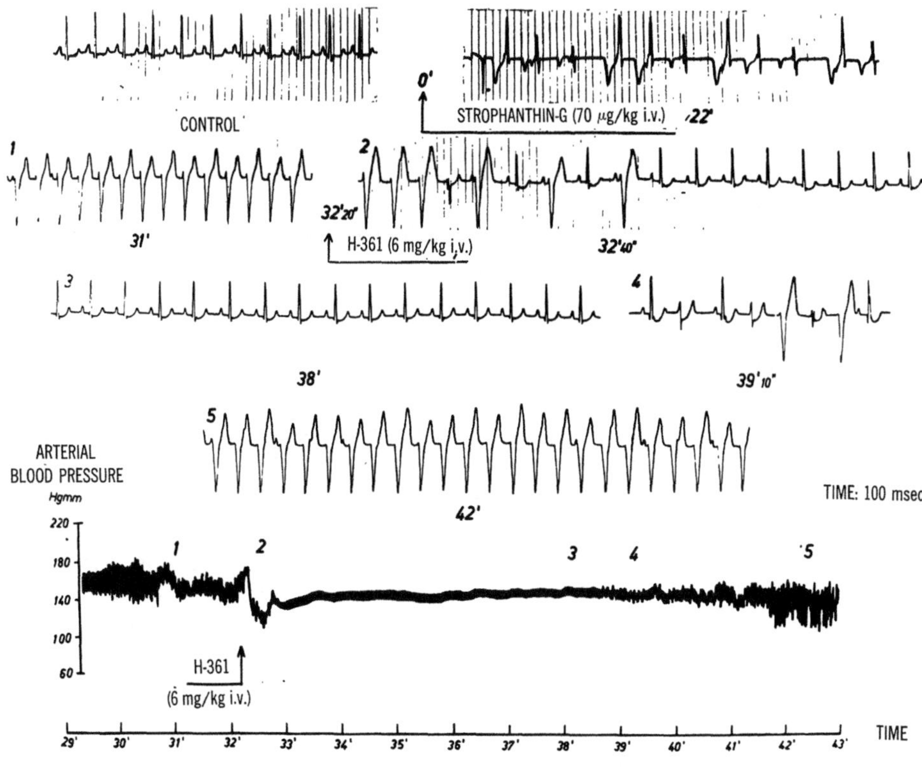

FIG. 3. Use of H. 361, a new antiarrhythmic agent, in the dog for suspension of ventricular tachycardia induced by 70 ug/kg i.v. strophanthin (ouabain). Upper curve: II lead ECG; lower curve: arterial blood pressure; numbers on the blood-pressure curve refer to the related ECG tracings. Time in minutes.

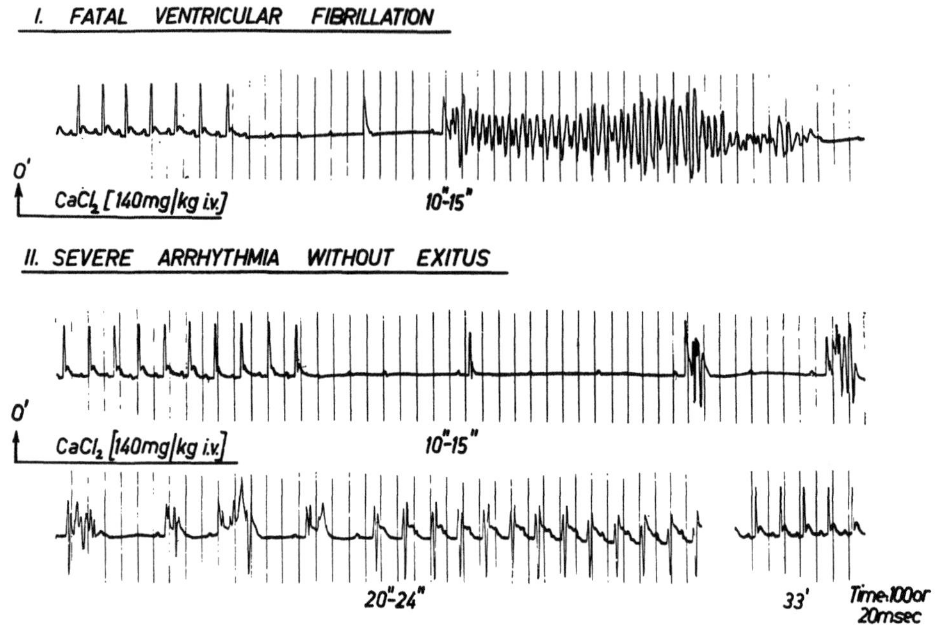

FIG. 4. The main types of action of rapid intravenous injection of $CaCl_2$ solution, 140 mg/kg, into anesthetized rats: I. Fatal ventricular fibrillation, II. Severe arrhythmia without exitus.

brought the heart to standstill. Furthermore, in about 15 percent of the cases, irreversible apnea ensued, and here the combined effect on the heart of asphyxia and of $CaCl_2$ appeared in the form of a transient tachycardia, followed by severe progressive bradycardia, and finally by ventricular fibrillation or asystole. Antiarrhythmic drugs injected intravenously two minutes prior to $CaCl_2$ administration could markedly reduce the incidence of lasting and fatal ventricular fibrillation, but even high doses of well-known, reliable antiarrhythmic agents were not able to abolish the heart rhythm disturbance completely. Thus, the method is of little practical value in the assay of antiarrhythmic agents. Similarly Winbury (1956) asserts that the $CaCl_2$ arrhythmia is far less sensitive for selecting active antiarrhythmic compounds than the two-stage coronary ligation procedure of Harris (1950).

As mentioned earlier, the great advantage of the coronary ligation method is that the heart rhythm disturbance produced is etiologically similar to that occurring in human coronary occlusion. Since the arrhythmia is long-lasting, testing of the same drug can be repeated many times. Furthermore, comparison with other drugs is possible and the duration of the antiarrhythmic action can be estimated. Another advantage of the method is that it enables one to perform the assay in the unanesthetized animal. Finally, besides the antiarrhythmic action, the procedure gives information on possible side effects. Antiarrhythmic action of the drugs to be tested is compared either by their action in reducing the rate of ventricular tachycardia or by the number of extra beats. The only inconvenience of the method is that it requires a sterile operative technique, and it may be accompanied in 16 to 20 percent of the cases by fatal ventricular fibrillation appearing at the time of total coronary ligation (Clark and Cummings, 1956).

Epinephrine injected intravenously in higher doses may also induce tachycardia and ventricular extrasystole, which can be readily antagonized not only by the beta receptor-blocking sympatholytics, but also by other antiarrhythmic agents. Thus, the method lends itself well to evaluation of antiarrhythmic drugs (Maling and Moran, 1957; Maling and Highman, 1958; Somani and Lum, 1965; Somani et al., 1966). A typical epinephrine arrhythmia is shown in Figure 5 (Papp, 1967) in which 100 mg/kg administered intravenously to dogs evokes ectopic activity reaching maximal effect 1.5 to 2 minutes after injection. Here about 90 percent of the total number of contractions appeared in the form of extrasystoles. Reproducible values were obtained only if a 30- to 60-minute pause was inserted between two epinephrine injections; otherwise subsequent epinephrine administration evoked progressively increasing ECG changes. The drug to be tested should be injected two minutes prior to the administration of epinephrine (Papp, 1967), and the dose sufficient to reduce by 50 percent the ectopic activity at the height of epinephrine action is estimated. Ectopic activity may be determined as the percent of extrasystoles calculated on the basis of the total number of systoles in a 30-second interval. Chloroform alone has recently been used for evaluating antiarrhythmic activity in the mouse (Lawson, 1968; Aviado and Reutter, 1969). The procedure consists of a rapid production of chloroform anesthesia leading to respiratory arrest and ventricular fibrillation. The difference between the slowest and fastest heart rate during anesthesia and the incidence of ventricular fibrillation is recorded. The method is not suitable for delayed analysis, but it might be of some use as a rapid screening method, especially when limited amounts of the compounds are available.

Having considered the strengths and deficiencies of the methods reviewed, I now want to recommend some further methods, which are partly new and partly modifications of known procedures. These were elaborated by us and found to possess practical value for assaying antiarrhythmic drugs.

In the first method, the antiarrhythmic drug in question is tested for its effect in suspending a lasting atrial fibrillation or ventricular tachycardia evoked in the dog by continuous electrical stimulation of the myocardium, using rectangular pulses of 1 msec duration and 20 cycles/sec frequency. It is essential that the lowest dose of the drug capable of suspending for a given time the arrhythmia produced by permanent electrical stimulation of the auricles and ventricles, respectively, should be estimated. Persistent stimulation of the myocardium at the same spot corresponds to a steadily firing ectopic focus, and since the arrhythmia produced lasts as long as stimulation is on, its spontaneous termination does not have to be taken into account, as with other methods (Ellis, 1956; Fekete and Borsy, 1964). Reliable results can be obtained not only as to the activity of the drug but also as to the duration of its action.

First, we tried to introduce the electrodes mounted on a catheter, according to Ellis (1956), through the femoral vein to the right auricle, without opening the

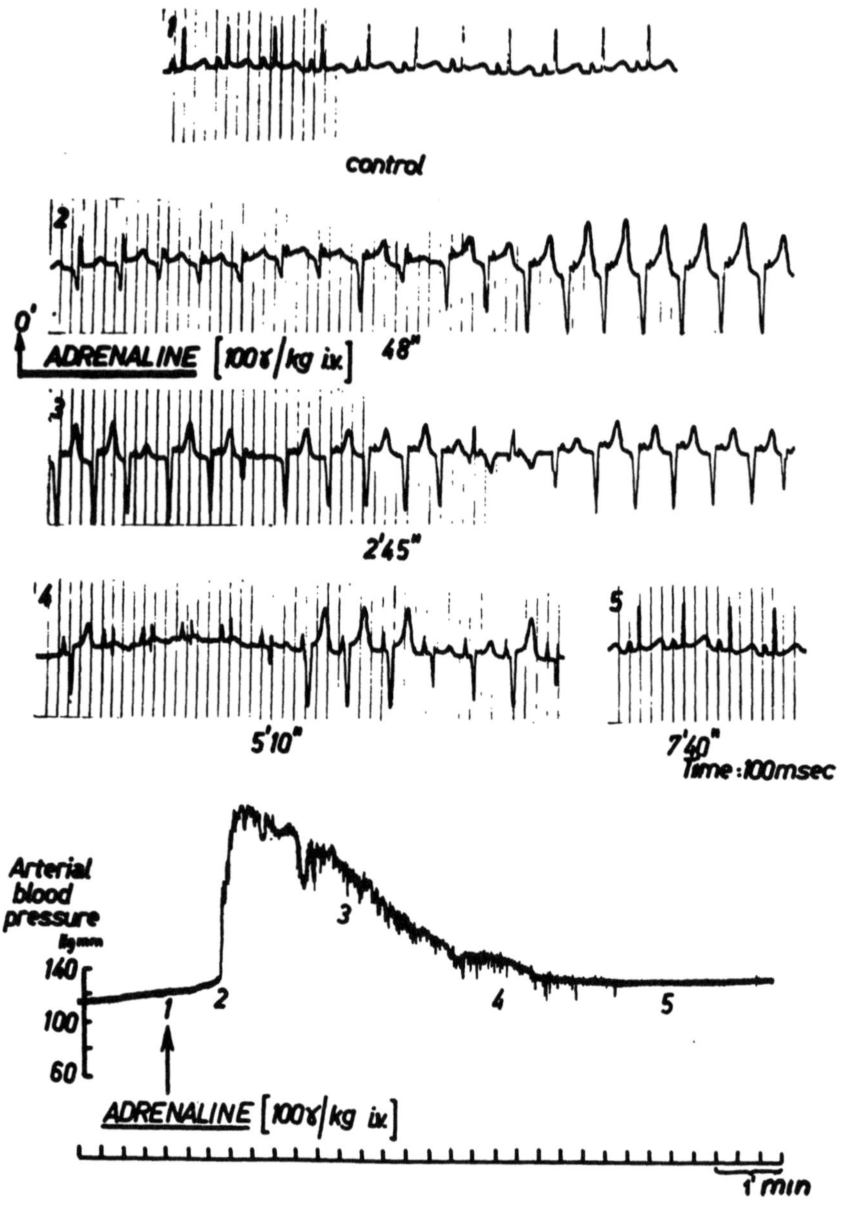

FIG. 5. Arrhythmia induced by i.v. injection of 100 μg/kg adrenaline (epinephrine) into the anesthetized dog. Numbers on the blood-pressure curve refer to the related ECG tracings.

chest. The main trouble with this procedure is that fixation of the electrodes is unreliable. Pressing the electrodes against the cardiac wall is not sufficient to exclude changes in position. In addition, our attempts to fix them by vacuum, using suction electrodes, did not prove to be entirely satisfactory.

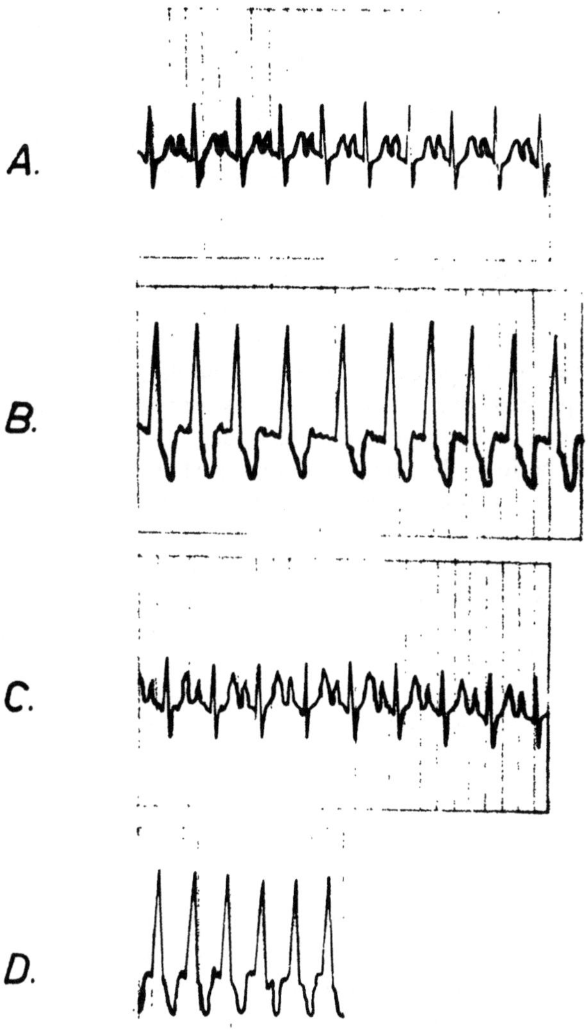

FIG. 6. Procaine-induced temporary abolishment of ventricular arrhythmia due to lasting electrical stimulation of the dog heart. (Rectangular impulses of 25 c/sec frequency and 1 msec duration were used. ECG was recorded in the II lead. Time signal: 100 msec.)

(A) Control

(B) Stimulation of the right ventricle—Ventricular arrhythmia.

(C) Procaine injection, I mg/kg i.v., during the stimulation of the ventricle—Complete abolishment of the ventricular arrhythmia for 6 min.

(D) Termination of the procaine effect-Reappearance of the ventricular arrhythmia.

Therefore, the following method was adopted: After introducing artificial respiration, the chest was opened and bipolar silver electrodes were stitched to the ventral surface of the right ventricle and auricle. The chest was then closed, the pneumothorax reduced, and spontaneous respiration restored. Stimulation was started and stimulus strength was raised until atrial fibrillation and ventricular tachycardia, respectively, could be observed in the ECG. The lowest concentration resulting in a temporary but complete suspension of arrhythmia and the highest concentration giving a partial suspension were estimated. Partial suspension means that arrhythmia repeatedly appears for the time of a few beats, then disappears again. The significance of the determination of this latter dose lies in the fact that it allows more exact definition of the threshold dose giving complete suspension. An example of this method is given in Figure 6.

Though we do not have enough experience with this method to be able to compare it with other methods, it represents in our opinion a very good supplementary test to the procedure based on the determination of the fibrillation threshold. It is possible that in the future this assay may be also applied in the unanesthetized animal with implanted electrodes.

The need to perform the assay in the unanesthetized animal stimulated us to modify the hitherto qualitative $BaCl_2$ test for a quantitative assay method. The $BaCl_2$ technique was recommended for screening of antiarrhythmic drugs by Van Dongen (1936), but since then it has not been frequently used for this purpose because of the low margin of safety, as only slightly higher doses than those required for production of ventricular extrasystole precipitated ventricular fibrillation. Comparing different forms of administration and using different dosages, the most reliable, reproducible $BaCl_2$ test arrhythmia was induced when 4 mg/kg of this substance in 2 percent solution was injected slowly, to avoid ventricular fibrillation, into the marginal ear vein of conscious rabbits (Papp et al., 1967). ECG tracings taken in the V-4 precordial position revealed a severe and long-lasting arrhythmia appearing as polytopic, predominantly ventricular extrasystole, often in form of bigeminy, which could be readily antagonized and reverted to normal rhythm by antiarrhythmic agents, as shown in Figure 7. After elimination of the drug, bigeminy reappeared, thus enabling comparison of the duration of antiarrhythmic action of different drugs. An interval of at least 24 hours is required between two subsequent $BaCl_2$ injections in the same animal to produce arrhythmias of identical severity and duration.

The dose abolishing arrhythmia for at least one minute in 50 percent of the animals can be used as a reference value for comparison of antiarrhythmic activities. The relative activities observed with the $BaCl_2$ method proved to be consistent with the data yielded by the fibrillation threshold method (Papp et al., 1967). The method possesses the advantages of being very simple and of allowing the use of a conscious animal, thereby eliminating the need for surgical intervention. Furthermore it yields data comparable with those given by other methods, and determinations can be repeated on different days in the same animal at will.

The desire to produce arrhythmias of predominantly atrial origin in the closed-chest animal led us to try intravenous administration of aconitine in rats (Szekeres, 1964a; Szekeres and Papp, 1970). Although it soon became clear that the developing heart rhythm disturbance is by no means restricted to the atria, it represents an easily producible, fairly long-lasting test arrhythmia which is suitable for evaluating antiarrhythmic action on a large series of animals.

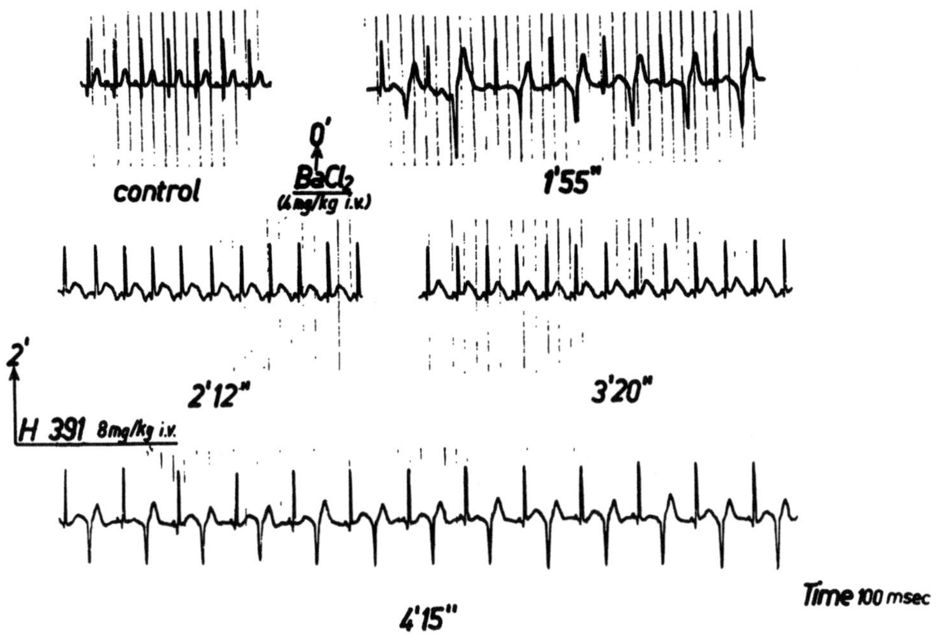

FIG. 7. Suspension by a new antiarrhythmic agent, H. 391., of the bigeminy produced by i.v. injection of 4 mg/kg $BaCl_2$ into conscious rabbits.

Intravenous administration of 40 μg/kg freshly prepared aconitine solution to anesthetized rats evokes, after an initial latency period of 30 to 60 seconds, the first arrhythmic phase which lasts from 16 to 130 seconds. This is followed by a second latency period which lasts 3 to 4 minutes with occasional appearance of some extra beats, short auricular flutter, or ventricular tachycardia. The third phase is the period of prolonged arrhythmia. This appears in various forms such as auricular flutter or fibrillation alone, or together with extrasystoles or tachycardia of ventricular origin; sometimes bigeminy; and with large doses, not infrequently, ventricular fibrillation. This phase is long enough, lasting in average 15 minutes, to enable determination of the antiarrhythmic action. Suspension of aconitine arrhythmia by quinidine is shown in Figure 8. Since arrhythmia returns after elimination of the antiarrhythmic agent, measurement of the duration of antiarrhythmic action of different drugs is possible. The dose normalizing the heart rhythm for at least one minute in 50 percent of the treated animals may be taken as a reference value for determination of antiarrhythmic potency.

As shown by us (Szekeres, 1964a; Szekeres and Papp, 1970), antiarrhythmic potencies determined by the intravenous rat aconitine test are in good agreement with those obtained by other methods for evaluation of antiarrhythmic activity. Thus, in our opinion, the proposed procedure based on suspension of existing aconitine arrhythmia seems to be more suitable for selecting active antiarrhythmic agents than that used by Fekete and Borsy (1964), who estimated the dose preventing the appearance of aconitine-induced heart rhythm disturbance.

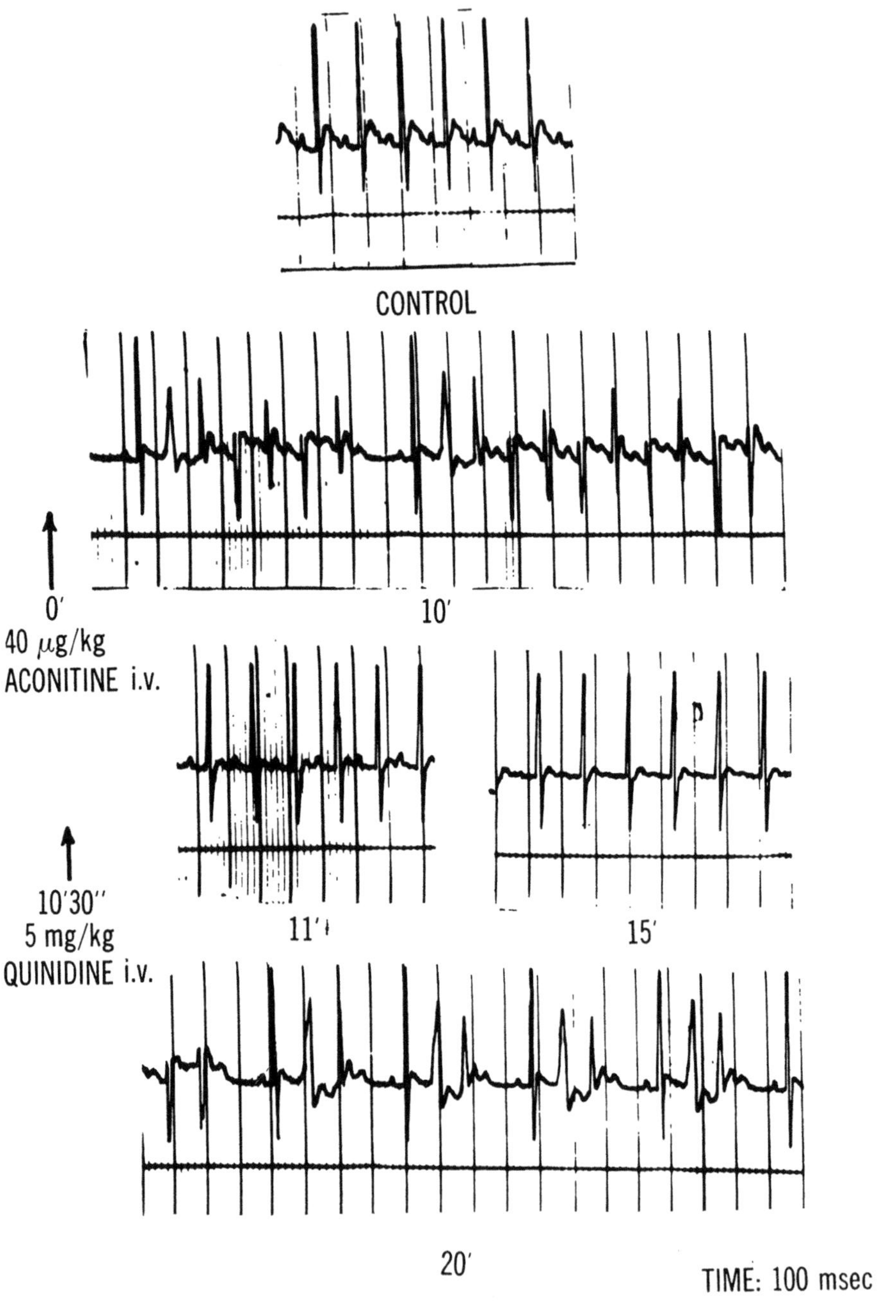

FIG. 8. Temporary suspension by quinidine of the aconitine-induced arrhythmia in the anesthetized rat.

We can now pass to the discussion of the antiarrhythmic assay techniques based on the principle of estimating the dose that just prevents the appearance of arrhythmia.

The idea of prevention is of great clinical importance. Therefore it is obvious that continuous effort is made to apply it in pharmacologic assays. Nevertheless, in spite of its unquestionable significance in therapy, it seems as if the preventive methods would be less suitable for estimation of antiarrhythmic potency of drugs than methods based on the principle of abolition of arrhythmias. This is mainly due to the fact that theoretically reliable and comparable values for the estimation of preventive doses could be obtained only if the maximum of the preventive effect coincides with the maximum of the arrhythmia evoked by some other agent. If two drugs of nearly equivalent antiarrhythmic activity but of different rates of cellular adsorption and elimination are compared, very different results can be obtained depending on whether administration of the drugs occurred immediately before injection of the arrhythmogenic agent or much earlier. In the first case, the drug which acts more rapidly seems to be more effective, since the other drug is not able to prevent the appearance of arrhythmia owing to its slow rate of adsorption to the cells. In the second case, the concentration of the rapidly acting and rapidly eliminated drug may have already sunk to a low ineffective level by the time arrhythmia reaches its maximum, so it is unable to prevent its appearance, whereas the slowly eliminated drug is still present in efficient concentration to successfully prevent the heart rhythm disturbance.

In spite of these difficulties, the methods founded on the principle of prevention of arrhythmia proved to be useful in practice. Moreover, this is the only possible procedure in all those cases when the animal has to be protected from some otherwise definitely fatal arrhythmia, such as from ventricular fibrillation due to coronary ligation or from that occurring in consequence of a combination of hypothermia and occlusion of venous inflow (Shumacker et al., 1956) and other similar measures used in attempts to imitate the human pathologic process or surgical intervention. In these cases, either the mortality rate or the percentage of successful protection is given as a measure of preventive activity of the drug in question. From the foregoing it is obvious that this procedure is less suitable for screening, but it can be used in the course of a more detailed analysis of drugs already selected for their antiarrhythmic activity, or it may be applied to prove the therapeutic value of some other nonpharmacologic intervention, such as denervation, etc.

Methods Based on Estimation of Changes in the Threshold Stimulus Required to Elicit Arrhythmia

The second fundamental principle enabling the study of factors both promoting and inhibiting arrhythmias is based on determination of drug-induced changes in the intensity of threshold stimulus required to precipitate arrhythmia. Among the methods belonging to this category are those based on the measurement of the electrical threshold for production of flutter and fibrillation, which have already been thoroughly discussed. Another possibility is to determine the minimum dose of an arrhythmogenic agent just sufficient to evoke arrhythmia before and after administration of antiarrhythmic drugs. Blumenthal and Oppenheimer (1939) found that in the presence of quinidine or other antiarrhythmic agents, much more $BaCl_2$ was needed to produce ventricular fibrillation in the isolated perfused cat heart than in the nontreated control hearts. Nevertheless, this latter method does not seem to have any advantage over the electrical threshold method. Moreover, it allows only one or two determinations in the same preparation. Therefore, it is not used for assay any longer.

The advantages of the electrical theshold methods can be summarized as follows:

1. The evoked change is reversible or can be easily made reversible, particularly if flutter threshold is determined.
2. The procedure is equally suitable for investigation of factors enhancing and inhibiting susceptibility to arrhythmias.
3. It enables nearly simultaneous determination of the auricular and ventricular susceptibility to arrhythmias.
4. The changes in susceptibility to arrhythmia can be continuously followed.
5. The development and cessation of the arrhythmic or antiarrhythmic action can be very accurately measured. Thus, a reliable picture as to the time of the maximal effect and also as to the duration of action of the drug in question can be obtained.
6. As a consequence of the reversibility and reproducibility of the changes measured, the method allows the estimation of the effect of the same drug in several dose ranges or even comparison of different drugs in the same animal, with the possibility of self-control. Rise of the electrical fibrilloflutter threshold induced by increasing doses of the antiarrhythmic drug to be tested (the changes being expressed as percentages of the initial value) serves as basis for the plotting of dose-response curves. Doses producing 25 to 50 or 100 percent elevation of the thresholds may be used for comparison of antiarrhythmic activity.

In the dog, unlike the cat, use of the fibrilloflutter threshold method involves the risk of a lasting, and not infrequently fatal, ventricular fibrillation. Therefore instead of applying the foregoing method, drug-induced changes in the ventricular multiple response threshold are determined. This is an equally satisfactory procedure for estimating antiarrhythmic activity.

Methods Based on Determination of Alterations in the Fundamental Properties of the Heart Influencing the Development or Perpetuation of Arrhythmias

Application of the third principle–namely, determination of drug-induced changes in the fundamental properties of the heart (automaticity, conductivity, refractoriness, and excitability), which are assumed to play an important role in the genesis and perpetuation of arrhythmias–seems to be theoretically simpler than the complex methods discussed previously. However, interpretation of the results requires great caution. The change of a single parameter is not enough to allow the conclusion that arrhythmia is influenced in the same direction as the parameter in question, since arrhythmia is brought about by simultaneous interdependent changes of several parameters. A fundamental criterion for the usefulness of these methods is a good correlation with the more adequate methods previously discussed.

To investigate the applicability of the different parameters in estimating antiarrhythmic activity, experiments were performed in the isolated artificially driven rabbit atria, comparing the action of five different drugs (with reputed antiarrhythmic activity) on conduction velocity, effective refractory period, and threshold for the production of fibrillation (Vaughan Williams and Szekeres, 1961). Dose-response curves were plotted for quinidine, papaverine, procaine, dibenamine, and procaine amide.

The rate of the artificial pacemaker was 180/min, which was in nearly every case faster than the spontaneous frequency. Increasing current was then passed until the atria began to follow the stimulator. The thresholds were in the range of 50 to 420 microamperes. The effective refractory period was estimated by raising the stimulus strength to 2 milliamperes and increasing the driving frequency until atria would no longer follow every stimulus. Conduction velocity was determined by photographing action potentials from left and right atria while the atria were being driven at frequencies from 180 to 464/min insofar as they would still follow. The change in conduction velocity after administration of the drug was then calculated separately at each frequency as a percentage of the control conduction velocity at that frequency. Thresholds for extrasystoles, flutter, and fibrillation were measured in the way already discussed; i.e., the strength of rectangular stimuli of 3-msec duration and 10 cycles/sec frequency was progressively increased until extrasystoles, flutter, and finally fibrillation appeared.

The refractory period is affected by a number of factors. These include the fundamental driving frequency and the strength of the conditioning stimulus. Measuring the maximum frequency at which atria will follow a stimulus is therefore not truly a test of the effective refractory period. Dawes (1946) showed, however, that it was of great practical value in testing synthetic substitutes for quinidine. The results of this test (Vaughan et al., 1961) showed that quinidine is the most, and procaine amide the least, active substance. The parallelism of the dose-response curves was reasonable. The measurements of the threshold for extrasystoles and for flutter put the drugs in the same order, but the dose-response curves were neither so straight nor so parallel as in the maximum frequency test. Measurements of the fibrillation threshold, on the other hand, gave results very similar to measurement of increase in effective refractory period in the maximum frequency test.

Conduction velocity was reduced by all drugs, and since the measurement of the distance between photographed action potential is easy, accurate, and entirely objective, it was hoped that conduction velocity measurements might afford a useful antifibrillatory test. The decreases in conduction velocity were relatively greater at the higher driving frequencies, which improved the discrimination.

Nevertheless, it turned out that dose-response curves for dibenamine, procaine, and papaverine have quite different slopes from those for quinidine and procaineamide. The implication is that, although all drugs with antifibrillatory action depress conduction velocity, the factors controlling conduction velocity are complex and are not necessarily affected to the same extent as the factors governing susceptibility to fibrillation. For this reason, measurements of the conduction velocity alone cannot be regarded as a satisfactory test for antifibrillatory activity.

On the other hand, the order of potency of the drugs investigated and also their relative activities obtained by determination of the fibrillation threshold and measurement of the effective refractory period, respectively, yielded very similar quantitative results. Since the latter is extremely simple and easy to perform, it is felt the quoted work vindicates its use as a standard test for screening of antiarrhythmic drugs. Also, observations of Winbury (1956) and of Ellis (1956) are in favor of the expressed opinion.

Although the problem is not entirely new, determination of the asynchronism of recovery of excitability at various points of the myocardium has been only very recently introduced by Han and Moe (1964) and Han et al. (1964, 1966) for characterization of changes in the tendency of the heart to arrhythmia. It is based upon the observation that duration of the action potential and of the refractory period is not uniform in all parts of the myocardium (Hoffman and Cranefield 1960; Han and Moe, 1964). This means that the recovery of excitability of the heart is different in various regions of the heart (see upper part of Fig. 11), suggesting that uneven propagation of impulses and asynchronous recovery of excitability lead to the development of arrhythmia, ending in complete disorganization of the cardiac action (Brooks et al., 1955). The technique recommended first by Han and Moe (1964) enables nearly simultaneous measurement of the duration of the refractory period at various points of the myocardium and estimation of changes in the difference between the extreme values, the so-called temporal dispersion or asynchronism of the recovery of excitability.

In the following, details of the procedure as adopted and modified by us (Papp and Szekeres, 1968) will be given: Experiments were performed in anesthetized, artificially respirated, thoracotomized dogs. The electrode holder, containing four testing bipolar electrodes arranged symmetrically around the central driving electrode pair at a 10-mm distance from this latter, was stitched to the right anterior ventricular surface. A further bipolar electrode located in the apical region at a distance of about 30 mm from the driving electrode served for detection of the propagated ventricular response (Fig. 9). Rectangular impulses of 2-msec duration and 200 to 240/min frequency delivered by channel I of a special two-channel stimulator applied through the central electrode, served for artificial driving of the ventricle. About 1.5 to 2 milliamperes current intensity, corresponding to about double the diastolic threshold, was used to ensure the dominance of the artificial pacemaker over the sinoatrial impulses. At position "A" of the selector switch of channel II, the test stimuli were delivered through electrodes 1-4 connected with the channel. The test stimulus was triggered by the driving impulse, and the very finely adjustable delaying of channel II enabled us to apply the test stimulus at any instant of the cardiac cycle with 1-msec accuracy. At position "B"

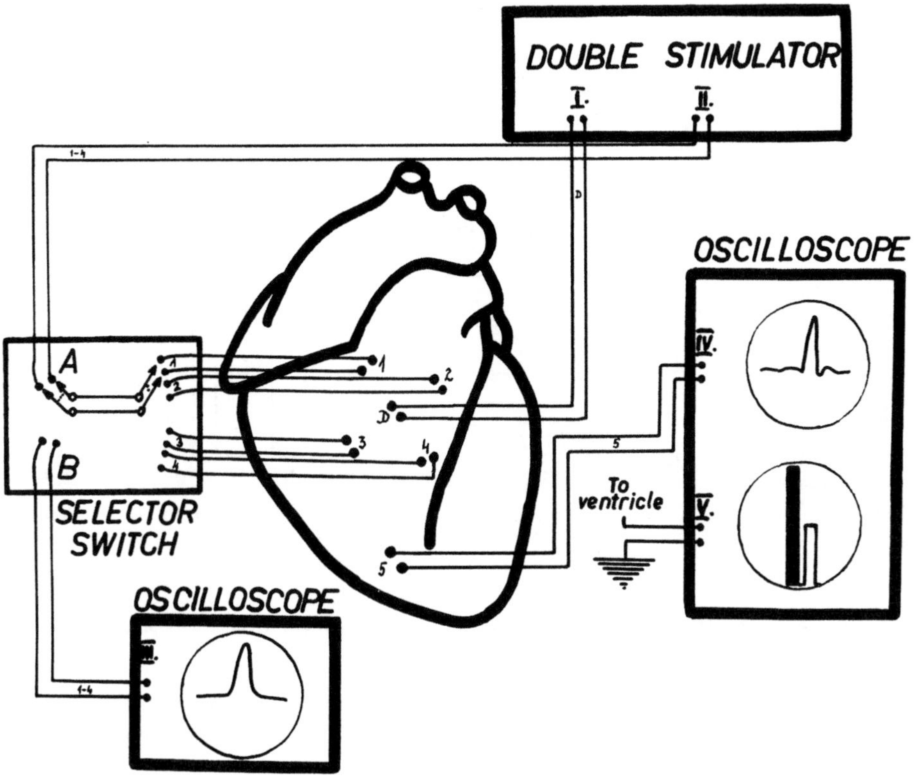

FIG. 9. Experimental arrangement for determination of asynchronous recovery of excitability. A and B: Selector switch positions; 1, 2, 3, and 4: Testing electrodes; D: Driving electrode; I: Driving stimulus; II: Test stimulus; III: Ventricular electrogram from points 1-4; IV: Ventricular electrogram from point 5; V: Record of stimulus intensity.

of the selector switch, ventricular potentials from test electrodes 1-4, further from electrode 5, appeared on channels III and IV. Occurrence of extrasystoles, indicating effectiveness of the test impulse, was displayed in II lead of the ECG. Determination of the test stimulus intensity was carried out on the calibrated screen of channel V. The schematic circuit diagram is given in Figure 10.

Determination of the ventricular refractory periods at four different points of the myocardium and subsequent estimation of the degree of asynchronism was carried out as follows: In position "B" of the selector switch, the site in the cardiac cycle of the action potential leading from electrodes 1-4, in the presence of artificial driving delivered by channel I, was displayed on oscilloscope screen III. After switching to selector position "A", the diastolic threshold was subsequently determined at each of the four measuring points of the myocardium by extra stimuli delivered by channel II applied in the late diastolic phase. Refractory periods were estimated on the basis of extrasystoles produced by the test stimuli at different times within the cycle by gradually shifting the delay of channel II from

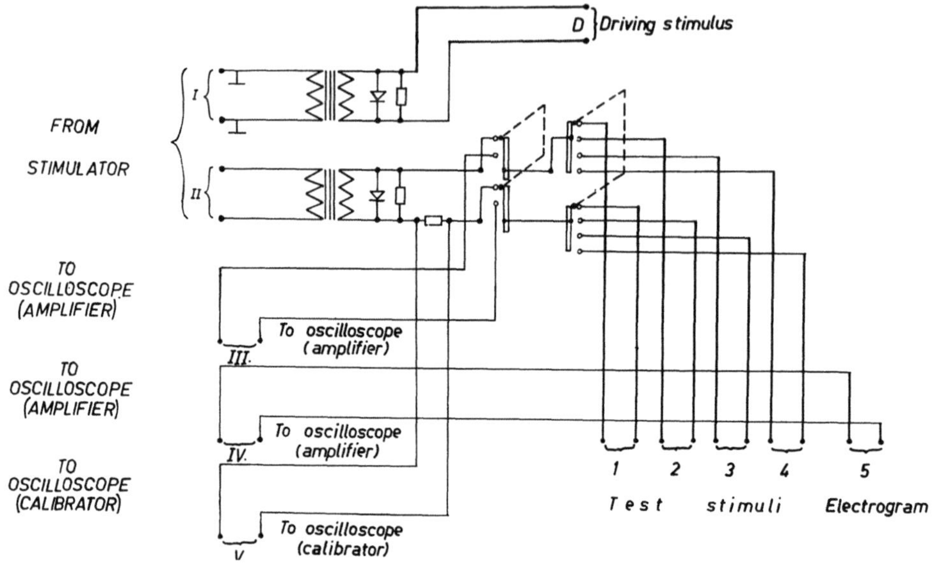

FIG. 10. Schematic circuit diagram of the experimental arrangement for determination of asynchronous recovery of excitability. (Abbreviations as in Fig. 9.)

the end toward the beginning of the cycle. The border between the last stimulus still evoking extrasystole and the first stimulus without response was determined within the cardiac cycle.

In order to carry out the measurement rapidly, the exact boundary of the relative refractory period and that of the absolute refractory period were not determined, since test stimuli with fixed parameters had to be used (stimulus intensity: double of the diastolic threshold; stimulus duration: 2 msec). Although simultaneous determination of the refractory period at the four measuring points was not possible, with some practice all refractory periods could be determined within 30 seconds if their approximate value was previously estimated. Since this intervention could be repeated at will and without delay, yielding reproducible results, changes in the refractory periods at the four different measuring points could be nearly continuously followed.

Evaluation of the results may be carried out in two ways, as described by Han and Moe (1964) and Han et al. (1964). Either the average value of the duration of refractory periods at the four measuring points was given, or the difference between the extreme values in msec was estimated, indicating the degree of asynchronism of recovery of excitability. An example of a drug (strophanthin) induced increase of asynchronism of recovery of excitability is shown in Figure 11. Since arrhythmia is a consequence of the uncoordinated function of several cardiac fibers, to get a deeper insight into the mode of action of antiarrhythmic drugs it seems to be indispensable to investigate changes in multicellular parameters. Therefore, in our opinion, the methods of measuring asynchronism of impulse

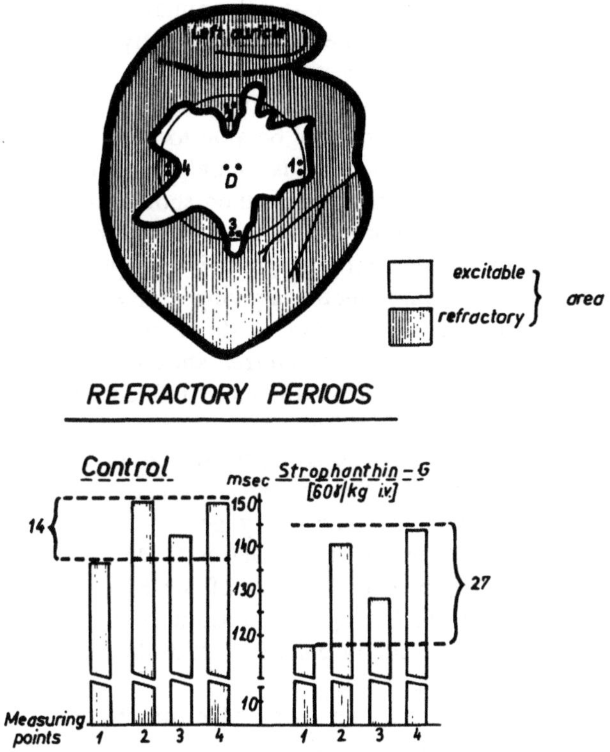

FIG. 11. (A) Schematic delineating of nonuniform recovery of excitability in the heart. (B) Change evoked by 60 μg/kg i.v. strophanthin-G during the refractory periods in the heart in situ of the anesthetized dog at the four measuring points. Temporal dispersion increases from 14 msec to 27 msec.

propagation and asynchronous recovery of excitability will be of great importance in the future for the analysis of antiarrhythmic drugs.

For the sake of completeness, it should be mentioned that there were attempts to estimate the antiarrhythmic action by comparison of other (nonantiarrhythmic) pharmacologic effects of the drugs in question, such as antihistaminic, local anesthetic, anticholinergic (Burn, 1956), and antiveratrinic (Arora and Das, 1956) action, but none of these effects proved to be satisfactory for determination of antiarrhythmic activity.

RATIONAL SCREENING PROGRAM FOR SELECTION OF EFFECTIVE ANTIARRHYTHMIC DRUGS

It has been shown in this survey that a systematic search for new antiarrhythmic agents is rendered difficult by the lack of generally accepted, adequate assay methods. This is mainly due to the fact that hardly any of the great number of model arrhythmias produced in experimental animals corresponds to the heart rhythm disturbances occurring in patients. Consequently, as Terry (1956) pointed out in his rather sceptical survey, it is understandable that current methods of screening have failed to yield results directly applicable to man. There is little hope that a single experimental procedure may be able to predict the therapeutic value of a drug in clinical practice. It is obvious, therefore, that for selecting effective antiarrhythmic agents more than one test method should be used. The procedures to be applied should be simple, reproducible, and, last but not least, inexpensive.

Careful planning of the screening program is indispensable. This involves a critical selection of a few adequate methods giving a maximum of information. In addition, a rational sequence of the use of these methods is necessary, which generally means that the simpler procedures should be used first for rough screening and the more elaborate ones for more refined analysis of the already selected, promising antiarrhythmic drugs.

With this in view, a three-stage program for screening of antiarrhythmic drugs was recommended by Ellis (1956). The *first stage* consists in determination of drug-induced changes in the effective refractory period on the isolated auricular preparation according to the technique of Dawes (1946); *second stage:* measurement of changes in the length of the P wave of the ECG, indicating changes in intraauricular conduction:*third stage:* estimation of the dose preventing or abolishing arrhythmias induced by electrical stimulation of the right auricle through intracardial electrodes.

In his comprehensive survey on assay of antiarrhythmic drugs, Winbury (1956) pointed out that consistent results can be obtained in the isolated rabbit auricle as well as in the cat papillary muscle preparation when estimating the effective refractory period determined by the maximum frequency followed. As to the assay in the intact animal, Winbury found that arrhythmias produced by injection of $CaCl_2$ in rats are much less suitable for selecting effective antiarrhythmic agents than the cyclopropane-epinephrine induced ventricular arrhythmia in the dog and the ventricular extrasystoles appearing after two-stage ligation of the coronary artery. The latter two methods generally yield reliable and comparable results. In his opinion, the use of the suspension of auricular flutter and fibrillation seems to be sufficient for antiarrhythmic assay when it is induced (1) by the Rosenblueth-Garcia-Ramos (1947) method and (2) by the Scherf aconitine technique, and (3) reduction to half the number of extrasystoles appearing after the two-stage coronary ligation according to Harris (1950).

Winbury recommends the following three-stage program for screening: The *first stage* consists in determination of the maximal tolerated dose in unanesthetized animals; whereas antiarrhythmic activity is measured only in the *second stage* by estimating the effect of the maximal tolerated dose administered at 30-minute intervals on the arrhythmia appearing in the dog after coronary ligation. Here the total dose reducing to half the number of extrasystoles is determined. According to the results obtained in this test, the drugs are divided into three groups: (a) effective drugs active in doses less then 21 mg/kg, (b) drugs of varying activity, and (c) inactive drugs. In the *third stage* of the screening program the drugs are tested in the foregoing order of potency against the Rosenblueth-Garcia-Ramos and Scherf-type auricular arrhythmias. This program has the great advantage that besides antiarrhythmic activity, allowance is made for toxicity and possible side effects of the drug in question.

Taking all this into consideration and on the basis of our own experience, we recommend a *two-stage screening program* which seems to be sufficient for selection of effective antiarrhythmic agents, yielding satisfactory quantitative data on the potency of the drugs under assay. Moreover, valuable hints on toxicity and possible side effects may also be obtained, since both tests are made in the more or less intact animal, anesthetized and unanesthetized, respectively.

The recommended tests are the *electrical fibrilloflutter threshold* test in the cat and the *$BaCl_2$ arrhythmia* test in the conscious rabbit. In spite of the need for thoracotomy and artificial respiration, the fibrilloflutter method should be used as the first step in screening. This is due to the great advantages of the method, amply discussed in previous chapters. In addition, this method, besides possessing the advantages of the techniques performed in the isolated auricle or papillary muscle (simplicity of measuring and the possibility of repeating measurements in the same preparation), yields more information than the latter techniques. It allows simultaneous determination of auricular and ventricular action of the drug under assay and thus renders unnecessary the separate estimation of these effects on auricular ventricular preparations (each involving the loss of an animal). Very low doses may be compared in the same animal, enabling a fine discrimination of the potencies and the plotting of dose-response curves of several drugs in the same animal. Finally, the continuous recording of blood pressure and pressure in the right auricular cavity may yield valuable data about possible side effects concerning the heart and circulation.

The second stage of our screening program, the $BaCl_2$ test in rabbits, fulfills further requirements not elicited by the first stage: i.e., it determines the ability of the drug to abolish a persisting heart rhythm disturbance and yields comparative data on the duration of the antiarrhythmic action. The test is very simple; it may be carried out in the unanesthetized animal and can be repeated days later in the same animal giving the possibility of a prolonged assay.

The preceding screening program may supply sufficient information with respect to the main problems concerning selection and evaluation of antiarrhythmic drugs. If, however, a more detailed analysis of a few selected drugs seems to be necessary, bearing in mind the requirements associated with clinical applicability, some further complementary tests may be used, such as the two-stage coronary ligation in the dog or suspension of persisting auricular fibrillation or of ventricular tachycardia produced by continuous electrical stimulation of the dog's auricle and ventricle, respectively. If the results of the accurate cat fibrilloflutter threshold method are to be checked in the very sensitive dog, the ventricular multiple-response threshold method should be applied. It is advisable to test the most promising drugs as to whether they act in arrhythmias evoked by toxic doses of cardiac glycosides.

Work still remains for the pharmacologist who is interested in the finer details of the mode of action of the drug. After selecting the most active antiarrhythmic substances, the drug-induced changes in the fundamental properties of the heart which play a part in the genesis and perpetuation of arrhythmias should be analyzed carefully. The methods described in this survey may be applied, including those measuring changes in multicellular parameters such as nonuniform spreading of excitation or asynchronism of recovery of excitability. Only the knowledge of these changes may help us to attain a theory-guided approach in the search for new, effective antiarrhythmic agents.

REFERENCES

Andersen, N., and Johansen, S.H. 1963. Incidence of catechol-amine-induced arrhythmias during halothane anesthesia. Anesthesiology, 24:51.

Andrus, E.C., and Carter, E.P. 1930. The refractory period of the normally beating dog's auricle; with a note on the occurrence of fibrillation following a single stimulus. J. Exp. Med., 51:357.

Arora, R.B., and Das, P.K. 1956. Antiveratrinic activity of antiarrhythmic drugs. Arch. Int. Pharmacodyn., 106:28.

Aviado, D. M., and Reutter, H. 1969. Antimalarial and antiarrhythmic activity of plant extracts. II. Acid extracts of plants. Med. Exp., 19:95.

Blumenthal, B., and Oppenheimer, E.T. 1939. Method for the study of ventricular fibrillation. Amer. Heart J., 18:363.

Boehm, R. 1875. Über die Wirkungen der Barytsalze auf den Tierkörper nebst Bemerkungen über die Wirkung des Wasserschierlings auf Frosche. Naunyn Schmiedeberg Arch. Pharm. Exp. Path., 3:216.

Brooks, C.Mc. C., Gilbert, J.L., Greenspan, M.E., Lange, G., and Mazella, H.M. 1960. Excitability and electrical response of ischaemic heart muscle. Amer. J. Physiol., 198:1143.

—Hoffmann, B.F., Suckling, E.E., and Orias, E. 1955. Excitability of the heart. New York, Grune and Stratton, Inc.

—Orias, O., Gilbert, J.L., Siebens, A.A., Hoffmann, B.F., and Suckling, E.E. 1951. Auricular fibrillation: relationship of "vulnerable period" to "dip" phenomenon of auricular excitability curve. Amer. J. Physiol., 164:301.

Burgen, A.S.V., and Terroux, K.G. 1953. On the negative inotropic effect in the cat's auricle. J. Physiol. (London), 120:449.

Burn, J.H. 1956. Functions of Autonomic Transmitters. Baltimore, The Williams and Wilkins Co.

—Vaughan Williams, E.M., and Walker, J.M. 1955. The effects of acetylcholine in the heart-lung preparation including the production of auricular fibrillation. J. Physiol. (London), 128:277.

Clark, B.B., and Cummings, J.R. 1956. Arrhythmias following experimental coronary occlusion and their response to drugs. Ann. N.Y. Acad. Sci., 64:543.

Dawes, G.S. 1952. Experimental cardiac arrhythmias and quinidine like drugs. Pharmacol. Rev., 4:43.

—1964. Synthetic substitutes for quinidine. Brit. J. Pharmacol., 1:90.

De Boer, S. 1921. On the fibrillation of the heart. J. Physiol. (London), 54:400.

Dreifus, L.S., Watanabe, Y., and McGarry, T.F. 1964. Clinical techniques for evaluating antiarrhythmic drugs. *In* Animal and Clinical Pharmacologic Techniques in Drug Evaluation. Nodine, J.H., and Siegler, E.P., eds. Chicago, Year Book Medical Publishers, p. 171.

—Rabbino, M.D., and Watanabe, Y. 1965. New antiarrhythmic drugs: Clinical evaluation. *In* Cardiovascular Drug Therapy. Brest, A.N., and Moyer, J.H., eds. New York, Grune and Stratton, Inc., p. 491.

Dresel, P.E., Hart, M.C., and Strömblad, B.C.R. 1963. Cardiac arrhythmias induced by injection of isoproterenol into the coronary arteries. J. Pharmacol. Exp. Ther., 140:67.
Dudel, J., and Trautwein, W. 1958. Elektrophysiologische Messungen zur Strophanthinwirkung am Herzmuskel. Naunyn Schmiedeberg Arch. Pharm. Exp. Path., 232:393.
Ellis, C.H. 1956. Screening of drugs for antiarrhythmic activity. Ann. N.Y. Acad. Sci., 64:553.
Fekete M., and Borsy, J. 1964. On the antiarrhythmic effect of some thymoleptics: Amitriptylene, Imipramine, Trimepropimine and Desmethylimipramine. Med. Exp., 10:93.
Garb, S., and Chenoweth, M.B. 1948. Studies on hydrocarbon-epinephrine induced ventricular fibrillation. J. Pharmacol. Exp. Ther., 94:12.
Gilbert, J.L., Lange, G.G., and Brooks, C.Mc.C. 1959. Influence of sympathomimetic pressor drugs on arrhythmias caused by multiple stimuli. Circ. Res., 7:417.
Greiner, T.H., and Garb, S. 1950. The influence of drugs on the irritability and automaticity of heart muscle. J. Pharmacol. Exp. Ther., 98:215.
Gross, E. 1903. Die Bedeutung der Salze der Ringer'schen Lösung für das isolierte Säugetierherz. Pflügers Arch. Ges. Physiol., 99:264.
Grumbach, L., Howard, J.W., and Merril, V.I. 1954. Factors related to the initiation of ventricular fibrillation in the isolated heart: Effect of calcium and potassium. Circ. Res., 2:452.
Han, J., Moe, G.K. 1964. Nonuniform recovery of excitability in ventricular muscle. Circ. Res., 14:44.
—Jalon, P.G., and Moe, G.K. 1964. Adrenergic effects on ventricular vulnerability. Circ. Res., 14:516.
—Jalon, P.G., and Moe, G.K. 1966. Fibrillation threshold of premature ventricular responses. Circ. Res., 18:18.
Harris, A.S. 1950. Delayed development of ventricular ectopic rhythms following experimental coronary occlusion. Circ. Res., 1:1318.
Hauswirth, O. 1969. Effects of halothane on single atrial, ventricular and Purkinje fibers. Circ. Res., 24:745.
Hoff, H.E., and Nahum, L.H. 1934. The role of adrenaline in the production of ventricular rhythms. J. Pharmacol. Exp. Ther., 52:235.
—and Stansfield, H. 1949. Ventricular fibrillation induced by cold. Amer. Heart J., 38:193.
Hoffman, B.F., and Cranefield, P.F. 1960. The Electrophysiology of the Heart. New York, McGraw-Hill Book Company.
—Suckling, E.E., and Brooks, C.Mc.C. 1955. Vulnerability of the dog ventricle and effects of defibrillation. Circ. Res., 3:147.
Holland, W.C. 1957. Potassium exchange in atrial fibrillation. Amer. J. Physiol., 19:63.
Katzung, B. 1968. Evaluation of drugs affecting the contractility and the electrophysiological properties of the heart. *In* Selected Pharmacological Testing Methods. Burger, A., ed. New York, Marcel Dekker Inc., p. 193.
Kleinfeld, M., Stein, W., and Myers, S. 1954. Effects of barium chloride on resting and action potentials of ventricular fibers of the frog. Circ. Res., 2:488.
Krayer, O., and Acheson, G.H. The pharmacology of the veratrum alcaloids. Physiol. Rev., 26:383.
Kruta, V.L. 1934. Sur l'activité automatique de l'oreilette gauche isolée du coeur du mammifère. Arch. Int. Physiol., 40:140.
Lawson, J.W. 1968. Antiarrhythmic activity of some isoquinoline derivatives determined by a rapid screening procedure in the mouse. J. Pharmacol. Exp. Ther., 160:22.
Levèque, P.E. 1964a. A simple repeatable standardized procedure for the production of auricular fibrillation in the intact dog. Arch. Int. Pharmacodyn., 149:297.
—1964b. Anti-arrhythmic action of guanethidine. Nature (London), 203:1389.
Levy, A.G. 1914. The genesis of ventricular extrasystoles under chloroform; with special reference to consecutive ventricular fibrillation. Heart, 5:299.
Lewis, T., Drury, A.M., Iliescu, C.C., and Wedd, A.M. 1921. Observations relating to the

action of quinidine upon the dog's heart: with special reference to its action on clinical fibrillation of the auricles. Heart, 9:55.
Lewis, R., Fil, H.S., and Stroud, W.D. 1930. Observations upon flutter and fibrillation. II. The nature of auricular flutter. Heart, 7:191.
Lorente de Nó, R., and Feng, T.P. 1946. Analysis of the effect of barium upon nerve with particular reference to rhythmic activity. J. Cell. Comp. Physiol., 28:396.
Maling, H., and Moran, N.C. 1957. Ventricular arrhythmias induced by sympathomimetic amines in unanesthetized dogs following coronary artery occlusion. Circ. Res., 5:409.
—and Highman, B. 1958. Exaggerated ventricular arrhythmias and myocardial fatty acid changes after large doses of norepinephrine and epinephrine in unanesthetized dogs. Amer. J. Physiol., 194:590.
Malinow, M.R., Battle, F.F., and Malamud, B. 1953. Nervous mechanisms in ventricular arrhythmias induced by calcium chloride in rats. Circ. Res., 1:554.
Meek, W.J., Hathaway, H.R., and Orth, O.S. 1937. The effects of ether, chloroform and cyclopropane on cardiac automaticity. J. Pharmacol. Exp. Ther., 61:240.
Melville, K.I., and Share, N.N. 1963. Cardiovascular responses following injection of picrotoxin into the lateral cerebral ventricle. Rev. Canad. Biol., 22:265.
Moe, G.K., and Mendez, C. 1964. Animal techniques for evaluating antiarrhythmic drugs. In Animal and Clinical Pharmacologic Techniques in Drug Evaluation. Nodine, J.H., and Siegler, P.E., eds. Chicago, Year Book Medical Publishers, p. 166.
Moran, N.C., Moore, J.I., Holcomb, H.K., and Mushet, G. 1962. Antagonism of adrenergically induced cardiac arrhythmias by dichloroisoproterenol. J. Pharmacol. Exp. Ther., 136:327.
Nahum, L.H., and Hoff, H.E. 1934. The mechanism of sudden death in experimental acute benzol poisoning. J. Pharmacol. Exp. Ther., 50:336.
—and Hoff, H.E. 1934. The experimental production of ventricular fibrillation and its prevention by acetyl-beta-methyl-choline chloride. Amer. J. Physiol., 109:78.
—and Hoff, H.E. 1940. Production of auricular fibrillation by application of acetyl-beta-methylcholine chloride to localized regions on the auricular surface. Amer. J. Physiol., 129:428.
Nickerson, M., and Nomaguchi, G. 1949. Mechanism of dibenamine protection against cyclopropane-epinephrine cardiac arrhythmias. J. Pharmacol. Exp. Ther., 95:1.
Nieschulz, O., Popendiker, K., and Hoffman, I. 1955. Weitere pharmakologische Untersuchungen über N-Methyl-piperidyl-(3)-methyl-phenothiazin. Arzneimittelforschung, 5:680.
Papp, J. (Gy.) 1967. Data concerning the adrenergic mechanism and pharmacotherapy of cardiac arrhythmias [In Hungarian]. C. Sc. thesis, Pécs.
—and Szekeres, L. 1968. Analysis of the mechanism of adrenergic actions on ventricular vulnerability. Europ. J. Pharmacol., 3:15.
—Szekeres, L., and Szmolenszky, T. 1967. The effects of quinidine, ajmaline, papaverine and adrenergic β-receptor inhibitors in experimental $BaCl_2$-arrhythmia developed for the quantitative assay of antiarrhythmic drugs. Acta Physiol. Acad. Sci. Hung., 32:365.
Rand, M.J., and Walker, J.M. 1958. A comparison of antifibrillatory drugs in the heart-lung preparation. Brit. J. Pharmacol., 13:107.
Rosenblueth, A., and Garcia-Ramos, J. 1947. Studies on flutter and fibrillation. II. The influence of artificial obstacles on experimental auricular flutter. Amer. Heart J., 33:677.
Rothberger, C.J., and Winterberg, H. 1911. Über die experimentelle Erzeugung extrasystolischer, ventriculärer Tachykardie durch Acceleranswirkung (Ein Beitrag zur Herzwirkung von Barium und Calcium). Pflügers Arch. Ges. Physiol., 142:461.
—and Winterberg, H. 1914. Über Vorhofflimmern und Vorhofflattern. Pflügers Arch. Ges. Physiol., 160:42.
Scherf, D. 1944. Experimental digitalis and strophanthin extrasystoles. Exp. Med. Surg., 21:70.

—1947. Studies on auricular tachycardia caused by aconitine administration. Proc. Soc. Exp. Biol. Med. 64:233.

—and Terranova, R. 1949. Mechanism of auricular flutter and fibrillation. Amer. J. Physiol., 159:137.

—and Chick, F.B. Experimental parasystole. Amer. Heart J., 42:212.

—and Schott, A. 1953. Extrasystoles and allied arrhythmias. London, William Heineman, Ltd.

—Blumenfeld, S., and Yildiz, M. 1963. Experimental study of ectopic impulse formation in the left atrium. Cardiologia (Basel), 43:133.

Schmidt, R.F. 1958. Versuche mit Aconitin zum Problem der spontanen Erregungsbildung im Herzen. Pflügers Arch. Ges. Physiol., 233:531.

Shumacker, H.B.J., Riberi, A., Boone, R.D., and Kajikuri, H. 1956. Ventricular fibrillation in the hypothermic state. IV. The role of extrinsic cardiac innervation. Ann. Surg., 143:223.

Somani, P., and Lum. B.K.B. 1965. The antiarrhythmic actions of beta adrenergic blocking agents. J. Pharmacol. Exp. Ther., 148:194.

—Fleming, J.G., Chan, G.K., and Lum, B.K.B. 1966. Antagonism of epinephrine-induced cardiac arrhythmias by 4-(2-isopropylamino-1-hydroxyethyl)-methansulfonanilide (MJ 1999). J. Pharmacol. Exp. Ther., 151:32.

Swain, H.H., and Curtis, G.P. 1966. The use of hypertonic solutions to produce atrial fibrillation in the dog heart-lung preparation. J. Pharmacol. Exp. Ther., 151:438.

Szekeres, L. 1964a. Auswertung von Flimmerwidrigen Substanzen, II. Conferentia Hungarica pro therapia et investigatione in pharmacologia. Budapest, Akadémiai Kiadó, p. 165.

—1964b. Discussion of Dr. West's paper. Pharmacology of cardiac function. Proc. of the Second Int. Pharmacol. Meeting Prag. Oxford, Pergamon Press, Vol. 5:143.

—and Papp, J. (Gy.) 1964. The influence of the autonomic nervous system on the mammalian heart's tendency to fibrillation. Acta Physiol. Acad. Sci. Hung. (Suppl.), 24:38.

—and Papp, J. (Gy.) 1970. Experimental cardiac arrhythmias and antiarrhythmic drugs. Budapest, Akademiai Kiado.

Takaori, M., and Loehnig, R.W. 1965. Ventricular arrhythmias during halothane anesthesia: Effect of isoproterenol, aminophylline and ephedrine. Canad. Anaesth. Soc. J., 12:275.

Terry, L.L. 1956. Correlation between pharmacological tests and clinical trial. Ann. N.Y. Acad. Sci., 64:574.

Trautwein, W., and Dudel, J. 1956. Aktionspotential und Kontraktion der Herzmuskels im Sauerstoffmangel. Pflügers Arch. Ges. Physiol., 263:23.

Turner, R.A. 1965. Screening Methods in Pharmacology. New York, Academic Press, Inc.

Van Dongen, K. 1936. The action of some drugs on fibrillation of the heart. Arch. Int. Pharmacodyn., 53:80.

Varma, D.R., Gillis, R.A., and Melville, K.I. 1963. On the relationship of catecholamines and thyroid activity to ventricular fibrillation during hypothermia in dogs. Canad. J. Biochem., 41:361.

Vassalle, M., Greenspan, K., and Hoffman, B.F. An analysis of arrhythmias induced by ouabain in intact dogs. Circ. Res., 13:132.

Vaughan Williams, E.M., and Szekeres, L. 1961. A comparison of tests for antifibrillatory action. Brit. J. Pharmacol., 17:424.

Vulpian, A.F.E. 1874. Note sur les effets de la faradisation directe des ventricules du coeur chez le chien. Arch. Physiol. Norm. Path., p. 975.

Walker, S.M. 1952. Ventricular fibrillation induced by ether inhalation in rat. Amer. J. Physiol., 169:50.

Wégria, R., and Nickerson, N.P. 1942. The effect of papaverine, epinephrine and quinidine on the fibrillation threshold of the mammalian ventricles. J. Pharmacol. Exp. Ther., 75:50.

—and Nickerson, N.D. 1943. The benzol-adrenaline test as a reliable method of estimating

changes in the sensitivity of the dog's ventricles to fibrillation. Application of the method to the study of quinidine sulfate. Amer. Heart J., 25:56.
West, T.C. 1964. Fibrillatory and antifibrillatory drugs. Pharmacology of cardiac function. Proc. of the Second Int. Pharmacol. Meeting. Oxford, Pergamon Press, 5:133.
—and Landa, J.F. 1962. Minimal mass required for induction of sustained arrhythmia in isolated atrial segments. Amer. J. Physiol., 202:232.
Wiggers, C.J., and Wégria, R. 1940. Quantitative measurement of the fibrillation thresholds of the mammalian ventricles with observation on the effect of procaine. Amer. J. Physiol., 131:296.
—and Wégria, R., Pinera, B. 1940. The effects of myocardial ischaemia on the fibrillation threshold – the mechanism of spontaneous ventricular fibrillation following coronary occlusion. Amer. J. Physiol., 131:309.
Williams, C.N., Deutsch, S., Linde, H.W., Bullough, J.W., and Dripps, R.D. 1961. Effects of intravenously administered succinyldicholine on cardiac rate rhythm and arterial pressure in anesthetized man. Anesthesiology, 22:947.
Winbury, M.M. 1956. Relation between atrial and ventricular antiarrhythmic assay methods, rationale for a screening program. Ann. N.Y. Acad. Sci., 64:564.
—and Hemmer, M.L. 1955. Action of quinidine, procaine amide and other compounds on experimental atrial and ventricular arrhythmias in the dog. J. Pharmacol. Exp. Ther., 113:402.
—Hausler, L.M., Prioli, N.A., and Zitowitz, L. 1962. Effect of epinephrine on cardiac rhythm in the miniature pig before and after coronary occlusion. J. Pharmacol. Exp. Ther., 138:287.

CHAPTER 7

Myocardial and Other Muscle Cell Cultures

Willi Halle and Albert Wollenberger

German Academy of Sciences, Institute of Circulation Research
Berlin-Buch, German Democratic Republic

INTRODUCTION

The General Principles of Cell Culture

The modern methods of cell culture were introduced almost twenty years ago by Dulbecco (1952) and Moscona (1952). It became possible then, with the aid of proteolytic enzymes, to isolate single cells en masse from compact tissues and organs (see Rinaldini, 1958, 1959). These isolated cells can be explanted into an artificial environment and may be cultivated there for various lengths of time. Cell culture may thus be defined as the maintenance and/or growth of initially discrete living cells outside the organism of origin. It differs from tissue and organ culture in that isolated cells constitute the starting material.

The authors appreciate the generosity of Professor Otto Bucher, Lausanne, Dr. Nick Sperelakis, Charlottesville, Virginia and of the copyright holders Akademische Verlagsgesellschaft Geest und Portig K.–G., Leipzig; American Heart Association, Inc., New York; S. Karger-Verlag, Basel, New York; Pergamon Press, Oxford; Rockefeller University Press, New York; and Springer-Verlag, Heidelberg; who granted permission for reproducing published materials. Mrs. Eva Janiszewski, nee Kallabis, made available to us some as yet unpublished results. Dr. Wolfgang Schulze, Berlin-Buch, supplied us with an original electron micrograph. To all of them we express our sincerest thanks.

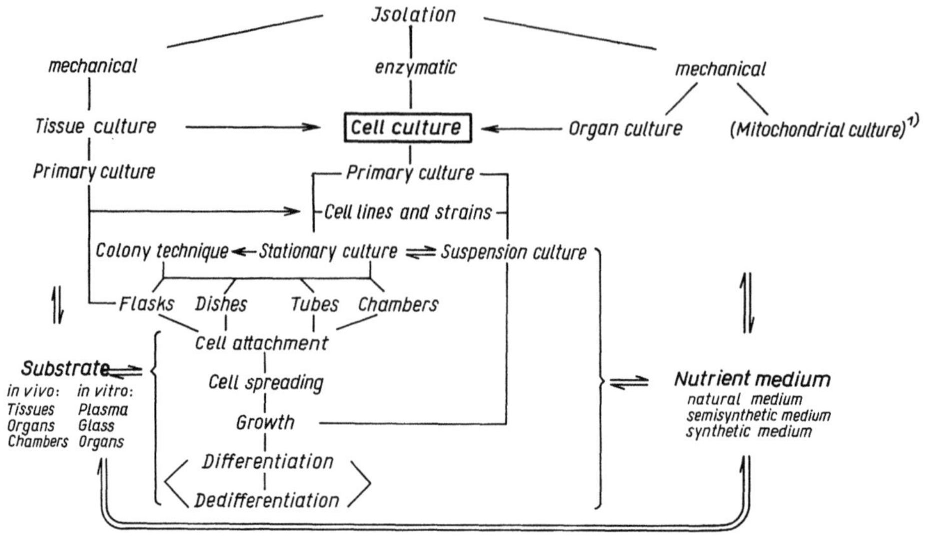

FIG. 1. Outline of the methods and principles of cell and tissue culture. (After Halle. 1967b. *Gegenbaurs Morph. Jahrb.*, 111:3. [1] Claimed by Vogel and Kemper, 1965.)

The working scheme shown in Figure 1 represents an outline of current methods of cell and tissue culture. It is presented for the purpose of briefly defining frequently used terms and to point out the position of cell culture within the framework of the known cultivating systems. According to the scheme, one may distinguish between cultures of organs, tissues, cells, and, possibly, subcellular structures such as mitochondria. Cell culture with single cells as the starting point is the method and object of choice for the study of many problems in cell biology. Tissue and cell cultures may exist as primary cultures, cell lines, and cell strains. In primary cultures we are dealing with cells, tissues, or organs that are obtained directly from the organism and in which usually several cell types exist side by side such as, for example, fibroblastlike and epitheliumlike cells. As a rule, primary cultures can be kept in a satisfactory state for about four weeks. Under favorable conditions this period can be extended to several months. The cultures then degenerate. But it is also possible for a cell type to become adapted to the new conditions of life in vitro. In this case cell division is accelerated. From such a culture, subcultures can be plated by serial passages: The primary culture becomes a cell line after the first subculture. Cell lines and strains, therefore, consist generally of only a single cell type and they can be cultivated for months and years.

In tissue culture proper, fragments of tissues or organs serve as the starting material. Explants, usually in the form of fragments less than 1 mm^3 in volume, with cells growing out of them, and pure cell cultures can be cultured in vitro on various substrates such as plasma, collagen, cellophane, polystyrene, and glass, and on living tissues or organs. They can also be cultured in vivo following implantation into the host organism. From the explants the cells may migrate and proliferate, becoming attached to, and spread out on the substrate. Such tissue cultures may develop into cell cultures. A detailed nomenclature for animal tissue and cell culture has recently been proposed and published by the Committee on Nomenclature of Tissue Culture Terminology in the Tissue Culture Association (Fedoroff, 1967).

In cell culture all cells at the start of cultivation are suspended in the nutrient medium before settling on the surface of the supporting substrate. As the single cells spread out on the surface, they often begin to reaggregate to clusters or layers which may take on tissue or organlike properties. Growth and proliferation and the processes of differentiation, dedifferentiation, and adaptation may then occur simultaneously, sequentially, or in retrograde procession.

The Maintenance of Organ-Specific Characteristics in Cell Culture

There are types of cells from normal tissues and organs that, at least for a certain time, do not lose in primary cell culture those properties they possessed in the tissue or organ of origin (see Halle, 1967b). As an example we may mention the behavior of isolated thyroid cells. Cells isolated from the thyroid glands of pig, sheep, and rat are capable of synthesizing, in the presence of ^{125}I or ^{131}I in the nutrient medium, labeled monoiodotyrosine and diiodotyrosine, triiodothyronine, thyroxine, and thyroglobulin for a period of three to seven days. TSH increases the iodine incorporation and stimulates the formation of glandlike structures (Kerkof and Chaikoff, 1966; Rabin et al., 1966).

However, organ-specific characteristics can be maintained, if at all, only for a few days or weeks in primary cell culture. After this period, organ-specific functions are no longer detectable in most cases. The cultivated cells begin then to show signs of dedifferentiation. Specific characteristics can also be maintained in cells cultured for longer periods, for example, in cell lines. Studies carried out by Green and collaborators (1965 and 1966) show that fibroblasts can still synthetize collagen and hyaluronate after 700 days in culture. Only few examples exist for the maintenance of specific characteristics in cell lines derived from normal cells. On the other hand, there are several reports describing the maintenance of such characteristics in tumor cells cultivated as cell lines or strains (see the reviews of Sato and Yasumura, 1966; Schindler, 1965; Yasumura et al., 1966).

Pharmacologic Studies of Cells Cultured In Vitro

The use of cultured cells and tissues in pharmacologic studies has been discussed in several reviews (Dawson and Dryden, 1967; Pomerat, 1954; Rosenoer and Jacobson, 1966). In most reports the interest centered on the influence of drugs on the growth and survival of normal and tumor cells and on related metabolic processes. The results obtained for the particular drugs studied are quite variable and not easily comparable, chiefly because of the heterogeneity of the cell material used as the test object. In general, less information is available on the influence of a drug on such cells in cell culture in which tissue or organ-specific characteristics are maintained for a greater length of time. But precisely these types of cells offer frequently more favorable conditions for studying the influence of drugs at the cellular level than does the study of growth processes common to many cell types. In the present chapter, attention will be focused chiefly on the maintenance of organ-specific function during cultivation.

Cells from the heart and from other muscles are isolated with the aid of proteolytic enzymes from organ fragments. The heart cells can be cultivated on glass for three to four weeks in a liquid nutrient medium. Many cells exhibit, during this period, the ability to contract spontaneously and rhythmically. Figure 2 shows an isolated heart ventricle cell spread out on glass. Figure 3 shows ventricular cells that have fused into a reticular cell layer. The cells were pulsating autorhythmically and synchronously. It is evident that cell cultures in which structural and functional changes can be registered and analyzed quantitatively in a pharmacologic experiment without affecting their viability may constitute a useful physiologic model. A good case in point is the cultured muscle cell, since it is available to quantitative functional investigation during growth and differentiation (Halle, 1963a, 1963b and 1967b; Wollenberger, 1964a).

Burrows (1910 to 1912) was the first to observe the contractions of heart cells in tissue culture. The contracting cells were present in cell monolayers on the periphery of the growth zone of explants of the embryonic chick heart. These results were taken as supporting evidence for the myogenic theory of muscle contraction. Without underrating these fundamental and important experiments, the disadvantages inherent in the method of explant culture should not be overlooked. In particular it is necessary to call attention to the following points: (1) Cultivation is possible only in natural nutrient media. These media are relatively

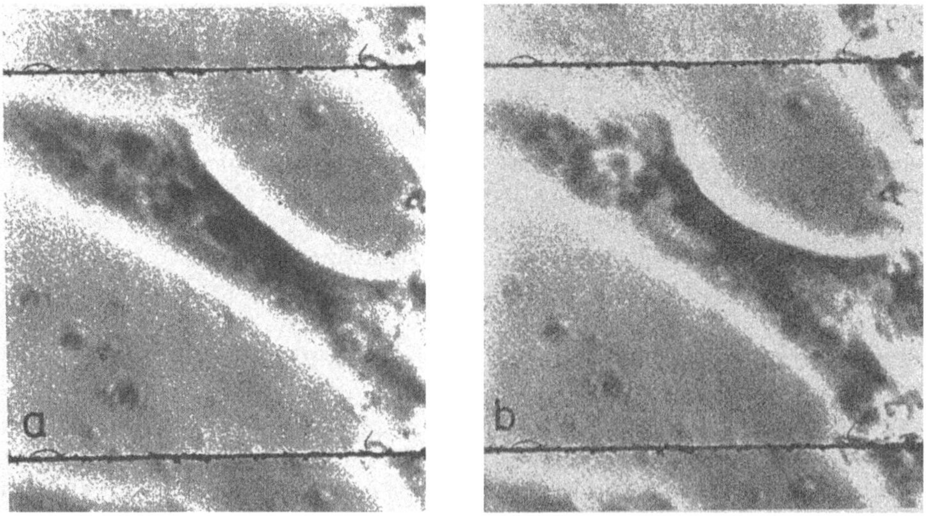

FIG. 2. An isolated spontaneously and rhythmically pulsating embryonic chick ventricle cell. Two-day culture in chemically defined nutrient medium SM 20. Cine frames. (a) in the relaxed state between two contractions and (b) in the contracted state. Final magnification × 2,000.

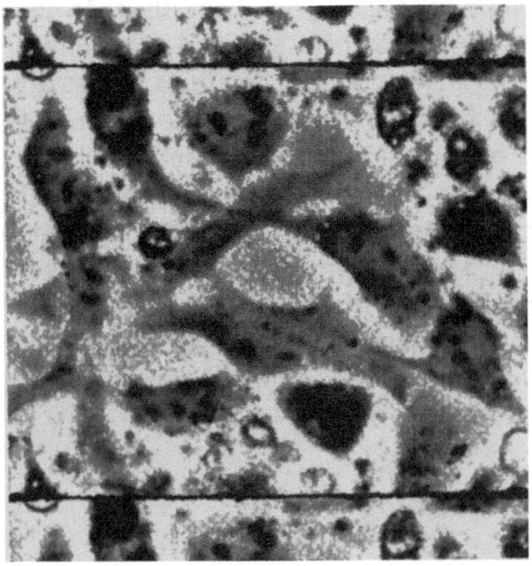

FIG. 3. A reticular cell layer formed by embryonic chick ventricle cells. Two-day culture in chemically defined nutrient medium SM 20. Cine frame. Final magnification × 600.

rich in undefined proteins and other undefined components. (2) Degenerating cells and cellular autolysis with necrotic regions in the interior of the explants can release undefined biologically active substances capable of affecting the cells (see Rinaldini, 1958). (3) Spontaneous pulsations of cells in the growth zone of muscle explants could conceivably originate in the body of the explant which may still harbor functionally intact nerve elements. (4) In such muscle cultures the number of pulsating cells is low, and quantitative evaluation of chronotropic, inotropic, and bathmotropic effects of a drug is hardly possible.

The isolated muscle cells in cell culture do not possess these drawbacks and are, therefore, better suited for the study of the action of drugs at the cellular level.

METHODS

The methods described in detail in this section have proved in our laboratory to be satisfactory for the cultivation of spontaneously pulsating heart and amnion muscle cells of chick embryos, and lately also for the cultivation of neonatal rat heart cells (see Appendix). They permit the establishment of standardized and readily reproducible conditions of cultivation. This is an essential requirement because the isolated cell in vitro is readily exposed to a large number of deleterious factors to which the cells in the intact organ in vivo are much less vulnerable.

The Laboratory

Penso and Balducci (1963) have described various types of tissue culture laboratories and presented examples of their layout. There are tissue culture laboratories that employ not more than one technician and a second laboratory helper and which occupy an area of not more than 25 m^2. Such a unit can house one large or two small sterile cabinets, a small lockchamber, a washing and rinsing unit, a table for preparatory work, and facilities for writing and microscopy. The remaining space serves for accommodating two incubators, a refrigerator, and a hot air sterilizer. It is not advisable to install an autoclave in this unit. Persons not belonging to the tissue culture laboratory should not be allowed to enter this unit. Needless to say, the washing and rinsing facility should be used exclusively for cleaning the glassware and equipment employed in the cell and tissue culture work. It is also generally known that histologic work, in particular the treatment of cultures with heavy metal fixatives, should never be conducted in a tissue culture laboratory. No glass equipment and apparatus used for cultivating cells should be used for other purposes.

Cleaning the Sterile Rooms

All surfaces and the floors in sterile rooms are to be cleaned daily; the walls are cleaned once a week. We use a 1 percent solution of the disinfectant Fesiamon, a product of VEB Fettchemie, Karl-Marx-Stadt (dimethylaminoacetic acid dodecyl-amidochlorobenzylate 10 g, sodium nitrite 1 g, sodium phosphate 2 g, water 87 g) and allow the cleaned surfaces to dry in the air. Prior to the start of an experiment, tables and similar surfaces are washed with 70 percent alcohol, and two ultraviolet lamps are turned on for 60 minutes. The sterile rooms need not be ventilated with germ-free air, unless the ultraviolet lamps have produced more than traces of ozone. This is usually not the case if the lamps are equipped with quartz glass impermeable to wavelengths of less than 220 nm.

The floors in the other rooms are cleaned daily with Fesiamon or a similar disinfectant.

Cleaning of the Glassware

Standard cleaning procedures have been described in detail in the monographs of Hanks et al. (1955), Penso and Balducci (1963), and in the review of Cahn et al. (1967). We are presently using them with only minor changes. In the following we present a list of cleaning instructions which have been followed for years in our laboratory. The washing detergent Fit (powder form) used in our laboratory is a product of VEB Fettchemie, Karl-Marx-Stadt, and is similar in its action to the anionic detergent Micro-Solv, an alkyl-aryl-sulfonate specifically prepared for use with tissue culture glassware by Microbiological Associates, Bethesda, Maryland, and to the anionic detergent 7X(Serva Entwicklungslabor, Heidelberg, and other sources).

1. CLEANING OF NEW GLASSWARE

a. Glassware without cover slips

(1) Remove obvious dirt (glass dust, etc.) with warm tap water.

(2) Brush vigorously in a 0.2 percent Fit solution.
(3) Rinse in running hot water.
(4) Rinse in running cold water.
(5) Place in a 1 percent HCl solution for 20 to 24 hours.
(6) Wash with a 0.2 percent Fit solution.
(7) Rinse in running hot water.
(8) Rinse in running cold water.
(9) Rinse twice with distilled water (double distilled water).*
(10) Dry in a drying oven at 100°C.
(11) Sterilize for 90 minutes at 190°C in a hot air sterilizer.

b. Cover slips. Use only new microscope cover slips (maximum thickness 0.17 mm) and discard after use.
(1) Preliminary cleaning–see 1a(1).
(2) Wash–see 1a(6).
(3) Place in concentrated sulfuric acid for 24 hours.
(4) Rinse–see 1a(3) to (4).
(5) Acid treatment–see 1a(5).
(6) Rinse–see 1a(3) to (4).
(7) Rinse for 5 hours in running tap water.
(8) Place in distilled water for 24 hours and change water three times.
(9) Dry–see 2a(7)–and place in petri dishes.
(10) Sterilize–see 1a(11). After repeated sterilization, the cover slips may become covered with a fine coat and should in this case be either discarded or cleaned once more.

2. CLEANING OF USED GLASSWARE.–The cleaning procedure is in principle the same, except that the acid treatment is not carried out; however, see 2a(5).

a. Culture and medium flasks, hollow ground slides
(1) Rinse with cold water after use, fill with water up to the rim, and allow to stand until the cleaning is started.
(2) Thoroughly remove the paraffin on the Thomas or other culture flasks and on the slides. If necessary, cook in Fit solution.
(3) Wash–see 1a(6).
(4) Rinse–see 1a(3) to (4).
(5) Rinse with 1 percent HCl solution and let stand for approximately 60 minutes in this solution.
(6) Proceed as described under 1a(7) to 1a(9).
(7) Dry the glass surface of the culture bottles onto which the cells stick with a clean linen cloth. Alternatively expose the vessels to water steam.
(8) Dry and sterilize–see 1a(10) to (11).

*The term "distilled water" used in this chapter always refers to water twice distilled in a quartz apparatus.

b. Pipettes
   (1) Rinse by rapid passage of cold water to remove adhering cells and/or protein-containing nutrient medium.
   (2) Treat with acid–see 1a(5).
   (3) Rinse with running water in a pipette cleaning apparatus for approximately 10 hours.
   (4) Rinse–see 1a(9).
   (5) Dry, place into pipette containers, and sterilize–see 1a(10) to (11).

c. Filters for sterilizing nutrient media and other solutions. We use the glass bacterial filters 117-G 5 (manufactured by Saale-Glas GmbH, Jena) for sterilizing nutrient media and other solutions by means of suction filtration. According to Bechhold, the filter plate has a maximum fictive pore diameter averaging 1.35μm.
   (1) Rinse the filter plate with a strong jet of cold water; do not brush.
   (2) Fill the space above the filter plate with distilled water and allow the water to drain through the filter plate for 24 hours.
   (3) Suck boiling distilled water several times through the filter plate.
   (4) Rinse the entire filter with cold distilled water.
   (5) Cover the filter and allow to dry in air.
   (6) Sterilize for 90 minutes at 180°C in the hot air sterilizer.

   After a longer period of use, the filter must be chemically cleaned with hot concentrated sulfuric acid and then subjected to treatment according to the instructions given by the manufacturer.

d. Rubber stoppers and sealing rings
   (1) Brush vigorously with a hot 1 percent Fit solution.
   (2) Rinse–see 1a(3).
   (3) Boil in water for 10 minutes.
   (4) Rinse–see 1a(9).
   (5) Boil in distilled water for 30 minutes.
   (6) Place on a linen cloth and let dry in the air for approximately 20 minutes.
   (7) Place in autoclave for 30 minutes at 2 atmospheres (132°C).

Glassware, such as beakers, graduated cylinders, Erlenmeyer flasks, etc., is cleaned as described under 2a, omitting, however, items 2a(2), (5), and (7).

Prior to sterilization the openings of bottles, flasks, pipettes, and filters are covered with aluminum foil. Slides and petri dishes with cover slips should be wrapped in aluminum foil before sterilization. Cotton stoppers are used in the usual manner only for the mouths of the pipettes and filters. The use of tissue paper and cheesecloth stoppers should be avoided in order to prevent contamination of the fluids and cultures. Tissue paper swabs are sterilized in the autoclave for 30 minutes at 2 atmospheres (132°C).

A quartz apparatus serves for making double-distilled water, which is used for rinsing, for nutrient media, and for other solutions to which the cells are exposed. In our experience, water treated with ion exchange resins is not suited for cultivating cells. Such water should additionally be subjected to double distillation.

Nutrient Media; Salt and Trypsin Solutions

SEMISYNTHETIC NUTRIENT MEDIA.—Various types of nutrient media are used for cultivating animal cells and may be classified, depending on their composition, into natural, semisynthetic, conditioned, or synthetic nutrient media. Table 1 lists the undefinable, biologically active body and cell components that

TABLE 1

The Various Classes of Media and Their Basic Components

Phase	Natural Media	Semisynthetic Media	"Conditioned" Synthetic Media	Synthetic Media
"Solid"	Plasma (or collagen)	–	–	Cellulose derivatives
Liquid	Salt solution Glucose Embryo extract Serum	Salt solution Carbohydrate Amino acids* Some vitamins Serum†	Salt solution Carbohydrate Amino acids Some vitamins Nondefined biologic factors coming out of masses of cultured cells	Salt solution Carbohydrate Amino acids Some vitamins Nonnutrient macromolecules‡

*Amino acids can be replaced by hydrolysates of lactalbumin and other proteins.
†Serum can be replaced by serum dialysate, protein fractions, and dialyzed serum.
‡Cellulose derivatives (methylcellulose, dinitrocellulose), dextran, polyvinylpyrrolidone.

constitute the bulk of the various so-called natural nutrient media and are not present in synthetic media. But a clear delineation, such as the one presented here, is not possible in every case. In general, however, a synthetic nutrient medium that contains not more than 15 percent serum and 5 percent embryo extract (diluted 1:1 with salt solution) can be still classified as a semisynthetic medium.

On account of the incomplete knowledge of the composition of plasma, embryo extract, and serum, whose components may be subject to wide fluctuations, it is difficult to rigidly standardize experimental conditions when using these fluids and to perform reproducible experiments aimed at discovering essential growth and differentiation factors (see Kopac, 1954; Puck et al., 1958; White and Waymouth, 1954).

For this reason attempts have been made, ever since the tissue culture technique came into being, to eliminate the uncontrollable factors and to prepare simple nutrient media. However, it was observed time and again, that only very complex nutrient media promote the maintenance, growth, and proliferation of cells in vitro. Some idea of the histroical development in this field is given by the sequential listing of the nutrient media in Table 1. As the understanding of the nutritive requirements of cultured cells and tissues increased with increasing knowledge of their metabolism (cf. Eagle, 1965a, 1965b; Eagle and Levintow, 1965; Lucy, 1965; Paul, 1965), it became possible to produce commercial synthetic basal and minimum essential media for mammalian cell lines. Of special value in this connection were the biochemical investigations of Eagle (1955, 1959), who established the requirements for specific amino acids and other substances. Rapid proliferation of cell lines and strains, however, usually requires the addition of about 1 percent serum or of 3 to 5 percent dialyzed serum.

Serum or serum components that are added to a synthetic nutritive medium are important not only for growth. They are also responsible for the fact that cells from various organs can keep their organ-specific characteristics in culture for a certain length of time.

It is beyond the scope of this chapter to go into a detailed discussion of this still largely unexplored function of serum and of the protein fractions (cf. the review of Halle, 1963c). Suffice it to state that serum proteins play a role in the nutrition of the cells and are necessary for their optimum growth. In addition they help to buffer the nutrient medium and promote the adhesion and spread of the cells on glass.

There are also certain sera that have a deleterious influence on cultured cells. The immunoglobins and, in particular, Cohn's plasma protein fraction II (γ-globulins) can be responsible for this effect. However, other components of sera have been isolated and partly characterized which can stimulate or inhibit the growth and the mutual adhesion of cultured cells as well as their attachment to the glass substrate (Curtis, 1965; see also DeHaan, 1967a). One of these substances is fetuin, an α_1-glycoprotein, which has been isolated from fetal calf serum and which promotes adhesion and growth of isolated cells on glass (c.f. Puck et al., 1968). Harary et al. (1966) reported that isolated rat heart cells incubated in a synthetic nutrient medium are able to attach themselves to polystyrene plastic dishes only in the presence of fetuin.

The semisynthetic nutrient medium M 12, which we used at first for spontaneously pulsating muscle cells, is the modified amino acid hydrolysate medium of Edlinger et al. (1958). Its composition is shown in Table 2. Adenosine, xanthine, hypoxanthine, and peptone were added to this medium on the basis of the studies of Cavanaugh (1955) and Cavanaugh and Cavanaugh (1957) on the cultivation of isolated beating chick embryo heart cells and of other studies, reviewed by Morgan (1958), on the nutrition, metabolism, and growth of fibroblastlike cells from explants of embryonic chick heart fragments in a synthetic nutrient medium.

The amino acids listed in Table 3 are added in the preparation of medium M 12 by dissolving 500 mg of the amino acid hydrolysate Aminovit (Boehringer, GmbH Mannheim,) in 1 liter of the otherwise complete nutrient medium. The amino acid composition of Aminovit has been determined by this firm through microbiologic assay (Table 3).

In order to simplify the preparation of the M 12, the individual components are pooled in different groups according to their solubility (Table 4). We usually weigh out an amount of each substance sufficient to prepare 100 liters of medium. The components making up each group are finely ground and thoroughly mixed in a mortar. The powders are placed in bottles and can be kept in a desiccator at 4°C for at least 6 months.

TABLE 2

*Compositions of the Semisynthetic Media M 12 and M 19 and of the Synthetic Medium SM 20**

	M 12	M 19	SM 20	Comments
NaCl	6,500	6,500	6,500	
KCl	350	350	64.9	
KH_2PO_4	60	60	60	
Na_2HPO_4 $12H_2O$	150	150	150	
$CaCl_2$	140	140	140	
$MgCl_2 \cdot 6H_2O$	200	200	200	
$NaHCO_3$	3,200	3,200	330	
D-Glucose	2,000	2,000	2,000	
Glutamine	70	70	70	
Cystine	5	5	5	
Tyrosine	9	9	9	
Cysteine-HCl	1	1	1	
Arginine†	13	21.5	21.5	
Histidine†	8	13	13	
Histidine	–	–	775	Buffer
Isoleucine†	22.5	45	45	containing 50%
Leucine†	42	84	84	D-allo-Isoleucine
Lysine†	25.5	34	34	
Methionine†	12	24	24	
Phenylalanine†	21.5	43	43	
Threonine†	15	30	30	
Tryptophan†	5	10	10	
Valine†	31	62	62	
DL-Serine	–	20	20	
Proline	–	10	10	
Hydroxyproline	–	5	5	
Thiamine-HCl	1	1	1	
Pyridoxine-HCl	1	1	1	
Ca-Pantothenate	1	1	1	
Niacinamide	1	1	1	
p-Aminobenzoic acid	1	1	1	
Choline chloride	1	1	1	
Biotin	1	1	1	
Folic acid	1	1	1	
Riboflavin	0.2	0.2	0.2	
meso-Inositol	1	1	1	
L-Ascorbic acid	2	2	2	
Adenosine	7	7	7	
Xanthine	0.8	0.8	0.8	
Hypoxanthine	1.2	1.2	1.2	
Hydrocortisone	–	1	1	
Peptone pr. bact.	5,000	5,000	–	
Streptomycin sulfate	100	100	100	
Penicillin G	100,000 IE	100,000 IE	100,000 IE	

*C.P. grade of all substances, where available. Unless otherwise stated, the amino acids are present in the L-form. Concentrations are listed in mg per liter.

†Present in "Aminovit;" see Table 3.

Prior to use, the required aliquots of each mixture of dry substances are dissolved in one of the solvents listed in Table 4, using small conical centrifuge tubes. When preparing 1 liter of medium, these solutions are transferred into a 1-liter flask containing approximately 500 ml of distilled water. More water is

TABLE 3

*Composition of the Amino Acid Mixture in 500 mg of the Casein Hydrolysate "Aminovit"**

Arginine	13 mg
Histidine	8 mg
Isoleucine	22.5 mg
Leucine	42 mg
Lysine	25.5 mg
Methionine	12 mg
Phenylalanine	21.5 mg
Threonine	15 mg
Tryptophan	5 mg
Valine	31 mg
Total	195.5 mg

*Product of Boehringer, Mannheim GmbH. All amino acids are present in the L-form.

TABLE 4

Grouping of Some of the Components of the Media of Table 2 According to Their Solubility

Group	Substances		Dissolve 1% of the Quantity Listed for Each Group in:
1	Ascorbic acid	0.20 g	5 ml distilled water
	Cysteine-HCl	0.10 g	
		0.30 g	
2	Thiamine-HCl	0.10 g	5 ml distilled water
	Pyridoxine-HCl	0.10 g	
	Ca-Pantothenate	0.10 g	
	Niacinamide	0.10 g	
	p-Aminobenzoic acid	0.10 g	
	meso-Inositol	0.10 g	
		0.60 g	
3	Tyrosine	0.90 g	0.2 ml 1 N HCl + 0.5 ml distilled water
	Cystine	0.50 g	
		1.40 g	
4	Hypoxanthine	0.12 g	0.1 ml NH_4OH + 1 ml distilled water
	Xanthine	0.08 g	
		0.20 g	
5	Biotin	0.10 g	3 ml distilled water, and adding slowly 3 ml of 2.8% $NaHCO_3$
	Folic acid	0.10 g	
	Riboflavin	0.02 g	
		0.22 g	
6	Amino acids without glutamine, cystine, thyrosine, cysteine-HCl, and histidine (buffer)	40.15 g	20 ml distilled water

added to bring the volume up to approximately 900 ml. Prior to filling up to 1,000 ml, glucose, glutamine, and bicarbonate are added in this sequence (see Morgan et al., 1955; Swim and Parker, 1958).

After filtration of the solution through a paper filter, it is sterilized by suction filtration through a 117-G5 filter. One can also use a Millipore, Gelman, or other vacuum filter holder with membrane filters of pore size 0.45 μm (see Cahn, 1967a; Cahn et al., 1967). All solutions destined for use in cultivation should be stored at 4°C for not more than 30 hours in the unsterilized state.

Calf serum, which has been inactivated in a water bath for 30 minutes at 56°C and been sterilized by filtration through a Seitz stainless steel pressure filter or by other means, is added to the M 12 to give a concentration of 10 percent serum.

Besides the M 12, we have mainly used in our laboratory the media M 18 (Halle, 1963b), M 19 (Table 2), and M 20. In these three media Aminovit is omitted. Hydrocortisone is added on the basis of the findings of Flückiger and Verzãr (1957a, 1957b), Grossfeld (1959), and Tanz (1960). M 19 likewise contains 10 percent serum. M 20 differs from M 19 in that serum is replaced by Cohn's protein fractions V (albumin, 0.32 percent) and/or IV_1 and IV_4 (α-globulin, each 0.02 percent) (Pentex, Inc., Kankakee, Illinois). Depending on the proteins added, M 20 is then designated as M 20-AGP (albumin, globulin, peptone), M 20-A (albumin), etc. The bicarbonate concentration in M 20 is reduced from 38.1 mM to 3.9 mM, which lowers the sodium concentration by 23 percent. The weak phosphate-bicarbonate buffer is supplemented by 5 mM histidine, which buffers from pH 7.2 downward. This buffer makes it possible to work in open systems in air atmosphere (see p. 216). Phosphate in higher concentration, imidazole, tris, and tes proved to be deleterious to heart cells (E. Kallabis, unpublished studies).

In the preparation of M 20 the procedure used for the preparation of M 12 is followed in principle. A solution of 775 mg histidine in 90 ml of water, adjusted to pH 9.6 with 1 N NaOH, is added before making up to the final volume. At the start of the cultivation the pH of the medium is 7.6 ± 0.2 and does not drop below 7.2 during cultivation.

More recently we have been using, in the preparation of M 20, 100-fold concentrated stock solutions of most of the groups of substances listed in Table 4. They are kept frozen at –20°C. Tyrosine and cystine are best kept as a substance mixture in the dry state. We have not as yet prepared our media in the form of dry powders (see Greene et al., 1965; Swim and Parker, 1958; Young et al., 1966).

As in the case of M 12, the serum or protein fractions, with the exception of peptone, are added shortly before the start of cultivation or before renewing the medium during cultivation.

THE SYNTHETIC NUTRIENT MEDIUM SM 20.—The cultivation of animal cells from multicellular organisms in primary cell culture or as cell lines or strains in a chemically defined nutrient medium is still difficult and problematic in the great majority of cases, but it offers many advantages (Halle, 1963c; Waymouth, 1965a, 1965b). Nevertheless, it is often preferable to culture a well-defined and morphologically clean cell type in an undefined or partly defined nutrient medium rather than a poorly definable cell type in a well-defined nutrient medium (see Konigsberg, 1963). However, in those cases in which the growth and differentiation of cells can be studied in a chemically defined nutrient medium, it is easier to specify the extracellular factors that promote and retard growth and differentiation.

The use of a synthetic nutrient medium may be of value in the study of the response of cultured cells to drugs or other small molecules which are bound to serum proteins, because fluctuations in the effective concentration of these molecules from test to test due to the use of different sera with varying protein content are avoided.

For cultivation studies in chemically defined media fibroblastlike (Dietel-Mauersberger and Tanneberger, 1964; Evans et al., 1964; Ham, 1965; Sanford et al., 1963) and epitheliumlike (DenBeste et al., 1966; Evans et al., 1964; Ham, 1965) cells of lines and strains were used which were adapted to the new conditions of cultivation. Cultivation of primary cells cultures in synthetic media is a more difficult task. Healy and Parker (1966a, 1966b) reported that mouse embryo cells freshly isolated with trypsin were multiplying in linear progression during cultivation in a chemically defined basal medium (CMRL-1415) which was supplemented with 7 percent of the nonnutrient macromolecule dextran (molecular weight 100,000 to 200,000). The second subculture could be seeded already 6 to 9 days after explantation in vitro, and cultivation was possible for several weeks.

Mouse embryo cells were also used by Andresen et al. (1967). These authors isolated by a mechanical procedure single cells and small aggregates of cells. The medium was renewed after 30 days. After having maintained the cultures for 500 days in the same culture flasks, i.e., without subcultivation, the authors observed an increased proliferation of the cells. Subcultures could be plated through the transfer of mechanically separated fragments of multilayered sheets of fibroblast-like cells into other culture flasks. In both studies whole embryos were used.

Since in such experiments several cell types of different organization and grade of differentiation are present at the start of cultivation, the chance for a successful cultivation is greater than if only a single tissue or organ is selected. A study by Waymouth (1965b) is of interest in this connection. Fibroblastlike cells were isolated with the aid of trypsin from the lungs of mouse embryos and were cultured in a chemically defined medium supplemented with insulin. The cells had to be kept in the phase of maintenance for almost 500 days in the culture flasks before the first subcultivation could be started. This lag phase preceding the phase of proliferative growth is unusually long. Long-term cultivation of masses of single cells in primary cell culture or as cell lines or strains in a chemically defined medium has not yet been achieved without loss of tissue- or organ-specific functions.

In the course of the development of a synthetic nutrient medium for the cultivation of isolated, spontaneously active heart cells in primary culture, which led to the formulation of the chemically defined medium SM 20, the amino acid hydrolysate was replaced by chemically defined substances (substitution method of Waymouth, 1965a). The "analytical" method proved to be the most suitable one; i.e., the cultivating conditions were simplified step by step by gradual elimination of undefined factors from semisynthetic media (see the note by Willmer, 1960). The composition of SM 20 is shown in Table 2. It contains neither peptone nor serum protein fractions and is therefore termed a fully defined nutrient medium. The SM 20 is simpler in its composition than other synthetic nutrient media, since it contains only 42 different components, in contrast to the media CMRL-1415 (Healy and Parker, 1966a) and MAB 87/3 (Waymouth, 1965b), which contain 50 and 51 components, respectively.

The Na^+ concentration in SM 20, like that in M 20, amounts to only 115.6 mM. In SM 20 the concentration of K^+ has been lowered to 1.3 mM. This is a favorable concentration for the spontaneous beating of cultured embryonic chick heart cells (Cahn, 1964; DeHaan, 1967a, 1967b).

The preparation of SM 20 is carried out in the same manner as that of M 20. When using distilled water having a pH of about 5.2, an additional 1.2 ml of 1 N NaOH must be added to the histidine solution in order to attain a pH of the medium of 7.6 at the outset of cultivation.

SALT AND TRYPSIN SOLUTIONS.—The composition of the buffered salt solution (BSS) free of Ca^{++} and Mg^{++} ions is shown in Table 5. The BSS serves

TABLE 5
Composition of the Ca^{++} and Mg^{++}-free Buffered Salt Solution (BSS)

Substance	Concentration (gram per liter)
NaCl	7.000
KCl	0.340
KH_2PO_4	0.060
$Na_2HPO_4 \cdot 12H_2O$	0.150
$NaHCO_3$	2.100
Streptomycin sulfate	0.100
Penicillin G	100,000 IE

for washing the fragments and the cell suspensions and for dissolving the trypsin.

A 0.1 percent solution of crude powdered trypsin (a product of Vitrum, Stockholm) gave good results in the preparation of single cell suspension from organ fragments. Aliquots of 5 or 10 ml of the enzyme solution are stored frozen at –20°C until use. Harary and Farley (1963a) used a 0.1 percent solution of trypsin 1-300 (obtained from Nutritional Biochemicals Corporation, Cleveland, Ohio). Trinkaus and Lentz (1964) used 3 percent trypsin plus 1 percent pancreatin. Other proteolytic enzymes such as collagenase (see Smith and Berndt, 1964) and pronase were not found to be superior to trypsin with respect to the cell yield or to the morphology of the cells obtained. Neither is the percentage of pulsating cells increased through the use of these enzymes (E. Kallabis, unpublished findings).

Schneider et al. (1965) added 0.1 percent methyl cellulose to a 0.25 percent solution of trypsin free of divalent ions. This solution dissociates the intact hearts of 6–day-old chick embryos into single cells. It is also used on the following day for washing the cell layers that have formed on the glass. The solution is very gently agitated over the cells for about 30 sec and is then poured off. A morphologically pure cell layer is obtained with this procedure.

The Cell Cultures

The preparation of a suspension consisting of individual heart cells is accomplished in two steps: (1) isolation of organ fragments; and (2) preparation of single cell suspensions by the trypsinization procedure. Eggs of chickens, usually White Leghorns, incubated at 37°C for 9 to 13 days, furnish the starting material.

1. PREPARATION OF THE ORGAN FRAGMENTS.

a. Rub eggs with 70 percent ethyl alcohol.
b. Using a pair of scissors, cut a hole in the egg shell at the blunt end of the egg in such a way that a calotte-shaped portion of the shell can be removed.
c. Transfer the embryo under sterile conditions to a petri dish with the aid of a pair of flat tweezers.
d. Open embryo on the ventral side with two scalpels, dissect the heart free, and remove the vessels.
e. Collect 10 hearts in a petri dish containing BSS.
f. Transfer the hearts to another sterile petri dish, 90 mm in diameter, and wash with fresh BSS.
g. Separate the atria from the ventricles in 2 ml BSS with a single cut.
h. Remove by aspiration the atria, vessel fragments, and other pieces of tissue that are not going to be processed further.
i. Add 2 ml BSS to the ventricles.
j Cut ventricles into fragments of approximately 1 mm^3 by shearing the ventricles between the cutting blades of two sharp scalpels.
k. Transfer the fragments to a 10-ml centrifuge tube.
l. Wash fragments twice, each time using 5 to 10 ml of BSS. The major portion of the residual blood can then be removed with a pipette after the sedimentation of the fragments.

2. TRYPSINIZATION PROCEDURE I

a. Remove the BSS by suction and add 4 ml of a 0.1 percent solution of trypsin.
b. Place at once the centrifuge tubes with the fragments to be digested in an incubator for 20 minutes at 37°C. Shake the tubes gently several times during this period.
c. Break up the fragments by repeated passage of the entire contents of the tubes through a narrow-bore pipette: individual cells become dissociated.
d. Dilute trypsin solution with 5 ml BSS.
e. Separate the cell suspension from the sedimented fragment residues and bigger cell clusters by pipetting or filtration through gauze.
f. Centrifuge at ~700 rpm = 50*g* for 4 minutes.
g. Suck off the diluted supernatant trypsin solution and the suspended cell debris.
h. Wash the cells by resuspending the pellets in BSS.
i. Centrifuge (see f).
j. Suck off the BSS.
k. Resuspend pellets in nutrient medium.

l. Remove 0.1 ml of the cell suspension with a pipette for cell count (see section "cell counting").
m. Start the cultivation by taking the cell suspension and placing equal aliquots in each culture vessel.
n. Incubate culture vessels in an incubator at 37°C.
o. Check the glass walls of the used centrifuge tubes with a microscope in order to make sure that only a relatively small number of cells is attached. Attachment is not possible on siliconized glass walls.

3. TRYPSINIZATION PROCEDURE II.—This procedure, used by Miss Eva Kallabis (unpublished studies), is a slight modification of the so-called fractionated trypsinization procedure described by others for the preparation of primary cultures of other cell types. It is similar to the procedures outlined by Harary and Farley (1963a) and by DeHaan (1967a, 1967b).

a. Prepare fragments from 35 ventricles as described under 1a to l.
b. Place fragments in a 25-ml Erlenmeyer flask containing 5 ml of a 0.1 percent trypsin solution.
c. Agitate solution at 37°C with a magnetic stirrer having a glass-covered magnet core weighing 1g (~200 rpm) for 8 to 10 minutes.
d. Remove the cell suspension formed completely with the aid of a pipette and discard.
e. Add 7.5 ml of fresh trypsin solution to the slightly digested fragments.
f. Stir with magnetic stirrer for 20 minutes at 37°C.
g. Switch off magnetic stirrer and allow the fragment residues to settle.
h. Pipette 3.75 ml of cell suspension into each of two 10-ml centrifuge tubes.
i. Dilute trypsin solution by placing 3.75 ml BSS into each tube.
j. Store the two cell suspensions in an ice bath at 0°C until fragments and larger cell clusters have settled.
k. Separate the cell suspension from the remains of the fragments and from the cell clusters (see 2e).
l. Centrifuge at 120_g.
m. Suck off the diluted trypsin solution (see 2g).
n. Wash by resuspending in BSS (see 2h).
o. Collect the two cell suspensions in one tube and store in an ice bath at 0°C for 10 to 20 minutes.
p. Repeat the trypsinization with the remaining fragment residues from 3g according to procedure 3e to h.
q. Treat the two cell suspensions according to 3i to o.
r. If a very high cell yield is desired, repeat once more the trypsinization and follow-up treatments according to 3e to o.
s. Centrifuge (see 3l) the cell suspensions obtained in the two or three trypsinizations.
t. Suck off BSS.
u. Resuspend each of the two or three pellets separately by pipetting in about one fifth of the amount of nutrient medium necessary for cultivation. Pool the suspensions in one tube.

v. Store the cell suspension in medium in the ice bath at 0°C for about 20 minutes.
w. Withdraw 0.1 ml of the cell suspension with a pipette for cell count (see section "cell counting").
x. Dilute the cell suspension with nutrient medium to obtain desired cell population density for cultivation and transfer to culture vessels.
y. Incubate (see 2n).
z. Inspect the glass walls of the centrifuge tubes with a microscope (see 2o).

A cell suspension is obtained more rapidly and easily using trypsinization procedure I, but procedure II has the advantage that cells damaged in the cutting process are apparently removed from the fragments by the preliminary trypsinization. Moreover, it avoids possible extensive damage of the cells caused by the mechanical breakup of the fragments during the repeated passage through the narrow-bore pipette (2c).

The yield of viable cells (without 3r) is about twice as high in procedure II as it is in procedure I. The number of dead cells amounts to only 5 to 8 percent in procedure II as compared to 20 percent in procedure I. On the basis of preliminary findings the use of procedure II cannot be recommended for cultivation in SM 20, since the number of pulsating cells obtained is significantly lower than after dissociation by procedure I.

In our experience the use of trypsin inhibitors following trypsinization (DeHaan, 1967a, 1967b) is of no visible advantage.

The procedures described in 1,2, and 3, with the exception of the trypsinizations, are carried out at room temperature, i.e., at 20° to 25°C. All procedures should be carried out under sterile conditions. For instance, each time the centrifuge tubes, culture flasks, and flasks containing sterile solutions are opened or closed, the mouths and the rubber stoppers should be flamed with a gas flame or other heat source. When following procedure 1, two sets of dissection instruments should be used. Following their use the instruments should be cleaned with sterile swabs and should then be immersed into 70 percent ethyl alcohol. Thereafter the wet instruments are flamed and transferred to a petri dish in which the remaining alcohol burns off. The work is then continued with the second set of instruments, which in the meantime has cooled and is ready for use.

An unused sterile pipette should be taken from the pipette jar for each operation requiring a pipette.

If these instructions are adhered to, there is a reasonable degree of assurance that exogenous infections of the cultures do not occur. However, it is necessary to check the cultured muscle cells or cell suspensions from time to time for mycoplasma or L forms of bacteria, either by means of electron microscopy or better still by culturing these organisms on specific nutrient media (see Buskirk, 1967; Hayflick, 1967; Macpherson, 1966).

Procedures 2 and 3 can also be used for dissociating pieces of heart atria from 11-day-old chick embryos or pieces of amnion from 8-day-old chick embryos into individual cells.

CELL COUNTING.—Various types of hemacytometer chambers, such as the counting chambers of Fuchs and Rosenthal or of Thoma, can be used for the visual determination of the number of viable and nonviable cells in the suspension after trypsinization, employing neutral red and trypan blue, respectively, for staining (see Girardi et al., 1956). In the trypan blue procedure the following components are mixed together about 5 minutes before starting the count: 0.1 ml of a 0.2 percent solution of trypan blue, 0.1 ml of the cell suspension in nutrient medium or BSS, and 0.1 ml BSS. The dead cells and cell debris can be distinguished from the unstained cells by their blue coloration, which indicates that these cells are impermeable to the dye. They are hence considered viable. Recommendations for the use of electronic cell counters, such as the Coulter electronic counter, are given in the paper by Smith and Berndt (1964).

CULTIVATION.—Primary cultures of ventricle cells are usually cultured in our laboratory in 1.5-mm-thick hollow ground slides, using M 12 and M 19; in small round culture flasks constructed according to Thomas (1937) (see Fig. 7); in modified Thomas flasks (Halle, 1960), using M 20 and SM 20; and in Bucher flasks (Bender et al., 1968), using M 20. But cultivation is also possible in Maximow slides (Rumery and Rieke, 1967), in other types of culture flasks, in test tubes, and in glass or plastic petri dishes, such as, for example, plastic Cooper dishes (Falcon, Plastics Division of B-D Laboratories, Inc., Los Angeles, California). It may sometimes be of advantage to incubate the cultures at 37.5°C in a humid atmosphere of 5 percent carbon dioxide, 40 percent oxygen, and 55 percent nitrogen, or in a mixture of 5 percent CO_2, 10 percent O_2 and 85 percent N_2 (DeHaan, 1967a).

Hollow Ground Slide Cultures.—We use hollow ground slides having a depression 0.4 mm in depth and 16 mm in diameter. The volume is approximately 4 mm^3. Cell suspension in nutrient medium, 0.1 ml, is placed on the slide and is covered with a cover slip in such a manner that a small air bubble, having a diameter of approximately 5 mm and a volume of about 1.0 mm^3, remains in the center of the cavity. Excess suspension is removed with sterile swabs, and an airtight seal is placed around the cover slip with sterile paraffin (melting point 60°C). Prior to incubating at 37°C the hollow ground slides are inverted so that the cover slips upon which the muscle cells are going to settle are facing downward.

Using trypsinization procedure I, 10 heart ventricles of 11-day-old chick embryos are necessary for obtaining 10 cultures in hollow ground slides. At the start of cultivation the cell density is approximately 150,000 cells per milliliter of nutrient medium.

An area of approximately 180 mm^2 is available for the adhesion and flattening of the cells on each hollow ground slide. There are several reasons for using a relatively low quantity of cells: (1) The volume of the cell suspension on the slide amounts to 0.1 ml, but the capacity of the hollow ground slide amounts to only about 0.004 ml. (2) Several minutes may pass before the cover slips are placed on the slides; many cells settle in the course of this time and then remain in the hollow ground slide when the cover slip is placed on it. (3) Cell layers grow primarily in the immediate vicinity of the air bubble, whereas the remaining glass surface remains vacant (Halle, 1963a).

Flask Cultures.–Cultivation studies in hollow ground slides show that a number of factors cannot be standardized. More favorable cultivation conditions have been attained in the aforementioned flasks.

Using the trypsinization procedure I, 9 to 10 ventricles or 29 auricles of 11-day-old embryos are required for cultivation in three Thomas flasks in M 20-AGP. The total yield of viable cells amounts to approximately 8×10^6 cells; about 20 percent of the cells are dead. The pellets are resuspended in 6 ml of nutrient medium. Two milliliters each of suspension are pipetted into the culture flasks, at the bottom of which (diameter 35 mm) lies a 24- by 24-mm cover slip. The number of cells seeded amounts to approximately 10^6 cells per ml of nutrient medium.

An area of 962 mm^2 plus ~ 200 mm^2 is available to the cells for adhesion and spreading; since the cover slips do not lie tightly on the bottom of the flask, the cells can also adhere and spread beneath the cover slip over an area amounting to 30 to 40 percent of that of the cover slip.

The preceding number of cells does not suffice for the successful cultivation of spontaneously pulsating ventricle cells in the low-protein M 20-P or in the chemically defined SM 20. It was found that the initial number of cells has to be increased to approximately 2.9×10^6 cells per 2 ml of nutrient medium, corresponding to about 2,500 cells per mm^2. In addition it was observed that it is necessary to coat the cover slips with a fine film of the nonnutrient substance celloidin (dinitrocellulose) in order to facilitate the adhesion and spreading out of the heart cells (Halle and Wollenberger, 1968).

Coating with celloidin is basically carried out by a method described by Romeis (1948) for other purposes. A 0.1-percent solution of celloidin in a 1:1 mixture of ethyl alcohol and ether is prepared from a commercial, highly concentrated celloidin block.

The cover slips are immersed in the solution for several minutes. Immediately after drying in the air and hardening in 80 percent ethyl alcohol, the celloidin film is washed with sterile distilled water. For subsequent sterilization both sides of the cover slips treated in this manner are exposed for one hour each to the rays of two ultraviolet lamps in the usual manner.

With the technique of the seated drop (see Fig. 7) it was shown that a celloidin film is not necessary for culturing the heart cells in SM 20. Using this technique the number of cells at the beginning of cultivation is kept around 3,900 per mm^2.

This is a higher count than that recommended with the technique described earlier. Only 7 ventricles or 18 to 19 auricles of r 11-day-old chick embryos are necessary for three culture flasks. The pellets are resuspended in 1.5 ml of SM 20; 0.5 ml of the cell suspension is placed on a 24-mm-square cover slip lying on the bottom of each flask.

According to semiquantitative cell counts, the number of cells on the cover slip after 28 to 38 hours is about 2,400 cells per mm^2 when the celloidin film technique is used and 3,800 cells per mm^2 with the seated drop technique.

A total area of 1,740 mm^2 is available for adhesion and spreading out in

Bucher flasks having a volume of 50 ml. The number of seeded cells per flask should be about 2.4 × 10^6 in 3 ml of nutrient medium M 20—AGP. Thirty-five ventricles of chick embryos of 11 to 13 days of incubation yield a sufficient quantity of cells for starting 24 cultures when using the trypsinization procedure II.

RENEWAL OF THE MEDIUM.—After a certain period of time the nutrient medium containing the cell debris, dead cells, and cells that do not adhere to the glass surface must be removed and replaced by fresh medium. The first renewal of the medium can be carried out after 20 to 24 hours when using M 19 or M 20-AGP; otherwise the renewal is effected 24 to 28 hours after starting the cultivation. If the seated drop technique is used, the 0.5 ml are sucked off and 2 ml of fresh nutrient medium are added to a flask. During the first 7 days the nutrient medium is changed every 24 hours; after the seventh day it is changed every other day, and after the fourteenth day every 3 to 4 days.

METHODS USED BY OTHER AUTHORS.—*Cultivation of Heart Cells.*— The fact that White (1946, 1949) succeeded 20 years ago in maintaining pulsating heart explants in a synthetic nutrient medium over a period of more than 80 days is of historical interest. Following the experiments of Rinaldini (1954), Cavanaugh (1955) described the behavior of isolated, spontaneously beating heart cells from auricular and ventricular fragments of embryonic chicks of 4 to 6 days of incubation in a natural nutrient medium, consisting of plasma and embryo extract. Rumery and co-workers (1961, 1964, and 1967) also cultivated ventricle cells isolated from 2- to 4-day-old chick embryos in plasma and embryo extract.

Lehmkuhl and Sperelakis (1963) and Sperelakis and Lehmkuhl (1964, 1966) used isolated cells from ventricles of 6- to 8-day-old chick embryos for electrophysiologic experiments. The cells were isolated from the ventricles with 0.1 percent trypsin. A magnetic stirrer was used for the mechanical isolation. The balanced salt solution of Hanks, free of Ca^{++} and Mg^{++} ions (see Puck et al., 1958), was used for dissolving the trypsin and for washing the fragments. The authors use the modified Puck nutrient medium (pH 7.2) for cultivation. It has the following composition: 15 percent horse serum, 45 percent modified Hanks solution, and 40 percent saline F containing the synthetic N 16 nutrient solution (see Puck et al., 1958). The ionic composition of the nutrient medium and of the Tyrode solution used is specified by Sperelakis and Lehmkuhl. Phenol red was not used as a pH indicator (cf. Halle, 1959). Various modifications of the nutrient medium are described in the original reports.

Harary and Farley (1963a, 1963b) described the following medium which they used in their work with spontaneously pulsating heart cells from 3- to 10-day-old postnatal Wistar rats. The growth medium is a modification of the medium used by Puck. It contains 30 percent Hanks saline solution (Marcus et al., 1956), 50 percent nutrient solution, 10 percent human serum, and 10 percent fetal calf serum. The nutrient solution consists of 10 ml of Eagle's amino acid mixture and 10 ml of Eagle's vitamin mixture (concentrated 100 times, supplied by Microbiological Associates), supplemented with 0.03 g L-aspartate, 0.075 g L-glutamate,

0.20 g L-glutamine, 0.100 g glycine, 0.025 g L-proline, 0.001 g inositol, and 0.025 g hypoxanthine. It is made up to 1 liter, using a modified Hanks solution which contains glucose, salts, antibiotics, and indicator, in the concentration present in Puck's nutrient solution (Marcus et al., 1956). After mixing all components the medium was sterilized by filtration through an Ertel filter.

The medium used by Gordon and Wilde (1965) was Eagle's Minimal Essential Medium (Microbiological Associates) to which were added nonessential amino acids. The initial osmolality of the medium was 301 to 307 milliosmoles. This synthetic nutrient medium was conditioned by outgrowing and spontaneously pulsating heart fragments of 7-day embryonic chick hearts. By adding 15 to 60 percent of the nutrient medium conditioned in this manner to a synthetic nutrient medium, the adhesion, the spreading out, and the formation of cross striations are promoted and the spontaneous contractions in primary cultures of 9-day chick embryo heart cells disaggregated with trypsin are maintained. The number of cells per mm^2 at the beginning of the cultivation was 40 to 50 percent lower in these experiments than in the synthetic nutrient medium SM 20 in the presence of celloidin.

As shown by the studies of Gordon and Wilde (1965), undefined factors that get into a synthetic nutrient medium as a result of conditioning are important for the processes of adhesion and flattening out of the heart cells on the glass substrate. But one cannot rule out the possibility that cells damaged by trypsinization can give off some of the undefined substances. However, it appears from the report of Gordon and Wilde that such substances do not suffice for the adhesion and spreading out of isolated heart cells. It is not known yet whether they are of importance for the cultivation in SM 20, at least during the first 24 hours. In view of the fact that the SM 20 nutrient medium is renewed every 24 hours during the first seven days, one can be reasonably certain that most cell debris and dead cells are removed from the culture flask not later than during the second medium renewal. Additional evidence exists that the contractions are not supported by appreciable amounts of as yet undefined substances produced by intact or degenerating cells (Halle and Wollenberger, 1968).

Cultivation of Skeletal Muscle Cells.—Skeletal muscle cells from fragments of various muscles have been isolated with the aid of trypsin or collagenase and have been cultivated in vitro. Konigsberg (1963) reported the formation of colonies from single cells and observed myogenesis (development of multinuclear myotubes) in a conditioned synthetic nutrient medium containing 5 to 10 percent of embryo extract. On the average only one cell was seeded per 9.80 mm^2. Between the seventh and tenth day of cultivation, spontaneous contractions of the multinuclear cells could be observed (Konigsberg, 1961). Konigsberg and Hauschka (1965) and Hauschka and Konigsberg (1966) could replace the undefined factors in the conditioned medium by reconstituted rat-tail collagen which was spread uniformly over the surface of Falcon plastic petri plates. According to these authors these results imply that the development of muscle cells requires the presence of a metabolic product of an associated cell type—the fibroblast. They point out that the development of a number of different cell types has been shown to be dependent upon the close proximity of connective tissue elements and that it is not unlikely that collagen plays a common role in a variety of differentiative events.

We cannot go into the details of these and similar studies on isolated skeletal muscle cells. The literature on this subject up to 1963 has been reviewed by Murray (1965). We merely wish to mention the numerous reports from the Department of Embryology of the Carnegie Institution of Washington (see Kaighn et al., 1966; Lee et al., 1966) and the studies of DeLaHaba et al. (1966), Okazaki and Holtzer (1965, 1966), Yaffe and Feldman (1964, 1965), and Yaffe and Fuchs (1967). DeLaHaba et al. (1966) investigated the influence of insulin and somatrotropin on myogenesis and on the accumulation of protein and DNA. Okazaki and Holtzer (1965, 1966) analyzed myogenesis with the aid of the immunologic antibody technique. They used rabbit antibodies prepared against chick myosin and conjugated with fluorescein isocyanate. The evidence for the specificity of the antibody and the details of the histologic techniques for reacting cells with the antibody have been presented elsewhere (Holtzer, 1961). Bischoff and Holtzer (1968) investigated the action of antimitotic drugs on myogenesis.

It is interesting in regard to the myogenic theory of the muscle contraction that spontaneous contractions of skeletal muscle cells from trypsinized thigh muscles of newborn rats were observed after differentiation to multinucleated fibers (Yaffe and Feldman, 1964; Yaffe and Fuchs, 1967). Eagle's essential medium supplemented with 7.5 to 10 percent calf serum was used in these experiments.

Apparatus and Equipment

MICROSCOPES.—The microscopic observation of the cultures is generally carried out in Thomas and Bucher flasks or in petri dishes with inverted phase-contrast microscopes. It is generally known that only low magnifications—e.g., achromates × 10 (numerical aperture 0.25)—can be used with flask cultures. Only general morphologic details can be examined in this manner. For microscopic examination with high-resolution objectives, the cover slips with the adhering muscle cells should be transferred to small chambers. The edges are covered with paraffin, thus ensuring an airtight seal, in a manner similar to that used in mounting the cover slips on the hollow ground slides. If the cover slips are washed twice in sterile nutrient medium or BSS before being transferred, cultivation can be continued under sterile conditions.

WARM STAGE.—It is recommended that one carry out all microscopic observations of the living cells as well as the determination of the number of contractions per minute (RP = rate of pulsation) at a temperature of 37°C. Counting of the RP is effected either conventionally with a stop watch or with the aid of electronic registration and recording equipment. Temperature tests have revealed that cultures of ventricular cells become increasingly more sensitive to lowered temperatures in the course of the cultivation process, especially when SM 20 is used. In a semisynthetic nutrient medium the first pulsations in 1- to 2-day-old cultures which were cooled to 10°C are observed at 15°C during the warming-up process. In SM 20, pulsation in cooled cultures of the same age starts at 24° to 25°C, and in 7- to 11-day-old cultures at 28°C; after 11 days the number of pulsating cells in SM 20 at 28° to 32°C is approximately 70 percent lower than at the same temperature at the beginning of cultivation (Halle, 1967b).

A microscope stage for warming and cooling is used for attaining temperatures lying above or below the room temperature. The stage is fastened to the table mounting of the microscope and consists, in the simplest case, of a metal coil located in the interior of the stage and firmly connected to its cover plate. Good heat transmission can be ensured by soldering the coil to the cover plate of the stage. The ends of the coil protruding from the stage are designed as connection pieces for rubber tubes. In this way the warming and cooling stage can be connected to thermostats.

The temperature fluctuation at the plane of the object and on the stage is not to exceed ± 0.5°C. For certain experiments, in particular for time-lapse cinemicrography with high-resolution objectives, the temperature variation in the culture chamber above the stage opening and in the plane of the object should be less than ± 0.3°C (Heunert, 1961, 1962). A novel heating and cooling system has been developed, in which the temperature fluctuation at the object plane amounts to less than ± .015°C, provided the room temperature remains relatively constant. A detailed description of the design is given by Halle (1965) and Halle and Ristau (1966). We merely wish to point out here that the preparation container, e.g., the culture chamber, is heatable both from below and from the objective above. The heating of the objective proved to be necessary, especially if immersion objectives are used. The reason for this is that the heat is conducted from the heating stage to the objective, which is always colder when a drop of immersion fluid is placed on the cover slip. As a consequence of this temperature gradient, the temperature in the plane of the object is lowered to such an extent that the ventricle cells attached to the cover slip may cease their pulsations. By attaching smaller thermistors on the centrally arranged stage opening and on the objective, it is possible to obtain constant control of the heating in direct and/or compensation circuitry with the aid of electronic components. In this manner the disadvantages described by Engel and Zerbst (1960) in the use of conventional commercial warming stages, such as the development of temperature gradients from the periphery of the stage toward the center, temperature fluctuations when changing from dry to immersion objectives, etc., are obviated.

Microscope thermostats have also been recommended and described for the cinemicrographic technique (see Heunert, 1961, 1962). However, these thermostats are hardly suitable for use in conjunction with perfusion apparatus and micromanipulators. In contrast, the warming and cooling system briefly described here has been used with good results in combination with this equipment.

PERFUSION APPARATUS.—For the observation of the reaction to a drug of selected single cells in a cell layer we recommend the use of a perfusion chamber. Hitherto we have mostly been using the chamber described by Robineaux and Barski (1956). It consists of plexiglas and is provided with two sidewaysconnecting pieces for the introduction and removal of the nutrient medium or other fluid. But we also wish to mention the well-known versatile and convenient multipurpose culture chamber designed by Rose (1954) and Rose et al. (1958). In the case of the chamber of Robineaux and Barski the cover slip with the cells is attached to the chamber with a paraffin seal around its edges. This kind of attachment has the disadvantage that the paraffin sealing can develop leaks as a result of the pressure exerted by the fluid column during passage of the fluid. In the Rose chamber a pure latex rubber gasket is placed between the two cover slips. Tight sealing of the chamber is guaranteed by four screws. The top cover slip in the Rose chamber can be replaced by a cover slip of polystyrene sheet plastic one hundredth of an inch in thickness instead of the conventional glass (Mark and Strasser, 1966). The plastic allows considerable gaseous diffusion of the surrounding air. In the gas experiments of Mark et al. (1967), chambers containing cell cultures were dismantled and reassembled with a perforated cellophane membrane directly over the cells, and a glass top cover instead of the plastic.

Both types of perfusion chambers and also other types of chambers can be used in conjunction with a perfusion system. In the simplest case such a system consists of a reservoir connected to the chamber by a rubber or similar tube. The effluent may be discarded or collected as desired. Buchsbaum and Kuntz (1954) described a system that permits the automatic continuous flow at known rates and under known gas tensions of liquid media past the cells in a perfusion chamber under microscopic observation, whereby the microscope is kept in a thermostatically controlled warm box.

If such a warm box is not used, it is recommended that one choose a type of chamber whose base plate lies in close contact flat on the cover plate of the warm stage. In this way the heat is conducted from the warm stage to the culture fluid and thus to the cells, even if insulating material such as Plexiglas is used instead of metal. The perfusion experiments with autorhythmically pulsating muscle cells have shown that greater temperature fluctuations should be avoided or kept at a minimum for the aforementioned reasons. This may be achieved either by adjusting the perfusion temperature to the incubation temperature of the cultures and insulating the inflow tube, or by maintaining the flow at such a rate that the temperature in the chamber does not fall. Moreover, the height of the chamber and hence the distance between the top condenser lens and the plane of the object must be adjusted to the working distance of the microscope condenser. For chambers in which the condenser cannot be adjusted according to the lighting method of Köhler on account of the chamber height, it is preferable to employ a long working distance phase-contrast condenser.

Various types of chambers have been designed and described, not only for short-term experiments, but also for extended perfusion with gases, such as O_2 and CO_2, as well as with fluids, permitting long-term cultivation also under sterile conditions. Thomas and Cramer (1966a, 1966b) described an interesting perfusion system for several perfusion chambers. This is a multipurpose inexpensive system. The cover slips of the perfusion chambers in this system consist of optically clear polystyrene.

Thus there exist a whole range of various types of perfusion systems, and one can select a system that meets the specific requirements of a given experiment.

MICRURGY.–Micrurgy (microsurgery) is an important method of analytical cell research. Thus the electrophsiologic study of individual cells requires micrurgical techniques. Other examples are the local application of drugs to selected cells by means of microinjection (Kopac, 1964) or microeletrophoresis (Curtis, 1964). Kopac (1964) has reviewed and described the modern apparatus available for micrurgical work on isolated cells. Further details of the micrurgical technique in the study of isolated cells are presented in this review and in the paper of Goldstein and Eastwood (1964).

A capillary drawing apparatus serves for making microtools from glass. A simple micrurgy chamber open on one side, which has proved reliable in its use, is depicted in Figure 4. In its simplest form it consists of a slide on which a glass wall is fixed with paraffin. The cover slip is placed on the wall with the cells facing downward. Another cover slip forms a sort of moist chamber. Such a chamber makes it possible to work with individual heart muscle cells for six to eight hours at a temperature of 37°C to ±0.15°C in a histidine-buffered medium without a significant change in the RP of the beating cells. Generally it is not necessary to renew the nutrient medium until three to four hours have passed.

Unlike the cells of lines or strains in long-term culture, the cells from the heart ventricles and amnion muscle of chick embryos and the heart ventricle cells of 2- to 3-day-old postnatal rats in the semisynthetic nutrient medium M 20-AGP are very sensitive to micrurgy. We have not been able to modify the extracellular milieu in such a manner as to be able to repeat the experiments of Goldstein et al. (1960) and of Munro and Daniel (1965) on cells in long-term culture with our autorhythmically pulsating muscle cells in primary culture. These authors were able to separate several large cytoplasmic pieces from isolated flattened cells. Thus far all muscle cells responded to this microsurgical manipulation with cessation of contraction and with cytoplasmic shrinkage. At the same time blebs are seen, which appear to have a dark-brown color in the phase contrast without color filter and which at first are hardly miscible with the nutrient medium. On the other hand, it has been found in electrophysiologic investigations of these cells that capillary microeletrodes with a tip diameter of about 0.5 μm can penetrate through the cell membrane without greatly injuring the cells (see Lehmkuhl and Sperelakis, 1967; Sperelakis, 1967).

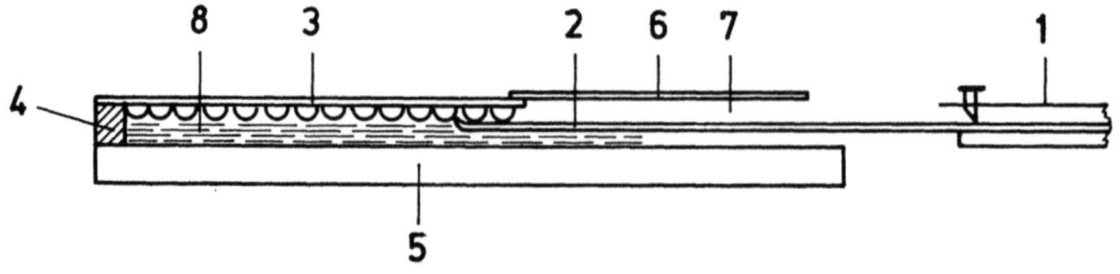

FIG. 4. Schematic cross-sectional view of a single micrurgy chamber opened on one side. (1) Needle holder. (2) Needle. (3) Cover slip with cells. (4) Glass wall. (5) Slide. (6) Cover slip. (7) "Moist chamber". (8) Medium.

CINEMICROGRAPHY—With the aid of the cinemicrography technique it is possible to detect, record, and analyze quantitatively movements of, and inside of, isolated cells which the human eye is not able to discern. Apart from the normal exposure frequency of 24 frames per second, we differentiate between time-lapse and speeded cinematography. The cytodynamics of isolated cells in the cell culture can generally be examined with an exposure frequency of 1 to 5 frames per minute. One may thus be able to study the effects of drugs on peripheral bubble formation and on the undulations of the ruffled cell membranes and to observe the earliest stages in the formation of vacuoles by the infolding of the ruffled cell border. These effects in connection with pinocytosis, movements of nuclei, mitochondria, and myofibrils and changes in size and shape of these cell structures may give a clue to the mode of action and the point of attack of a drug. Speeded cinematography helps in the analysis of rapid movements such as the twitching of muscle cells and the movements of sarcomeres and of cilia. Various aspects of the cinemicrography of cultured cells are discussed in the monograph by Rose (1963).

A 16-mm film camera has been used in our laboratory for monitoring changes in contractile activity of cultured muscle cells under various experimental conditions. The attachment of the camera to the microscope and other details of the technique are described in the monographs of Heunert and Philipp (1957) and Rose (1963). In some of our experiments the exposure frequency was greater than 24 frames per second, necessitating a technique differing from that used for making time-lapse exposures. The light source was connected to a DC outlet. The camera had to be mounted on a vibration-free stand to avoid blurred exposures. A 10-ampere carbon arc lamp was required for phase-contrast exposures of an 18°DIN film with the phase-contrast objective Phv HI ×100 /n.a. 1.25 when the exposure frequency was 32 frames per second. A 500-watt xenon lamp with an operating current of 20 amperes allowed the taking of phase-contrast pictures at 96 frames per second, using a 19°DIN (38 ASA) film with the objective Phv HI ×100/n.a. 1.25. To avoid damaging the cells with ultraviolet and infrared light, a 65-mm-deep glass cuvette filled with distilled water, a 4.1-mm-thick BG 17 and a 2-mm-thick GG 13 filter, and in certain cases a 2-mm-thick VG 4 filter, arranged in that order, were interposed in the light path (Halle and Wollenberger, 1959; Wollenberger and Halle, 1963a).

The frame-to-frame analysis technique developed mainly by Kuhl (1949) is used for detailed and quantitative examination of the motion picture. The records by Mark and Strasser (1966) of heart cell beating rates were made during film projection with a strip-chart recorder connected to a manually operated microswitch. Noguchi et al. (1966) recorded the responses of heart cells by cinematography at scanning speed. The resulting film sequences were analyzed with a Vanguard film analyzer and cadmium sulfide photoconductors (see Pomerat et al., 1964).

Mercer and co-workers (1966, 1967) used an inverted phase-contrast microscope and a closed-circuit television system. The heart cells were observed as they appeared on the television screen during passage of the culture dish across the objective on the movable stage.

MEASUREMENT OF THE CONTRACTION AMPLITUDE.—Bucher and Kolb (1962) have described an apparatus that permits the recording of the contracting amplitude of an isolated pulsating cell. The contractile movements of a portion of a cell cause slight fluctuations of the light intensity in a phase contrast and can be recorded photoelectrically. One of the records made by the authors and representing the rhythmic beat of an isolated cell obtained from the heart of a 10-day-old chick embryo is shown in Figure 5. It is now possible in single muscle cell cultures to measure quantitatively the inotropic action of drugs.

ELECTROPHYSIOLOGIC STUDIES.—The resting and action potentials of cultured, spontaneously pulsating heart cells were recorded for the first time by Fänge et al. (1956) and Crill et al. (1959) with the aid of capillary microelectrodes. Sperelakis and Lehmkuhl (1964, 1966), Lehmkuhl and Sperelakis (1967), and Sperelakis (1967) determined, in addition, other electrophysiologic parameters in such cells, such as membrane resistance and capacity. They were able to classify the pulsating cells, on the basis of their electrophysiologic properties, into pacemaker cells and driven cells and to characterize them in detail. Figure 6 shows an example of the transformation of pacemaker cells into nonpacemaker cells by increasing the K^+ concentration in the medium to more than 10 mM. Results obtained to date indicate that the electrophysiologic properties of monolayer cultures of chick ventricular cells are similar to those of cells in intact adult hearts (Lehmkuhl and Sperelakis, 1967; Sperelakis, 1967). Lieberman (1967) examined the influence of cell density and potassium concentration on the action potentials of cultured embryonic chick heart cells.

Kaufmann and Tritthart (1967) succeeded in measuring simultaneously the electrical activity and the contraction amplitude in single beating heart cells cultured on glass.

METABOLIC MEASUREMENTS.—The respiratory metabolism of pulsating heart cell layers and of single cell suspensions containing 10^3 to 10^5 cells can be measured with the Cartesian diver microrespirometer (see Holter et al., 1956). With this respirometer it is also possible to determine quantitatively the rate of glycolysis of single cell suspensions and of cell layers in bicarbonate-containing nutrient medium and to measure other reactions that are causing changes in the gas phase of the diver. For experiments with cell layers the cells should be cultivated on mica strips instead of on cover slips. The size of the pieces to be cut from the mica strip will depend on the size of the opening of the diver vessel.

Danes (1955) determined the rate of respiration of cultured fibroblasts from explants of 7-day embryonic chick hearts. One to 3 $\times$ 10^3 cells were required per diver for these measurements. The average rate of respiration was 1.7 $\times$ 10^{-5} μl/hr $\times$ cell at 37.5°C and 3.4 $\times$ 10^{-6} μl/hr $\times$ cell at 20.2°C.

Isolated ventricle cells of chick embryos of 11 days of incubation were used in our first respiration experiments. The cells were cultured in semisynthetic nutrient medium M 20-AGP on optically clean mica strips 100 μm in thickness, which were placed in Thomas flasks. The mica strips are washed according to the instructions

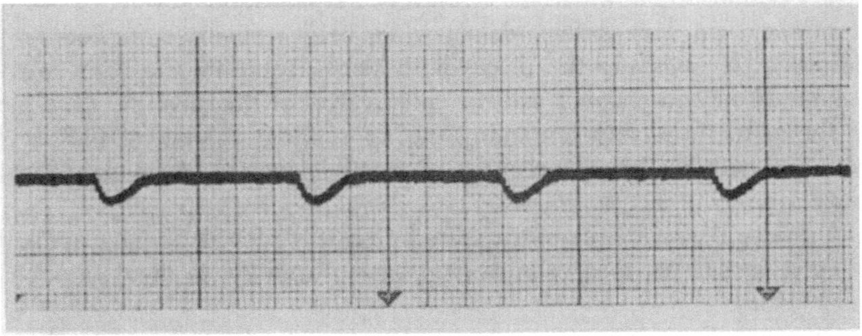

Fig. 5. Photoelectrically recorded pulsation curve of a single heart cell attached to glass. Contraction is indicated by a downward deflection of the tracing. The frequency of pulsation was 56 per minute. (From Bucher and Kolb. 1962. *Med. Exp.*, 6:14, Fig. 1.)

given for washing cover slips (see p. 197). However, depending on the type of nutrient medium and its protein content, it may be advisable to treat the strips with 12 N NaOH for 18 hours instead of with acid [p. 197, 1b(3), (5)]. After marking

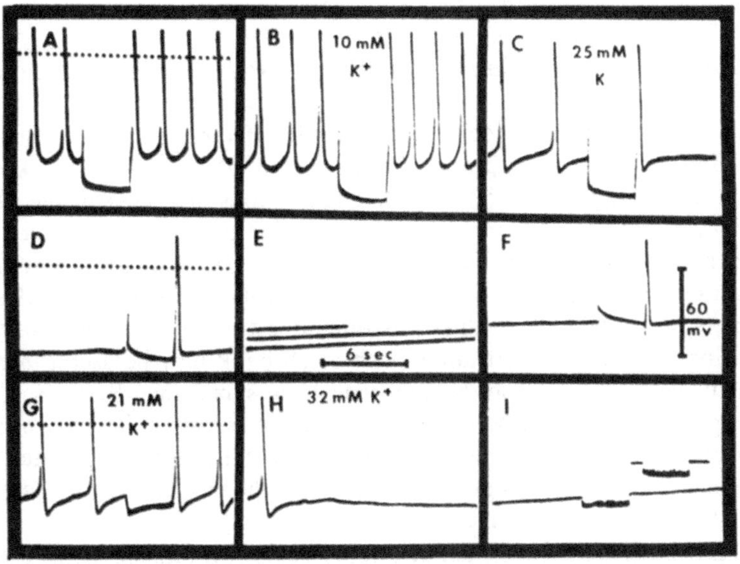

FIG. 6. Conversion of pacemaker cells into nonpacemaker cells by K^+. Voltage and time calibrations apply to all photos. The zero potential level is marked by the dotted lines in A, D, and G. The photographs A to F were taken from one impalement. (A) Control in Tyrode's medium; $[K^+]_0$ is 2.7 mM. (B) 1.5 min postinjection of KCl into culture medium; total K^+ concentration 10 mM. (C) 4 min, (D) 5 min, (E) 6 min, and (F) 7 min after elevation of $[K^+]_0$ to 25 mM; three sweeps superimposed in E. Hyperpolarizing pulses of 4.8 na applied in all photos except E; microelectrode resistance change in D and F. G, H, and I from an impalement in another culture; control in 2.7 mM K^+ and activity in 9 mM K^+ not illustrated. (G) 4 min after elevation of $K^+{}_0$ to 21 mM. (H) 1 min after elevation of $K^+{}_0$ to 32 mM. (I) 1.5 and 5 min (inset) later. Hyperpolarizing pulses of 2.4 na applied in G and I. (From Sperelakis and Lehmkuhl. 1966. *J. Gen. Physiol.*, 49:867, Fig. 10.)

the sites on the strip at which the cell layers are pulsating, they are cut off from the rest of the strip with a fine scalpel while being immersed in BSS or nutrient medium. After washing the pieces with sterile solution and after microscopic checking of the morphology and the contractions of the cells, the mica pieces are transferred to the divers containing the appropriate volume of BSS or nutrient medium. Another microscopic check of the cell layers is recommended after the completion of the measurements.

Utilizing the technique of the seated drop it is possible to have approximately 2,400 cells settled per mm^2 of mica strip, in conformity with the data published by Danes (1955).

The oxygen uptake of freshly isolated and still spherically shaped and suspended ventricle cells from chick embryos of 11 days of incubation was found to be, at 37°C, 13.0 μl O_2/hour $\times$ mg protein in aerated saline solution containing 11.1 mM glucose (Wollenberger, 1967). The cell density in the diver was 5×10^4 cells per μl, corresponding to 3.7 μg protein per μl. The rate of oxygen uptake of ventricle cells cultured for 1 to 2 days on mica strips in M 20-AGP was 10 to 20 μl O_2/hour $\times$ mg protein (B. Kleitke, unpublished experiments). Guidotti et al. (1969, see Appendix) found the oxygen consumption of isolated, suspended heart cells from 7-day-old chick embryos at 37.5°C to be 14.2 μl per mg of dry weight.

The Preservation of Cell Suspensions at Low Temperatures

The tissue- or organ-specific characteristics of various types of cells are not lost by cooling the cells under proper precautions to -78° to -196°C and keeping them at these temperatures (Stowell, 1965). The methods described in the literature for freezing and preserving living cells of primary cultures and of cell lines and strains in the frozen state are also suited for preserving the faculties of automaticity and contractility of suspensions of single ventricle cells (Wollenberger, 1967; Wollenberger et al., 1967). It is thus possible to establish a "bank" of heart cells possessing the capacity of beating. Such a cell bank may be useful in experiments in which the cells cannot all be cultured at the same time. Portions of the frozen cell suspensions can then be used at different times, and uniformity of the starting material is thus assured. The frozen heart cells are also better suited for transportation and shipment than unfrozen heart cells, which are relatively sensitive to shaking and vibrations.

Dissociated cells (see pp. 206-208) from 13 ventricles of 11-day-old chick embryos are suspended, following washing in BSS, in 0.5 to 1 ml of M 20-AGP nutrient medium containing 1 M dimethyl sulfoxide (DMSO). The suspension is kept for 30 minutes at room temperature, with occasional gentle agitation. Aliquots of 0.5 ml are transferred each to small glass ampules under sterile conditions. The ampules are sealed and cooled to -50°C at a constant rate of 1° to 2°C per minute before being placed in a liquid nitrogen refrigerator. Commercial instruments, such as the Linde BF 3 biologic freezer, are available for automatic cooling at chosen rates.

For quick thawing the ampules are placed at once for 1 minute in an agitated

37°C water bath. The thawed cell suspension is diluted with an equal volume of M 20-AGP, being gently agitated in the process. A few minutes later more M 20-AGP is added until a dilution of 1:10 is reached, corresponding to a DMSO concentration of 0.1 M. This concentration has no noticeable effect on isolated and cultured embryonic chick heart cells. The cells are cultured in the presence of 0.1 M DMSO until the first renewal of the medium, which is usually effected after 24 to 30 hours, using DMSO-free nutrient medium.

Following this procedure 13 heart ventricles of 11-day-old chick embryos yield 6 ml of cell suspension for three Thomas flasks. To compensate for the loss of living cells due to freezing and thawing, about 30 percent more of ventricular muscle tissue is needed than is normally the case (see pp. 206-213). The number of living cells at the start of the cultivation on cover slips in Thomas flasks is about 10^6 per ml of nutrient medium.

At the beginning of and during cultivation the majority of the cells do not differ from unfrozen cells in control cultures with respect to their morphology as observed with the phase-contrast and the electron microscope. There are, however, considerably more cell debris, ghosts, and cells with protruding blebs than in the control cultures. The damaged and dead cells and the cell debris are largely removed from the culture flask by the first change of the nutrient medium.

The intact heart cells from the frozen-thawed suspension flatten out on the glass more slowly than unfrozen heart cells. After 24 to 28 hours, quite a few of the frozen-thawed cells attached to the glass still have a more or less spherical shape. Nevertheless, they form compact, rhythmically and synchronously pulsating layers. No significant difference in RP is observed between frozen and unfrozen cells at the end of the first day of cultivation. In both groups of cells the RP falls continually during the course of the cultivation and reaches a value ranging between 40 and 50 beats on the fifth day. The contractions are maintained for a period of two to three weeks.

Although the procedure described may not insure maximum recovery and may not yield the highest quota of viable cells, survival of a good part of the frozen heart cells has been achieved without loss of pacemaker function and capacity for growth after storage at -190°C for as long as three months (Wollenberger, 1967).

Summary of the Cultivation Technique

A schematic view of the technique of cultivation of heart cells is given in Figure 7. The figure illustrates the various phases of the cultivation process. After separation of the atria from the ventricles and after the mechanical isolation of the fragments (I) and their trypsinization in centrifuge tubes or in small flasks with a magnetic stirrer (II), the fragment residues are removed and the cell suspension is washed in BSS (III). Following resuspension of the pellets in the nutrient medium (IV), the cells are seeded for cultivation by conventional techniques or utilizing the technique of the seated drop in Thomas flasks (V), in which physiologic and pharmacologic studies can be conducted (VI). Transfer of

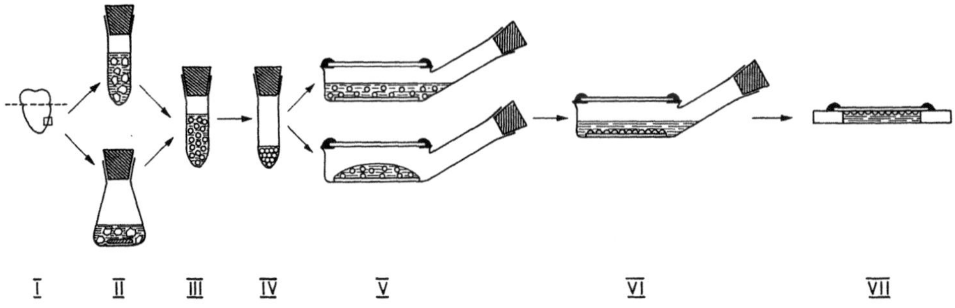

FIG. 7. Schematic view of the cultivation technique. Alternatively, Petri dishes may be used for phase V and VI. (See text for details.)

the cover slips and the attached cells to smaller culture chambers (VII) permits the observation of the cells with a phase-contrast microscope equipped with high-resolution immersion objectives for micrurgy, cinematography, and direct visual examination of morphology and contractile activity.

Definitions of the Principal Terms

The terms "single cells" and "isolated cells" as used here refer to cells disaggregated (dissociated) from the organ fragments by means of trypsinization. These cells are present in the form of a cell suspension at the beginning of cultivation. This nomenclature is usually adhered to regardless of whether these cells lie isolated as individual cells on the glass substrate or whether they are connected with one another in a cell layer after explantation or cultivation in vitro. When determining the RP, we generally cannot well differentiate between isolated cells, cells that are in slight contact with neighboring cells via cell appendages, and cells that lie in dense monolayers. The synchronous pulsation of a cell layer in a field of vision is recorded as an individual value in the determination of the RP. When we use the terms "spontaneously pulsating cells" or "autorhythmically active cells," we cannot visually distinguish between "driven" cells and real pacemakers. This is only possible by recording the action potential (Sperelakis and Lehmkuhl, 1964, 1966). However, using nutrient medium enriched with serum and embryonic extract, one can keep the number of cells at the beginning of cultivation so low that the cells do not establish contact with one another, at least not during the first 24 hours. Under these conditions the behavior of pacemaker cells lying as isolated individuals can be studied by visual observation (see DeHaan, 1967a, 1967b).

When we culture isolated cells under in vitro conditions, we are dealing, by definition, with cell cultures. These so-called primary cell cultures differ from long-term cultured "heart fibroblasts" in that the latter can be cultured as cell lines or cell strains for years. During this time profound changes occur in the karyotype of these cells. According to the available evidence such cells do not possess the faculties of autorhythmicity and contractility. Consequently they are not to be defined as heart muscle cells.

Some authors use the terms "heart myoblasts," "heart cells," and "heart muscle cells" in their primary cultures without having convinced themselves that spontaneously active and contracting cells are present. In order to preclude misunderstandings we propose to define the inactive cells as fibroblastlike heart cells. It can easily be decided in a heart cell culture whether or not the cells are capable of spontaneous action by exposing them at 37°C to 0.2 mM Ba^{++} (Halle, 1967a; Halle and Wollenberger, 1968). This treatment stimulates the presumptive heart muscle cells to beat. Thus a functional property is used to characterize heart muscle cells.

Electron microscopic observations of cells that have proliferated from heart explants indicate that these cells can be morphologically defined either as fibroblasts (Schwarz et al., 1962) or as muscle cells (Meyer and Queiroga, 1959). In such cultures it may be difficult to decide whether the pulsating cells in the growth zone are spontaneously active or whether they are merely stimulated by impulses arising in the body of the explant. The disadvantages of tissue cultures as opposed to cell cultures were pointed out above (see pp. 193-195).

The Addition of Drugs

In the study of the responses of the isolated explanted and cultured muscle cells to drugs, some of the same precautions have to be observed as in more conventional pharmacologic tests. When solubilizers are used for dissolving substances, their possible action must be tested separately on control cultures. Attempts to determine the action of drugs on isolated heart cells may fail if the solubilizer exerts injurious effects. Such injuries are usually visible in the microscope and consist of vacuole formation, changes in cell shape, changes in contractility and excitability, and other alterations. When ethyl alcohol is used for dissolving drugs, its concentration in the medium should not exceed 0.02 to 0.04 volume percent, since higher concentrations affect the RP (Halle, 1963a).

Either BSS or a nutrient medium lacking serum proteins is used for preparing stock solutions. The dilution of the stock solutions to the desired concentration is accomplished, as usual, with a complete nutrient medium.

As pointed out previously, in many instances the binding of small molecules to serum proteins must be regarded as an important factor contributing to the reduction of the effective drug concentration. The binding of certain drugs to glass may have the same effect (cf. Stouffer and Lipscomb, 1963; Wollenberger, 1964b). This fact is of special importance if the nutrient medium containing such a drug is sterilized by passage through a glass bacterial filter.

SOME REPRESENTATIVE RESULTS

This section deals with important characteristics of cells isolated from the hearts of 9- to 13-day-old chick embryos and from the amnion of 8-day-old chick embryos and cultured in vitro. Only those points will be discussed that appear necessary for an understanding of the behavior of the cells in pharmacologic experiments.

Cytology and Enzyme Pattern

It has been reported that the enzyme pattern of the heart cells undergoes certain changes during exposure to proteolytic enzymes (Table 6). Trypsin also acts

TABLE 6

Changes in the Activities of Some Enzymes Following the Isolation of Myocardial Cells

I. Specific enzyme activities in percent after treatment with various proteolytic enzymes. The specific enzyme activity in the organ is set at 100 percent.

II. Percentage loss of enzyme quantity cells kept in the disaggregated state for 60 minutes at 37°C (II a) and for 40 minutes at 25°C (II b), respectively.

Animal Species, Enzyme	Age (Days)	Enzyme	I	II	Authors
Chick embryo, Trypsin	15	Succinic dehydrogenase	−26	–	Leslie and Yarnell (1960)*
		Cytochrome oxidase	+7	–	
	19	Succinic dehydrogenase	−44	–	
		cytochrome oxidase	−66	–	
Rat, Trypsin	3-10	Ca^{++}-ATPase	+43	–	Harary et al. (1964)
		Isocitric dehydrogenase	+8	–	
		Glucose-6-phosphate dehydrogenase	+30	–	
		Malic dehydrogenase	−13	–	
Chick embryo, Ventricle Elastase	11	Lactic dehydrogenase	−5	−19[a]	Levinson and Green (1965)
Chick embryo, Ventricle Trypsin	11	Lactic dehydrogenase	–	−50[b]	Wollenberger (1967)
		Malic dehydrogenase	–	42[b]	

*The values of Leslie and Yarnell (1960) are referred to 1 μg of cellular DNA phosphorus, those of the other authors to 1 mg of cell protein.

on the structural elements of the heart muscle cells: the myofibrillar structure is largely dissolved, and remnants of Z-lines with disorderly arranged individual myofilaments and groups of myofilaments are left over after the trypsin treatment (Schulze et al., 1966; Wollenberger, 1964a, 1967) (Fig. 8).

Biochemical changes likewise accompany the disaggregation process. Thus the activity of lactic dehydrogenase of freshly isolated embryonic chick heart cells suspended in Hanks salt solution declines in 5 hours by about 45 percent owing to lysis of the cells (Levinson and Green, 1965). Wollenberger (1967) found that 40 to 50 percent of the malic and lactic dehydrogenase activity in embryonic chick heart cells following disaggregation by trypsin were released within 40 minutes into the suspension medium. In spite of the occurrence of such changes, a portion of the

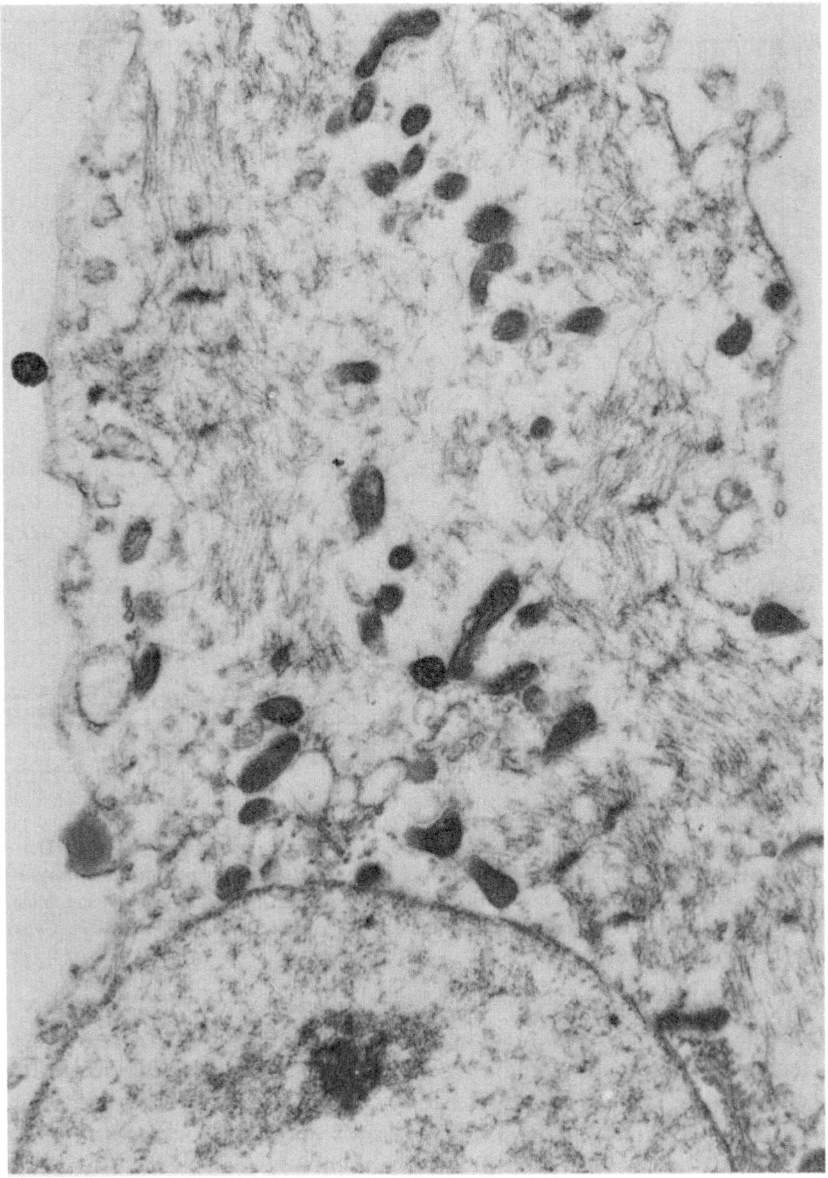

FIG. 8. Section through an isolated heart ventricle cell from a single cell suspension. The myofibrillar structure has largely been lost. Remnants of Z-bands and numerous myofilaments or fragments of them, running in different directions, are located in various parts of the cytoplasm. Electron micrograph courtesy of Dr. Wolfgang Schulze. Final magnification × 25,000.

suspended heart cells is capable of autorhythmic contraction both in the semisynthetic and in synthetic nutrient media 3 to 5 hours after the start of cultivation, when the cells still have a spherical shape. Cahn (1967b) found that heart cells

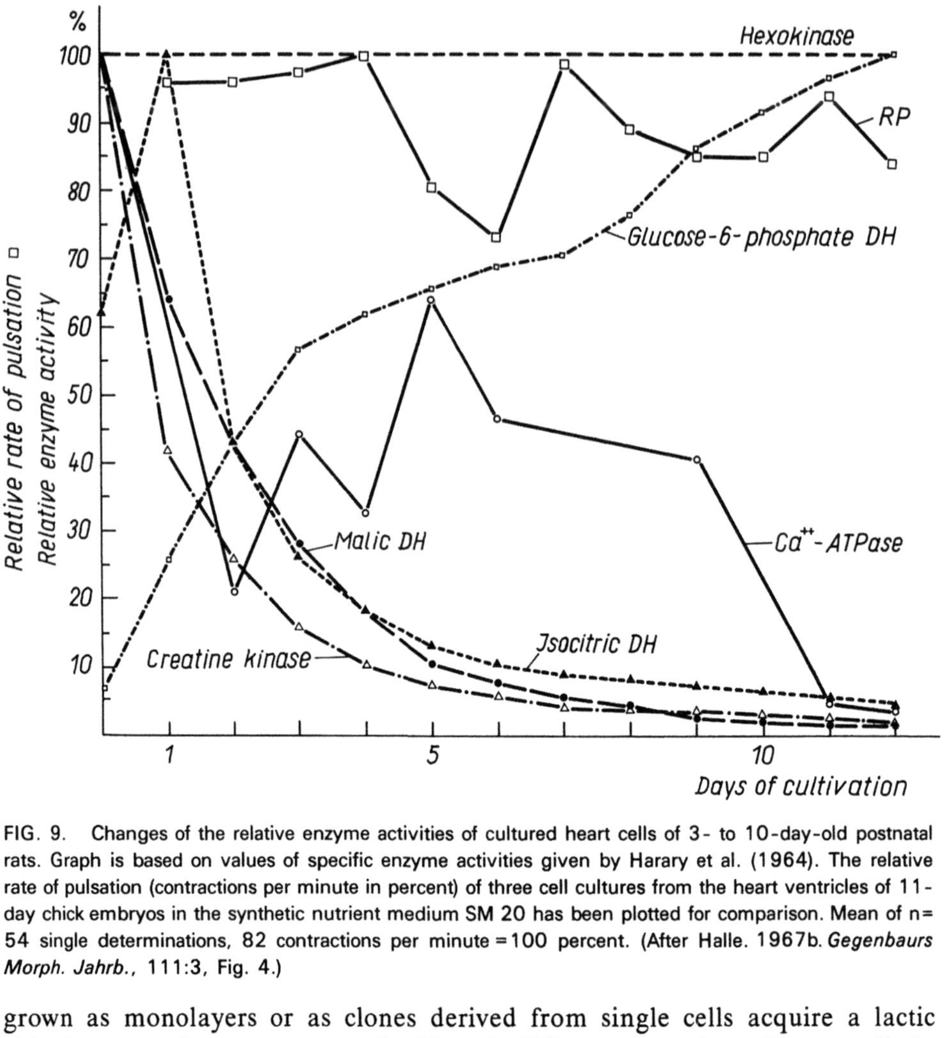

FIG. 9. Changes of the relative enzyme activities of cultured heart cells of 3- to 10-day-old postnatal rats. Graph is based on values of specific enzyme activities given by Harary et al. (1964). The relative rate of pulsation (contractions per minute in percent) of three cell cultures from the heart ventricles of 11-day chick embryos in the synthetic nutrient medium SM 20 has been plotted for comparison. Mean of n = 54 single determinations, 82 contractions per minute = 100 percent. (After Halle. 1967b. *Gegenbaurs Morph. Jahrb.*, 111:3, Fig. 4.)

grown as monolayers or as clones derived from single cells acquire a lactic dehydrogenase isozyme pattern significantly different from that of heart cells in vivo. Heart cells, originally containing almost exclusively H-LDH subunits when placed into culture, rapidly begin within 4 to 5 days to synthesize predominantly the M-LDH subunit. The shift in LDH pattern is not due to overgrowth and is not correlated with a so-called dedifferentiation of the cells, because the clones originating from beating cardiac myoblasts develop the same isozyme subunit composition as those derived from nonbeating cardiac myoblasts or from fibroblasts, and because beating and nonbeating monolayer networks of cardiac cells have an identical isozyme composition. In agreement with the results of biochemical investigations on various types of cells in primary cell culture, which showed that the cells soon develop the uniform enzyme pattern of dedifferentiated cells, Harary et al. (1964) found that rat heart cells likewise undergo such changes in culture. The activity of most of the enzymes examined diminishes in the course of 10 to 12 days, and the cells assume the simple enzyme pattern of dedifferentiated cells in long-term culture (Fig. 9).

THE BEHAVIOR OF THE HEART CELLS IN SEMISYNTHETIC AND SYNTHETIC NUTRIENT MEDIA.—We call a heart cell culture "normal" when all cells look morphologically clean, i.e., when they are free of vacuoles and of a greater amount of fat droplets and when the cells and cell layers exhibit rhythmic pulsations. Approximately 3 hours after the start of cultivation, some of the isolated heart cells have become attached to the glass surface and begin to flatten out there. Both the still spherically shaped and the flattened cells are pulsating rhythmically at this time. Semiquantitative determinations show that in M 20-AGP and SM 20 about 1 percent of the total number of cells are pulsating 6 to 10 hours after the start of cultivation. Cell contact increases with the continued spread of the cells and a loose cell reticulum, and then a dense monolayer is formed in 24 to 48 hours, containing smaller or larger areas of usually synchronously beating cells.

Several types of contractions can be observed (Fig. 10): (1) Only a single pulsation center is present in a cell. (2) The cell contracts simultaneously at opposite ends of its periphery. (3) The cell "extends" during contraction; i.e., the peripheral portion on one side or on two sides recedes from the center of the cell.

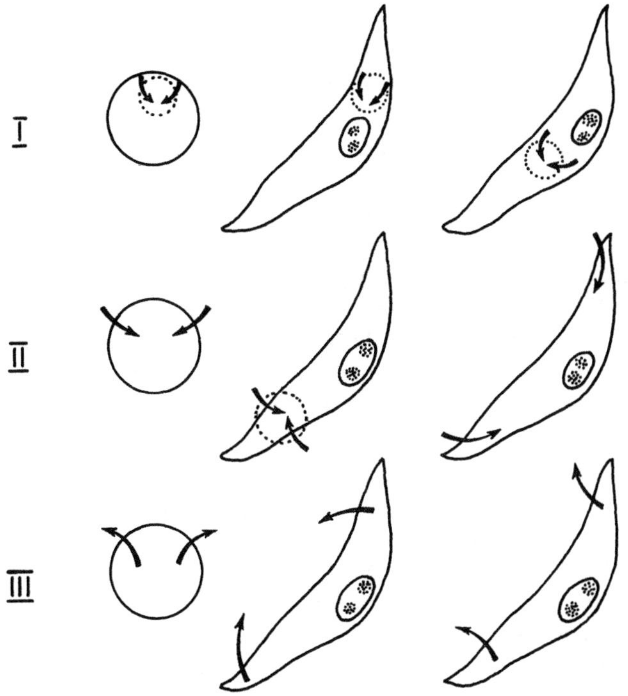

FIG. 10 Schematic presentation of different kinds of contractions of spherically shaped and of flattened heart cells in cell culture (see text for details). (From Halle and Wollenberger. 1968. *Z. Zellforsch.*, 87:292, Fig. 1.)

This type of contraction, which occurs not very frequently, can probably be explained by contractile activity of peripheral cell regions.

In most cases the contractions are neither of the pure isotonic nor of the pure isometric type. A method of registering changes in cell profile (amplitude of contraction) was mentioned above (see p. 218). No technique has been worked out for the measurement of tension in single cultured muscle cells.

The pulsations are rhythmic. Arrhythmically beating cells are not normally encountered in greater number. Three main types of arrhythmias can be distinguished: (1) There are intervals of varying duration between the individual pulsations. (2) The irregular pulsation is accompanied by a constantly changing intensity of contraction. (3) Secondary pulsation sites (ectopic foci) appear in the cells.

Pulsating ventricle cells can be cultured for 16 to 18 days in M 19 and M 20-AGP and for about 30 days in M 20-P, if these semisynthetic nutrient media contain 5.1 mM K^+. The RP declines in all these media in the course of the cultivation.

In SM 20 the atrial and ventricular cells flatten out on the glass more slowly than they do in a semisynthetic nutrient medium. But otherwise the ventricle cells behave in a manner similar to that seen in the semisynthetic media.

Pulsating heart cells can be cultured for more than 30 days in SM 20. In contrast to what was seen in semisynthetic nutrient media, the RP increases steadily in the course of cultivation. Up to the sixteenth day of cultivation there is a statistically significant difference ($P < 0.001$) between the RP of atrial and of ventricular cells, comparable to the difference in frequency between nomotopic and heterotopic pacemaker parts.

Isolated cells and cell layers begin to exhibit arrhythmic contractions after the second day of cultivation. Luciani periods occur quite frequently–repeated fibrillatory contractions alternating with longer periods of standstill. These arrhythmias are observed only up to the ninth to twelfth day of cultivation. Thereafter entire layers pulsate rhythmically and synchronously.

Kopac (1954) and White and Waymouth (1954) have emphasized the desirability of using chemically defined media in pharmacologic studies on cultured tissues and cells (see p. 199). This requirement can now be met in the case of pulsating heart cells by the use of the medium SM 20 (see Halle and Wollenberger, 1968).

CELL TYPES IN THE HEART CELL CULTURES.–On the basis of a number of findings it can be taken for granted that heart cell cultures contain no viable nerve cells (cf. Halle, 1963b; Sperelakis, 1967). However, inactive fibroblastlike cells, differing morphologically from the potentially pulsating cells, may be present in these cultures in SM 20. The fibroblastlike cells appear more flattened and cell components such as cytogranules and nuclei are more clearly visible than in the pulsating cells, which have a greater thickness and are optically more dense. Attempts at separating the two types of cells in culture have met with little success (cf. Refson, 1959). Mark and co-workers (1966, 1967) found, in addition to the pulsating heart cells, non-pulsating endotheliumlike cells in their cell cultures. Cahn (1964) reported that a few fibroblastlike and epitheliumlike cells were always present in his heart cell cultures, but that they were beating in the same way as the spindle-shaped cells. We could confirm this finding in experiments using semisynthetic media.

It has hitherto not been possible in passage experiments to obtain a line or strain of pulsating heart cells from primary pulsating heart cells. The work of Konigsberg (1963), Konigsberg and Hauschka (1965), and Hauschka and Konigsberg (1966), who succeeded in culturing typical muscle cell colonies from single isolated skeletal muscle cells (see pp. 212-213). has not yet fully been duplicated with heart muscle cells. Cahn (1967b) and Cahn et al. (1967) reported on experiments in which clones were derived from single beating and nonbeating heart cells. A clone was on one occasion seen to grow into a beating clone.

The Behavior of Amnion Muscle Cells in Semisynthetic Nutrient Media

It is difficult to isolate single cells of smooth muscle for physiologic studies by teasing them out of the tissue (see Stave, 1954, and Walls, 1960). Cells isolated from smooth muscle by trypsinization are especially well suited for observing the contractile process in the isolated cell.

Amnions of chicken eggs of 7 to 8 days of incubation offer a particular advantage, because the organs at this age yield a high percentage of isolated and pulsating cells. The cells were cultivated in hollow ground slides in M 12.

The amnion muscle cells, which are rounded at the beginning of the cultivation, do not pulsate. The first pulsations can be observed only after the cells have begun to adhere to and flatten out on the glass surface.

The contractions, which are quite different from those of the heart muscle cells, are accompanied by pronounced changes in the shape of the cells and are not always rhythmic. Some cells exhibit a sudden, stepwise mode of contraction and relaxation. The RP after 7 hours in culture is 9 and declines after 28 hours to about 6 to 7 per minute.

After 24 hours the number of pulsating amnion cells decreases steadily. Pulsating cell layers were never observed. After 48 hours most of the cells are flattened out on the glass and only a few of them are pulsating.

When the amnion muscle cells are cultured in medium M 20-AGP in Thomas flasks, the RP after 18 to 24 hours lies between 7 and 10 per minute. A comparison of the maximum frequency of the heart and of the amnion during embryogenesis of the chick (see Bautzmann et al., 1954; Preyer, 1885; Romanoff, 1944) with the RP in 24-hour cultures of atrium cells in SM 20, ventricle cells in SM 20, and amnion cells in M 20-AGP, yields the following organ frequency/RP quotients: 2.8, 3.2, and 2.4, respectively.

Pharmacologic Studies

The first pharmacologic studies of isolated heart cells in cell culture were conducted by Cavanaugh and Cavanaugh (1957), Halle (1959), Halle and

Wollenberger (1959), and Wollenberger and Halle (1960). The results demonstrated that the cultured heart cells respond to quinidine and to digitoxin in a manner similar to that of the intact heart. The question arose: Are the isolated cultured heart muscle cells a representative system for testing cardioactive drugs at the cellular level?

In answer to this question it is necessary to point out, first of all (see pp. 224-227) that the heart cells undergo profound functional and structural changes as a result of trypsinization and during cultivation. But sufficient information is available today on the behavior of these cells to warrant their use as a model test object in the study of the action of cardioactive drugs (see Halle, 1963a, 1963b, 1967b, and 1969; Wollenberger, 1964a). A few examples will be presented of effects of drugs and ions on heart cell cultures which are observable with the phase-contrast microscope.

CARDIAC GLYCOSIDES.—Cardiac glycosides bring about a concentration-dependent increase in the RP of cultured ventricle cells. The concentration-effect curve covers the range of 10^{-9} to 10^{-7} M (approximately 10^{-3} to 10^{-1} μg/l) and is linear in the semilogarithmic coordinate system (Fig. 11). The action of higher concentrations on the automaticity is marked by a steeper rise (Fig. 11) or, in a few cultures, by a fall of the RP. Previously quiescent cells may be stimulated to beat. This effect is observed at glycoside concentrations as low as 10^{-9}M.

The contractions of the cultured cardiac cells are visibly strengthened by 10^{-8} to 10^{-7}M glycoside. The processes of shortening and relaxation are speeded up. These inotropic effects are recognized by following the changes in the cell profile and the passive movements of cytogranules. Another observed change is that bigeminal and trigeminal beats occur more frequently than in control cultures. The number of arrhythmically pulsating cells increases sharply after addition of 10^{-7}M and, even more so, 10^{-6}M glycoside. The arrhythmias manifest themselves as irregularly spaced contractions of the entire cell body and as asynchronous contractions of two or more pulsation centers in the same cell, occurring independently of each other and at varying frequencies (see Fig. 12). Undulatory pulsations, fibrillatory movements, and cessation of contractile activity often characterize the terminal stage of glycoside poisoning.

The glycoside effects can be washed away quickly. The contractions become rhythmic again and the RP returns to values recorded prior to the application of glycoside. In this respect the behavior of the isolated cultured embryonic chick heart ventricle cells differs from that of the intact postnatal heart of various species to which many glycosides, especially digitoxin, are rather strongly bound. Possible reasons for this difference are discussed by Wollenberger (1964a).

Cell culture in a perfusion chamber permits the observation of the reactions described here on selected single cells. The glycoside effects have been recorded by cinemicrography (see Halle and Wollenberger, 1959). Details are given by Wollenberger and Halle (1963a) and Halle (1967c). Suggestions concerning the use of heart cell cultures for standardization and bioassay of cardiac glycosides are discussed in the latter paper.

Studies carried out in several laboratories under widely varying conditions of cultivations have confirmed the observations previously described. We are dealing

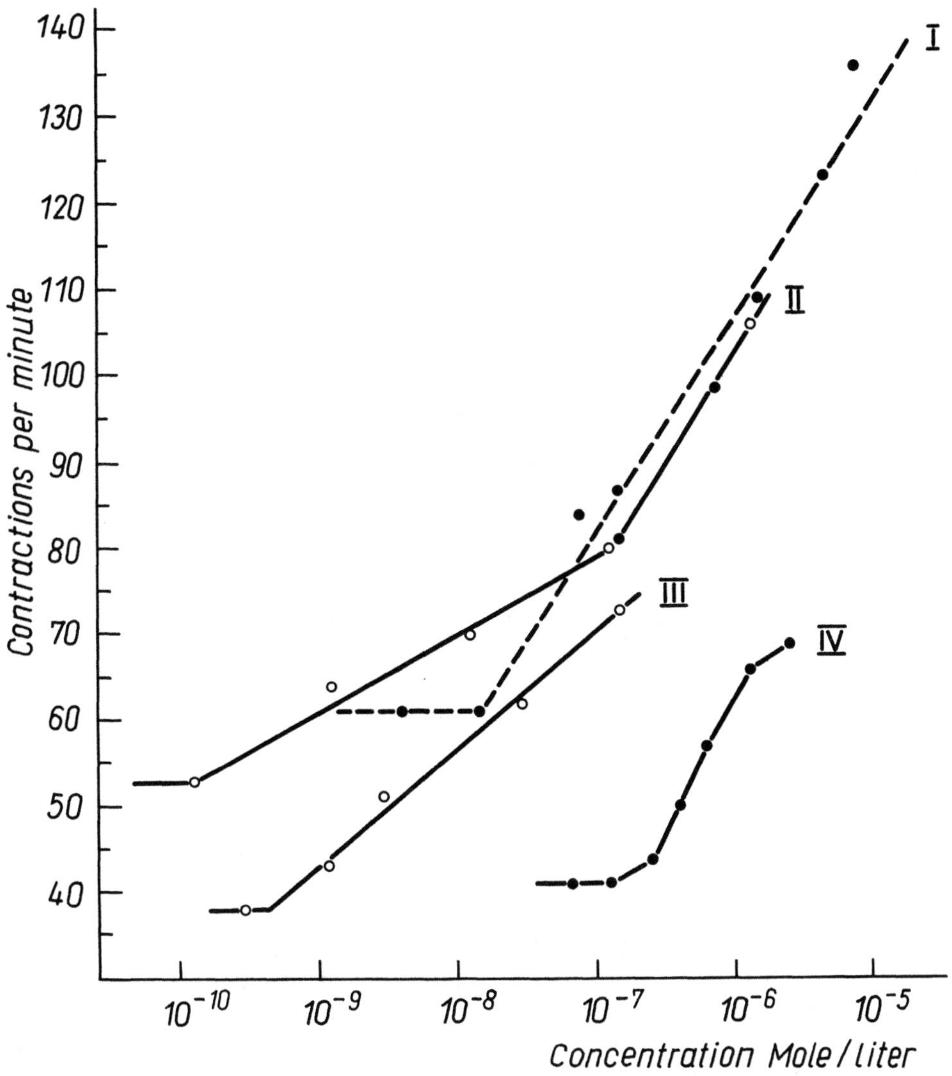

FIG. 11. Positive chronotropic action of aconitine (I), digitoxin (II), β^{1-24}-corticotropin (III), and L-Triiodothyronine (IV) on the pulsation of cells isolated from the heart ventricles of 10- to 12-day-old chick embryos after 1 to 2 days of incubation in semisynthetic media. (After Halle. 1967b. *Gegenbaurs Morph. Jahrb.*, 111:3, Fig. 5.)

here with a characteristic case of organ-specific reactions of cultured cells to a group of drugs (see DeHaan, 1964; Halle, 1959 and 1967c; Harary and Farley, 1960; Harary and Slater, 1965; Mercer and Dower, 1966; Mercer et al., 1967; Omura, 1966; Omura et al., 1964; Pankey and Mogabgab, 1965; Wollenberger and Halle, 1963a).

Amnion cells are less sensitive to cardiac glycosides than are heart ventricle cells. Their RP is not affected by 10^{-8}M digitoxin, but is increased by 10^{-7}M and

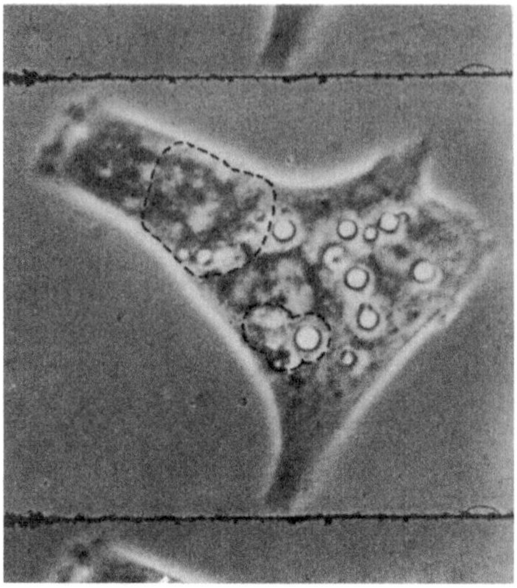

FIG. 12. Isolated ventricle cell poisoned with digitoxin. Two independently operating centers of spontaneous contractile activity, marked off by the broken lines, are located on each side of the cell nucleus. Motion picture frame; final magnification × 1,700. (From Wollenberger and Halle. 1963a. *Proc. First Internat. Pharmacol. Meeting,* Oxford, Pergamon Press, Vol. 3, p. 87, Fig. 7.)

lowered by 10^{-6}M glycoside. At 10^{-7} M the number of pulsating cells increases and the pulsations become more vigorous. The glycoside effect is not, or not easily, reversed by washing with glycoside-free medium.

OTHER DRUGS AND HORMONES.—The RP of cultured heart ventricle cells is increased by the pituitary polypeptides corticotropin and α-MSH in concentrations as low as 10^{-9}M (Wollenberger, 1964a), by triiodothyronine (Wollenberger, 1964b), by 5×10^{-8} to 5×10^{-7} M epinephrine (Wollenberger, 1964b; Wollenberger and Halle, 1963b), and by 10^{-7} M aconitine (Halle, 1967a); it is lowered by 1 to 5×10^{-6} m quinidine (Halle, 1967a) and reserpine (Wollenberger and Halle, 1963b). Figure 11 shows the increase in RP as a function of the concentration of some of these compounds. Figure 13 depicts the time course of action of synthetic β^{1-23}-corticotropin on the adult dog heart and on cultured embryonic chick heart ventricle cells. The two responses are practically identical, both with regard to the percentage increase in the rate of beat and with regard to the transient nature of the increase. The positive chronotropic effects of epinephrine and digitoxin on the cultured heart cells are inhibited by β-adrenergic blocking agents and reserpine (Wollenberger, 1964b; Wollenberger and Halle, 1963b). The suppression of the isoproterenol effect by propranolol was studied by Harrison et al. (1967). The action of ATP and phosphocreatine on beating heart

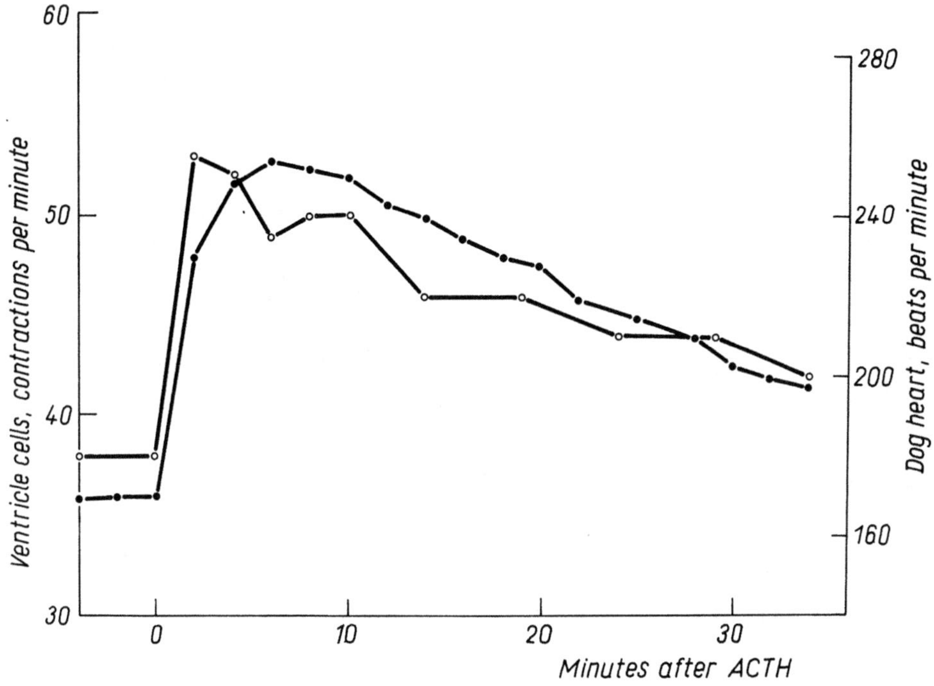

FIG. 13. The positive chronotropy of corticotropin on the adult dog heart in the heart-lung preparation (Solid circle) and on single cultured chick embryonic ventricle cells (Open circle); 0.09 μg of natural β-corticotropin per ml blood was used in the heart-lung preparation, and 0.02 μg of synthetic β^{1-24}-corticotropin added per ml culture medium. (After Wollenberger. 1964a. *Circ. Res.,* 14 (Suppl. 2), and 15:184, Fig. 12.)

cells was described by Blomquist (1964). Other pharmacologic investigation on heart cells were carried out by Bovis et al. (1966), Kallabis (1966), Kroon and Jansen (1968), Mulder and Wit (1966), Noguchi et al. (1966), and Sperelakis and Lehmkuhl (1965, 1967).

IONS.—Isolated heart cells exhibit positive chronotropic, inotropic, and bathmotropic reactions to 0.15 to 0.3 mM Ba^{++} (Fig. 14). The positive bathmotropic action of barium is impressively demonstrated in heart cell cultures in which all cells are at rest (Halle, 1967a; Halle and Wollenberger, 1968). The action of various K^+ concentrations on the bathmotropy of pacemaker cells (DeHaan, 1967a, 1967b) and on the chronotropy of cell layers in heart cell cultures (Halle and Wollenberger, 1968) has been described. Extensive electrophysiologic studies of the action of various ions on spontaneously pulsating cultured ventricle cells were carried out by Lehmkuhl and Sperelakis (1967), Sperelakis (1967), and Sperelakis and Lehmkuhl (1966).

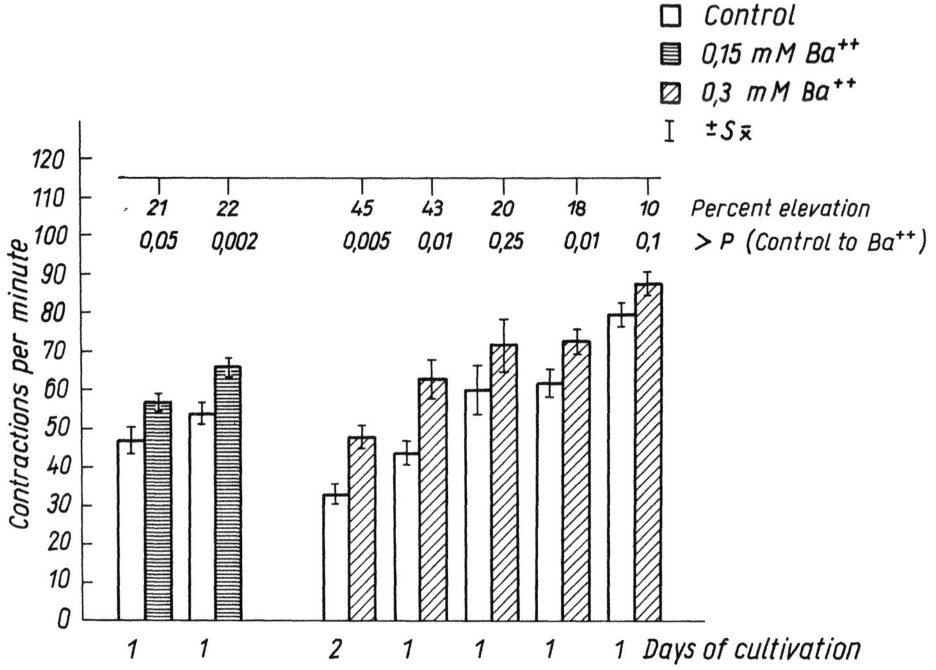

FIG. 14 Increase in the rate of contractions after addition of Ba^{++}. Slowly beating cultures were more strongly stimulated by Ba^{++} than faster beating ones. $S_{\bar{x}}$ = standard error of the mean. From Halle, 1969).

CONCLUSION

The question raised above–are the isolated heart muscle cells a representative system for testing cardioactive drugs at the cellular level?–can now be answered as follows: On the whole, the effects of drugs on isolated myocardial cells in culture which have been described in the literature resemble closely the actions of these drugs on the intact heart or its pacemaker parts. Similarly, the responses of single cultured amnion cells to drugs are comparable to those of the intact amnion. The isolated cultured muscle cells as living (not merely surviving), homogeneous, and well-defined biologic systems are thus model test objects for the analysis of the action of drugs and other biologically active substances at the cellular level. In view of the observed biochemical changes which are taking place in the myocardial and possibly other muscle cells during their isolation and cultivation it is advisable to carry out pharmacologic tests in the course of the first days of cultivation. It has been shown that during this period at least the autorhythmically pulsating muscle cells behave with respect to excitation and contraction in a manner similar to that of the intact organ of origin or its pacemaker parts in the absence of nervous influences.

Finally, a great advantage of single heart cell cultures, from the point of view of the economy of the experimental work in pharmacologic testing, is the fact that each isolated cell carries the same statistical weight as a whole heart or an animal (Wollenberger and Halle, 1963a).

This chapter has presented a detailed description of methods which may be employed in the cultivation of heart and other muscle cells under standardized conditions in semisynthetic, conditioned, and synthetic nutrient media. The cultured myocardial cells represent a useful biologic model for the study of the action of a variety of cardiac drugs and of other cardioactive substances at the cellular level. Functional differentiation (automaticity, excitability, contractility), biochemical differentiation (specific enzyme pattern, synthesis of contractile proteins), and structural differentiation (myogenesis) may be analyzed in a controlled milieu in conjunction with growth and proliferation and their regulation. Inductor effects for these processes may be examined independently of the influences of complex tissue and organ systems. For these reasons cultures of cells derived from various tissues and organs are being employed on an increasing scale in biochemical, physiologic, and pharmacologic studies.

The isolated cultured heart cells may be regarded as "microhearts" which are particularly useful in the testing of cardioactive drugs when it appears desirable to widen the range of assay methods employed and when there is only a very small amount of drug available.

The methods for isolating and culturing heart cells that are described or refered to in this chapter provide a reasonable guarantee, when properly employed, that the isolated cells keep their property of spontaneous pulsation in the culture for a minimum of two weeks and frequently for much longer. No particular nutrient medium is required for the maintenance of the spontaneous pulsations of isolated myocardial and other muscle cells. The problem of how processes of differentiation or dedifferentiation in these cells are influenced by specific constituents of the various nutrient media remains to be explored.

APPENDIX

A number of relevant publications which appeared or came to our attention following completion of this chapter deserve brief mention. Spontaneously pulsating, isolated heart cells of 1- to 4-day-old hamsters (Andrus and Strasser, 1967) and of 15- to 16-day-old mouse embryos (Goshima, 1969) have been cultured in semisynthetic nutrient media. Beating, neonatal rat heart ventricle cells could be cultured for 20 days in a chemically fully defined nutrient medium (Halle and Wollenberger, 1970). Additional morphologic characteristics of embryonic chick heart cells in the synthetic nutrient medium SM 20 have been described (Halle, 1969b). Heart cells cultured in a nutrient medium enriched with agglutinin-free serum were seen to pulsate for six months (Gross et al., 1969) and for more than a year (Gross, 1969).

Dower and Ziegler (1968) described a balloon isolator for working in a sterile environment. Capillary tubes were used as perfusion chambers for heart cells

(Savageau and Steward, 1967). A spin-filter culture system was developed (Himmelfarb et al., 1969) which permits the study of the action of drugs upon cells in suspension. Langer et al. (1969) studied $^{45}Ca^{++}$ exchange in heart cells attached to a surface consisting of glass scintillator material. Karapetyan et al. (1969) described a new system for measuring the contraction amplitude of heart cells. Offerijns et al. (1969) and Yaffe (1968) reported the long-term storage of myocardial cells and skeletal muscle cell lines of neonatal rats at −196°C and −80°C, respectively, without loss of viability and of differentiation potentiality.

Fujisawa (1969) found that the lactic dehydrogenase isozyme pattern shifts from a predominantly H type to the M type in the course of cultivation of heart and skeletal muscle cells. Coleman and Coleman (1968) studied muscle cytodifferentiation as manifested by myosin synthesis and creatine kinase activity in cell cultures to which 5-fluorodeoxyuridine was added at the time of muscle cell fusion for prevention of overgrowth by non-muscle cells. Bischoff and Holtzer (1969) and O'Neill and Strohman (1969) presented evidence that processes of differentiation in skeletal muscle cell cultures, such as the formation of myotubes, occur in the G_1 phase of the cell cycle. Bischoff and Holtzer (1970) and Coleman et al. (1969) suppressed differentiation in cultures of skeletal muscle cells by the use of 5-bromodeoxyuridine. The relationship between differentiation and proliferation in muscle cell cultures was discussed by Halle and Wollenberger (1970).

The following substances were tested in pharmacologic and biochemical studies on pulsating muscle cell cultures: Oligomycin and 2-deoxyglucose (Seraydarian et al., 1969), cortisol acetate (McCarl and Margossian, 1969), actinomycin D (McCarl and Shaler, 1969), cyclic 3′,5′-adenosine monophosphate and its dibutyryl derivative (Krause et al., 1970), insulin (DeLaHaba et al., 1968; Guidotti et al., 1969; Ziegler and Lippmann, 1970; Ziegler et al., 1969), diphtheria toxin (Bonventre and Imhoff, 1967), and calcium chloride (Olivo and Basa, 1967).

The electrophysiologic behavior of beating heart cells cultured in media of varying composition continued to be the subject of extensive investigation (Sperelakis and Lehmkuhl, 1968; Pappano and Sperelakis, 1969a, 1969b, 1969c; Sperelakis and Pappano, 1969a, 1969b; Kaufmann et al., 1968, 1969a, 1969b; DeHaan and Gottlieb, 1968; Girardier et al., 1968). Some of these authors, in contrast to Krause et al. (1970), could not reproduce the positive chronotropic effect of catecholamines described in this chapter. Possibly the adrenergic receptor system was inactivated or destroyed in these experiments, perhaps as a result of trypsinization (Kaufmann et al., 1968 to 1969b).

REFERENCES

Andresen, W. F., Price, F. M., Jackson, J. L., Dunn, T. B., and Evans, V. J. 1967. Characterization and spontaneous neoplastic transformation of mouse embryo cells isolated and continuously cultured in vitro in chemically defined medium NCTC 135. J. Nat. Cancer Inst., 38:169-183.

Andrus, W. De W., and Strasser, F. F. 1967. Beating hamster heart cells in tissue culture. Exp. Cell Res., 47:613-616.

Bautzmann, H., Dunker, E., and Schröder, R. 1954. Registrierung der Motorik des Amnions und des embryonalen Herzens beim Hühnchen mittels des Kathodenstrahl-Oszillographen. Anat. Anz., 101:317-321.

Bender, E., Schramm, T., Bierwolf, D., and Herrmann, G. 1968. Geräte zur Erleichterung und Verbesserung der Arbeit in der Zell- und Gewebezüchtung. Z. Med. Labortechn., 9:90-95.

Bischoff, R., and Holtzer, H. 1968. The effect of mitotic inhibitors on myogenesis in vitro. J. Cell Biol., 36:111-127.

—and Holtzer, H. 1969. Mitosis and the processes of differentiation of myogenic cells in vitro. J. Cell Biol., 41:188-200.

—and Holtzer, H. 1970. Inhibition of myoblast fusion after one round of DNA synthesis in 5-bromodeoxyuridine. J. Cell Biol., 44:134-150.

Blomquist, C. H. 1964. Studies of embryonic chick heart cells in tissue culture. Doctoral Thesis, University of Minnesota, 149 pp.

Bonventre, P. F., and Imhoff, J. G. 1967. Studies on the mode of action of diphtheria toxin. II. Protein synthesis in primary heart cell cultures. J. Exp. Med., 126:1079-1086.

Bovis, R., Kasten, F. H., and Okigaki, T. 1966. Electron microscopic study of the toxic effect of sodium fluoroacetate on rat myocardial cultures. Exp. Cell Res., 43:611-621.

Bucher, O., and Kolb, I. 1962. Zur photoelektrischen Registrierung der Pulsationen isolierter und in vitro explantierter Herzmuskelzellen. Med. Exp., 6:14-20.

Buchsbaum, R., and Kuntz, J. A. 1954. The effects of certain stimulants and depressants on individual fibroblasts in a perfusion chamber. Ann. N.Y. Acad. Sci., 58:1303-1310.

Burrows, M. T. 1910. The cultivation of tissues of the chick embryo outside the body. J. Amer. Med. Assoc., 55:2057-2058.

—1911. The growth of tissues of the chick embryo outside the animal body, with special reference to the nervous system. J. Exp. Zool., 10:63-84.

— 1912. Rhythmische Kontraktionen der isolierten Herzmuskelzelle ausserhalb des Organismus. München. Med. Wschr., 59:1473-1475.

Buskirk, H. H. 1967. Control of pleuropneumonia-like organisms in cell culture. Appl. Microbiol., 15:1442-1446.

Cahn, R. D. 1964. Developmental changes in embryonic enzyme patterns: The effect of oxidative substrates on lactic dehydrogenase in beating chick embryonic heart cell cultures. Develop. Biol., 9:327-346.

—1967a. Detergents in membrane filters. Science, 155:195-196.

—1967b. Changes in enzyme patterns in functional heart, cartilage, and pigmented retina cells in culture. *In* Factors Influencing Myocardial Contractility. Tanz, R. D., Kavaler, F., and Roberts, J., eds. New York, Academic Press, Inc., pp. 293-299.

—Coon, H. G., and Cahn, M. B. 1967. Cell culture and cloning techniques. *In* Methods in Developmental Biology. Wilt, F., and Wessells, N., eds. New York, Thomas Y. Crowell Company, pp. 493-530.

Cavanaugh, M. W. 1955. Pulsation, migration and division in dissociated chick embryo heart cells in vitro. J. Exp. Zool., 128:573-589.

—and Cavanaugh, D. J. 1957. Studies on the pharmacology of tissue cultures. I. The action of quinidine on cultures of dissociated chick embryo heart cells. Arch. Int. Pharmacodyn., 110:43-55.

Coleman, J. R., and Coleman, A. W. 1968. Muscle differentiation and macromolecular synthesis. J. Cell. Physiol. (Suppl. 1), 72:19-34.

—Coleman, A. W., and Hartline, E. J. H. 1969. A clonal study of the reversible inhibition of muscle differentiation by the halogenated thymidine analog 5-bromodeoxyuridine. Develop. Biol., 19:527.

Crill, W. E., Rumery, R. E., and Woodbury, Y. W. 1959. Effects of membrane current on transmembrane potentials of cultured chick embryo heart cells. Amer. J. Physiol., 197:733-735.

Curtis, A. S. G. 1965. Some interactions between cell and medium in culture. Arch. Biol. (Liège), 76:209-215.

Curtis, D. R. 1964. Microelectrophoresis. *In* Physical Techniques in Biological Research. Nastuk, W. L., ed. New York, Academic Press, Inc., Vol. 5, Part A, pp. 144-190.
Danes, B. S. 1955. Metabolism of cells grown in tissue culture. Adaptation of the cartesian diver method for the measurement of metabolic activity. C. R. Trav. Lab. Carlsberg, Sér. Chim., 29:209-221.
Dawson, M., and Dryden, W. F. 1967. Tissue culture in the study of the effects of drugs. J. Pharm. Sci., 56:545-561.
DeHaan, R. L. 1964. Pacemaker cells in the embryonic heart. *In* Annual Report of the Director, Dept. of Embryology, Carnegie Institution of Washington, Year Book, Vol. 63, pp. 531-535.
—1967a. Regulation of spontaneous activity and growth of embryonic chick heart cells in tissue culture. Develop. Biol., 16:216-249.
—1967b. Introduction: Spontaneous activity of cultured heart cells. *In* Factors Influencing Myocardial Contractility. Tanz, R. D., Kavaler, F., and Roberts, J., eds. New York, Academic Press, Inc., pp. 217-230.
—and Gottlieb, S. H. 1968. The electrical activity of embryonic chick heart cells isolated in tissue culture singly or in interconnected cell sheets. J. Gen. Physiol., 52:643-665.
DeLaHaba, G., Cooper, G. W., and Elting, V. 1966. Hormonal requirements for myogenesis of striated muscle in vitro: Insulin and somatotropin. Proc. Nat. Acad. Sci., U.S.A. 56:1719-1723.
—Cooper, G. W., and Elting, V. 1968. Myogenesis of striated muscle in vitro: Hormone and serum requirements for the development of glycogen synthetase in myotubes. J. Cell. Psysiol., 72:21-27.
DenBeste, H. E., Fjelde, A., Jackson, J. L., Andresen, W. F., Kerr, H. A., and Evans, V. J. 1966. Adaptation, growth, and chromosomal analysis of HEp-2 cells in chemically defined medium. J. Nat. Cancer Inst., 36:1075-1088.
Dietel-Mauersberger, B., and Tanneberger, S. 1964. Zellzüchtung in proteinfreien Nährmedien. I. Zellstamm L (Earle): Wachstum und Chromosomen. Acta Biol. Med. German., 13:254-263.
Dower, G. E., and Ziegler, W. G. 1968. A balloon isolator for culture of heart cells without antibiotics. Exp. Cell Res., 51:335-346.
Dulbecco, R. 1952. Production of plaques in monolayer tissue cultures by single particles of an animal virus. Proc. Nat. Acad. Sci., U.S.A. 38:747-752.
Eagle, H. 1955. Nutrition needs of mammalian cells in tissue culture. Science, 122:501-504.
—1959. Amino acid metabolism in mammalian cell cultures. Science, 130:432-437.
—1965a. Growth-regulatory effects of cellular interaction. Israel J. Med. Sci., 1:1220-1228.
—1965b. Metabolic controls in cultured mammalian cells. Science, 148:42-51.
—and Levintow, L. 1965. Amino acid and protein metabolism. I. The metabolic characteristics of serially propagated cells. *In* Cells and Tissues in Culture. Willmer, E. N., ed. New York, Academic Press, Inc., Vol. 1, pp. 277-296.
Edlinger, E., Dietel, S., Gao Dchang Liä and Spies, K. 1958. Zellkultur des Mäusefibroblastenstammes "L" in einem semisynthetischen Medium. Naturwissenschaften, 45:295-296.
Engel, H. J., and Zerbst, E. 1960. Untersuchungen zur Präparattemperatur auf Mikroskopheiztischen. Z. Wiss. Mikr., 64:384-394.
Evans, V. J., Bryant, J. C., Kerr, H. A., and Schilling, E. L. 1964. Chemically defined media for cultivation of long-term cell strains from four mammalian species. Exp. Cell Res., 36:439-474.
Fänge, R., Persson, H., and Thesleff, S. 1956. Electrophysiologic and pharmacological observations of trypsin-disintegrated embryonic chick hearts cultured in vitro. Acta Physiol. Scand., 38:173-183.
Fedoroff, S. 1967. Proposed usage of animal tissue culture terms. J. Nat. Cancer Inst., 38:607-611.

Flückiger, E., and Verzár, F. 1957a. Vergleichende Untersuchungen über die Wirkung von Desoxycorticosteron und Hydrocortison auf den Kohlehydrat-, Natrium- und Kaliumstoffwechsel des isolierten Muskels. Helv. Physiol. Pharmacol. Acta, 15:293-303.
—and Verzár, F. 1957b. Glykogen-, Natrium- und Kaliumstoffwechsel des überlebenden Muskels bei sukzessiver oder simultaner Wirkung von Corticosteroiden. Helv. Physiol. Pharmacol. Acta, 15:304-314.
Fujisawa, H. 1969. Changes in the isozyme patterns of lactate dehydrogenase (LDH) in the in vitro cultured muscle cells. Embryologia, 10:256-272.
Girardi, A. J., McMichael, H., Jr., and Henle, W. 1956. The use of HeLa cells in suspension for the quantitative study of virus propagation. Virology, 2:532-544.
Girardier, L., Forssmann, W. G., Hyde, A., and Matter, A. 1968. Ultrastrukturelle und elektrophysiologische Untersuchungen zur Frage der interzellulären Erregungsausbreitung am Rattenherzmuskel. Anat. Anz., 121:57-65.
Goldstein, L., and Eastwood, J. M. 1964. Micrurgy of tissue culture cells. *In* Methods in Cell Physiology. Prescott, D. M., ed. New York, Academic Press, Inc., Vol. 1, pp. 403-416.
—Cailleau, R., and Crocker, T. T. 1960. Nuclear-cytoplasma relationships in human cells in tissue culture. Exp. Cell Res., 19:332-342.
Gordon, H. P., and Wilde, C. E., Jr. 1965. "Conditioned" medium and heart muscle differentiation: Contrast between explants and disaggregated cells in chemically defined medium. Exp. Cell Res., 40:438-442.
Goshima, K. 1969. Synchronized beating of and electrotonic transmission between myocardial cells mediated by heterotypic strain cells in monolayer culture. Exp. Cell Res., 58:420-426.
Green, H., and Goldberg, B. 1965. Synthesis of collagen by mammalian cell lines of fibroblastic and nonfibroblastic origin. Proc. Nat. Acad. Sci., U.S.A. 53:1360-1365.
—Todaro, G. J., and Goldberg, B. 1966. Collagen synthesis in fibroblasts transformed by oncogenic viruses. Nature (London), 209:916-917.
Greene, A. E., Silver, R. K., Krug, M. D., and Coriell, L. L. 1965. A premixed powder for preparation of tissue culture media. Proc. Soc. Exp. Biol. Med., 118:122-128.
Gross, W. O. 1969. Über fortgesetzte Schlagtatigkeit isolierter Herzmuskelzellen während der Mitose und in den Tochterzellen. Meeting of the European Tissue Culture Society, Žinkovy, ČSSR, May 9.
—Schöpf-Ebner, E., and Bucher, O. M. 1968. Technique for the preparation of homogeneous cultures of isolated heart muscle cells. Exp. Cell Res., 53:1-10.
Grossfeld, H. 1959. Action of adrenalcortical steroids on cultured cells. Endocrinology, 65:777-784.
Guidotti, G. G., Luneburg, B., and Borghetti, A. F. 1969. Amino acid uptake in isolated chick embryo heart cells. Effect of insulin. Biochem. J., 114:97-105.
Halle, W. 1959. Über die Züchtung von Herzmuskelzellen in einem semisynthetischen Medium und ihr Verhalten gegenüber Digitoxin. Naturwissenschaften, 46:267.
—1960. Eine neue Flasche für Zellkulturen. Z. Med. Labortechn., 1:128-129.
—1963a. Wachstum und Pulsation isolierter Muskelzellen in einem semisynthetischen Nährmedium und ihr Verhalten gegenüber Herzglykosiden. 216 pp., Dissertation, Math. Nat. Fakultat der Humboldt-Univ. Berlin.
—1963b. Über die Kultivierung und das Verhalten spontan pulsierender Herzventrikelzellen in semisynthetischen Nährmedien unter in vitro-Bedingungen. Acta Biol. Med. German., 10:387-413.
—1963c. Die Bedeutung makromolekularer Substanzen für die Kultivierung tierischer Zellen in synthetischen Nährmedien. Z. Arztl. Fortbild. (Jena), 57:756-768.
—1965. Heiz- und Kühleinrichtung für mikroskopische Präparatehalter. DDR-Patentschrift 36160.
—1967a. Beitrag zur Wirkung verschiedener Ionen und Pharmaka auf die Automatie von Herzventrikel- and Amnionmuskelzellen in der Zellkultur. Naunyn-Schmiedebergs Arch. Pharm. Exp. Path., 256:322-332.

—1967b. Die in vitro kultivierte Zelle als Modell für morphologische und physiologische Untersuchungen. Gegenbaurs Morph. Jahrb., 111:3-30.
—1967c. Wirkung von Herzglykosiden auf die Automatie isolierter Herzzellen in vitro. Arzneimittelforschung, 17:1254-1258.
—1969b. Beitrag zur Morphologie von Herzzellen in einem chemisch definierten Nahrmedium. Z. Wiss. Zool., 180:34-45.
—1969a. Die in vitro kultivierte Muskelzelle als Modell fur Untersuchungen der Function und Stuktur: Habilitationsschrift, 214 pp., Humboldt-Univ. zu Berlin.
—and Ristau, O. 1966. Heiz- und Kühlsystem für mikroskopische Präparatehalter. DDR-Patentschrift 51459.
—and Wollenberger, A. 1959. Rhythmic contraction of single cultured cardiac muscle cells and their response to digitoxin. Research Film HF 326 with Booklet, 13 pp., Berlin, German Central Institute for Teaching Aids.
—and Wollenberger, A. 1968. Die Differenzierung isolierter Herzzellen in einem chemisch definierten Nährmedium. Z. Zellforsch., 87:292-314.
—and Wollenberger, A. 1970. Differentiation and behavior of isolated embryonic and neonatal heart cells in a chemically defined medium. Amer. J. Cardiol. (in press).
Ham, R. G. 1965. Clonal growth of mammalian cells in a chemically defined, synthetic medium. Proc. Nat. Acad. Sci., U.S.A., 53:288-293.
Hanks, J. H., Scherer, W. F., Fawcett, D. W., Leighton, J., and Porter, K. R. 1955. An Introduction to Cell and Tissue Culture. Minneapolis, Burgess Publishing Co., 123 pp.
Harary, I., and Farley, B. 1960. In vitro studies of single isolated beating heart cells. Science, 131:1674-1675.
—and Farley, B. 1963a. In vitro studies on single beating rat heart cells. I. Growth and organization. Exp. Cell Res., 29:451-465.
—and Farley, B. 1963b. In vitro studies on single beating rat heart cell. II. Intercellular communication. Exp. Cell Res., 29:466-474.
—and Slater, E. C. 1965. Studies in vitro on single beating heart cells. VIII. The effect of oligomycin, dinitrophenol, and ouabain on the beating rate. Biochim. Biophys. Acta, 99:227-233.
—Fujimoto, A., and Kuramitsu, H. 1964. Enzyme changes in cultured heart cells. Nat. Cancer Inst. Monogr., 13:257-275.
—McCarl, R., and Farley, B. 1966. Studies in vitro on single beating rat heart cells. IX. The restoration of beating by serum lipids and fatty acids. Biochim. Biophys. Acta, 115:15-22.
Harrison, D. C., Kleiger, R. E., and Merigan, T. C. 1967. Action of isoproterenol on heart cells in tissue culture. Proc. Soc. Exp. Biol. Med., 124:122-126.
Hauschka, S. D., and Konigsberg, I. R. 1966. The influence of collagen on the development of muscle clones. Proc. Nat. Acad. Sci., U.S.A. 55:119-126.
Hayflick, L., consult. ed., 1967. Biology of the mycoplasma. Ann. N. Y. Acad. Sci., 143:1-824.
Healy, G. M., and Parker, R. C. 1966a. An improved chemically defined basal medium (CMRL-1415) for newly explanted mouse embryo cells. J. Cell Biol., 30:531-538.
—and Parker, R. C. 1966b. Cultivation of mammalian cells in defined media with protein and nonprotein supplements. J. Cell Biol., 30:539-553.
Heunert, H. H. 1961. Präparationsmethoden für mikrokinematographische Vitaluntersuchungen an Bakterien. Research Film, 4:59-65.
—1962. Methoden zur Verhinderung von Schärfenschwankungen bei Zeitrafferaufnahmen von Agarkulturen. Research Film, 4:382-387.
— and Philipp, K. 1957. Grundlagen der Schmalfilmtechnik. Leitfaden für die wissenschaftliche Kinematographie. Berlin, Springer-Verlag, 200 pp.
Himmelfarb, P., Thayer, P. S., and Martin, H. E. 1969. Spin filter culture: The propagation of mammalian cells in suspension. Science, 164:555-557.

Holter, H., Linderstrom-Lang, K., and Zeuthen, E. 1956. Manometric techniques for single cells. *In* Physical Techniques in Biological Research. Oster, G., and Pollister, A. W., eds. New York, Academic Press, Inc. Vol. 3, pp. 577-625.

Holtzer, H. 1961. Aspects of chondrogenesis and myogenesis. *In* Synthesis of Molecular and Cellular Structure, 19th Growth Symposium. Rudnick, D., ed. New York, The Ronald Press Company, pp. 35-87.

Kaighn, M. E., Ebert, J. D., and Stott, P. M. 1966. The suspectibility of differentiating muscle clones to Rous sarcoma virus. Proc. Nat. Acad. Sci., U.S.A. 56:133-140.

Kallabis, E. 1966. Wirkung von Halothan und Chloroform in Verbindung mit Adrenalin auf die Spontanrhythmik isolierter und in vitro kultivierter Herzmuskelzellen. Acta Biol. Med. German., 17:327-333.

Karapetyan, A. E., Gevorkyan, R. A., Lvov, M. V., and Manukyan, G. A. 1969. Ustanovka dlya fotoelektricheskoy registratsii amplitudy sokrashcheniya kletok i eksplantatov miokarda kurinogo embriona. Bull. Eksp. Biol. No. 9, 124-125.

Kaufmann, R. and Tritthart, H. 1967. Registrier-Einrichtung zur gleichzeitigen Erfassung der mechanischen und elektrischen Aktivität einzelner Herzmuskelzellen aus Zellkulturen. Pflügers Arch. Ges. Physiol., 294:R 2.

—Rodenroth, S., and Tritthart, H. 1968. Trypsinbedingte Inaktivierung adrenergischer β-Receptoren bei kultivierten Herzmuskelzellen. Pflügers Arch. Ges. Physiol., 300:R 57.

—Tritthart, H., and Rodenroth, S. 1969a. Das mechanische und elektrische Verhalten isolierter embryonaler Herzmuskelzellen in Zellkulturen. Pflügers Arch. Ges. Physiol., 311:25-49.

—Tritthart, H., and Rost, B. 1969b. Trennung der Ca^{++}-antagonistischen Wirkungskomponente von den β-aandrenolytischen Effekten herzhemmender Pharmaka an Kulturen embryonaler Herzmuskelzellen. Naunyn-Schmiedebergs Arch. Pharmakol. Exp. Pathol., 264:252-253.

Kerkof, P. R., and Chaikoff, I. L. 1966. Follicular reorganization and ^{131}I utilization by cultured rat thyroid cells implanted into thyroidectomized rats. Endocrinology, 78:1177-1188.

Konigsberg, I. R. 1961. Some aspects of myogenesis in vitro. Circulation, 24:447-457.

—1963. Clonal analysis of myogenesis. Science, 140:1273-1284.

—and Hauschka, S. D. 1965. Cell and tissue interactions in the reproduction of cell type. *In* Reproduction: Molecular, Subcellular, and Cellular. Locke, M., ed. New York, Academic Press, Inc., pp. 243-290.

Kopac, M. J. 1954. Tissue culture: Past, present, and future. Ann. N. Y. Acad. Sci., 58:973-975.

—1964. Micromanipulators: Principles of design, operation, and application. *In* Physical Techniques in Biological Research. Nastuk, W. L., ed. New York, Academic Press, Inc., Vol. 5, Part A, pp. 191-233.

Krause, E. G., Halle, W., Kallabis, E., and Wollenberger, A. 1970. Positive chronotropic response of cultured isolated rat hearts cells to N^6, 2′-O-dibutyryl-3′,5′-adenosine monophosphate. J. Molec. Cell. Cardiol., 1 (in press).

Kroon, A. M., and Jansen, R. J. 1968. The effect of low concentrations of chloramphenicol on beating rat-heart cells in tissue culture. Biochim. Biophys. Acta, 155:629-632.

Kuhl, W. 1949. Die technischen Grundlagen der kinematischen Zellforschung. Berlin, Springer-Verlag, 185 pp.

Langer, G. A., Sato, E., and Seraydarian, M. 1969. Calcium exchange in a single layer of rat cardiac cells studied by direct counting of cellular activity of labeled calcium. Circ. Res., 24:589-597.

Lee, H. H., Kaighn, M. E., and Ebert, J. D. 1966. Viral antigens in differentiating muscle colonies after infection with Rous sarcoma virus in vitro. Proc. Nat. Acad. Sci. U. S.A., 56:521-525.

Lehmkuhl, D., and Sperelakis, N. 1963. Transmembrane potentials of trypsin-dispersed chick heart cells cultured in vitro. Amer. J. Physiol., 205:1213-1220.
—and Sperelakis, N. 1967. Electrical activity of cultured heart cells. *In* Factors Influencing Myocardial Contractility. Tanz, R. D., Kavaler, F., and Roberts, J., eds. New York, Academic Press, Inc., pp. 245-278.
Leslie, I., and Yarnell, M. 1960. Succinic dehydrogenase and cytochrome oxidase activities in cell cultures. J. Biophys. Biochem. Cytol., 7:265-272.
Levinson, C., and Green, J. W. 1965. Cellular injury resulting from tissue disaggregation. Exp. Cell Res., 39:309-317.
Lieberman, M. 1967. Effects of cell density and low K on action potentials of cultured chick heart cells. Circ. Res., 21:879-888.
Lucy, J. A. 1965. Amino acid and protein metabolism. II. Further aspects of the amino acid and protein metabolism of tissues in culture. *In* Cells and Tissues in Culture. Willmer, E. N., ed. New York, Academic Press, Inc., Vol. 1, pp. 297-315.
Macpherson, I. 1966. Mycoplasmas in tissue culture. J. Cell Sci., 1:145-168.
Marcus, P. I., Cieciura, S. J., and Puck, T. T. 1956. Clonal growth in vitro of epithelial cells from normal human tissues. J. Exp. Med., 104:615-628.
Mark, G. E. and Strasser, F. F. 1966. Pacemaker activity and mitosis in cultures of newborn rat heart ventricle cells. Exp. Cell Res., 44:217-233.
—Hackney, J. D., and Strasser, F. F. 1967. Morphology and contractile behavior of cultured heart cells, and their response to various oxygen concentrations. *In* Factors Influencing Myocardial Contractility. Tanz, R. D., Kavaler, F., and Roberts, J., eds. New York, Academic Press, Inc., pp. 301-315.
McCarl, R. L., and Margossian, S. S. 1969. Restoration of beating and enzymatic response of cultured rat heart cells to cortisol acetate. Arch. Biochem. Biophys., 130:321-325.
—and Shaler, R. C. 1969. The effects of actinomycin D on protein synthesis and beating in cultured rat heart cells. J. Cell Biol., 40:850-854.
Mercer, E. N., and Dower, G. E. 1966. Normal and arrhythmic beating in isolated cultured heart cells and the effects of digoxin, quinidine, and procaine amide. J. Pharmacol. Exp. Ther., 153:203-210.
—Ziegler, W. G., Wickland, G. F., and Dower, G. E. 1967. The effect of diphenylhydantoin upon beating of heart cells grown in vitro. J. Pharmacol. Exp. Ther., 155:267-270.
Meyer, H., and Queiroga, L. T. 1959. An electron microscope study of embryonic heart muscle cells grown in tissue culture. J. Biophys. Biochem. Cytol., 5:169-170.
Morgan, J. F. 1958. Tissue culture nutrition. Bact. Rev., 22:20-45.
—Campbell, M. E., and Morton, H. J. 1955. The nutrition of animal tissues cultivated in vitro. I. A survey of natural materials as supplements to synthetic medium 199. J. Nat. Cancer Inst., 16:557-567.
Moscona, A. 1952. Cell suspensions from organ rudiments of the early chick embryo. Exp. Cell Res., 3:535-539.
Mulder, A. H., and Wit, J. G. 1966. The inhibitory action of 2,6-dichloro-3-hydroxybenzonitrile and 2,6-dichloro-4-hydroxybenzonitrile on the beating of heart cells in tissue culture. Antagonism of oligomycin. Biochim. Biophys. Acta, 128:391-393.
Munro, T. R., and Daniel, M. R. 1965. The effects of micro-operations on the morphology, survival, and lysosomes of Chinese hamster fibroblasts. Exp. Cell Res., 38:483-494.
Murray, M. R. 1965. Muscle. *In* Cells and Tissues in Culture. Willmer, E. N., ed. New York, Academic Press, Inc., Vol. 2, pp. 311-372.
Noguchi, T. T., Ohnuki, Y., and Okigaki, T. 1966. Effect of sodium fluoroacetate on myocardial cells in vitro. Nature (London), 209:1197-1198.
Offerijns, F. G. J., Freud, G. E., and Krijnen, H. W. 1969. Reanimation of myocardial cells preserved in the frozen state. Nature (London), 222:1174-1175.
Okazaki, K., and Holtzer, H. 1965. An analysis of myogenesis in vitro using fluorescein-labeled antimyosin. J. Histochem. Cytochem., 13:726-739.

—and Holtzer, H. 1966. Myogenesis: Fusion, myosin synthesis, and the mitotic cycle. Proc. Nat. Acad. Sci., U.S.A. 56:1484-1490.

Olivo, O. M., and Basa, M. 1967. L'azione del $CaCl_2$ su cellule dissociate di miocardio embrionale coltivate in vitro. Boll. Soc. Ital. Biol. Sper., 43:1085-1087.

Omura, Y. 1966. Optimal serum concentration for obtaining spontaneously beating tissue-cultured cardiac cells, and classification of cells from direct effect of cardiac glycoside. Fed. Proc., 25:621.

—Hoffman, B. F., and Herter, F. P. 1964. Pacemaker localization and conduction block in beating cardiac cells treated by cardiac glycoside. Circulation (Suppl. 3), 30:134-135.

O'Neill, M., and Strohman, R. C. 1969. Changes in DNA polymerase activity associated with cell fusion in cultures of embryonic muscle. J. Cell. Physiol., 73:61-68.

Pankey, G. A., and Mogabgab, W. J. 1965. Contracting chicken embryo heart cells in tissue culture. Effect of viruses and other agents. Amer. Heart J., 70:94-109.

Pappano, A. J., and Sperelakis, N. 1969a. Spike electrogenesis in cultured heart cells. Amer. J. Physiol., 217:615.

—and Sperelakis, N. 1969b. Low K^+ conductance and low resting potentials of isolated single cultured heart cells. Amer. J. Physiol., 217:1076.

—and Sperelakis, N. 1969c. Spontaneous contractions of cultured heart cells in high K^+ media. Exp. Cell Res., 54:58-68.

Paul, J. 1965. Carbohydrate and energy metabolism. *In* Cells and Tissues in Culture. Willmer, E. N., ed. New York, Academic Press, Inc., Vol. 1, pp. 239-276.

Penso, G., and Balducci, D. 1963. Tissue cultures in biological research. Amsterdam, Elsevier Publishing Company, 468 pp.

Pomerat, C. M., consult. ed., 1954. Tissue culture technique in pharmacology. Ann. N. Y. Acad. Sci., 58:971-1325.

—Rounds, D. E., and Huff, W. 1964. Optical scanning and electronic recording of cellular activity. J. Roy. Micr. Soc., 83:265-270.

Preyer, W. 1885. Specielle Physiologie des Embryo. Leipzig, Th. Grieben's Verlag (L. Fernau), 644 pp.

Puck, T. T., Cieciura, S. J., and Robinson, A. 1958. Genetics of somatic mammalian cells. III. Long-term cultivation of euploid cells from human and animal subjects. J. Exp. Med., 108:945-956.

—Waldren, C. A., and Jones, C. 1968. Mammalian cell growth proteins. I. Growth stimulation by Fetuin. Proc. Nat. Acad. Sci., U.S.A., 59:192-199.

Rabin, B. S., Kite, J. H., Jr., and Rose, N. R. 1966. Loss of organ specific characteristics of hog thyroid cells during growth in vitro. Proc. Soc. Exp. Biol. Med., 121:888-894.

Refson, C. M. 1959. A method for the separation of chick heart muscle cells from heart fibroblasts and the determination of their growth rates on glass substrates. Doctoral Thesis, Rutgers The State University, New Brunswick, New Jersey, 131 pp.

Rinaldini, L. M. 1954. A quantitative method for growing animal cells. Nature (London), 173:1134-1135.

—1958. The isolation of living cells from animal tissues. *In* International Review of Cytology. Bourne, G. H., Danielli, J. F., eds. New York, Academic Press, Inc., Vol. 7, pp. 587-647.

—1959. An improved method for the isolation and quantitative cultivation of embryonic cells. Exp. Cell Res., 16:477-505.

Robineaux, R., and Barski, G. 1956. Chambres pour la perfusion des cultures de tissu et l'observation en microscopie à contraste de phase. Mikroskopie, 11:65-69..

Romanoff, A. L. 1944. The heart beat of avian embryos. Anat. Rec., 89:313-316.

Romeis, B. 1948. Mikroskopische Technik. München, Leibniz-Verlag, p. 256, 695 pp.

Rose, G. G. 1954. A separable and multipurpose tissue culture chamber. Texas Rep. Biol. Med., 12:1074-1083.

—Ed. 1963. Cinemicrography in Cell Biology. New York, Academic Press, Inc., 516 pp.

—Pomerat, C. M., Shindler, T. O., and Trunnel, J. B. 1958. A cellophane-strip technique for culturing tissue in multipurpose culture chambers. J. Biophys. Biochem. Cytol., 4:761-764.

Rosenoer, V. M., and Jacobson, W. 1966. Tissue culture in pharmacology. *In* Cells and Tissues in Culture. Willmer, E. N., ed. New York, Academic Press, Inc. Vol. 3, pp. 351-396.

Rumery, R. E., and Blandau, R. J. 1964. The cytodifferentiation of myocardial cells from 4-day embryonic chick hearts grown in culture. Acta Anat. (Basel), 58:116-130.

—Blandau, R. J., and Hagey, P. W. 1961. Observations on living myocardial cells from cultured 48-hour chick hearts. Anat. Rec., 141:253-261.

—and Rieke, W. O. 1967. DNA synthesis by cultured myocardial cells. Anat. Rec., 158:501-507.

Sanford, K. K., Dupree, L. T., and Covalesky, A. B. 1963. Biotin, B_{12}, and other vitamin requirements of a strain of mammalian cells grown in chemically defined medium. Exp. Cell Res., 31:345-375.

Sato, G. H., and Yasumura, Y. 1966. Retention of differentiated function in dispersed cell culture. Trans. N. Y. Acad. Sci., Ser. 2, 28:1063-1079.

Savageau, M. A., and Steward, J. P. 1967. Contraction rate of rat cardiac cells in culture: Responses to prolonged perfusion. Curr. Mod. Biol., 1:159-164.

Schindler, R. 1965. Die tierische Zelle in Zellkultur. Recent results in cancer research. Berlin, Springer-Verlag, Vol. 1, 88 pp.

Schneider, H., Shaw, M. W., Muirhead, E. E., and Smith, A. 1965. The in vitro culture of embryonic chicken heart cells. Exp. Cell Res., 39:631-636.

Schulze, W., Wollenberger, A., and Halle, W. 1966. Feinstrukturelle und zytochemische Untersuchungen an embryonalen Hühnerherzzellen. *In* Probleme der Zell- und Gewebezüchtung. Lohmann, K., ed. Verhandl. der Gesellsch. für exp. Med. der DDR. Dresden und Leipzig, Th. Steinkopff-Verlag, Vol. 9, pp. 170-171.

Schwarz, W., Merker, H. J. and Kutzsche, A. 1962. Elektronenmikroskopische Untersuchungen über die Fibrillogenese in Fibroblastenkulturen. Z. Zellforsch., 56:107-124.

Seraydarian, M. W., Sato, E., Savageau, M., and Harary, I. 1969. In vitro studies of beating heart cells in culture. XII. The utilization of ATP and phosphocreatine in oligomycin and 2-deoxyglucose inhibited cells. Biochim. Biophys. Acta, 180:264-270.

Smith, T. E., Jr., and Berndt, W. O. 1964. The establishment of beating myocardial cells in long-term culture in fluid medium. Exp. Cell Res., 36:179-191.

Sperelakis, N. 1967. Electrophysiology of cultured chick heart cells. *In* Elektrophysiology and Ultrastructure of the Heart. Sano, T., Mizuhira, V., and Matsuda, K., eds. Tokyo, Bunkodo Company, Ltd., pp. 81-108.

—and Lehmkuhl, D. 1964. Effect of current on transmembrane potentials in cultured chick heart cells. J. Gen. Physiol., 47:895-927.

—and Lehmkuhl, D. 1965. Insensitivity of cultured chick heart cells to autonomic agents and tetrodotoxin. Amer. J. Physiol., 209:693-698.

—and Lehmkuhl, D. 1966. Ionic interconversion of pacemaker and nonpacemaker cultured chick heart cells. J. Gen. Physiol., 49:867-895.

—and Lehmkuhl, D. 1967. Effects of temperature and metabolic poisons on membrane potentials of cultured heart cells. Amer. J. Physiol., 213:719-724.

—and Lehmkuhl, D. 1968. Ba^{2+} and Sr^{2+} reversal of the inhibition produced by ouabain and local anesthetics on membrane potentials of cultured heart cells. Exp. Cell Res., 49:396-410.

—and Pappano, A. J. 1969a. Depolarization of cultured heart cells by a lipid-soluble acetylcholine analogue. Amer. J. Physiol., 217:625.

—and Pappano, A. J. 1969b. Increase in P_{Na} and P_K of cultured heart cells produced by veratridine. J. Gen. Physiol., 53:97-114.

Stave, U. 1954. Beiträge zum Studium der Bewegungsformen glattmuskeliger Organpräparate. Naunyn-Schmiedebergs Arch. Exp. Path. Pharm., 223:294-305.

Stouffer, J. E., and Lipscomb, H. S. 1963. Reversible binding of ACTH to a glass surface. Endocrinology, 72:91-94.

Stowell, R. E., ed. 1965. Cryobiology. A conference sponsored by the American Cancer Society. Fed. Proc. (Suppl. 15), 24:1-324.

Swim, H. E., and Parker, R. F. 1958. Stable tissue culture media prepared in dry form. J. Lab. Clin. Med., 52:309-311.

Tanz, R. D. 1960. Studies on the action of cortisone acetate on isolated cardiac tissue. J. Pharmacol. Exp. Ther., 128:168-175.

Thomas, F. L. X., and Cramer, L. M. 1966a. A chamber and perfusion system for general and specialized in vitro studies. Part I. Texas Rep. Biol. Med., 24:700-711.

—and Cramer, L. M. 1966b. A chamber and perfusion system for general and specialized in vitro studies. Part II. Biaxially oriented polystyrene: An inert substrate and diffusion membrane for use in tissue culture. Texas Rep. Biol. Med., 24:712-719.

Thomas, J. A. 1937. Un flacon nouveau pour la culture des tissus sur une lamelle amovible. Arch. Exp. Zellforsch., 20:68-72.

Trinkaus, J. P., and Lentz, J. P. 1964. Direct observation of type-specific segregation in mixed cell aggregates. Develop. Biol., 9:115-136.

Vogel, F. S., and Kemper, L. 1965. Structural and functional characteristics of deoxyribonucleic acid-rich mitochondria of the common meadow mushroom, Agaricus campestris. II. Extracellular cultures. Lab. Invest., 14:1868-1893.

Walls, E. W. 1960. The microanatomy of muscle. *In* The Structure and Function of Muscle. Bourne, G. H., ed. New York, Academic Press, Inc., Vol. 1, Structure, pp. 21-61.

Waymouth, C. 1965a. Construction and use of synthetic media. *In* Cells and Tissues in Culture. Willmer, E. N., ed. New York, Academic Press, Inc., Vol. 1, pp. 99-142.

—1965b. The cultivation of cells in chemically defined medium and the malignant transformation of cells in vitro. *In* Tissue Culture. Ramakrishnan, C. V., ed. The Hague-The Netherlands, Dr. W. Junk, Publisher, pp. 168-179.

White, P. R. 1946. Cultivation of animal tissues in vitro in nutrients of precisely known constitution. Growth, 10:231-289.

—1949. Prolonged survival of excised animal tissues in vitro in nutriments of known constitution. J. Cell. Comp. Physiol., 34:221-236.

—and Waymouth, C. 1954. Chemically defined synthetic nutrients for tissue cultures for pharmacological studies. Ann. N. Y. Acad. Sci., 58:1023-1028.

Willmer, E. N. 1960. Tissues in culture and in the body. Sympos. Soc. Exp. Biol., 14:28-40.

Wollenberger, A. 1964a. Rhythmic and arrhythmic contractile activity of single myocardial cells cultured in vitro. Circ. Res. 14 (Suppl. 2), and 15:184-201.

—1964b. Akute Wirkung von Trijodthyronin auf die Spontanrhythmik isolierter, in vitro kultivierter Herzzellen. Naunyn-Schmiedebergs Arch. Exp. Path. Pharm., 249:288-294.

—1967. Survival of potentially beating single heart cells in the frozen state. *In* Factors Influencing Myocardial Contractility. Tanz, R. D., Kavaler, F., and Roberts, J., eds. New York, Academic Press, Inc., pp. 317-327.

—and Halle, W. 1960. Specificity of the effects of cardiac glycosides on the rhythmic contraction of single cultured cardiac muscle cells. Nature (London), 188:1114-1115.

—and Halle, W. 1963a. Action of cardiac glycosides on automaticity and contractile activity in single cardiac muscle cells grown in vitro (a slow motion picture). *In* New Aspects of Cardiac Glycosides. Wilbrandt, W., ed. Proc. First Intern. Pharmacol. Meet., New York, Pergamon Press, Inc., Vol. 3, pp. 87-110.

—and Halle, W. 1963b. Einfluss von Reserpin und Dichlorisoproterenol auf die durch Adrenalin und Digitoxin hervorgerufenen Wirkungen an Kulturen spontan schlagender isolierter Zellen des embryonalen Hühnerherzens. Monatsberichte der Deutsch. Akad. Wiss. (Berlin), 5:38-42.

—Halle, W., Kallabis, E., Kleitke, B., Hinterberger, U., and Schulze, W. 1967. Cultivation of beating heart cells from frozen heart cell suspensions. Naturwissenschaften, 54:174.

Yaffe, D. 1968. Retention of differentiation potentialities during prolonged cultivation of myogenic cells. Proc. Nat. Acad. Sci. U.S.A., 61:477-483.

—and Feldman, M. 1964. The effect of actinomycin D on heart and thigh muscle cells grown in vitro. Develop. Biol., 9:347-366.

—and Feldman, M. 1965. The formation of hybrid multinucleated muscle fibers from myoblasts of different genetic origin. Develop. Biol., 11:300-317.

—and Fuchs, S. 1967. Autoradiographic study of the incorporation of uridine-^{3}H during myogenesis in tissue culture. Develop. Biol., 15:33-50.

Yasumura, Y., Tashjian, A. H., Jr., and Sato, G. H. 1966. Establishment of four functional clonal strains of animal cells in culture. Science, 154:1186-1189.

Young, F. B., Sharon, W. S., and Long, R. B. 1966. Preparation and use of dry powder tissue culture media. Ann. N. Y. Acad. Sci., 139:108-110.

Ziegler, B., and Lippmann, H. G. 1970. Zur Charakterisierung von Wachstum, Glukoseverbrauch und Laktatproduktion kultivierter, pulsierender Rattenherzzellen. Acta Biol. Med. German. (in press).

—Lippmann, H. G., Mehling, R., and Jutzi, E. 1969. Proteinzuwachs und Glukoseaufnahme isolierter Myokardzellen von Huhnchenembryo und Ratte in der Primarkultur. Experientia, 25:781-782.

CHAPTER 8

The Mitochondrion

Louis A. Sordahl, Carl Johnson, Zack R. Blailock and Arnold Schwartz

Division of Myocardial Biology, Baylor College of Medicine
Houston, Texas

INTRODUCTION

Mitochondria are the organelles primarily responsible for the major source of energy for most cells. It is not surprising that for many years there has been a great deal of research concerning their structure and function. The effects of a variety of substances, including pharmacologic agents, on mitochondria have captured the interest of investigators. The purpose of this chapter is to describe several isolation methods of selected types of mitochondria and the assay of their oxidative phosphorylation capacities. The concepts of electron transport and oxidative phosphorylation have been amply reviewed (Lehninger, 1967; Sanadi, 1965; Racker, 1965; Lehninger and Wadkins, 1962; Estabrook and Pullman, 1967; Pullman and Schatz, 1967; Tager et al., 1966), and the reader is referred to these references for further information. Other methods of isolation and assay are also

Some of the studies reported herein were supported by grants from U.S. Public Health Service (HE 07906 and HE 05435), the National Science Foundation (GB 6895), the National Cystic Fibrosis Foundation, and the Houston and Texas Heart Association.

Dr. Schwartz is a recipient of a USPHS Career Development Award (K_3HE 11875).

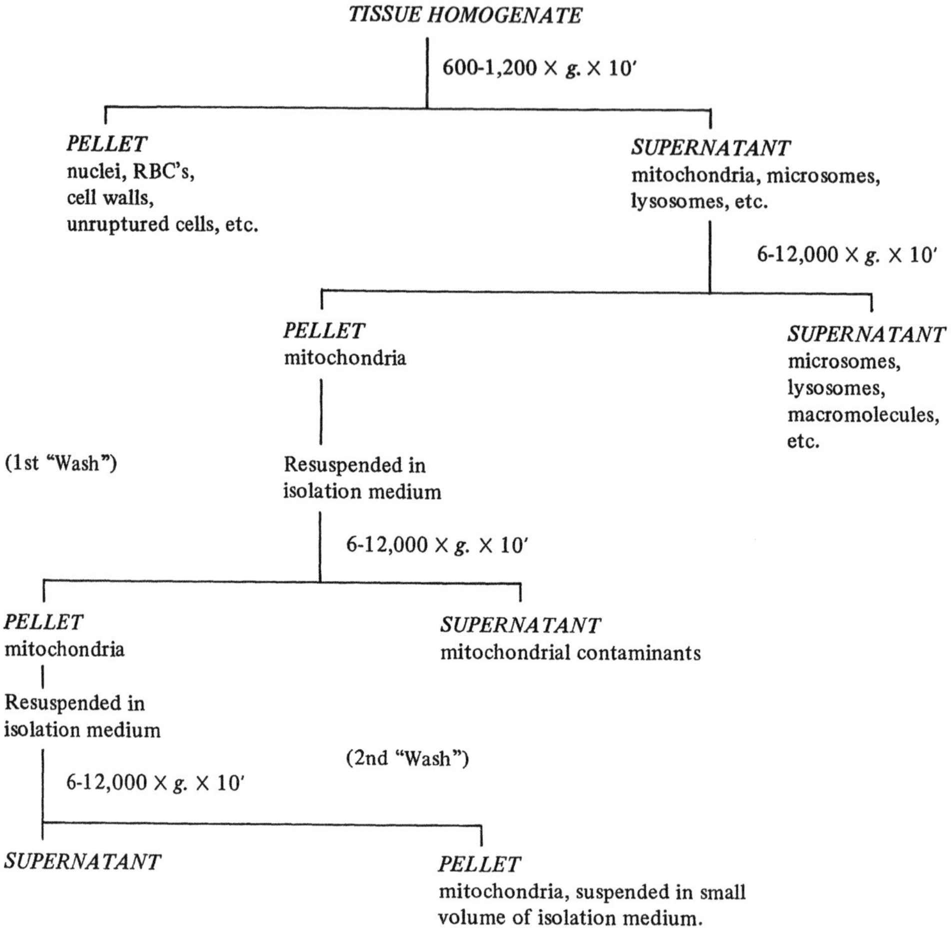

FIG. 1. Flow diagram for general mitochondrial isolation procedure.

available in the excellent compilation by Estabrook and Pullman (1967). Examples of the in vitro effects of a pharmacologic agent on mitochondria are discussed.

Other aspects of mitochondrial function such as ion translocation and low amplitude swelling-contraction are considered to be energy-linked (Packer et al., 1966; Lehninger et al., 1967). Consequently, the measurement of these important processes is detailed. In analyzing possible mechanisms of drug action on mitochondria, specific reactions of the electron transport chain can be studied using submitochondrial particles. Accordingly, the discussion of the preparation and assays of these particles is included. Since mitochondrial ultrastructure and biochemical function may be intimately related, a brief description of the preparation of electron micrographs has also been included.

The descriptions of these procedures are detailed with the intent of giving the investigator who might be relatively unfamilar with this field a working knowledge of relevant techniques.

ISOLATION OF MITOCHONDRIA

All procedures are carried out at 0° to 4°C. Glassware, solutions, and other materials that are used should be kept ice cold. All solutions used for preparation and assay should be made up in glass-distilled water. A composite flow sheet for mitochondrial preparation is shown in Figure 1.

Liver

This method is a modification of the method described by Schneider and Hogeboom (1950). The isolation medium (STE medium) consists of

0.25 M sucrose
1 mM tris–HCl (never use tris-SO_4)
1 mM ethylenediaminetetraacetate (EDTA)
ph 7.2-7.4

PROCEDURE:

1. The animal is decapitated and bled. The liver is quickly excised and placed in a beaker of ice-cold STE medium. In some cases it might be desirable to perfuse the liver in vivo through the portal vein, with ice-cold medium.
2. The liver is blotted dry, weighed, and placed in fresh STE medium.
3. The tissue is minced with sharp scissors and transferred to a homogenizing vessel (A. H. Thomas, size C). An alternative procedure is to put the liver through a tissue press (1-mm holes) and the resulting "paste" transferred to the homogenizing vessel. A standard garlic press makes an excellent, inexpensive device.
4. Ten volumes of STE medium per gram of tissue are added to the homogenizing vessel (10 percent homogenate; w/v).
5. The suspension is homogenized with a motor-driven, tight-fitting Teflon pestle until no whole particles of tissue are seen. Approximately six to seven strokes are necessary for 8 grams of tissue.
6. The homogenate is centrifuged at 600 × *g* for 10 minutes in a refrigerated centrifuge. The resulting pellet is discarded.
7. The supernatant is centrifuged at 8,500 × *g* for 12 minutes.
8. The resulting mitochondrial pellet is resuspended in approximately half the volume of STE medium used for the initial homogenate and centrifuged at 8,500 × *g* for 10 minutes. This "washing" procedure is repeated once or twice to remove microsomal and other cellular contamination. Quite often the mitochondrial pellet will appear with a light tan layer surrounding a darker pellet. This loose packing or "fluffy" layer should be removed by gentle agitation with STE medium over the packed pellet, prior to resuspension of the mitochondria during the "washing" process.
9. The pellet is finally resuspended in STE medium (approximately 1 ml per gram of original tissue). This will yield a suspension containing 20 to 30 mg of protein

per ml. Mitochondrial protein determinations are usually made by a biuret method. (Jacobs et al., 1956).

Heart

A number of methods have been described for both small and large scale preparation of heart mitochondria (Estabrook and Pullman, 1967). The following is a method of choice for the isolation of heart mitochondria from laboratory mammals (rat, guinea pig, rabbit, mouse and hamster). This method is a modification (Sordahl and Schwartz, 1967) of that suggested by Von Korff (1965). The isolation medium (KEA medium) consists of

0.18 M KCl
10 mM ethylenediaminetetraacetate (EDTA)
0.5 percent bovine serum albumin (Sigma, Fraction V)
pH 7.2-7.4

When heart mitochondria are prepared for potassium ion transport studies, the following isolation medium should be used:

0.18 M choline-Cl
20 mM tris-Cl
10 mM ethylenediaminetetraacetate (EDTA)
1.0 percent bovine serum albumin
pH 7.4

The STE medium previously described under "Liver" has also been used to isolate heart mitochondria. However, the concentration of EDTA is increased to 10 mM. KEA and choline-Cl media are equally good in obtaining adequate mitochondrial preparations. Mitochondria prepared in the STE medium have lower oxidative phosphorylation values compared to those isolated in KEA or choline-Cl.

PROCEDURE:

1. Animals are killed; the hearts are quickly excised below the atria and placed in ice-cold KEA medium.
2. The hearts are weighed, placed in a glass homogenizing vessel (A. H. Thomas, size C), and homogenized (12 volumes KEA medium per gram of tissue) for three to four seconds with a Polytron, PT-20* tissue processor at a rheostat setting of two. Two quick passes through the homogenate with a motor-driven Teflon pestle are then made to ensure complete cellular disruption. The latter, however, may not be necessary since similar results are obtained when the Polytron is used alone and homogenization is carried out directly in a centrifuge tube.

*Polytron, PT-20 (Brinkmann Instruments, Westbury, New York) exerts a shearing force on the tissue by rapidly driven blades encased in a fluted housing. At high speeds it also produces a sonication effect.

3. The homogenate is centrifuged at, 1,200 × *g* for 10 minutes.
4. The supernatant is strained through several layers of cheesecloth and centrifuged at 10,000 × *g* for 15 minutes.
5. The resulting mitochondrial pellet is resuspended in KEA medium (approximately half the volume used in the initial homogenization) and centrifuged at 10,000 × *g* for 8 minutes. This "washing" procedure is repeated once or twice to remove cellular contaminants adhering to the mitochondria.
6. The mitochondria are finally suspended in KEA medium (approximately half a ml medium per gram of original tissue) to yield a suspension containing 20 to 30 mg mitochondrial protein per ml. Protein concentration is determined by a biuret method (Jacobs et al., 1956).

COMMENTS: Heart mitochondria can be isolated in 0.18 M KCl-10 mM EDTA without bovine serum albumin, and they do exhibit adequate oxidative phosphorylation values. However, bovine serum albumin is required to maintain integrity for protracted periods. Several types of bovine serum albumin have been used with similar results. Ovalbumin cannot be used. Cesium chloride and RbCl have been used in place of KCl with equally good results, but NaCl and LiCl are detrimental. Hearts from animals larger than rats require some dicing with sharp scissors prior to homogenization.

Brain

Rat brain mitochondria are isolated by a modification of the method of Ozawa et al. (1966). The isolation medium (ME medium) consists of

0.3 M mannitol
0.1 mM ethylenediaminetetraacetate (EDTA)
adjusted to pH 7.4 with KOH.

PROCEDURE:

1. The rat is decapitated, the brain *rapidly* removed and placed in chilled ME medium.
2. Cerebellum and brainstem are removed while in the chilled medium.
3. Two brains are homogenized in 10 volumes of ME medium with a motor-driven Teflon pestle (homogenizing vessel as described under "Liver").
4. The homogenate is centrifuged at 600 × *g* for 8 minutes.
5. Supernatant is centrifuged at 10,000 × *g* for 10 minutes.
6. The resulting pellet is resuspended in 40 ml of ME medium and centrifuged at 5,000 × *g* for 10 minutes. The supernatant is decanted and saved.
7. A loosely packing, white sediment surrounding a brown pellet (mitochondria) should result. Remove the white sediment by gentle swirling with ME medium and combine with decanted supernate from step 6.
8. Suspend the brown mitochondrial pellet in ME medium (F_1 fraction).
9. Centrifuge the combined supernate and wash solution from steps 6 and 7 at 5,000 × *g* for 10 minutes.

10. A second mitochondrial pellet (brown) is obtained and combined with the F_1 fraction.
11. The two fractions are finally suspended in a small volume (approximately 0.8 ml per two rat brains) of ME medium, yielding a suspension of 10 to 20 mg mitochondrial protein per ml.

COMMENTS: Ozawa et al., (1966) have indicated the necessity for rapid removal of the brain from the calvarium after decapitation. They have demonstrated a marked decrease in oxidative phosphorylation values if the brains remain for more than one minute in the skull. These authors suggest that ischemia, caused by the decapitation, gives rise to the release of endogenous uncoupling factors. In our laboratory, we have found holding the rat head securely by the nose with a large forceps, making a posterior to anterior cut through the lateral sides of the calvarium and scooping out the entire brain with a small, spoon-type spatula, is most expeditious for rapid removal.

Tumor

The importance of the isolation medium in obtaining tumor mitochondria with adequate oxidative phosphorylation capacities has recently been emphasized (Mintz et al., 1967; Sordahl and Schwartz, 1967). The isolation medium is the STE medium previously described under the section for liver mitochondria, with the addition of 1 percent bovine serum albumin (Sigma, Fraction V). This medium is designated STEA.

PROCEDURE:

1. Animals are killed by cervical dislocation (mice) or decapitation (rats). The tumors are quickly dissected away from surrounding tissues and placed in chilled STEA medium.
2. The remaining steps in the isolation are identical with those described under "Liver," steps 2 through 9.

COMMENTS: Inclusion of bovine serum albumin in the *isolation medium* has been shown to be beneficial in obtaining mitochondrial preparations, with respiration control, from tumor (Sordahl and Schwartz, 1967). This is true for a variety of tumors, although a great deal of variability exists. The assay conditions can also influence (discussed in following section) the quality of values obtained for oxidative phoshorylation. Devlin (1967) has reported a beneficial effect of bovine serum albumin in either the isolation or assay medium. Since the serum albumin may be binding certain endogenous uncoupling factors (fatty acids), we recommend its inclusion in the isolation medium (STEA). Human serum albumin works as well as bovine, but ovalbumin is detrimental to mitochondria.

Other

Mitochondria have been isolated from a variety of tissues, both plant and animal. Among these are housefly flight muscle (Peron et al., 1965), thymus gland

(Tyler and Gonze, 1967), amphibian adrenal glands (Psychoyos et al., 1966), corn (Kenefick and Hanson, 1965), mammalian kidney (Weinbach, 1961), gastric mucosa (Forte et al., 1967), brown adipose tissue (Smith et al., 1966), skeletal muscle (Dow, 1967), developing red blood cells (Guggenheim et al., 1967) and sheep thyroid (Lamy et al., 1967). The reader is referred to these and other sources (Estabrook and Pullman, 1967) for detailed information.

Preparations of mitochondria from fetal tissues have generally relied on the techniques developed for respective adult organs. The biochemical characteristics of fetal mitochondria at a given stage of development have not been clearly defined, and further investigation and modification of techniques are necessary.

ASSAY OF OXIDATIVE PHOSPHORYLATION

Warburg Technique

The initial studies that defined mitochondrial oxidative phosphorylation were carried out with this procedure. Today the more rapid and less laborious polarographic procedure (to be discussed) is preferred by most investigators. However, many laboratories still use the Warburg apparatus, especially when prolonged incubations or in vitro exposure of mitochondria to certain agents is desired.

Figure 2 is a photograph of a typical Warburg apparatus. It consists of a constant temperature bath (A), thermoregulator (B), stirring motor (C) to ensure even temperature throughout the bath, heating element (D), shaker-motor (E) for manometers, and slots (F) for attachment of manometers to instrument. Some Warburg instruments are available with a compressor so that bath temperatures below ambient may be obtained.

The principle of Warburg manometry is based on the law of partial pressures of gases and on Henry's law, which states: The concentration of dissolved gas is directly proportional to the concentration above the fluid. When the manometer (with attached vessel) is closed, the change in gas pressure in the Warburg flask as oxygen is consumed is recorded as a change in the level of fluid in the manometer. A filter paper saturated with 20 percent KOH is placed in the center well of the flask to absorb the CO_2 given off. Figure 3 is a diagram of a Warburg manometer and flask. Flasks are attached to the manometer with the stopcock open and placed in the Warburg bath. The flasks are allowed to equilibrate approximately 8 to 10 minutes and then the level of fluid in the right arm of the manometer is set to a predetermined height by the turnscrew at the bottom. The stopcock is then closed and a reading taken of the fluid level in the left arm of the manometer. As oxygen is consumed, the fluid level on the right side rises. Usually, every 10 minutes the fluid on the right side is readjusted to its initial position, and a reading of the drop in pressure is recorded from the left arm of the manometer. During the entire incubation time in the bath, the vessels are shaken (100 to 125 oscillations per min) to ensure adequate mixing of the gas and liquid phases in the flask.

The total differential change in gas pressure is expressed in millimeters as recorded from the manometers. This figure is converted to the actual amount of

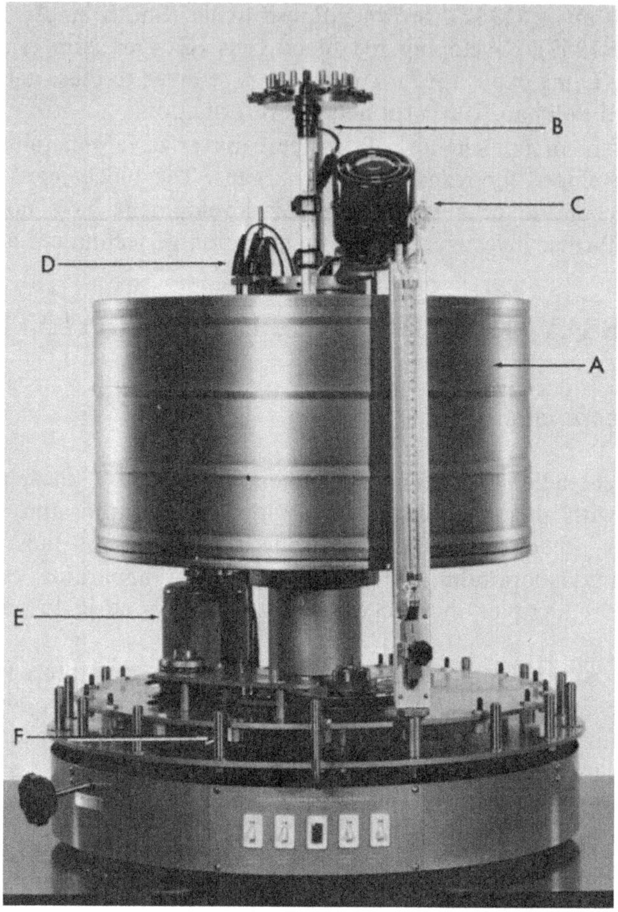

FIG. 2. Warburg constant temperature bath. (A) Constant temperature bath. (B) Thermoregulator. (C) Stirring motor. (D) Heating element. (E) Shaker motor. (F) Manometer slots.

oxygen consumed using the appropriate flask constant for each Warburg vessel. This constant takes into account temperature and pressure (of the manometer fluid), volume of gas in the flask and connecting manometer tube down to the reference point, volume of fluid in the flask, partial pressure of the gas involved in the assay, solubility of gas in the reaction mixture, and vapor pressure of the fluid involved in the determination. For a full description of the derivation of the flask constant the reader is referred to *Manometric Techniques* (Umbreit et al., 1964). Today many manufacturers offer precalibrated manometers and flasks. The uptake of oxygen is usually expressed as μ atoms oxygen per min per mg mitochondrial protein.

Since the determinations are based on pressure changes, which are sensitive to temperature, a thermobarometer is run concurrently with the reaction flasks during

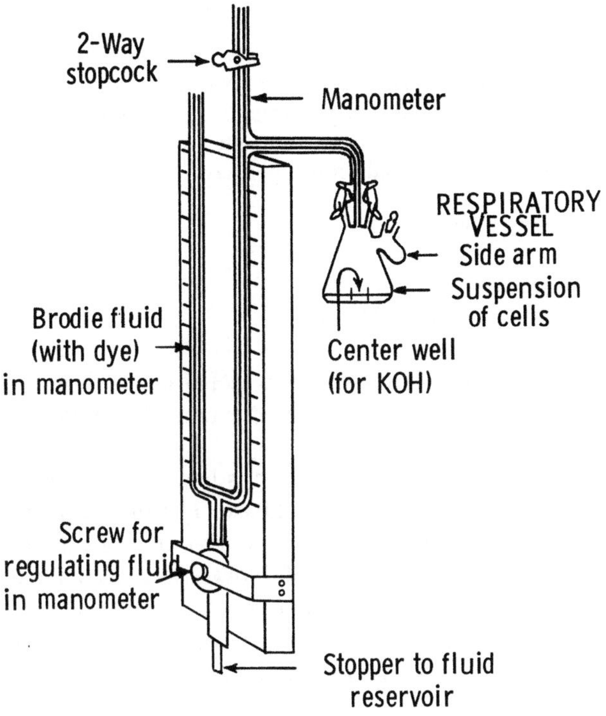

FIG. 3. Diagram of Warburg manometer and flask. (From Bresnick and Schwartz. 1968. *In* Functional Dynamics of the Cell, p. 111. Courtesy of Academic Press, Inc.)

an assay. This consists of a Warburg flask containing only the exact volume of water or the assay medium as used in the reaction vessels. It is run along with the other vessels and records changes in temperature and barometric pressure that might occur. Appropriate corrections in the manometer readings for the reaction vessels can then be made.

ASSAY MEDIUM:

Due to the prolonged incubation (20 to 30 min) employed in the Warburg assay, the reaction mixture is fortified to offset mitochondrial "aging" which leads to swelling and uncoupling of the mitochondria. Assay media vary somewhat with different laboratories, but most contain essentially the same ingredients. The following is the assay medium used in this laboratory (final concentrations):

MAIN FLASK:

70 mM sucrose
50 mM KCl (pH 7.4)
12 mM NaF
0.15 mM NAD^+

5 mM $MgCl_2$
0.3 mM EDTA
0.015 mM cytochrome c
2.5 mM ATP (Na salt)
900 to 1,200 μg inorganic phosphate (Na, K, or tris salt)
15 mM substrate (glutamate, pyruvate. β-hydroxybutyrate, citrate, α-ketoglutarate or succinate as the Na^+ or tris salts are usually employed
4 to 6 mg of mitochondrial protein per flask

SIDE ARM: ("Trap")

24 μ M glucose
5 mg hexokinase (750 K-M units)

The final volume is 2.2 ml and the pH 7.4. Sodium malate at a final concentration of 0.52 mM is usually added when glutamate or pyruvate is the substrate.

The initial pH of the ATP stock solution is low and must be adjusted to 6.8 to 7.0. Sodium fluoride is added to inhibit ATPase. The inorganic phosphate must be added in precise amounts since this enters into the calculation for phosphate esterification. The number of μmoles of inorganic phosphate that are removed during the reaction are equated with the number of μmoles of ATP formed. The "trap" is tipped in from the side arm after temperature equilibration, and the stopcock is closed. ATP generated by the mitochondria catalyzes the reaction:

$$\text{glucose} + \text{ATP} \xrightarrow[\text{Mg}^{++}]{\text{hexokinase}} \text{glucose-6-phosphate} + \text{ADP}$$

The inorganic phosphate is removed from the reaction medium by this "trapping" mechanism, and the ADP recycled to the mitochondria.

ASSAY PROCEDURE:

1. Vessels and side arms are loaded with the reaction medium and "trap" at room temperature or in ice. Mitochondria are added last.
2. A fluted filter paper, 1.7 to 2.0 cm^2, is placed in each center well, and 0.1 ml of 20 percent KOH is added. The center well rims are pregreased with petrolatum to prevent the alkali from "creeping" over into the reaction chamber.
3. The flasks are attached to the pregreased manometers (stopcocks open), placed in the bath, and the shaker turned on. A temperature equilibration time of 8 to 10 minutes is allowed. (Most determinations are carried out at 30° or 37°C.)
4. The shaker is turned off, the manometer fluid on the right side set to its reference point (usually 150 or 250 mm), a reading is made of the fluid level in the left manometer arm, and the stopcocks are closed. The contents of the side arm are tipped in to initiate the reaction.
5. The flasks are allowed to shake for 10 minutes. The fluid in the right arm of

the manometer is then returned to its reference point and a reading taken from the left manometer arm. Readings are taken every 10 minutes for a period of 20 to 30 minutes.

6. To terminate the reaction, the manometer stopcocks are opened after the last reading, the vessels quickly removed, and an ice-cold solution of 10 percent trichloroacetic acid (or perchloric) added to the vessels.
7. The contents of the flasks are removed, diluted to an appropriate volume, and centrifuged to precipitate the protein.
8. An aliquot from the supernate is analyzed for inorganic phosphate by a colorimetric method (Lowry and Lopez, 1946; Fiske and Subba Row, 1925; or see Section IV). The time elapsed from opening of the stopcocks (end of respiratory measurements) to the addition of the trichloroacetic acid to terminate the phosphorylation reaction is taken into account when calculating the uptake of inorganic phosphate. The number of μmoles of inorganic phosphate esterified can be equated to the μmoles of ATP formed and is usually expressed as μmoles ATP per min per mg mitochondrial protein.
9. Mitochondrial protein is usually determined by a biuret method (Jacobs et al., 1956).
10. The ratio of μatoms of oxygen consumed to the μmoles of ATP formed is expressed as the phosphorous to oxygen ratio or P:O ratio.

$$\mathrm{P{:}O} = \frac{\mu\text{moles ATP/min/mg}}{\mu\text{atoms } O_2\text{/min/mg}}$$

Experimentally this ratio falls between 2.8 to 3.4 for NADH-linked substrates or 1.8 to 2.2 for succinate.

COMMENTS: Warburg manometry yields accurate measurements of oxidative phosphorylation when carried out with care and attention to detail. Proper temperature equilibration must be allowed before beginning measurement of respiration. Filter papers in the center wells must all be the same size so that an equal absorptive surface for CO_2 is available in all vessels. Various stopcock greases change their viscosity with temperature and do not allow the flasks to seat properly on the manometers. The result is a "pulling-on" of the vessels during the course of the incubation, resulting in a change in pressure in the manometer tube and flask. This gives rise to low oxygen uptake readings. A 1:1 mixture of petrolatum and Lubriseal (A. H. Thomas) has been found to be reliable as a grease for the manometer heads. A thorough discussion of the factors involved in proper Warburg respirometry has been published by Slater (1967).

Polarographic Technique

This technique utilizes the properties of current-potential curves in conjunction with a specific type of electrode. The electrode is a polarized platinum electrode

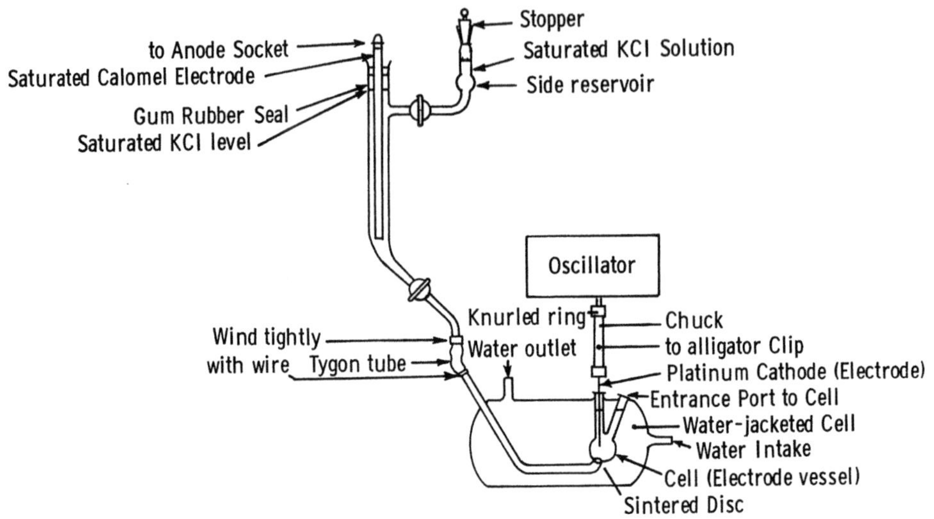

FIG. 4A. Vibrating platinum electrode and cell assembly. (Courtesy of Gilson Medical Electronics, Middleton, Wis.)

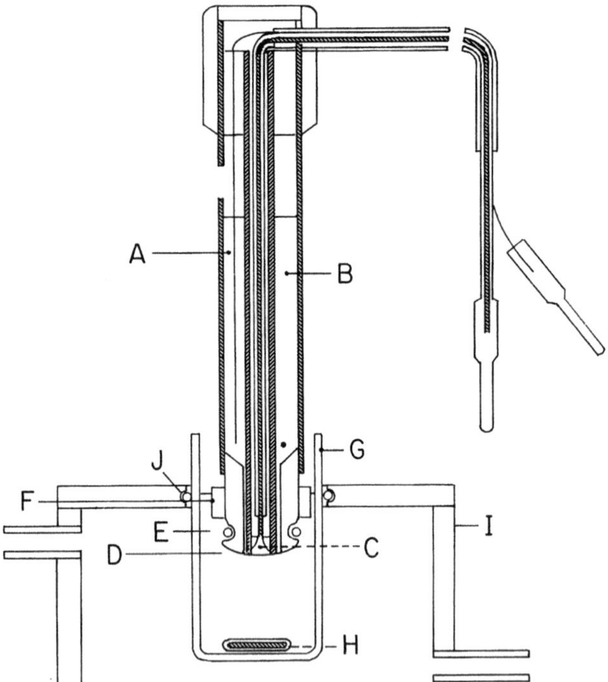

FIG. 4B. Arrangement of the Clark oxygen electrode. (A) Silver electrode. (B) Saturated KCl. (C) Platinum electrode. (D) Polyethylene membrane. (E) Rubber O ring. (F) Rubber gasket. (G) Reaction vessel. (H) Magnetic stirring bar. (I) Lucite water jacket. (J) Rubber O ring. (From *Methods in Enzymology,* 6:274., 1963. Courtesy of Academic Press, Inc., New York.)

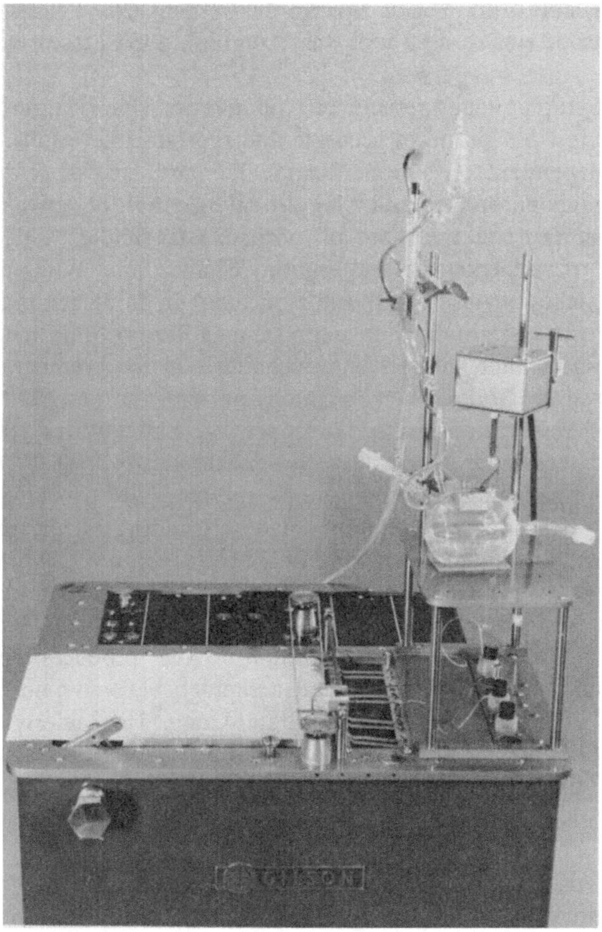

FIG. 5. Oxygraph. Complete unit with vibrating platinum electrode assembly. (Courtesy of Gilson Medical Electronics, Middleton, Wis.)

(cathode) and a nonpolarized, saturated calomel electrode (anode) coupled to a KCl salt bridge. At a constant applied voltage (0.6 to 0.8 volts) the change in current is recorded as a direct measure of the change in oxygen tension in a given solution. Two types of electrode systems employing this principle are available and are shown in Figure 4: (1) the vibrating platinum electrode (Fig. 4A), where the platinum cathode is placed directly in the assay medium separate from the anode, and relies on its oscillation to create a diffusion potential at the cathode; (2) the Clark electrode (Fig. 4B), where the cathode, anode, and KCl bridge are contained in a single housing and separated from the assay solution by a Teflon membrane. The membrane is permeable to oxygen, and the diffusion potential is created by a magnetic stirring bar. Both types of electrodes have been found to work with equal sensitivity in this laboratory. The entire amplifier and recorder assembly for the vibrating platinum electrode is available (Oxygraph, Gilson Medical Electronics, Middleton, Wisconsin). The Oxygraph is shown in Figure 5. The Clark electrode is available from Yellow Springs Instrument Co., Yellow Springs, Ohio. The Clark electrode can be used with the Oxygraph apparatus or with component parts.

The polarographic measurement of oxidative phosphorylation is a rapid and sensitive technique that produces accurate and reproducible results. Mitochondrial respiration is dependent on several factors. The presence of oxygen, oxidizable substrate, inorganic phosphate, and ADP are all essential for active respiration and phosphorylation. The concentrations of inorganic phosphate, ADP, and ATP can affect the rate of mitochondrial respiration. Chance and Williams (1956) have described five steady states of respiratory activity in mitochondria, which is the generally accepted terminology in expressing polarographic measurements of oxidative phosphorylation. *State 1* is mitochondria in the presence of oxygen, but no ADP or substrate. *State 2* the substrate is present, but not ADP. *State 3* is the active state of respiration in the presence of ADP. When all the ADP is phosphorylated, respiration returns to a slower rate, i.e., *State 4*. *State 5* is when all reactants are present, but the system is anaerobic.

Generally, most measurements are made by adding all the reactants except ADP and mitochondria to the oxygen-electrode chamber. The base line for maximum oxygen concentration is established on the recorder and the mitochondria are added. Since all reactants except ADP are now present, the mitochondria are essentially in State 4. Subsequent addition of ADP produces the active State 3 "burst" of respiration, and when all the acceptor (ADP) is phosphorylated, the mitochondrial respiration returns to the State 4 rate. The underlying principle in polarographic determinations is that the rate of mitochondrial respiration is under the control of phosphorylation; i.e., the system is tightly coupled. When no acceptor (ADP) is present (State 4) the respiratory rate is low, and in the presence of ADP (State 3) the rate is rapid. The ratio of State 3 to State 4 respiration is called the *respiratory control index* (RCI) and is an indication of the "tightness of coupling" in mitochondria. High respiratory control ratios are considered to be the primary measure of the intactness of mitochondrial function (Lehninger, 1965).

ASSAY MEDIA:

Unlike the fortified media used for Warburg determinations, media used for polarographic measurements are usually much simpler. Since the assays are carried out over shorter time periods, mitochondrial "aging" is not so much of a problem. We have found that 20- to 30-minute incubations of heart mitochondria, in media employed for oxygen-electrode studies, show very little deterioration.

Several types of media are used for oxygen-electrode studies and have been found to be optimal for the particular type of mitochondria being assayed. Heart, brain, and some types of tumor (Sordahl and Schwartz, 1967) mitochondria have yielded maximal values in the "sucrose-tris" medium to be described. The "choline-Cl" medium described is equally as good as the "sucrose-tris" medium for heart mitochondria. The "choline-Cl" medium is also used for potassium-ion transport studies. Liver mitochondria respire better in the "KCl-tris" medium described. This medium contains $MgCl_2$, which has been shown to be essential in sustaining respiration in liver mitochondria (Baltscheffsky, 1957; Chance, 1956). The medium described for brain is that suggested by Ozawa et al., (1966). Inclusion of one mg per ml of bovine serum albumin in this "brain medium" improves oxidative phosphorylation values.

HEART:

10 mM substrate (glutamate, β-hydroxybutyrate, or succinate as Na or tris salt)
10 mM K_2HPO_4
in: 0.25 M sucrose-10 mM tris-HCl, pH 7.4
or 0.125 M choline-Cl-10 mM tris-HCl, pH 7.4

LIVER:

75 mM KCl
50 mM tris-HCl
12.5 mM K_2HPO_4
5 mM $MgCl_2$
1 mM ethylenediaminetetraacetate (EDTA)
10 mM substrate (same as heart)
pH 7.4

BRAIN:

0.3 M mannitol
10 mM KCl
10 mM tris-HCl
5 mM K_2HPO_4
0.2 mM EDTA
pH 7.4

Depending on the size of the oxygen-electrode chamber, 1 to 3 ml constitute the final volume of the reaction mixture. Approximately 1.0 to 1.5 mg of mitochondrial protein per ml are added to the reaction mixture.

ASSAY PROCEDURE:

1. The amplifier and recorder are turned on. Voltage is applied to the electrode (0.6 to 0.8 volts). The oscillator is turned on in the case of the vibrating platinum electrode and the magnetic stirrer for the Clark.
2. The reaction chamber is thoroughly rinsed with water and then filled with the complete reaction mixture (buffer, inorganic phosphate, and substrate). The range for total oxygen concentration is established on the recorder.
3. Figure 6A is an oxygen-electrode tracing of rat heart mitochondria measured by the vibrating platinum electrode. The recorder pen is set at full range (R), which represents 960 nanoatoms oxygen in the reaction chamber. (The volume in the reaction chamber is 2 ml. Assuming 240 nanomoles atmospheric oxygen per ml in solution at 25°C, the total oxygen present is 240 nanomoles O_2/ml $\times$

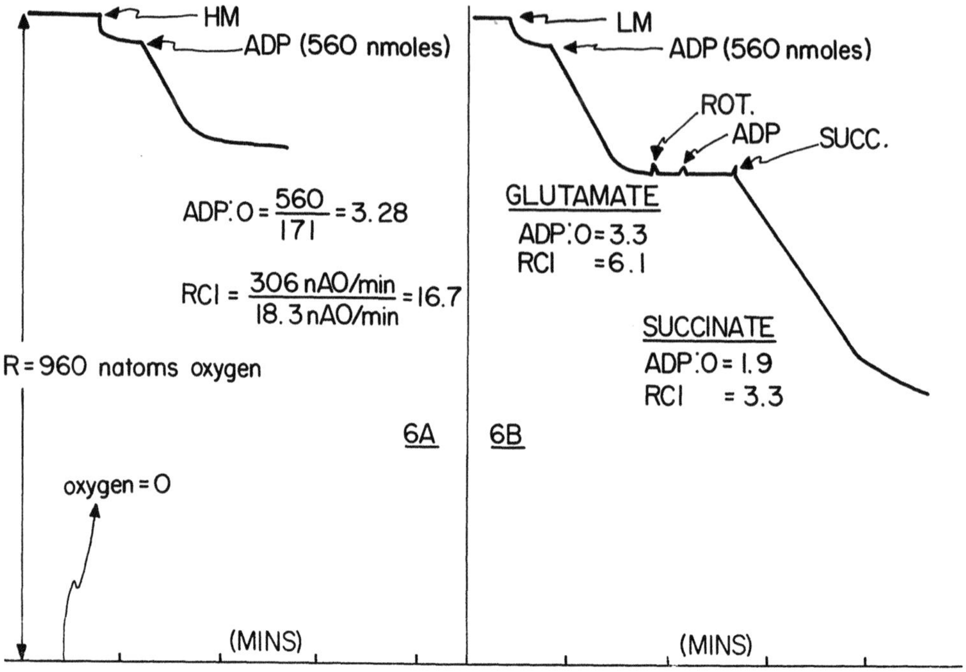

FIG. 6. Oxygen-electrode tracings of rat heart (A, left) and liver (B, right) mitochondria. Glutamate is the initial substrate in both traces. See text for details. Abbreviations: heart mitochondria (HM); liver mitochondria (LM); adenosine diphosphate (ADP); rotenone (Rot); succinate (Succ); respiratory control index (RCI).

2 = 480 nanoatoms 0/ml × 2 ml = 960 nanoatoms 0/2 ml.) The bottom of the tracing at zero current is equal to zero oxygen concentration.

4. Rat heart mitochondria (HM), 2 mg, are now added to the reaction chamber (Fig. 6A) and mixed to insure an even suspension. (In the case of the vibrating electrode, the recorder is momentarily turned off while making additions and stirring. This is not necessary with the Clark assembly because of the magnetic stirrer.) A downward deflection is seen, indicating oxygen uptake (and a slight dilution effect) with the addition of the mitochondria (HM, Fig. 6). The respiratory rate then equilibrates to a steady state. The mitochondria are in State 4 respiration. Glutamate is the substrate.
5. A 0.1-ml aliquot of ADP containing 560 nanomoles is added to produce the State 3 "burst" of respiration. When all the ADP is phosphorylated to ATP, the State 3 respiratory rate ceases and the mitochondria are again at State 4.
6. From these data, the ADP:O ratio (which is equivalent to the P:O ratio), the respiratory control index (RCI), and the rate of oxygen consumption (QO_2) in States 3 and 4 can be calculated.
7. ADP:O ratio: The amount of oxygen consumed during the State 3 "burst" is calculated from the chart paper as 171 nanoatoms (Fig. 6A). The ADP added was 560 nanomoles, the ADP:O ratio is calculated to be

$$\text{ADP:O} = \frac{560 \text{ nmoles ADP}}{171 \text{ natoms oxygen}} = 3.28$$

The exact concentration of the ADP solution is determined by reading the optical density (OD) in a spectrophotometer at 259 mμ and using a millimolar extinction coefficient of 15.4. An enzymatic analysis (Kornberg and Pricer, 1951) can also be carried out to determine concentration. The latter is a more sensitive method. We have found the direct OD readings and the enzymatic determinations to be in good agreement.

8. Respiratory control index (RCI): The ratio of respiratory rate in State 4 to that in State 3 is expressed as the RCI and is the primary measure of the "tightness" of coupling of the mitochondria. The RCI as calculated from Figure 6A:

$$\text{RCI} = \frac{\text{State 3; 306 natoms } O_2/\text{min}}{\text{State 4; 18.3 natoms } O_2/\text{min}} = 16.7$$

Since the RCI is a pure number, it can be determined quickly by computing the slopes of the State 3 and State 4 rates without having to calculate actual oxygen consumption rates.

9. Rate of oxygen consumption (QO_2): This value is usually computed for State 3 respiration and is an expression of the activity of the enzymatic protein. It is expressed as nanoatoms oxygen per min per mg mitochondrial protein. The (QO_2) for State 3 respiration in Figure 6A is 153.

10. Figure 6B is an oxygen-electrode tracing of rat liver mitochondria with glutamate and succinate as substrates. The RCI values obtained with rat liver mitochondria are generally not as high as those obtained with heart. After State 4 respiration is reached with glutamate as substrate, the inhibitor, rotenone (1 μg per mg protein), is added. Rotenone inhibits electron transport at the region of the flavoprotein (Fp_n) associated with NADH-linked respiration. ADP is then added to insure that rotenone inhibition is complete, at which time succinate is subsequently added. Succinate bypasses the rotenone block (see Fig. 7A), and since ADP is already present, the mitochondria are in State 3 respiration. When the ADP is used up, the State 4 rate is reached. Since one of the phosphorylation sites (site I) is not involved with coupled succinate oxidation, the maximum ADP:O ratio attainable is two. The State 4 rate of respiration with succinate as substrate is always higher due to some oxidation of the substrate in the absence of phosphorylation. Usual RCI values for succinate are from 3 to 5. Table 1 gives some representative values obtained in this laboratory for rat liver and heart mitochondria from several species.

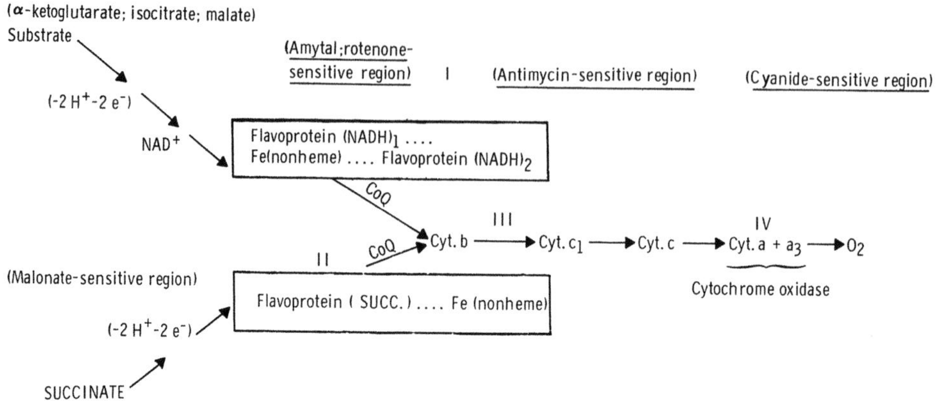

FIG. 7A Schematic representation of the electron transport chain, indicating the approximate loci of action of various inhibitors. The three coupling sites of phosphorylation are indicated by roman numerals I, III, and IV.

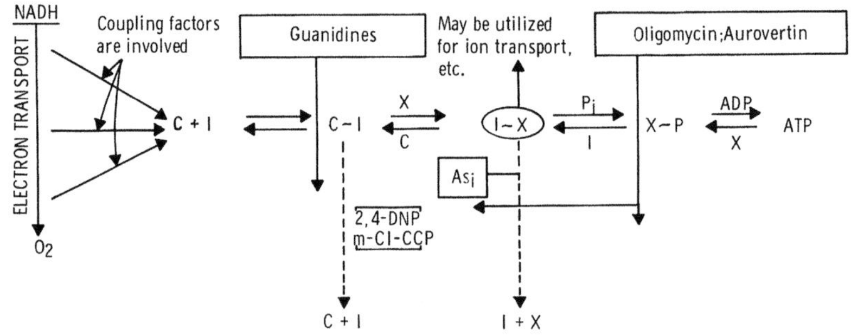

FIG. 7B. Hypothetical representation of the chemical coupling mechanism of phosphorylation. Inhibitors of phosphorylation are indicated in the boxes. The proposed point of action of uncouplers such as 2,4-dinitrophenol (2,4-DNP), *Meta*-chlorophenylhydrazone (*m*-CCP), and arsenate (As_i) are also indicated. C represents a reduced or oxidized carrier such as NADH, Co Q, or cytochromes. (Adapted from Bresnick and Schwartz. 1968. *In* Functional Dynamics of the Cell; pp. 115 and 126. Courtesy of Academic Press, Inc.)

The oxygen-electrode chamber is surrounded by an outer chamber through which water can be circulated to maintain a constant temperature. Most determinations are carried out at 25°, 30°, or 37°C. Compensation for the decrease in oxygen solubility at higher temperatures must be made.

A variety of compounds are used as "tools" to inhibit portions of the electron transport chain and the phosphorylation mechanism so that certain reactions can be studied. Figure 7A is a diagrammatic representation of the electron transport chain indicating the approximate locus of action of several of the more commonly used inhibitors and uncouplers. Rotenone, Antimycin A, and cyanide are relatively specific inhibitors of electron transport. Oligomycin (Fig. 7B) is an inhibitor of terminal phosphate transfer, but does not prevent the formation of "high-energy

TABLE 1

Representative Values for Oxidative Phosphorylation as Measured Polarographically With Heart and Liver Mitochondria. Glutamate is the Substrate.

	Heart		Liver	
Species	*ADP:O*	*RCI*	*ADP:O*	*RCI*
Rat	2.8-3.4	12-20	2.7-3.0	6-8
Guinea pig	2.8-3.4	8-16	2.7-3.0	6-8
Rabbit	2.8-3.2	12-22	–	–
Mouse	2.9-3.3	15-24	2.8-3.1	6-10
Human	2.9-3.2	9-30	–	–

ADP:O = amount of adenosine diphosphate esterified per oxygen consumed.
RCI = respiratory control index (see text).

intermediates" of phosphorylation, which are postulated to provide the energy for ion translocation, low-amplitude swelling, and contraction. The uncouplers (Fig. 7B), like 2,4-dinitrophenol (DNP), release respiration from phosphorylation producing rapid, uncontrolled respiration. The uncoupler 2,4-dinitrophenol also activates a mitochondrial ATPase. Most inhibitors are used in a concentration of 1 to 2 μg per mg protein. Concentrations for uncouplers vary. Dinitrophenol is usually used at a final concentration in the reaction chamber of 10^{-5}M. A new group of uncouplers, the salicylanilides (Williamson and Metcalf, 1967), are reported to be 1,000 to 10,000 times more potent than dinitrophenol as uncouplers and in stimulating mitochondrial ATPase.

It is important that both NADH-linked and succinate-linked respiration be studied, especially when mitochondria are prepared from pathologic or experimental animals. Both segments of the electron transport chain should be studied when the in vitro effects of various agents are being examined. Inhibitors, such as those previously cited, are used as a method of comparison when the in vitro effects of an experimental agent are being studied. An example of the assay of a pharmacologic agent upon mitochondria is given on pp. 269 ff.

SUBMITOCHONDRIAL PARTICLES

Keilin and Hartree (1938) were probably the first investigators to use a fragmented particle from whole tissue to study the enzymes later identified with mitochondria. Today a variety of procedures are used to break whole mitochondria down into subunits. The enzymatic properties of these submitochondrial particles tend to vary according to the method of preparation. Interest has been directed primarily to the preparation of phosphorylating submitochondrial particles with the aim of further elucidating the energy-linked reactions of electron transport. Employing such particles, a number of specific enzymatic reactions of electron transport and phosphorylation can be studied.

Beef heart mitochondria are the primary source for preparation of submitochondrial particles because of the availability of this material, the need for large amounts of mitochondria in order to obtain appreciable yields of particles, the ease with which beef heart mitochondria can be ruptured, and the relative stability of the preparations. Beef heart particles have been prepared by three basic techniques: (1) digitonin fragmentation (Wadkins and Lehninger, 1963), (2) mechanical rupture (Pullman and Penefsky, 1963), and (3) sonication (Green and Ziegler, 1963). A recent compilation (Estabrook and Pullman, 1967) describes a number of these techniques, properties of the particles, and assays of specific activities.

The preparation of sonic particles (SP) from beef heart described here is a modification of the method of Lam et al., (1966) adapted from Linnane and Ziegler (1958). Sonic particles from rat liver are prepared by a modification of the method of Gregg (1967). Beef heart mitochondria are easily disrupted by sonic oscillation. The preparations exhibit adequate enzymatic activity and remain stable upon storage at –70°C for several weeks. Liver mitochondria require more drastic treatment for rupture and do not have either the enzymatic activity or stability that beef heart particles possess.

PREPARATION OF BEEF HEART SONIC PARTICLES:

1. Mitochondria are prepared in 0.25 M sucrose, 10 mM tris-HCl, 10 mM EDTA at pH 7.4 (STE-10 medium). Fifty grams of ground beef heart are suspended in 500 ml of STE-10 medium and homogenized in a large Waring blender for 45 sec. If the pH of the homogenate is below 7 after homogenization, it should be readjusted to 7 with 1 M tris base.
2. The homogenate is centrifuged at 1,200 × *g* for 15 min. The supernate is poured through cheesecloth and centrifuged at 10,000 × *g* for 15 min.
3. The resulting mitochondrial pellets are resuspended in 200 ml of STE-10 medium and centrifuged at 10,000 × *g* for 10 minutes.
4. The mitochondrial pellets are suspended finally, in 0.25 M sucrose, to a concentration of 25 mg per ml.*
5. Thirty-ml aliquots of the mitochondrial suspension are sonicated at 20 kc at a power output of 8.5 to 9.0 amps for one minute with a Branson Sonifier.† The sonication procedure is done in two 30-sec intervals, with one minute cooling allowed between intervals, to prevent excess heating of the suspension.
6. The pH of the sonicated suspension is again adjusted, if necessary, to 7.4 with 1 M tris base. The sonicated suspension is then centrifuged at 20,000 × *g* for 15 min.
7. The supernate is centrifuged at 100,000 × *g* for 30 min. The resulting pellets of sonic particles (SP) are suspended in a small volume of 0.25 M sucrose. Particles not used immediately can be stored at –70 °C.

*Mitochondria can be sonicated in a solution of 1 mM succinate (K^+), 1 mM ATP, 5 mM $MgCl_2$ 10 mM $MnCl_2$. This Mg-Mn particle usually has higher activity and greater stability on storage.

†Branson sonifier, Model LS-75, Heat Systems, Inc., Great Neck, New York.

PREPARATION OF SONIC PARTICLES FROM RAT LIVER:

1. Rat liver mitochondria are prepared as previously described in this chapter. The final suspension of mitochondria is made with cold water, to a concentration of 25 mg mitochondrial protein per ml. The pH is adjusted to 7 with 1 M tris base.
2. Thirty-ml aliquots of the mitochondrial suspension are sonicated for one minute at 20 kc at a power output of 8.5 to 9.0 amps with a Branson Sonifier. The sonication is carried out in two 30-sec intervals with a minute in between to allow for cooling of the suspension.
3. The remaining steps are identical to those described for beef heart particles (steps 6 and 7).

Liver particles have more variable activities than the heart preparations and rapidly lose their activity on storage.

ASSAY: The energy-linked reduction of NAD^+ by succinate ("succinate-reversal") and the nonenergy-linked anaerobic oxidation of NADH by fumarate, as described by Sanadi and Fluharty (1963), will be outlined. By inhibiting the electron transport chain at the terminal oxidation step with cyanide, supplying electrons with succinate and ATP to drive the reaction, the reduction of NAD^+ through the electron transport chain can be monitored spectrophotometrically. This reaction is energy-requiring and can be inhibited by oligomycin, 2,4-dinitrophenol, and direct inhibition of electron transport with rotenone (see Fig. 7A, B). The oxidation of NADH catalyzed by fumarate does not require energy and thus is not inhibited by either oligomycin or 2,4-dinitrophenon. It has been suggested (Sanadi and Fluharty, 1963), that NADH oxidation by fumarate is an energy-producing reaction. These two reactions allow for study of the site 1 phosphorylation and electron transport region. Schatz and Racker (1966) have suggested that the reduction of exogenous coenzyme Q_1 by NADH in submitochondrial particles is a better measure of the "forward" reaction at the first coupling site (Fig. 7A). The sonic particles used for these assays are capable of other energy-linked reactions, and coupled oxidative phosphorylation can be measured manometrically. The values obtained are much lower than those with intact mitochondria.

Liver sonic particles also catalyze these reactions, but not with as high an activity as beef heart particles. The liver particles have an apparent high ATPase activity which causes the ATP-requiring reaction to terminate rapidly. Due to this ATPase activity, the "succinate-reversal" reaction is initiated with ATP instead of NAD^+ as in the case of beef heart particles. The following description is based on beef heart particles, and the activities expressed are those obtained with heart particles.

Reduction of NAD^+ by Succinate

PROCEDURE:

1. The assay medium consists of (final concentration):

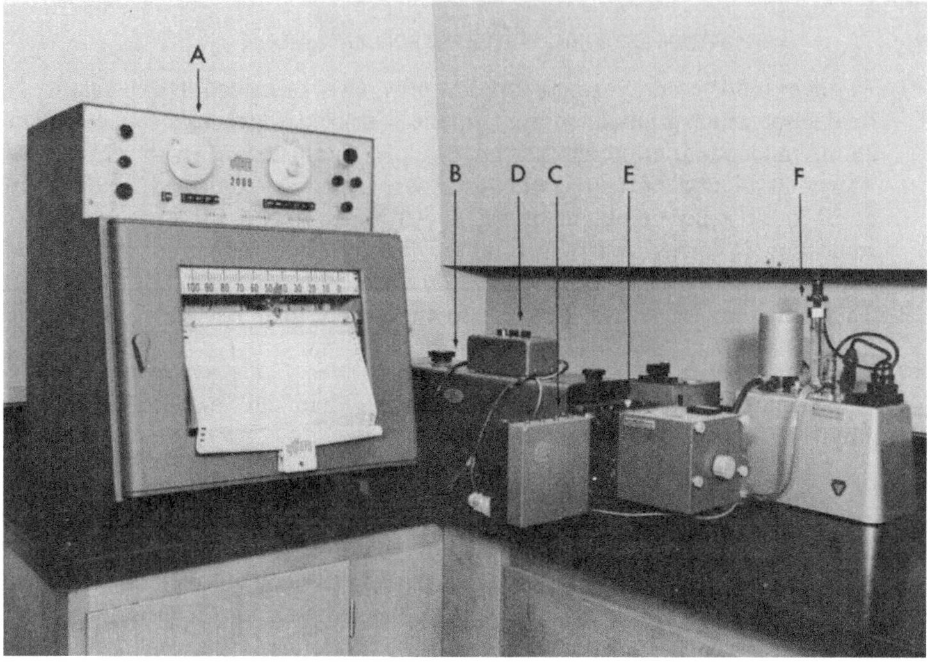

FIG. 8. Gilford multiabsorbance recorder and spectrophotometer. (A) Multiple absorbance recorder. (B) Beckman DU spectrophotometer. (C) Automatic cuvette changer. (D) Multi-channel offset control. (E) Water-jacketed cuvette chamber. (F) Constant temperature water bath and pump attached to cuvette chamber.

50 mM tris-SO_4 buffer, pH 7.5
0.1 mM EDTA
3.3 mM $MgCl_2$
6.7 mM succinate (Na salt)
1 mM NAD^+
2 mg crystalline bovine serum albumin
1 mM KCN
2 mM ATP
0.75 mg sonic particle protein

2. The reaction mixture is made up to a total volume of 2.9 ml with all ingredients except NAD^+. The mixture is incubated at 30° or 37°C for three minutes. The NAD^+ is added in a volume of 0.1 ml, and the increase in optical density (OD) at 340 mμ is measured with a Gilford multiple absorbance recorder attached to a Beckman DU spectrophotometer. The spectrophotometer cuvette chamber has thermospacers connected to a circulating water bath to maintain temperature during the course of the reaction (Fig. 8).
3. The chart speed on the recorder is set at 0.25 inch per minute, and the reactions in the cuvettes are measured at 4-second intervals. The increase in absorbance is usually expressed as Δ OD per 4 minutes. This value can be converted to actual specific activity by utilizing the millimolar extinction coefficient for NADH of

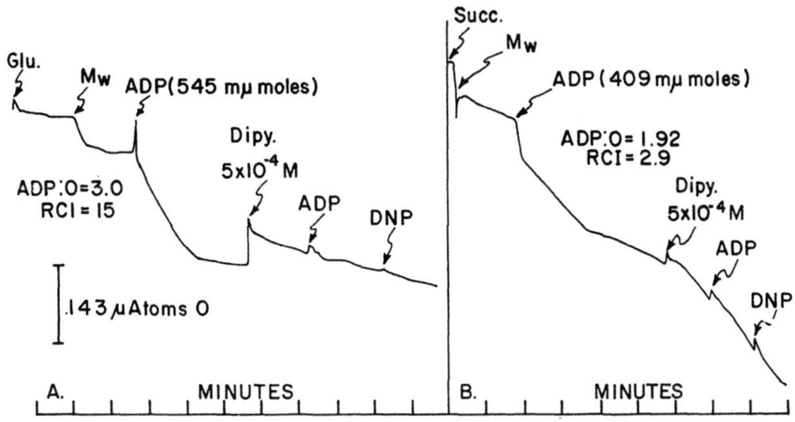

FIG. 9. Effect of high concentrations of dipyridamole on mitochondrial respiration with glutamate and succinate as substrates. Oxygen-electrode tracings of normal mitochondria with subsequent additions of dipyridamole Assay medium, ADP:O and RCI described in text. Dipyridamole additions are indicated as final concentrations in reaction chamber. Abbreviations: glutamate (Glu.), succinate (Succ.), mitochondria (Mw), dipyridamole (Dipy.), 4.75×10^{-5} M 2,4-dinitrophenol (DNP). (From Sordahl and Schwartz, *Molec. Pharmacol.,* 3:513, 1967. Courtesy of Academic Press, Inc.).

6.25. The values are expressed as nanomoles NADH formed per min per mg protein.

Under the conditions described, the reaction usually remains linear for at least 15 minutes. The rates of NAD^+ reduction are generally from 30 to 100 nanomoles per minute per mig (Δ OD/4 min from 0.1 to 0.6).

Oxidation of NADH by Fumarate

1. The reaction mixture is the same as that just described for "succinate-reversal" except the medium contains no succinate or ATP, and 0.56 μmoles of NADH instead of NAD^+
2. The reaction mixture is incubated at 30° or 37°C and then initiated by addition of 0.1 ml of 0.1 M fumarate. A control without fumarate should be run to account for the NADH oxidized by the particles in the absence of fumarate.
3. The change in absorbance is followed at 340 mμ as previously described. Fumarate-dependent NADH oxidation tends to be somewhat slower than the "succinate-reversal" reaction. The change in optical density is expressed as before. The actual nanomoles of NADH oxidized per minute per mg protein can be calculated in the same manner as described for energy-linked reduction.

ASSAY OF A PHARMACOLOGIC AGENT ON MITOCHONDRIA

The central role that mitochondria play in energy production makes these organelles possible loci of action for many agents. Furthermore, the mitochondrion

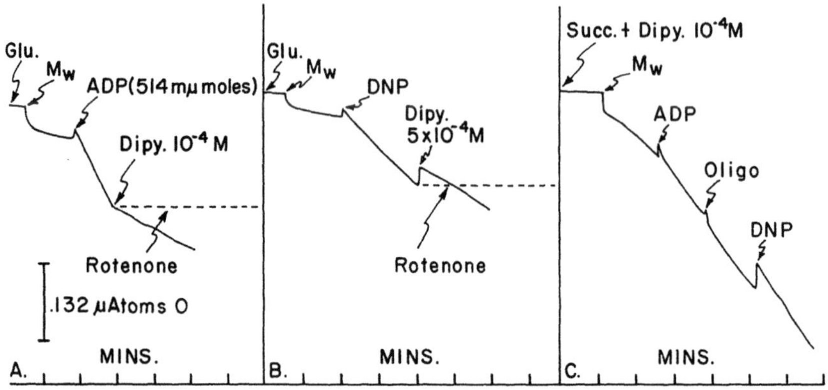

FIG. 10. Inhibitory effects of dipyridamole on active glutamate-supported respiration and uncoupling of succinate-supported respiration. Tracings A and B show active mitochondrial respiratory states produced by ADP and 2,4-DNP, respectively, and the effect of subsequent additions of inhibitory amounts of dipyridamole with glutamate as substrate. The inhibition of respiration if rotenone were added is indicated by the dotted lines. Tracing C demonstrates the uncoupling effect of dipyridamole on succinate-supported respiration. Dipyridamole additions are expressed as final concentrations in the reaction chamber. Assay conditions are described in text. Abbreviations: glutamate (Glu.), succinate (Succ.), dipyridamole (Dipy.), mitochondria (Mw), 4.75×10^{-5} M 2,4-dinitrophenol (DNP), 1 μg/mg protein oligomycin (Oligo.). Protein concentrations were the same in A, B, and C. (From Sordahl and Schwartz, *Molec. Pharmacol.*, 3:513, 1967. Courtesy of Academic Press, Inc., New York).

may be employed as a type of "model" membrane system upon which one can study drug-membrane interaction. The effects of dipyridamole,* a coronary vasodilator, on mitochondrial oxidative phosphorylation are described here as an example of how the assay of a drug is undertaken. The data shown have been previously reported (Sordahl and Schwartz, 1967).

Heart mitochondria were prepared and assayed polarographically as described earlier in this chapter. At in vitro concentrations below 10^{-5}M, dipyridamole had little effect on oxidative phosphorylation.

Figure 9A is an oxygen-electrode tracing, with glutamate as substrate, of normal mitochondrial respiration and the subsequent addition of an "inhibitory" amount of dipyridamole. It can be seen that the addition of dipyridamole slightly increases the State 4 rate. Subsequent additions of ADP and 2,4-dinitrophenol, however, cause no further increase in oxygen consumption. In Figure 9B the addition of dipyridamole with succinate as substrate causes a marked *increase* in respiratory rate, and subsequent additions of ADP and 2,4-dinitrophenol do not further increase the rate. It appears that dipyridamole produces both an inhibition of NADH-linked electron transport and an uncoupling with succinate-supported respiration. Figure 10A shows the inhibitory effect of dipyridamole addition during a glutamate-supported State 3 "burst" of respiration. Dipyridamole does not completely inhibit respiration as would rotenone (indicated by dotted line).

*Dipyridamole: 2,6-bis(diethanolamino)-4,8-dipiperidinopyridimo-(5,4*d*) pyrimidine (Persantin), Geigy Pharmaceuticals, Ardsley, New York.

However, the system loses respiratory control, and subsequent additions of ADP have no further effect, as shown in Figure 9A. Addition of dipyridamole to succinate-linked State 3 respiration has no inhibitory effect; the system becomes uncoupled and subsequent additions of ADP have no further effect. When 2,4-dinitrophenol is used to uncouple glutamate-supported respiration, dipyridamole addition inhibits the respiratory rate slightly, but not completely as would rotenone (Fig. 10B). Figure 10C shows the uncoupling effects of dipyridamole when succinate is used as substrate. Subsequent additions of ADP, oligomycin, and 2,4-dinitrophenol do not increase or reduce this rapid respiratory rate.

The possible in vivo effects of dipyridamole were tested by injecting rats with 20 mg per kg daily for ten days. Heart and liver mitochondria were isolated and assayed. No differences in the mitochondria from these animals as compared to controls were found.

The different effects of dipyridamole on NADH-linked and succinate-supported respiration emphasize the necessity of assaying both segments of the electron transport chain. In one case (NADH-linked) an "inhibitory" effect was observed, and in the other (succinate-linked) an uncoupling effect was recorded. Further studies can be undertaken to elucidate the effects of dipyridamole or oxidative phosphorylation by using submitochondrial particles.

A direct extrapolation as to the mechanism of action of this drug at therapeutic levels cannot be made. However, these results provide evidence for a reexamination of other reported effects (Laudahn, 1961) which suggested a beneficial effect of this agent on mitochondria from failing or damaged hearts. Recently, a chemically and pharmacologically unrelated drug, disulfiram,* has been reported (Hassinen and Hallman, 1967) to have in vitro effects on liver mitochondria similar to those of dipyridamole on heart mitochondria.

ENERGY-LINKED POTASSIUM TRANSPORT

Mitochondria will transport potassium under a variety of conditions. In a low-salt (less than 1 mM potassium) medium, a combination of the energized state and a facilitating agent is usually required to induce rapid potassium transport. The antibiotic valinomycin causes the active *uptake* of potassium (Moore and Pressman, 1964; Safer and Schwartz, 1967). Basic proteins, such as histones or parathyroid hormone, cause an energy-linked *efflux* of potassium from the mitochondrion (Johnson et al., 1967).

PROCEDURE:

1. Mitochondria are prepared as described earlier in this chapter and suspended at a protein concentration of 40 to 50 mg per ml.
2. Any buffer medium in the absence of monovalent cations may be used. We have employed the following:

*Disulfiram: tetraethylthiuram disulfide (Antabuse).

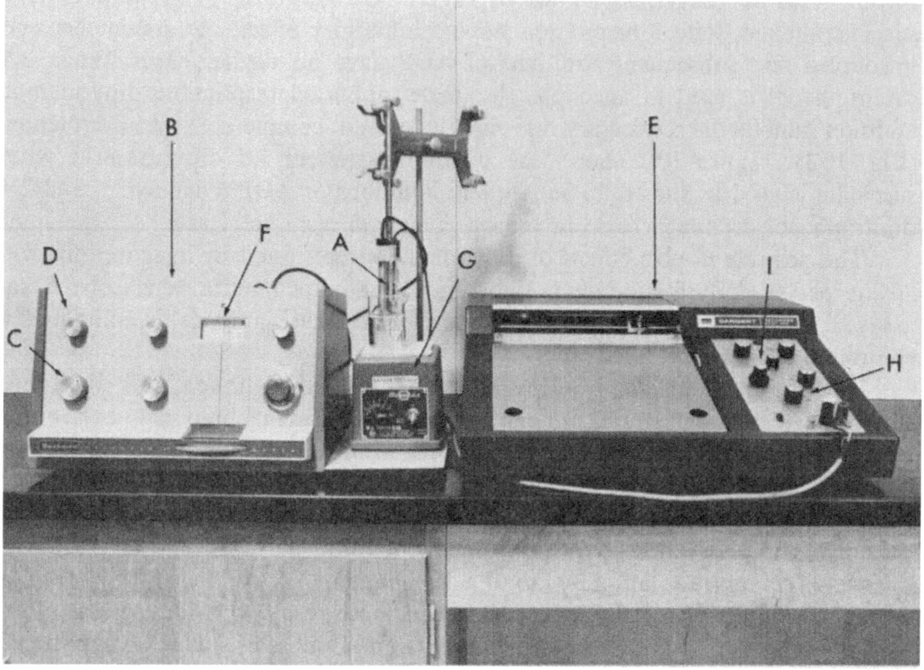

FIG. 11. Apparatus for measuring K^+ movements. (A) Beckman cation sensitive electrode (No. 39137) and reference electrode. (B) Beckman Research pH meter. (C) Function switch. (D) Sensitivity dial. (E) Sargent SRG recorder. (F) pH meter galvonometer. (G) Magnetic stirrer. (H) Recorder range plug. (I) Recorder zero knob.

a. 0.125 M choline-Cl-20 mM tris, pH 7.4
b. 0.25 M sucrose-10 mM tris, pH 7.4
c. 0.225 M mannitol-75 mM sucrose-20 mM tris, pH 7.4
1-10 mM substrate (tris salt)
5-10 mM tris-phosphate

Small amounts of K^+ (up to about 1 mM) may be added when measuring K^+ uptake.

3. Changes in the potassium ion concentration of the medium are detected by a cation-sensitive electrode with a standard reference electrode connected to a sensitive pH meter and potentiometric recorder (Pressman, 1965) (Fig. 11). Since the cation electrode is sensitive to all monovalent cations, it is essential that no monovalent cations other than potassium be present in the medium.
4. The electrodes are immersed in the basic assay medium (4 to 10 ml), which is stirred by a small magnetic flea. (It is advantageous to use a water-driven stirrer to eliminate electronic noise.) With the recorder disconnected from the pH meter, the solution is allowed to stand for several minutes until the mv reading stabilizes (usually between +30 to +70 mv for solutions containing no

potassium). The initial mv reading is noted; the recorder is connected to the pH meter and turned to "record." A small volume of the concentrated mitochondrial suspension is added to yield a final concentration of 1 to 2 mg per ml. An initial "jump" in the mv reading usually occurs due to the presence of ions in the mitochondrial suspension. Following this "jump," the curve should stabilize at a very slow, passive potassium efflux; and after a one- to two-minute equilibration period, agents that induce potassium-ion movement may be added. At the end of the recording, the recorder is quickly disconnected from the pH meter and the mv reading is immediately determined. The initial and final mv readings are used to calibrate the recorder chart in terms of mv changes.

5. To convert the chart mv readings to changes in potassium concentration, the electrode system may be calibrated by repeating the above procedure; but in place of the mitochondria, exact small volumes of a standard KCl solution are added in succession (8 to 10 additions of 0.01 ml each of a 0.01 M KCl standard are sufficient for an adequate calibration curve). Half a minute between additions should be allowed so that the electrode can stabilize. Since the output of the pH meter is logarithmic, it is necessary to construct a calibration curve by plotting the mv readings against the log of the potassium concentration. The mv readings at various intervals along the experimental trace may be converted to the actual potassium concentration.

EXAMPLE EXPERIMENT: Although the exact experimental details will depend on the equipment utilized to measure and record potassium concentration changes, the following experiment is included as a demonstration of the basic tehnique involved. This experiment was designed to measure histone-induced potassium efflux and was carried out in a potassium-free medium.

A Beckman cation-sensitive electrode (No. 39137) and reference electrode were connected to the Beckman Research pH meter. The function switch of the pH meter was set at "+mv" and the sensitivity dial was set at "low." The following reagents were added to a small plastic beaker: 2.0 ml of 0.5 M sucrose, 0.075 ml of 0.5 M tris-phosphate (pH 7.4), 0.025 ml of 0.5 M tris-succinate (pH 7.4), and 1.7 ml of water. The electrodes were immersed in this medium and the solution stirred with a small magnetic flea.

After a two-minute equilibration period, the pH meter galvanometer was nulled and a Sargent SRG recorder was connected and turned to "record." The range plug of the recorder was set at 5 mv span and the recorder zero knob was adjusted so that the pen trace was near the bottom (right side of recorder span) of the chart. The initial mv reading of the pH meter was noted, and 0.2 ml of mitochondria was added. At this point the assay medium had the following composition: 0.25 M sucrose, 9.4 mM tris-phosphate, 3.1 mM tris-succinate (pH 7.4), 1.85 mg mitochondrial protein per ml in a final volume of 4.0 ml. The electrode trace is shown in Figure 12B. One and half minutes after the addition of the mitochondria, 75 μg of a purified histone fraction was added. At the end of the recording, the recorder was disconnected and the final mv reading noted by renulling the pH meter galvanometer.

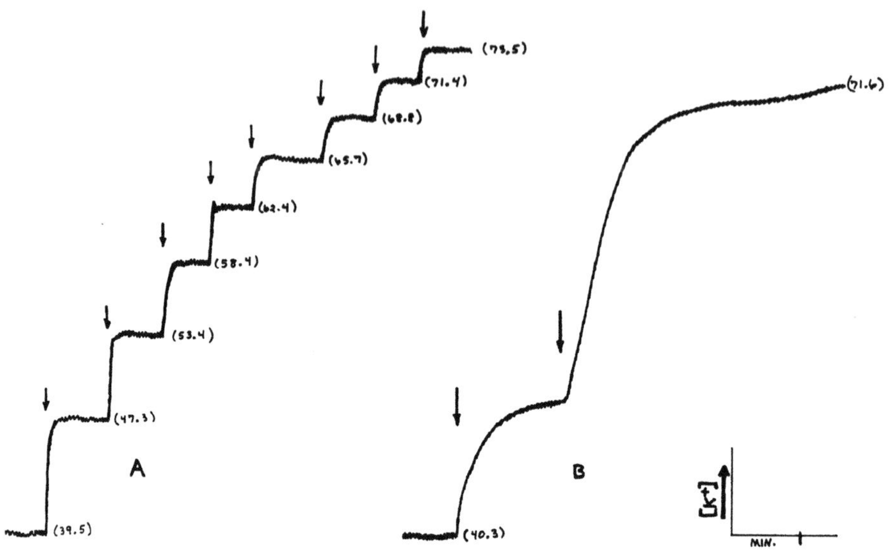

FIG. 12. (A) Calibration data for the cation-sensitive electrode. The medium is identical to that used in Figure 12(B). The additions were 0.1 μmoles KCl. The figure represents the recorder trace of the cation-sensitive electrode. (B) Induction of K^+ efflux by histone. The medium contained 0.25 M sucrose, 9.4 mM tris-phosphate, 3.1 mM tris-succinate, pH 7.4, in a final volume of 4.0 ml. At the first arrow, 7.4 mg mitochondrial protein was added; at the second arrow 75 μg β6-histone was added. The figure represents the recorder trace of the cation-sensitive electrode. The essay was conducted at room temperature.

To calibrate the electrode system, the exact same procedure as the foregoing was followed except that 0.2 ml water was added in place of the 0.2 ml of mitochondria. After equilibration, 0.01-ml additions of a standard 0.01 M KCl solution were added. The electrode response is shown in Figure 12A. The calibration data are replotted in Figure 13 on a semilog graph. Figure 14 is a replot of the data of Figure 12B based on the calibrated curve in Figure 13. Although this replot is necessary for accurate calculation of efflux rates, qualitative changes are easily noted in the direct electrode trace.

A similar procedure is followed in the case of valinomycin-induced potassium uptake from a medium containing low concentrations of potassium. In this case, the pen trace should be set with the recorder zero point near the top of the chart so that decreases in mv readings may be recorded.

MITOCHONDRIAL "SWELLING-CONTRACTION"

When mitochondrial suspensions are treated with various agents and under a variety of conditions, changes in the optical density of the suspension occur. In the case of relatively large decreases in optical density, these changes have to some extent been correlated with actual increases in mitochondrial water and volume

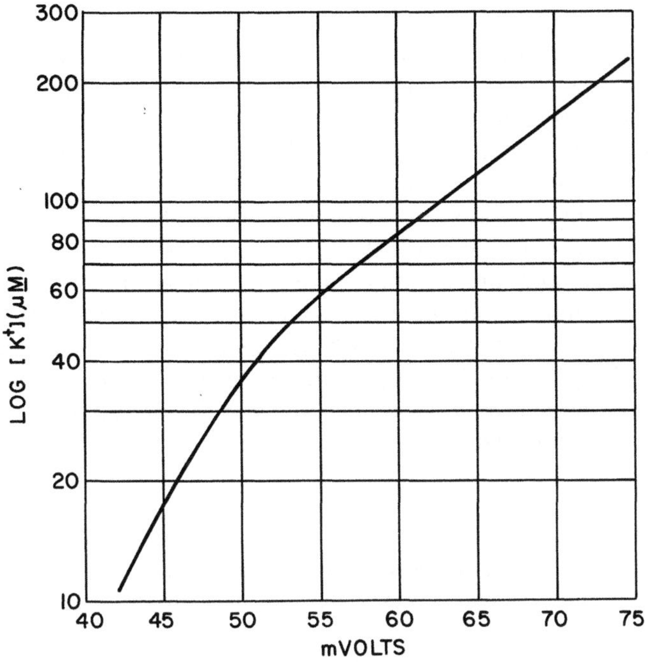

FIG. 13. Calibration curve for the cation-sensitive electrode. The data of Figure 12A were replotted on a semilogarithmic graph. The abscissa represents the potentials registered by the pH meter at the concentrations of K^+ shown on the ordinate.

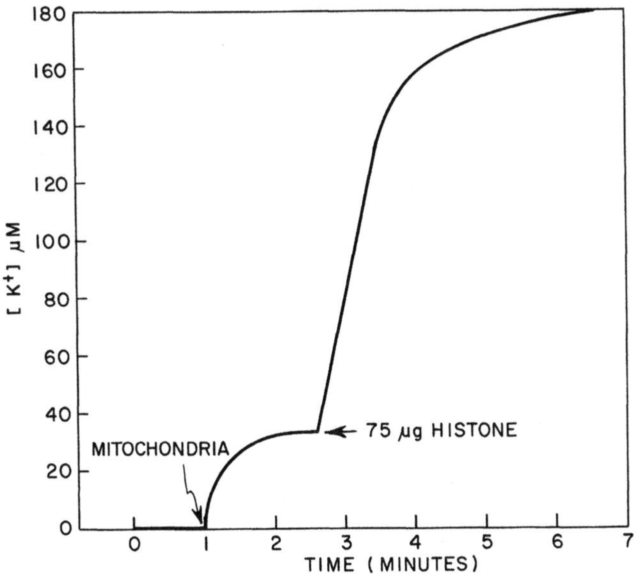

FIG. 14. Histone-induced K^+ efflux. This figure represents the data of Figure 12B, recalculated on the basis of the calibration curve of Figure 13. The ordinate gives the concentration of K^+ in the external solution.

(Lehninger, 1962). These "large-amplitude" absorbancy changes have thus been interpreted in terms of mitochondrial swelling. In many cases this large amplitude swelling is nonenergy-linked, and the physiologic role of this process has been questioned (Hunter and Smith, 1967). Under certain conditions, relatively small optical density changes are noted which cannot conveniently be correlated with actual volume changes because of the insensitivity of the mitochondrial water and volume measurements (Packer, 1967). In general, these "low-amplitude" changes are energy-linked and presumably have physiologic function. It should be mentioned that relatively large, energy-linked optical density changes can be obtained under certain conditions. Thus the distinction between large- and low-amplitude "swelling" is not clear at present. In any event, optical density change of a mitochondrial suspension is a convenient way of examining various energy-linked functions in mitochondria.

Methods

MITOCHONDRIAL ISOLATION: The mitochondria are isolated as described earlier in this chapter ("Liver") and suspended at a protein concentration of 30 to 50 mg per pml.

ASSAY MEDIUM: A variety of both ionic and nonionic media may be employed. We have utilized 0.25 M sucrose or 0.125 M KCl or NaCl (or combinations of sucrose and salt) buffered with tris at pH 7.4. For energy-linked swelling, either substrate or ATP is required. In many cases, a permeant anion such as phosphate facilitates the swelling.

In general, nonenergy-linked, large-amplitude swelling is measured at low mitochondrial protein concentrations (0.1 to 0.3 mg per ml). Since these changes can usually not be correlated with other mitochondrial functions, they are of somewhat limited use. To measure energy-linked swelling it is usually necessary to increase the protein concentration to about 1 to 2 mg per ml.

MEASUREMENT OF SWELLING: At high protein concentration (1 to 2 mg per ml), the ordinary laboratory spectrophotometer is not adequate because of the insensitivity of these instruments at high optical density. They may be utilized, however, by decreasing the cuvette path length by a factor of about 10. Alternatively, a spectrophotometer having a linear absorbance slide wire from 0 to 3.0 optical density units (Gilford multiple absorbance recorder, Fig. 8) may be used. Swelling is usually measured at 520 mμ.

EXAMPLE EXPERIMENT: The following experiment was designed to demonstrate low-amplitude, energy-linked swelling induced by basic proteins such as histones or parathyroid hormone. We have found the Gilford* 2000, recording spectrophotometer (Fig. 8) to be the most convenient for continuous measurement of swelling at high protein concentration. Standard 1 cm^2 glass cuvettes were used. Optical density changes were measured at a wavelength of 520 mμ.

The recorder portion of the Gilford is first calibrated to give a full-scale

*Gilford Instruments Co., Oberlin, Ohio.

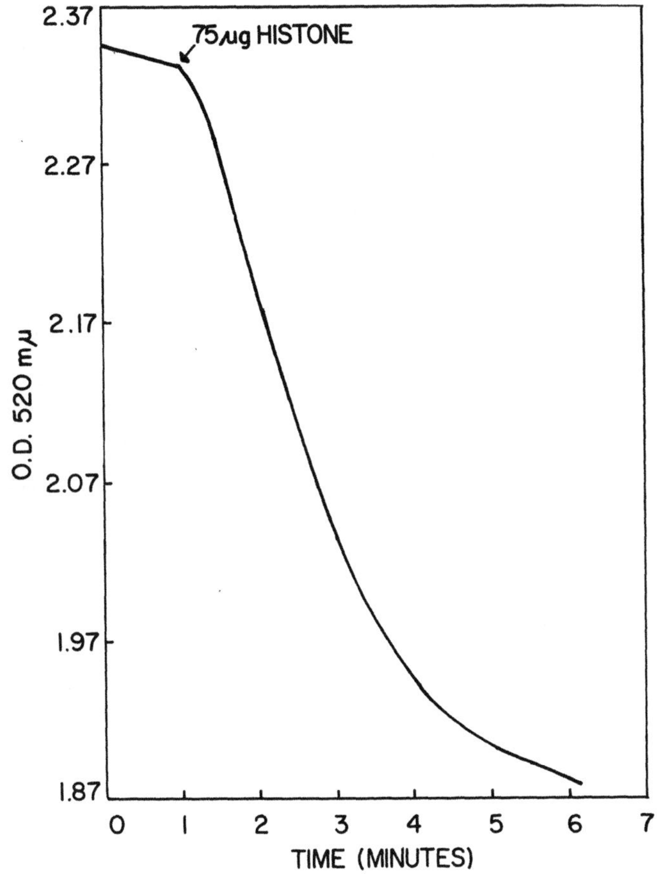

FIG. 15. Induction of low-amplitude swelling by histone. The medium contained 0.25 M sucrose, 9.4 mM tris-phosphate, and 3.1 mM tris-succinate, pH 7.4, in a final volume of 4.0 ml. At zero time, 7.4 mg mitochondrial protein was added. At the arrow, 75 μg β6-histone was added. The ordinate represents the optical density of the suspension at 520 mμ.

absorbance of 0.5 OD units. The assay medium consisted of 0.25 M sucrose, 9.4 mM tris-phosphate, 3.1 mM tris-succinate (pH 7.4), and 1.85 mg mitochondrial protein per ml in a final volume of 4 ml. Immediately after addition of the mitochondria, the cuvette was placed in the spectrophotometer and the pen trace was adjusted to the top of the recorder chart by means of the absorbance dial (with the function switch in the "read" position). The reading on the absorbance scale gives the recorder base-line optical density. The initial optical density of the suspension is then obtained by adding 0.5 OD units to the base-line absorbance. In this particular experiment, the base-line reading was 1.87 OD units and the initial optical density 2.37. After the scale is set, the recorder is turned on. The foregoing manipulations take approximately 15 seconds. After recording for one minute, 75 μ g of a purified histone fraction was added to the cuvette and the decrease in optical density followed continuously. A tracing of the reaction is shown in Figure 15.

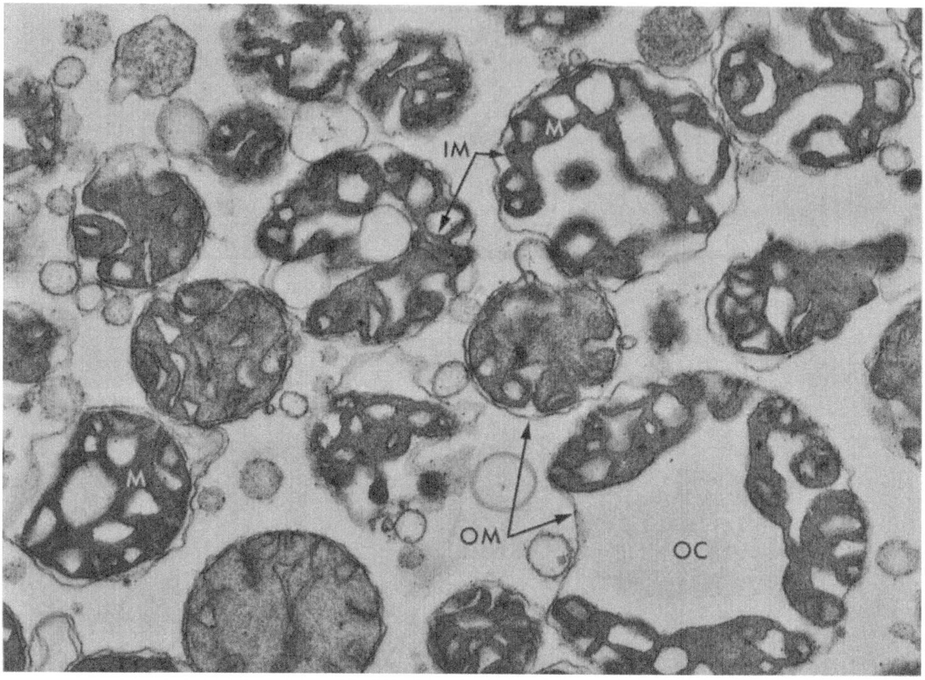

FIG. 16. Rat liver mitochondria fixed during State three respiration, illustrating condensed conformation. Matrix density is increased and the inner membrane is greatly infolded. The volume of the matrix space (inner compartment) is decreased in relation to the volume of the outer compartment (intracristal space) which is increased. (OM) Outer membrane. (IM) Inner membrane. (OC) Outer compartment. (M) Matrix space (inner compartment). × 28,000.

Recently, a multiparameter device has been developed by Drs. Pressman and Mayer at the Johnson Research Foundation of the University of Pennsylvania. Simultaneous measurements of oxygen consumption, pyridine nucleotide oxidation and reduction, ion movements, and light scattering may be made. A complete description can be found in volume 10 of *Methods in Enzymology* (Pressman, 1967).

ELECTRON MICROSCOPY OF ISOLATED MITOCHONDRIA

Thin-section electron microscopy is a valuable adjunct to the investigation of biochemical and pharmacologic reactions in mitochondrial suspensions. It provides a visual record of the purity or degree of contamination of such suspensions, as well as an indication of the intactness of the mitochondria in general. In addition, it enables one to investigate possible relationships between mitochondrial configurational changes and biochemical functions. Recent studies indicate that mitochon-

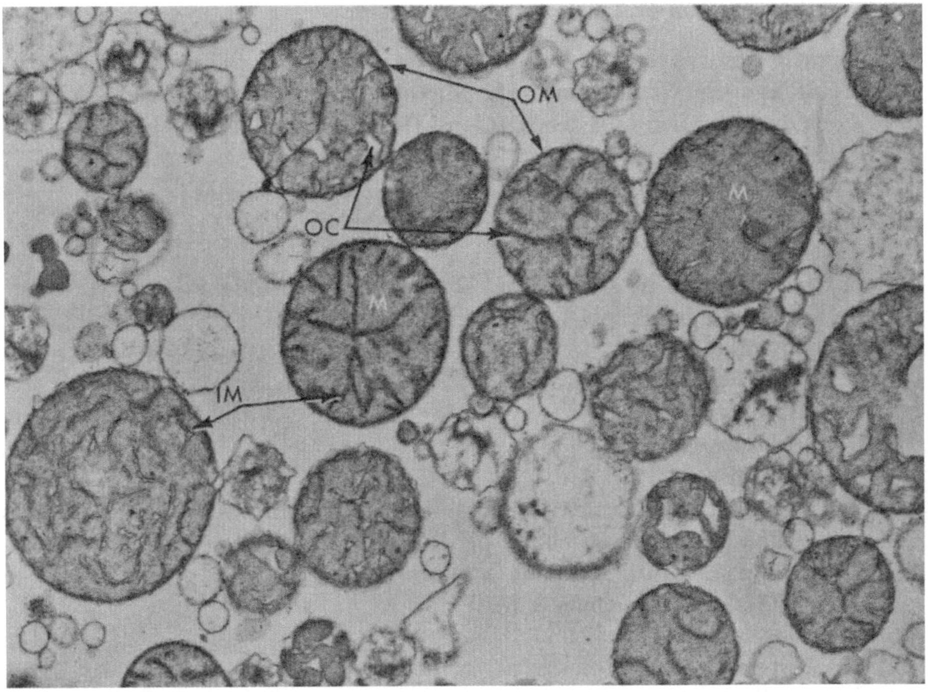

FIG. 17. Rat liver mitochondria fixed after fifteen minutes incubation in State four respiration, illustrating orthodox conformation. The mitochondria resemble those seen in intact tissue. The volume of the matrix space is great in relation to that of the outer compartment and intra-cristal space. Matrix density and infolding of the inner membrane are less than in the condensed conformation. (OM) Outer membrane. (IM) Inner membrane (cristae mitochondriales). (OC) Outer compartment. (M) Matrix space. × 21,000.

drial configuration is altered under various conditions of isolation and metabolic activity (Mintz et al., 1967; Hackenbrock, 1966; Weinbach et al., 1967). The configurational changes may be passive and secondary to the biochemical phenomena. Conversely they may somehow institute these reactions through a shift in the geometric arrangement of the inner membrane subunits. Which of these interpretations is correct is not yet clear.

Mitochondria in stock suspensions are usually in a condensed morphology. The volume of the intracristal space appears increased, the matrix space appears decreased, and there is marked infolding of the inner membrane. These features are more marked during State 3 respiration (Fig. 16). After 15 minutes incubation in State 4 respiration, liver mitochondria in 0.25 M sucrose assume an "orthodox" morphology which is similar to that of mitochondria as usually seen in intact tissue (Fig. 17). Heart mitochondria appear to resist this change to the orthodox conformation (Sordahl et al., 1969). Such conformational changes in mitochondria are easily studied by the method of Hackenbrock (1966), which is a modification of that of Malamud (1963).

PREPARATION OF A MITOCHONDRIAL PELLET:

1. Equipment and reagents:
   a. Centrifuge–Beckman/Spinco 152 Microfuge or Coleman Model 6-811
   b. Polyethylene Microfuge tubes, 0.4 ml (Beckman Inst. cat. #314326)
   c. Millonig's phosphate buffer:
      83 ml monobasic sodium phosphate, 2.26 percent (140 mM)
      17 ml sodium hydroxide, 2.52 percent (108 mM)
   d. Fixatives:
      (1) For fixation in suspension: 2 percent glutaraldehyde in Millonig's phosphate buffer, pH 7.4, 300 mOsM/liter.

glutaraldehyde (50%W/W [biological grade], Fisher Scientific Co.)*	1 ml
phosphate buffer	2 ml
1 M sucrose	1.7 ml
distilled water	20.3 ml

      (2) For fixation of centrifuged pellets: 2 percent osmium tetroxide in Millonig's phosphate buffer, pH 7.4, 320 mOsM/liter†.

4 percent osmium tetroxide in water (Matheson, Coleman & Bell)	2.5 ml
phosphate buffer	0.4 ml
1 M sucrose	1.1 ml
distilled water	1.0 ml

2. Fixation after formation of a pellet:
   a. An aliquot from the mitochondrial suspension is centrifuged for 10 seconds. Concentration of the suspension and/or volume of the aliquot is adjusted to obtain a pellet thickness of 0.2 to 0.3 mm (about 0.1 mg protein/0.1 ml aliquot).
   b. The supernate is quickly withdrawn and replaced by 2 percent osmium tetroxide in 10 mM phosphate buffer. Complete fixation occurs in a few seconds and is signaled by a blackening of the pellet.
3. Fixation in suspension:
   a. Mix the aliquot of mitochondria with an equal volume of 2 percent glutaraldehyde in the centrifuge tubes. By this method, fixation is immediate and centrifugation may be delayed until several tubes have been prepared.
   b. The fixed suspensions are then centrifuged for 30 to 60 seconds and the supernate is withdrawn and replaced with three changes of buffer.‡ For

*Various commercial glutaraldehyde preparations have a high content of impurities resulting in osmolalities much higher than the theoretical predicted value (Maser et al., 1967). The product by Fisher Scientific Co. is recommended. It should be adsorbed on activated charcoal or $BaCO_3$ until the pH is above 6.5, and the final osmolality of the buffered fixative should be checked with an osmometer.

†Osmium fumes are very toxic to mucous membranes. Therefore all steps involving osmium tetroxide fumes should be carried out under a hood.

‡At this point the pellets may be stored at 4°C for convenience before embedding. No deterioration in mitochondrial ultrastructure has been noted after 10 days storage in this manner. The stored pellets are postfixed in 2 percent osmium tetroxide just prior to embedding.

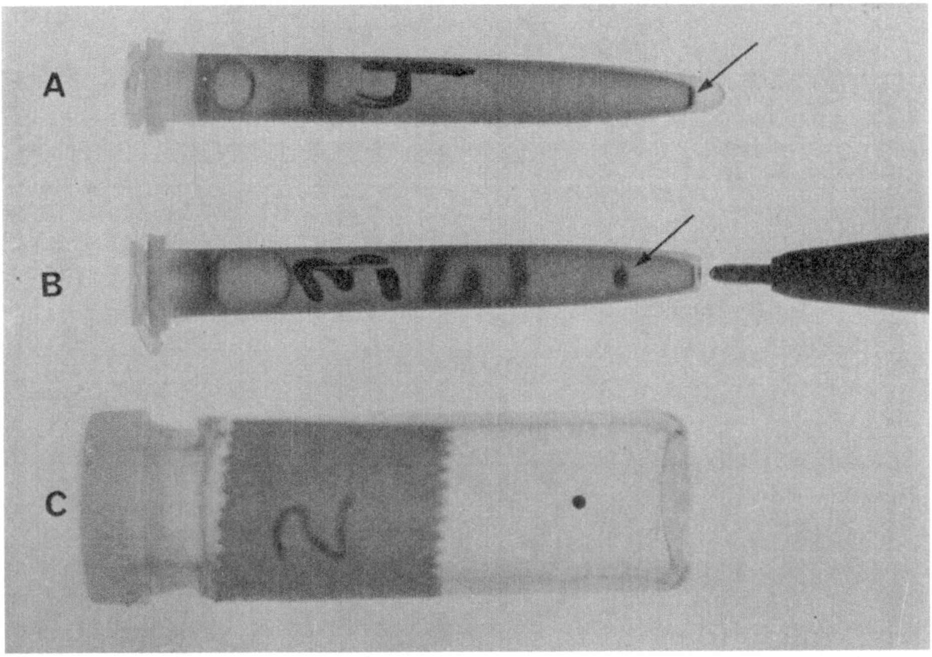

FIG. 18. Dehydration of a mitochondrial pellet. (A) Pellet (arrow) in tip of polyethylene centrifuge tube prior to dehydration. (B) Partially dehydrated pellet (arrow) which has been dislodged from the bottom of the centrifuge tube by pressing inward with a ball-point pen as shown. (c) Dehydrated pellet in vial containing absolute alcohol.

better contrast, these glutaraldehyde-fixed mitochondrial pellets may be postfixed in 2 percent osmium tetroxide.

4. Fifteen minutes to two hours after addition of osmium the fixative is removed and the pellet is dehydrated in graded concentrations of ethanol (30, 50, 70, 90 percent, absolute).
5. The pellet may then be dislodged from the bottom of the tube by cutting the tip off the tube just below the pellet and then pressing inward on the resulting flat surface with a dull pencil (Fig. 18).

EMBEDDING OF A MITOCHONDRIAL PELLET:

1. Fixed mitochondrial pellets may be handled like intact tissue and may be embedded in a variety of materials. Araldite 502 has been satisfactorily used in the author's laboratory according to the method of Luft (1961), which is summarized as follows:
2. Prepare an embedding mixture containing:

Resin-Araldite 502	27.0 ml
Hardener-DDSA (dodecenyl succinic anhydride)	23.0 ml
Accelerator-DMP-30 (tridimethylaminomethylphenol)	0.75-1.0 ml

The resin and hardener may be mixed in advance and stored frozen in an

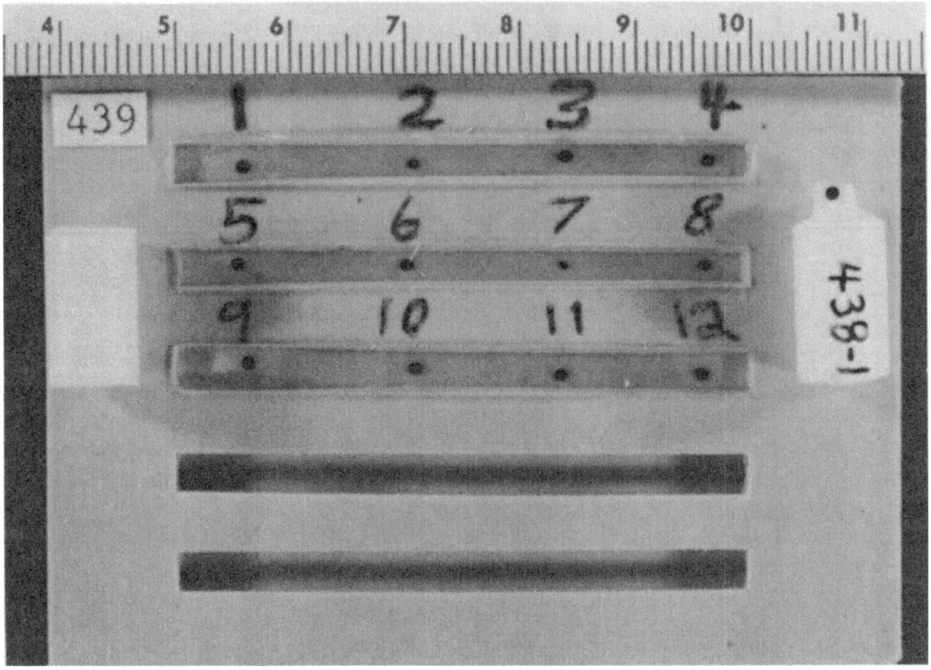

FIG. 19. Embedded mitochondrial pellets in strip mold of silastic rubber. The strips are 1/8 inch wide. After the araldite resin has hardened, the pellets are mounted at the ends of Plexiglas rods for sectioning. At left is a rod before a pellet has been mounted. At right is a pellet mounted on edge so that complete cross-sections of the pellet may be obtained.

airtight container until use. When ready to use, thaw the mixture to room temperature and add accelerator, being careful to mix well.

3. Transfer the fixed and partially dehydrated pellet to a small vial and complete dehydration with absolute ethanol for 15 minutes.
4. Replace absolute ethanol with propylene oxide* (two changes of 15 minutes each).
5. Replace the propylene oxide with a 50 percent solution of the embedding mixture (accelerator added) in propylene oxide. Let stand for one hour at room temperature.
6. Add an equal volume of the Araldite embedding mixture and let stand at room temperature for 3 to 6 hours (overnight is acceptable).
7. Transfer the pellets to undiluted Araldite embidding mixture† (accelerator added). This is conveniently done in one-eighth-inch-wide strip molds of silastic rubber (Fig. 19).

*Changes of propylene oxide should be done rapidly so that drying of the specimen does not occur. Care should also be taken to avoid contamination of the propylene oxide with water vapor.

†The accelerator should be thoroughly but gently mixed with the Araldite and hardener. After mixing, it is convenient to deaerate the mixture in a dessicating jar with a vacuum pump. This takes only a few seconds and avoids air bubbles in the final hardened block.

8. Polymerization is carried out in a 60°C oven for 12 hours.
9. When polymerization is complete, the Araldite strips are cut so that the pellets may be mounted on Plexiglas rods with epoxy resin (Fig. 19). The pellets are oriented so that they may be sectioned perpendicular to the plane of the pellet (which is a very thin disc).
10. Sections may be cut with glass or diamond knives on any quality ultramicrotome. If staining of the sections is desired, Reynolds lead citrate is satisfactory.
11. Sections should be large enough to include both top and bottom surfaces of the pellet. The composition of the mitochondrial population should be closely examined at all levels of the pellet. As many photographs as practicable should be taken and studied from enlarged prints.

As pointed out by Sjostrand (1967), studies of this kind require large numbers of photographs, and consequently a great deal of time is required in the developing and printing of pictures. Baudhin and Berthet (1967) have recently published a method for statistical study of populations of mitochondria from suspensions. This method may permit more objective, accurate conclusions from a fewer number of specimens and photographs. For details of this method, one should consult their original report.

REFERENCES

Baltscheffsky, H. 1957. Mitochondrial respiratory control and phosphorylative activities in a magnesium-free medium. Biochim. Biophys. Acta, 25:382-388.

Baudhuin, P., and Berthet, J. 1967. Electron microscopic examination of subcellular fractions II. Quantitative analysis of the mitochondrial population isolated from rat liver. J. Cell Biol., 35:631-648.

Chance, B. 1956. On possible mechanisms for the control of electron transport in the respiratory chain. Proc. Int. Cong. Biochem. Third Meeting. New York, Academic Press, Inc., pp. 300-303.

—and Williams, G. R. 1956. The respiratory chain and oxidative phosphorylation. Advances Enzym., 17:65-134.

Devlin, T. M. 1967. Neoplastic tissue mitochondria. *In* Methods in Enzymology. Estabrook, R. W., and Pullman, M. E., eds. New York, Academic Press, Inc., Vol. 10, pp. 110-114.

Dow, D. S. 1967. The isolation of skeletal muscle mitochondria showing tight coupling, high respiratory indices, and differential adenosine triphosphatase activities. Biochemistry, 6:2915-2922.

Estabrook, R. W., and Pullman, M. E. 1967. Oxidation and Phosphorylations, Methods in Enzymology. New York, Academic Press, Inc., Vol. 10.

Fiske, C. H., and Subba Row, Y. 1925. The colorimetric determination of phosphorous. J. Biol. Chem., 66:375-400.

Forte, J. G., Forte, G. M., Gee, R., and Saltman, P. 1967. Oxidative phosphorylation and the effects of SCN on mitochondria isolated from rabbit stomach. Biochem. Biophys. Res. Commun., 28:215-221.

Green, D. E., and Ziegler, D. M. 1963. Electron transport particles. *In* Methods in Enzymology. Colowick, S. P., and Kaplan, N. O., eds. New York, Academic Press, Inc., Vol. 6, pp. 416-424.

Gregg, C. T. 1967. Preparation and assay of phosphorylating submitochondrial particles:

particles from rat liver prepared by drastic sonication. *In* Methods in Enzymology. Estabrook, R. W., and Pullman, M. E., eds. New York, Academic Press, Inc., Vol. 10, pp. 181-185.

Guggenheim, S. J., Bonkowsky, H. L., Harris, J. W., and Webster, L. T., Jr. 1967. The preparation and characterization of mitochondria from developing red blood cells. J. Lab. Clin. Invest., 69:357-369.

Hackenbrock, C. R. 1966. Ultrastructural basis for metabolically linked mechanical activity in mitochondria. J. Cell Biol., 30:269-297.

Hassinen, I., and Hallman, M. 1967. Comparison of the effects of disulfiram and dimercaptopropanol arsenite on mitochodrial structure and function. Biochem. Pharmacol., 16:2155-2161.

Hunter, F. E., Jr., and Smith, E. E. 1967. Measurement of mitochondrial swelling and shrinking—high amplitude. *In* Methods in Enzymology. Estabrook, R. W., and Pullman, M. E., eds. New York, Academic Press, Inc., Vol. 10, pp. 689-696.

Jacobs, E. E., Jacob, M., Sanadi, D. R., and Bradley, L. B. 1956. Uncoupling of oxidative phosphorylation by cadmium ion. J. Biol. Chem., 223:147-156.

Johnson, C. L., Mauritzen, C. M., Starbuck, W. C., and Schwartz, A. 1967. Histones and mitochondrial ion transport. Biochemistry, 6:1121-1127.

Keilin, D., and Hartree, E. F. 1938. Cytochrome oxidase. Proc. Roy. Soc. (Biol.), B125:171-186.

Kenefick, D. G., and Hanson, J. B. 1966. Contracted state as an energy source for calcium binding and calcium plus inorganic phosphate accumulation by corn mitochondria. Plant Physiol.,41:1601-1609.

Kornberg, A., and Pricer, W. E., Jr. 1951. Enzymatic phosphorylation of adenosine and 2,6-diaminopurine riboside. J. Biol. Chem., 193:481-490.

Lam, K. W., Warshaw, J. B., and Sanadi, D. R. 1966. Studies on oxidative phosphorylation XIII. Relationship of coupling factors to stimulation by oligomycin of energy-linked reactions. Arch. Biochem. Biophys., 117:594-598.

Lamy, F. M., Rodesch, F. R., and Dumont, J. E. 1967. Action of thyrotropin on thyroid energetic metabolism. Exp. Cell Res., 46:518-532.

Laudahn, G. 1961. Die wirkung von persantin auf herzmuskel sarkosomen. Experientia, 17:415-416.

Lehninger, A. L. 1962. Water uptake and extrusion by mitochondria in relation to oxidative phosphorylation. Physiol. Rev., 42:467-517.

—1965. The Mitochondrion. 2d ed. Baltimore, W. J. Benjamin.

—and Wadkins, C. L. 1962. Oxidative phosphorylation. Ann. Rev. Biochem., 31:47-78.

—Carafoli, E., and Rossi, C. S. 1967. Energy-linked ion movements in mitochondrial systems. Advances Enzym., 29:259-320.

Linnane, A. W., and Ziegler, D. M. 1958. Studies on the mechanism of oxidative phosphorylation. Biochim. Biophys. Acta, 29:630-638.

Lowry, O. H., and Lopez, J. A. 1946. The determination of inorganic phosphate in the presence of labile phosphate esters. J. Biol. Chem., 162:421-428.

Luft, J. 1961. Improvements in epoxy resin embedding methods. J. Biophys. Biochem. Cytol., 9:409.

Malamed, S. 1963. Use of a microcentrifuge for preparation of isolated mitochondria and cell suspensions for electron microscopy. J. Cell Biol., 18:696-700.

Maser, M. D., Powell, T. E., and Philpott, C. W. 1967. Relationships among pH, osmolality, and concentration of fixative solutions. Stain Techn., 42:175-182.

Mintz, H. A., Yawn, D. H., Safer, B., Bresnick, E., Liebelt, A. G., Blailock, Z. R., Rabin, E. R., and Schwartz, A. 1967. Morphological and biochemical studies of isolated mitochondria from fetal, neonatal, and adult liver and from neoplastic tissues. J. Cell Biol., 34:513-523.

Moore, C., and Pressman, B. C., 1964. Mechanism of action of valinomycin on mitochondria. Biochem. Biophys. Res. Commun., 15:562-567.

Ozawa, K., Seta, K., Takeda, H., Ando, K., Handa, H., and Araki, C. 1966. On the isolation of mitochondria with high respiratory control from rat brain. J. Biochem., 59:501-510.

Packer, L. 1967. Energy-linked low amplitude mitochondrial swelling. *In* Methods in Enzymology. Estabrook, R. W., and Pullman, M. E., eds. New York, Academic Press, Inc., Vol. 10, pp. 685-689.

—Utsumi, K., and Mustafa, M. G. 1966. Oscillatory states of mitochondria I. electron and energy transfer pathways. Arch. Biochem., 117:381-393.

Péron, F. G., McCarthy, J., and Guerra, F. 1965. Further studies on the effect of calcium ions and corticosteroidgenesis. Biochim. Biophys. Acta, 110:277-289.

Pressman, B. C. 1965. Induced active transport of ions in mitochondria. Proc. Nat. Acad. Sci. U.S.A. 53:1076-1083.

—1967. Biological applications of ion-specific glass electrodes. *In* Methods in Enzymology. Estabrook, R. W., and Pullman, M. E., eds. New York, Academic Press, Inc., Vol. 10, pp. 714-726.

Psychoyos, S., Tallan, H. H., and Greengard, P. 1966. Aldosterone synthesis by adrenal mitochondria. J. Biol. Chem., 241:2949-2956.

Pullman, M. E., and Penefsky, M. S. 1963. Preparation and assay of phosphorylating submitochondrial particles: mechanically ruptured mitochondria. *In* Methods in Enzymology. Colowick, S. P., and Kaplan, N. O., eds. New York, Academic Press, Inc., Vol. 6, pp. 277-284.

—and Schatz, G. 1967. Mitochondrial oxidations and energy coupling. Ann. Rev. Biochem., 37 (II): 539-610.

Racker, E. 1965. Mechanisms in Bioenergetics. New York, Academic Press, Inc.

Safer, B., and Schwartz, A. 1967. Active transport of potassium ion in heart mitochondria. Circ. Res. 21:25-31.

Sanadi, D. R. 1965. Energy-linked reactions in mitochondria. Ann. Rev. Biochem., 34:21-48.

—and Fluharty, A. L. 1963. On the mechanism of oxidative phosphorylation VII. The energy-requiring reduction of pyridine nucleotide by succinate and the energy-yielding oxidation of reduced pyridine nucleotide by fumarate. Biochemistry, 2:523-528.

Schatz, G., and Racker, E. 1966. Partial resolution of the enzymes catalyzing oxidative phosphorylation VII. J. Biol. Chem., 241:1429-1438.

Schneider, W. C., and Hogeboom, G. H. 1950. Intracellular distribution of enzymes V. Further studies on the distribution of cytochrome c in rat liver homogenates. J. Biol. Chem., 183:123-128.

Sjostrand, F. 1967. Electron microscopy of cells and tissues. *In* Instrumentation and Techniques. New York, Academic Press, Inc., Vol. 1, pp. 436-447.

Slater, E. C. 1967. Manometric methods and phosphate determination. *In* Methods in Enzymology. Estabrook, R. W., and Pullman, M. E., eds. New York, Academic Press, Inc., Vol. 10, pp. 19-29.

Smith, R. E., Roberts, J. C., and Hittelman, K. J. 1966. Nonphosphorylating respiration of mitochondria from brown adipose tissue of rats. Science, 154:653-654.

Sordahl, L. A., and Schwartz, A. 1967a. Effects of dipyridamole on heart muscle mitochondria. Molec. Pharmacol., 3:509-515.

— and Schwartz, A. 1967b. Oxidative phosphorylation of tumor mitochondria isolated in albumin-containing media. J. Cell Biol., 35:128A.

—Blailock, Z. R., Kraft, G. H., and Schwartz, A. 1969. The possible relationship between ultrastructure and biochemical state of heart mitochondria. Arch. Biochem. Biophys., 132:404-415.

Tager, J. M., Papa, S., Quagliariello, E., and Slater, E. C., eds. 1966. Regulation of Metabolic Processes in Mitochondria. Biochim. Biophys. Acta Library, Amsterdam, Elsevier, Vol. 7.

Tyler, D. D., and Gonze, J. 1967. The preparation of thyroid and thymus mitochondria. *In* Methods in Enzymology. Estabrook, R.W., and Pullman, M. E., eds. New York, Academic Press, Inc., Vol. 10, pp. 101-103.

Umbreit, W. W., Burris, R. H., and Stauffer, J. F. 1964. Manometric Techniques. 2d ed. Minneapolis, Burgess Publishing Co.
Von Korff, R. W. 1965. Metabolic characteristics of isolated rabbit heart mitochondria. J. Biol. Chem. 240:1351-1358.
Wadkins, C. L., and Lehninger, A. L. 1963. Preparation and assay of phosphorylating submitochondrial particles. *In* Methods in Enzymology. Colowick, S. P., and Kaplan, N. O., eds. New York, Academic Press, Inc., Vol. 6, pp. 265-272.
Weinbach, E. C. 1961. A procedure for isolating stable mitochondria from rat liver and kidney. Anal. Biochem. 2:335-343.
—Garbus, J., and Sheffield, H. G. 1967. Morphology of mitochondria in coupled, uncoupled, and re-coupled states. Exp. Cell Res., 46:129-143.
Williamson, R. L., and Metcalf, R. L. 1967. Salicylanilides: a new group of active uncouplers of oxidative phosphorylation. Science, 158:1694-1695.

CHAPTER **9**

Liver Smooth Endoplasmic Reticulum "Microsomal" Drug-Metabolizing Enzyme System

James R. Fouts

Department of Pharmacology, The University of Iowa College of Medicine, Iowa City, Iowa

IN VIVO STUDIES OF DRUG METABOLISM

Attempts to Assess Rate of Metabolism of Drugs by Liver Microsomes

The metabolism of a drug by liver microsomal enzymes can lead to an increase, a decrease, or no change in the pharmacologic activity of that drug. There are processes other than metabolism that can affect the duration and intensity of drug action. These other processes include absorption, distribution, and excretion. In order to use duration of drug action, biologic half-life of a drug, or rate of excretion of metabolites as a measure of the rate of drug metabolism in vivo, several criteria must therefore be assessed. The methods to be described depend largely for their popularity upon more or less firm evidence that the parameters being measured and the drugs being used are chosen to minimize the

Studies, from the author's laboratory, referred to herein were supported by grants from the National Institutes of Health, GM–06034, GM–12675, and CA–05648.

effects of all changes except those in rate of metabolism. At this point it is probably sufficient to state that in vivo studies of the rate of metabolism of drugs by liver microsomal enzymes can only be suggestive and should be followed whenever possible by further experiments that assess the function of other processes like distribution and excretion, and/or directly measure liver microsomal enzyme activity in vitro, as will be described later (see p. 302 ff.).

Three types of studies are widely used as in vivo indicators of the status of liver microsomal drug-metabolizing enzyme activity. All three types of experiments depend on the fact that the metabolism of a drug by liver microsomes can lead to its inactivation and an increase in the rate of its elimination from the blood or body. The drug metabolites produced by liver microsomal enzymes can also sometimes be used to quantify or at least to estimate the enzyme activity, by assay of these metabolites in either body fluids or excreta. The three methods most widely used are, therefore, (1) duration of drug action, (2) biologic half-life of the drug, and (3) rate of excretion of metabolites.

DRUG METABOLISM AS ESTIMATED FROM DURATION OF DRUG ACTION.—In order for duration of drug action to serve as an indicator of liver microsomal enzyme activity, several questions must be answered. First, is the pharmacologic action one that has a sharp end point? Second, is the duration of this drug action dependent in most instances almost exclusively on rate of metabolism? Finally, are small changes in rate of metabolism sufficient to change duration of action to a measurable extent? As will soon be evident, none of these questions is completely answered by any of the techniques currently used, but these are still used because better techniques have yet to be developed. The two methods now to be described depend upon the righting reflex, and the two drugs chosen, hexobarbital and zoxazolamine, cause its loss.

a. Hexobarbital Sleeping Time. The duration of loss of the righting reflex after hexobarbital administration correlates well in most cases with the rate at which hexobarbital is metabolized by the liver microsomal enzyme systems. As with any generality, there may be exceptions to this statement, and an examination of the possibility of such exceptions is called for by anyone who uses hexobarbital sleeping times as a routine screen for liver microsomal enzyme activity. Some possible approaches to such an examination will be described shortly. First of all, though, there are some drawbacks to the hexobarbital sleeping time "screen." Thus, its use has been confined almost exclusively to rodents, especially mice and rats. In larger animals, barbiturate sleeping times are hard to quantify, probably because the much slower rate of barbiturate metabolism in larger animals leads to prolonging the period between wakefulness and sleep. The sharpness of the end point of hexobarbital sleeping time thus seems to depend on the rate of disposition of the drug. If this is very slow, the end point will be difficult to determine. As a practical matter, then, hexobarbital sleeping times are used to assess rates of drug metabolism in animals known to normally metabolize hexobarbital at a rapid rate—rats, mice, and occasionally rabbits, guinea pigs, or hamsters.

Then, there are a number of "tricks" that must be admitted to be necessary in measuring "sleeping times." Even with those species where hexobarbital sleeping times are often used, the end point is frankly subjective. Even with rats and mice, there is a period at the end of sleep where decision as to whether the animal is yet awake or asleep depends on the investigator. Each laboratory must set its own criteria for this decision, and it is best that the number of people running sleeping times be kept to a minimum. Ideally, a single person should run all sleeping times when two or more groups of animals (treated versus control) are to be compared. In order to obtain a reasonably acceptable sleeping time variability within a single group of animals, it is usually necessary for the investigator to apply some kind of stimulus to the animal near the end of its sleep. This can be a mild pinching of the tail, a sharp clap of the hands or a repositioning of the body of the mouse or rat, etc., at regular intervals. This is done to all animals in the group. Unless such stimuli are applied, the variability in sleeping time among animals in any one group will be quite high and will markedly increase as the mean sleeping time of the group increases.

It is also necessary to provide an environment of constant temperature, free of drafts or loud noises not initiated by the investigator. Ideally, sleeping times should be done in a way that also minimizes changes in body temperature of the animals. Hypothermia can result from barbiturate administration or be caused by prior treatment of animals with a test drug. Various heat lamps or ovens can be used to counteract this hypothermia, but their effects on body temperature should be monitored (e.g., by rectal thermistors). Generally, hexobarbital sleeping times are increased if body temperature falls and are decreased if body temperature rises. Ways to control these temperature fluctuations must be devised if hexobarbital sleeping times are to have primary relation to liver microsomal enzyme activity.

PROCEDURE. Hexobarbital can be administered by various routes. The two most common are intravenous and intraperitoneal. The latter is most often used because it is simpler and because the rate of injection and volume of solution, buffer, or ion composition of the vehicle are less critical than with intravenous injection. Another important point in favor of the intraperitoneal route is that drugs so administered are presented to the liver first and in almost quantitative amounts, whereas intravenous administration presents only a fraction of the total drug to the liver at any time. Since we are interested in assessing hepatic enzyme activity when we run hexobarbital sleeping times, the intraperitoneal route would seem to do this less ambiguously than the intravenous route. Generally speaking, most people inject 0.1 ml of the hexobarbital solution per 10 grams of mouse or rat when the intraperitoneal route is used. Deviation from such a prescription is possible, but can be ill-advised. Too concentrated solutions of hexobarbital (greater than 20 mg/ml) are irritating to muscosa and delay absorption from the peritoneum. Too dilute solutions of hexobarbital require excessive volumes being absorbed from the peritoneum, again resulting in delayed absorption.

Hexobarbital is generally made available as the sodium salt and is marketed in sealed ampules by Winthrop Laboratories (Special Chemicals Division, 90 Park Avenue, New York, New York). Weighing out hexobarbital for injection is a frustrating job, since it is a very sticky substance when exposed to air. It is usually best to take the manufacturer's word that each ampule contains 1.00 gram of hexobarbital sodium, and use the whole ampule for your experiment–making appropriate dilutions thereof with water or isotonic saline as you prefer. Once the solution is made it should be used as quickly as possible and always be kept tightly stoppered until the experiment is finished. Hexobarbital solutions pick up CO_2 from the atmosphere, and this leads to loss of hexobarbital from the solution. Tightly stoppered solutions of hexobarbital are stable for several hours, but those kept in open beakers or test tubes lose pharmacologic activity relatively quickly. In our laboratory, we make hexobarbital solutions up in saline and package them in rubber-sealed ampules of small capacity so that the amount of air in contact with the solution during our experiment remains small at all times. If large numbers of animals are to be treated, we divide our stock solution into several ampules rather than a single large container.

The dose-response curve for hexobarbital in mice and rats is fairly steep. Small changes in dose can markedly change duration of action. The desired duration of action depends on the purpose of the experiment. If one wishes to compare control sleeping times with groups where sleeping times will be longer than controls, the control group sleeping time can be relatively short (20 minutes); whereas if the treated group will have a shorter sleeping time than controls, the latter should sleep about 40 to 50 minutes. Thus, one chooses the hexobarbital dose so that the shortest sleeping time expected will be about 20 minutes, and the longest no more than two hours. Deviations from these limits usually lead to large variability about the mean, and this makes statistical evaluation difficult. Since hexobarbital sleeping times can vary with strain of animal, sex, age, or body weight of the animal, it is really of little value here to give typical doses of hexobarbital to use. The best technique is to determine for yourself what dose gives the desired sleeping time lying within the aforementioned rough limits. With most strains of rats and mice we have used, a dose of 100 to 125 mg/kg could be a starting point for such a dose-range study.

If one wishes to minimize variability, it is important to carefully monitor the environment in which the animals are kept before they are used for sleeping time studies, or any other in vivo and in vitro measures of drug metabolism to be made. These will be referred to again, but cannot be overemphasized. Control and treated groups must be housed in identical environments (preferably in randomized cages within the same room). Sleeping times can be affected by such diverse things as bedding. Ferguson (1966) reported that mice housed in cages with cedar-chip bedding sleep for shorter times after hexobarbital than mice kept on corncob bedding. Gillette (National Heart Institute, Bethesda), in a personal communication, says that this cedar-chip bedding phenomena has also been noted with sawdust. The in-group weight range of animals should also be kept as small as possible. Normally we limit this in mice to 2 grams and in rats to 20 to 25 grams. If weights range beyond these limits, in-group variability in sleeping times can be very large. One final point–if two groups of animals are to be compared, they must be treated as much alike as possible in one other way: they should be slept as nearly as possible at the same time of day. Thus the control group should not be run in the morning and the treated group in the afternoon. It is not enough that control and treated groups are always run on the same day, they must be run as nearly as possible at the same time. Circadian periodicity in drug response and toxicity has been reported for some drugs, among them a barbiturate (see Lindsay and Kullman, 1966, and Lutsch and Morris, 1967). Two very useful references for further reading concerning hexobarbital sleeping time as a technique are Rumke et al. (1963), and Winne (1964).

Zoxazolamine Paralysis Time.—As with hexobarbital sleeping time, the duration of loss of the righting reflex after zoxazolamine administration correlates well with the rate at which zoxazolamine is metabolized by liver microsomal enzymes. The same could be said for a number of drugs, and so one must at least offer some reason why zoxazolamine paralysis time may be a useful supplement to, or alternative to, hexobarbital sleeping times. Several workers have found that alterations in zoxazolamine paralysis time have occurred after drug treatments that have not affected hexobarbital sleeping times (see Conney et al., 1960). The most recent example of this occurred with DDT pretreatment in mice. DDT pretreatment did not affect hexobarbital sleeping time, but did shorten zoxazolamine paralysis time (Cram and Fouts, 1967). Thus, if one is interested in using in vivo measurements, such as hexobarbital sleeping times, to screen for inducers of hepatic microsomal drug-metabolizing enzymes, knowledge of the fact that zoxazolamine paralysis time can pick up changes not detected by hexobarbital sleeping time can be useful.

Inducers of hepatic microsomal enzymes can be classed into at least three major groups: (1) the anabolic steroids, (2) polycyclic hydrocarbons, and (3) phenobarbital and other barbiturates, chlorinated insecticides, chlorcyclizine, etc. (see Gillette, 1963). Of these three groupings, the most important, in terms of applicability to several species and preclinical drug screening, would seem to be the polycyclic hydrocarbons and the class to which phenobarbital belongs. Zoxazolamine metabolism is affected by all known members of the polycyclic hydrocarbon group and most of the members of group 3 (phenobarbital-like), while hexobarbital metabolism is seldom affected by any except drugs in group 3. The use of both hexobarbital sleeping time and zoxazolamine paralysis time should, therefore, be a reasonable attempt, at the in vivo level, to detect most important inducers of liver microsomal enzymes.

PROCEDURE. The method of assessing zoxazolamine paralysis time is quite analogous to that used in hexobarbital sleeping time. Again the same limitations and drawbacks apply, with the exception that zoxazolamine solutions are not unstable when exposed to air for any reasonable period of time. Zoxazolamine is not the easiest drug to get into solution in volumes reasonable for injection at the doses needed. In mice and rats, a dose of 100 to 200 mg/kg given intraperitoneally is a good starting point. For such doses, one can suspend zoxazolamine in something like carboxymethyl cellulose (1 percent). Attempts to dissolve zoxazolamine in water will be unsuccessful, and pH must be quite low to keep the drug in solution at reasonable concentrations for use in mice (20 mg/ml).

Solutions at such low pH are sometimes erratically absorbed, probably because they are so irritating. We suggest using zoxazolamine suspensions.

All other conditions, such as control of room temperature, animal body temperature, paralysis time end-point determinations, animal weight range, animal environment prior to test, time of day of experiment, duration of paralysis time (desirable limit is 20 minutes to 2 hours), apply equally to zoxazolamine paralysis time and hexobarbital sleeping time.

Having thus laid the basis for determining hexobarbital sleeping times or zoxazolamine paralysis times, what might be expected from the scientific community in terms of further experimentation? For example, if hexobarbital sleeping time is changed from control levels, what else might (still confining our studies to the in vivo situation) be asked for? I think the following might be minimal: (1) a determination of the amount of hexobarbital or zoxazolamine in the brain of the animal at the time of awakening or arousal, (2) determination of the rate of decline of whole-body levels of hexobarbital or zoxazolamine. Hexobarbital sleeping time or zoxazolamine sleeping time could be shifted by changes in rate of penetration of these drugs into the central nervous system, sequestration in body tissues, or excretion. If rate of hepatic metabolism is the only factor changing, then brain levels of hexobarbital or zoxazolamine should be the same, at time of awakening, in control and treated groups. On the other hand, changes in metabolism will change rate of disappearance of drug from whole body plus pooled excreta, while redistribution or changed excretion will not cause such changes. These latter, substantiating experiments will now be described.

ESTIMATES OF DRUG METABOLISM BY DETERMINATION OF DRUG LEVELS IN BLOOD OR WHOLE BODY.—The disappearance of drug from the whole body can be taken as a reliable estimate of rate of metabolism, if a few simple facts are not overlooked. All excreta must be collected and added to the final pool of material being assayed, and the method of assay must be reliably quantitative. Methods that give quantitative recovery from blood or urine may not work on homogenates of whole body and should be revalidated. Generally speaking, determinations of whole-body drug levels are limited to small species, e.g., mice and rats, though the only real limitation is the size of blendor available. In outline form the following would represent a typical protocol.

PROCEDURE. A known amount of drug is administered to each of a group of animals. Certain numbers (usually three to five animals) of animals are killed at various times after drug administration. Each animal and its collected excreta are ground up in a specified volume of water, saline, or buffer (e.g., a 20-gram mouse is ground up with 60 or 70 ml of saline). The homogenized mixture is made up to a convenient volume (e.g., with the mouse, dilution to 100 ml), and mixed thoroughly again, filtered through cheesecloth, and an aliquot of the filtrate assayed for drug content. A calculation can be made of the rate of disappearance of the drug from the body, and this can be related to the liver microsomal enzyme activity, if the drug was properly chosen—i.e., its metabolism occurs almost exclusively in liver microsomes. Thus, the rate of disappearance of hexobarbital, zoxazolamine, and aminopyrine from the body is a good index of hepatic microsomal enzyme activity in mice and rats. Changes in rate of these drugs' disappearance from the body occur when hepatic microsomal enzyme activity is raised or lowered (see, for example, Conney and Garren, 1961, Fig. 1 and Table 3, as well as Conney et al., 1960, Figs. 4 and 5).

Similar types of study using only blood or plasma levels of drug, and measuring rate of decline with time, can also reflect liver microsomal enzyme activity if certain questions can be answered. Such studies are always open to more criticism than measurements of whole-body levels of drugs, since plasma decay curves can be altered by many factors besides rate of removal of drug by liver enzymes. In order to equate plasma decay of a drug to its metabolism, one must establish that processes of absorption, distribution (including plasma binding of the drug), and excretion of the drug are not equally important to metabolism (ideally are not involved at all). This is particularly necessary when changes from normal are studied. Thus an increase in rate of disappearance of a given drug from blood may be due to an increase in its rate of metabolism by liver microsomal enzymes. But this could also result from displacing the drug from its plasma protein binding sites, changing the rate at which it was absorbed from its site of administration, or increasing its rate of excretion (by kidney, bile, lung, etc.). A carefully drawn study should include estimates of changes of each of these factors before statements correlating rate of drug decline in plasma with rate of metabolism in liver are made. Finally, one should not overlook the fact that changes from normal in plasma drug half-life can result from changes in rate of metabolism by extrahepatic tissues. Certain inducers of liver microsomal enzyme activity can also increase drug metabolism in other tissues as well (see Gelboin and Blackburn, 1964; Wattenberg and Leong, 1965).

Nevertheless, in large animals and humans, the rate of disappearance of drug from blood may be one of the few methods available to assess liver microsomal drug-metabolizing enzyme activity. With proper precautions, as mentioned, these studies can give us much valuable information. One of the most important precautions must be choice of drug to use in determining biologic half-life. Ideally this drug should be one that can be given intravenously (avoiding problems of absorption and the possibility of changing rates of absorption), is not extensively bound to plasma protein (avoiding problems of debinding as an influence on rate of disappearance), and is not excreted unchanged by liver or kidney (avoiding changes in execretion of unmetabolized drugs). Other practical considerations in the choice of the drug are obvious, but might be mentioned: (1) the drug must be nontoxic enough so that quantifiable blood levels can be maintained for several hours (preferably four to six hours); (2) methods must be available by which the drug can be separated from metabolites and preferably both drug and metabolite quantified; these methods must also be able to recover reproducibly, and preferably quantitatively, any drug present in blood; and (3) the drug should be metabolized exclusively by liver microsomes.

Among drugs whose biologic half-life (from plasma decay curves) has been used to estimate liver microsomal drug-metabolizing enzyme activity are several that do not fulfill all the foregoing requirements. The use of such imperfect compounds is not necessarily bad, but the results obtained must be scrutinized more closely than if more of the preceding criteria were met. Thus, both phenylbutazone and coumarin derivatives have been used in studies wherein shifts of their biologic half-lives accompanying various treatments were documented. Some of these changes in biologic half-life could be related to changes in rate of metabolism by the liver, but others have been shown to be related to changes in plasma binding of the phenylbutazone or coumarin drug used (see Aggeler et al., 1967, and Weiner et al., 1967; cf. Burns et al., 1965). The strong binding of coumarin and phenylbutazone derivatives to plasma proteins thus complicates the interpretation of shifts in their biologic half-life (plasma decay curve) accompanying other treatments.

For these and other reasons, the author recommends that measurement of hepatic microsomal drug-metabolizing enzyme activity by plasma decay curve (biologic half-life) be made with drugs like aminopyrine, antipyrine, or any other such compound having little plasma binding, little or no excessive tissue depot, little or no extrahepatic metabolism, and little or no renal or biliary excretion of the unchanged drug. Either aminopyrine or antipyrine can be administered intravenously, and methods are available for quickly and easily quantifying both parent drug and metabolites. In addition, the metabolic pathways entered by aminopyrine, at least, do not seem to differ qualitatively among most species studied, including man. Finally, most inducers or inhibitors of hepatic microsomal enzyme systems will affect aminopyrine metabolism and biologic half-life.

PROCEDURE: In practice, aminopyrine is administered intravenously in a dose of 10 to 15 mg/kg, and blood samples are drawn at periods of several hours thereafter. A typical protocol would call for sampling at 30 minutes, 1 hour, 2 hours, 3 hours, and 6 hours after dosing. Sample volume can range from 1 ml in the early time periods, to 5 ml at the later times. The same sample can be analyzed both for unchanged drug (aminopyrine) and for the principal metabolite thereof (4-aminoantipyrine) by the methods of LaDu et al. (1955) or Brodie and Axlerod (1950).

Antipyrine can be used similarly, though the dose is usually higher and adjusted to give a blood level of about 8 mg percent in the first sample (30 minutes). Antipyrine-^{14}C is now available commercially and, once purified, can be used to simplify the quantification procedure for determining the rate of disappearance of drug from the blood. A very rapid assay procedure, using antipyrine-^{14}C to estimate hepatic microsomal enzyme activity in control and phenobarbital pretreated rabbits, was recently demonstrated at the Workshop on Biochemical Approaches to Clinical Pharmacology, held at Vanderbilt University. Dr. William Pettinger and Dr. James V. Dingell, of the Department of Pharmacology at Vanderbilt, have written this procedure for the Workshop, but it has not yet been published. The author suggests that persons interested in using plasma half-life determinations as estimates of liver microsomal drug metabolism seriously consider use of this radioactive antipyrine, and write Dr. Dingell at Vanderbilt in Nashville, Tennessee, for further details.

ESTIMATION OF RATE OF DRUG METABOLISM BY EXCRETORY PRODUCTS.—If a drug metabolized by liver microsomes produces a metabolite that is rapidly and completely cleared from the body, preferably by the kidney, then measurement of this metabolite in the excreta, e.g., urine, may be used to estimate the activity of the liver drug-metabolizing enzymes. There are many possible pitfalls in this approach, and most of these are obvious but should be mentioned. If changes in rate of excretion of metabolite are documented, these can be due to changes in hepatic enzyme activity, but might also result from changes in renal function, plasma binding of the metabolite, or production by the liver of unusual metabolites of the drug which are not excreted as in the normal animal or human. Changes in renal function can include such less obvious things as uptake of the metabolite and/or metabolic alteration thereof, as well as the obvious changes such as decreased filtration and/or secretion rates. Thus, as with plasma decay curves, the use of metabolite excretion, as a measure of hepatic drug metabolism, is open to criticism, and the investigator using such methods has extra work to do as compared with someone who can measure whole-body levels.

To this author's knowledge, there are not very many drugs that can fit the criteria needed to satisfy most people that excretory metabolite measurements accurately reflect liver drug-metabolizing enzyme activity. One of those that has been used this way is aminopyrine, and the urinary metabolite measured is 4-aminoantipyrine. The test, as commonly used, is a simple one and has been applied to man. Remmer (1962) describes the experiment.

PROCEDURE. Some 0.8 to 1.0 gram of an aminopyrine analogue is administered intravenously (in man), and urine collections are made at 6 hours and at 24 hours (e.g., all urine voided between 0 and 6 hours is pooled, and an aliquot analyzed for 4-aminoantipyrine). In a series of 13 normal humans, some 53 $\pm$ 11 mg of 4-aminoantipyrine is excreted in 6 hours. This is increased markedly if the patient has ingested any of a number of drugs that are known from studies in animals to induce hepatic microsomal drug-metabolizing enzymes (e.g., barbital, glutethimide). The aminopyrine analogue, used in this test by Remmer, is called Novalgin, and has a methylaminomethane sulfonate group instead of the dimethylamino group in aminopyrine. Remmer states that Novalgin was used in his studies because it "is demethylated more easily than aminopyrine." Another name for Novalgin is dipyrone.

Pretreatment of Animals with Stimulators (Inducers) or Inhibitors of Drug Metabolism

CONSIDERATIONS IN THE USE OF INDUCERS OF DRUG METABOLISM.—Hepatic microsomal drug-metabolizing enzymes can be induced by pretreating animals with a variety of drugs or chemicals. These same phenomena have been demonstrated in some cases in man (see Remmer, 1962, and Burns et al., 1965). As already mentioned, inducers of drug-metabolizing enzymes can be divided into at least three groups on the basis of mechanism of action (see Gillette, 1963a). Such a diversity of mechanism of action suggests the possibility that optimal conditions, in terms of animal treatment, may vary for induction by one group of compounds versus another. Such has been found to be true. Unfortunately, we still do not know enough about many of the most practical aspects of these phenomena, and what will follow should be emphasized as only places to begin a study. Each investigator who wishes to study induction of liver microsomal enzymes in a new species of animal, or who wishes to use a new inducer, will have to determine for himself what the optimal conditions for this will be.

Routes of Administration, Frequency of Administration, and Dose of Inducers.

ROUTES OF ADMINISTRATION. Most compounds that have been shown to induce hepatic microsomal drug-metabolizing enzymes have been given intraperitoneally. Such a route would seem to allow maximum exposure of the liver to the inducer. Since most evidence suggests that inducers can exert their action directly on the liver (without needing the help of hormones, etc., released from other sites), it would seem reasonable to suggest that the intraperitoneal route be the one chosen first in any experiments dealing with new animal species or new inducers. This is not to suggest that effects cannot be obtained by other routes–indeed, effects of various inducers have been seen when these were given orally or injected subcutaneously or intramuscularly. How the amount or frequency of dosing with the inducer needs to be changed in order to achieve maximal induction, as compared with the intraperitoneal route, has not been systematically studied with any inducer as far as this author knows. It would seem obvious that preclinical drug testing for enzyme induction should at least compare the intraperitoneal route with the routes to be used clinically (e.g., orally). It should also be mentioned that whatever vehicle the inducer is dissolved or suspended in should also be administered to the control animal. Thus, if one is administering 3-methylcholanthrene in corn oil to the treated group, corn oil alone, in the same volume, should be given the control group. Some anomalous results with certain vehicles have been reported. Thus, Fujimoto (1965) has reported that gum tragacanth can block the shortening of hexobarbital sleeping time induced by phenobarbital and urethane in mice.

FREQUENCY OF ADMINISTRATION AND DOSE OF INDUCER. Frequency of administration and dose of inducer are really interrelated, since both are adjusted primarily for one purpose–to provide the liver with a continuous supply of the inducer during the time needed for induction to occur. Thus, a rapidly eliminated chemical or drug will have to be given either more frequently or in higher dose than another that is persistent, when attempts are made to use these chemicals as inducers. Induction of hepatic microsomal enzymes, either by polycyclic hydrocarbons like benzpyrene or by drugs and chemicals like phenobarbital or DDT, occurs maximally, in all species so far studied, within one week of continued treatment. This is not so with the anabolic steroids, which seem to require much longer for maximal effects, at least in some species. For example, Booth and Gillette (1962) and Gillette (1963a) have treated rats for two to four weeks with various anabolic steroids—this time period presumably being necessary for maximal effects. We have found that 14 days of treatment with methyltestosterone gives maximal stimulation of hepatic microsomal enzymes in rats (Mullen et al., 1966). While anabolic steroids have been shown to stimulate hepatic microsomal enzymes only in mice and rats, the frequency or duration of treatment needed to cause such enzyme induction may differ markedly between mice and rats. In all reports so far made, anabolic steroids work very slowly in rats, as already mentioned. However, in mice, steroid stimulation of microsomal drug metabolism may occur quickly. Thus, Novick et al. (1966) report that several anabolic steroids (19-nortestosterone derivatives) acted, in the mouse, within 12 hours after administration, with peak effects seen 12 to 24 hours after treatment. These same inducers were effective in rats only after prolonged (several weeks) treatment.

The evidence so far available, therefore, suggests that with any new inducer or new species of animal, the duration of treatment needed for optimal effect will have to be established empirically. So far, no inducer has failed, in any species tested, to exert its effects within two weeks of continued treatment, but these effects may not be those maximally obtainable. As a rough rule of thumb, such a two-week period of repeated administration might serve as a starting point.

With known inducers, the following represent the author's experience: (a) Benzpyrene and 3-methylcholanthrene exert maximal effects after a single dose in mice, rats, rabbits, and monkeys. (b) Phenobarbital and barbital exert maximal effects after three to four days of continued treatment (once or twice each day) in mice, rats, and rabbits. (c) The chlorinated, hydrocarbon insecticides, such as chlordane and DDT, exert maximal effects in five to seven days of continued treatment (injections once each day) in mice, rats, rabbits, and squirrel monkeys. In all cases, the route of injection was intraperitoneal.

Doses of inducers needed to exert maximal effects vary from one species to another. The only suggestion made as to why this is so seems to be that species differ in the rate at which they get rid of the inducer. If the inducer has a long half-life in a given species, then the dose and frequency of administration can be less than in a species where the inducer is eliminated rapidly. The major problem here, though, is that there really are very few studies, in any animal species, of what constitutes either a threshold or maximally effective dose of any given inducer. Since most people to date have concentrated almost entirely on obtaining maximal effects, our information is greatest in that area. Nevertheless, even with well-established inducers, such as benzpyrene or phenobarbital, the investigator should run his own pilot studies to assure himself where he is on the dose-response curve. With all inducers yet studied, there is increased response with increased dose up to a certain point, after which a plateau occurs. The following represent the author's experience: (a) Benzpyrene and 3-methylcholanthrene have exerted maximal effects after doses of 20 mg/kg in mice, rats, and rabbits. (b) Phenobarbital stimulates maximally in rats at doses of 75 mg/kg per day; in rabbits, maximal stimulation is seen at about 15 to 20 mg/kg per day; in mice, maximal stimulation is seen somewhere between 75 and 100 mg/kg per day. (c) γ-Chlordane stimulates maximally, in rats and mice, at doses of 100 mg/kg. Again all inducers were administered intraperitoneally.

It is perhaps germane at this point to at least suggest that, even within a given species, there may be differences between strains of animals in amount of an inducer needed for optimal effect. This has not been investigated by anyone to the author's knowledge. Yet we do know that strains vary widely in their rate of metabolism of drugs, and presumably would, therefore, differ greatly in the rapidity with which they get rid of inducers.

Species, Sex, Age, Environment (Care), and Physiologic State of the Animal, as These May Affect Induction of Microsomal Enzymes.

SPECIES, SEX, AND AGE. Hepatic microsomal enzyme induction can vary both quantitatively and qualitatively among species. Drug metabolism by liver microsomes can be stimulated by anabolic steroids in mice and rats, but not in rabbits. DDT can stimulate hexobarbital metabolism in rats but not in mice (Cram and Fouts, 1967). The list could be made longer, and the interested reader is referred to review articles for further information (e.g., Burns et al., 1965; Remmer, 1962; Gillette, 1963b). Qualitative differences in response to inducers can also occur within a given species—as, for example, among different strains of animals, or even among individuals of a given population. We have found that among six strains of rabbits there were both qualitative and quantitative differences in response of various drug metabolisms to pretreatment of these rabbit strains with phenobarbital (Cram et al., 1965). Burns (1965) has noted that among a series of mongrel dogs treated with phenobarbital, a few individual animals did not respond by increased hepatic drug metabolism.

Among rats, there is also a marked difference in the response of adult male versus female rats to phenobarbital as an inducer. Kato and his co-workers have made extensive studies of this phenomenon, and in one paper stated: "The administration of phenobarbital increased the activities of all enzymes (microsomal drug-metabolizing enzymes) tested in both female and male rats, although the activities in female rats were generally more markedly stimulated than in male rats" (Kato and Takayanaghi, 1966). In this same paper, it is pointed out that the induction of hepatic microsomal enzymes by methylcholanthrene can be both qualitatively and quantitatively different in male versus female rats. Such marked differences between sexes in response to inducers have not been seen in rabbits, but whether they occur in other species than the rat is simply not known to the author at this time.

In rats, the age of the animal also seems to affect the degree of response to inducers such as methylcholanthrene and phenobarbital. Conney et al. (1956) noted that it took much larger quantities of methylcholanthrene to cause similar increases in hepatic demethylase activity in adult than in three-week-old rats; on a body-weight basis, approximately ten times as much methylcholanthrene was required in adults as compared with weanling rats. This suggested that very young rats might be more appropriate for studies of enzyme induction than adult animals, and several groups of investigators have limited their studies of such enzyme responses to the very young (weanling) animal. In a recent paper, Chiesara et al. (1967) report studies suggesting that during growth, the liver is particularly sensitive to drug induction of microsomal enzymes. These workers used both phenobarbital and phenoglycodol as inducers in rats of varying age, and also in rats whose livers were rapidly regenerating after hepatectomy. This increased sensitivity of the liver to inducers seemed to apply to liver both during development after birth and during regeneration after partial hepatectomy. These authors (Chiesara et al., 1967) make the further statement that "In the adult animal [rat] it is almost impossible to obtain a similar result [enzyme induction and morphologic change in liver cells], except with a very high dose [of the enzyme inducer]."

Such results would, therefore, suggest that young animals would be the best candidates for studies on unknown or only-suspected microsomal enzyme inducers. We do not know if these results can be applied to any species except the rat. With rats, the best results seem to be obtained with the weanling animal (60 to 80 grams body weight).

ENVIRONMENT (CARE) AND PHYSIOLOGIC STATE OF THE ANIMAL. The experience of several laboratories suggests that the animals' environment may markedly affect response to microsomal enzyme inducers. In any given animal quarters, endogenous stimulators and inhibitors of hepatic microsomal drug-metabolizing enzymes may abound. An animal that has been exposed to an insecticide like DDT or chlordane (to rid the animal quarter of insects) will not respond, or will respond only minimally, to injections of phenobarbital (Hart and Fouts, 1965a).

The animals' diet may also contain stimulators of microsomal enzymes. These may be in the form of residual herbicides or insecticides, or may be contributed by endogenous sterols that have been peroxidized during extended storage. Brown et al. (1954) reported that livers of mice fed a commercial diet had twice the microsomal demethylase activity of those livers from mice fed purified diets. These workers concluded that the dietary stimulatory substance was probably a sterol peroxide, formed during processing or storing of the commercial feed. Such endogenous steroid materials would probably modify the ability of anabolic steroids, and polycyclic hydrocarbons, to stimulate drug metabolism by liver microsomes.

If the environment contains stimulators of microsomal enzymes, our control animals would be, in reality, already treated, and instead of assessing the effects of an inducer alone, we will be studying the interaction of inducers—our experiment will be confounded, and our results hard to interpret. The variety of chemicals capable of affecting hepatic microsomal enzymes, either as inducers or as blockers of induction, is becoming so large that this aspect of controlling animal care cannot be overemphasized.

Starvation and stress have both been shown to affect hepatic microsomal drug-metabolizing enzyme activity. Kato et al. (1962) present evidence suggesting that starvation of rats may enhance the response of hepatic microsomal enzymes to induction by phenobarbital. Driever and Bousquet (1965) show that stress can itself act to induce hepatic microsomal enzyme systems. Although the author knows of no one who has studied enzyme induction by phenobarbital, benzpyrene, etc., in stressed animals, it is reasonable to expect that such induction might be different from that in the unstressed animal.

Thus, it is my opinion that much of the interlaboratory variability in results with liver drug-metabolizing activity, both before and after inducers and inhibitors, will ultimately be shown to be caused by preexperiment handling and exposure of the animals. It is particularly in this area that the author feels most laboratories have not taken enough care, and where there is yet too little experimentation on which to base recommendations.

Determination of Inducer Effects In Vivo.—Whether or not hepatic microsomal drug-metabolizing enzymes have been stimulated by a given inducer can be assessed in vivo by any of the tests previously recommended (see pp. 000-000), as long as a few facts are considered: (1) Not all inducers affect the metabolism of all drugs by liver microsomes in any species. (2) Some inducers can act in one species, strain, or sex of animal, and not another. (3) Therefore, for these and all other reasons already discussed, it is best not to rely on a single test as the criterion for deciding whether induction has occurred or not. The author recommends the following battery of tests, since these will pick up all the currently known inducers, and are therefore likely to continue to be effective for new inducers: (a) *Hexobarbital and zoxazolamine* sleeping times in mice and rats. Zoxazolamine paralysis time will pick up polycyclic hydrocarbon inducers that are not detected by hexobarbital sleeping times. Rats will pick up inducers like DDT that do not affect mice, or do so very slightly. (b) *Biologic half-lives of aminopyrine in blood* (large animals) or whole body (small animals). Aminopyrine metabolism is affected by most anabolic steroids in those species (rats and mice) where induction by steroids has been demonstrated. Aminopyrine metabolism is also affected by phenobarbital and members of the phenobarbital-like group of inducers, e.g., the insecticides. (c) *Excretion of 4-aminoantipyrine in urine* after intravenous dosing with dipyrone. This can take place of, or supplement, the information obtained from biologic half-life if blood sampling is impractical.

Any such battery of tests, recommended by any given "expert," can be criticized for being incomplete or at least theoretically imperfect. The foregoing is offered as a guide, and no more.

Generally speaking, one tests for inducer effects at some time removed from the last dose of inducer. With most inducers, this is 24 to 72 hours after the last dose. This time lag, between testing for effect and last dose of inducer given, is generally agreed to be for the purpose of allowing for clearance of inducer from the liver tissue. Most inducers, if present in the liver at the time another drug is given (e.g., hexobarbital administered for the hexobarbital sleeping time assay), can act as inhibitors (competitive or noncompetitive) of the hepatic microsomal enzymes, and thus mask any enzyme induction that has occurred. Most of the microsomal enzyme inductions that have been studied last far beyond the time that significant amounts of the inducer can be detected in the liver tissue. Thus, one can test for enzyme induction following most steroids and polycyclic hydrocarbons within 72 hours after the last dose; within 24 hours after the last dose of phenobarbital and most drugs; and within 72 hours after the last dose of most chlorinated hydrocarbon insecticides, such as chlordane.

CONSIDERATIONS IN THE USE OF INHIBITORS OF DRUG METABOLISM.—Just as not all microsomal drug-metabolizing enzymes are stimulated by any given inducer, no inhibitor yet studied (with the possible exception of those that destroy microsomal structure and/or enzymes) affects all drug metabolism either equally or even at all. Again, there are species differences in susceptibility of any given drug metabolic pathway, and there are sex differences, at least in the rat. Some of the species, strain, and sex differences could be due to the fact that the drug administered as an inhibitor must be metabolized to the actual, active material, and such metabolism may vary both quantitatively and qualitatively among species.

Most inhibitors of hepatic microsomal enzyme systems act either immediately or at least within a few hours of administration (providing the absorption of the inhibitor is not the limiting factor). However, this is not an ironclad rule, and we have documented the prolonged delay with *p*-aminosalicylic acid (PAS) as a liver drug metabolism inhibitor. This compound (PAS) exerted effects on hexobarbital sleeping time only after it had been fed for about one week to rats. Single large doses of PAS (up to 3 g/kg given intraperitoneally) had no effect on hexobarbital sleeping time for periods from 3 to 48 hours after administration. Correlated with changes in hexobarbital sleeping times were changes in rate of drug metabolism by isolated liver microsomes (Rogers et al., 1963). This example is merely added to emphasize that, as with inducers, some inhibitors may act very slowly. Such slow action may suggest indirect effects, but whatever the mechanism, it is worth checking, particularly if the drug being studied as a possible microsomal inhibitor will be used chronically (e.g., therapeutically).

Most of the in vivo tests used to assess rate of hepatic microsomal drug metabolism can be used to detect compounds acting as inhibitors of these enzymes, if a few sources of error are recognized: (a) When using duration of drug effect (hexobarbital sleeping time or zoxazolamine paralysis time) as a screen, investigate the possibility that the shift in duration of action could be due to the "inhibitor" lowering body temperature, increasing the permeability of the blood-brain barrier, or blocking uptake of the barbiturate or zoxazolamine by the liver. Among tests to be run for these possibilities should at least be a determination of the levels of barbiturate or zoxazolamine in the animal's brain at various times after administration and at the time of awakening. (b) If using urinary excretion of drug metabolites as the method chosen to screen for inhibitors, you should determine whether the "inhibitor" has in any way interfered with the rate of clearance of metabolites by the kidney. This might be approached by a study of rate of urinary clearance of intravenously injected metabolite (e.g., 4-aminoantipyrine) in control versus inhibitor-treated animals.

Again, as with inducers, the environment, diet, etc., of the animal can markedly affect whether one will detect enzyme inhibition or not. Just as there are certain insecticides and dietary components that can stimulate drug metabolism, there are also materials that can inhibit these hepatic enzymes. Thus, many organophosphate insecticides are potent inhibitors of microsomal drug metabolism (Neubert, 1962), as are some insecticide synergists like safrol, isosafrol, sesamex, piperonyl butoxide, etc. (see Philleo et al., 1965; and Fine and Molloy, 1964). Animals exposed to such environmental (endogenous) inhibitors may not be affected further by addition of other inhibitors. At least the response of such exposed animals is likely to be far different from animals shielded from such materials.

IN VITRO STUDIES ON HEPATIC MICROSOMAL DRUG-METABOLIZING ENZYMES

Preparation of Tissue and Isolation of Enzymes for Study

EXCISION AND MINCING OF TISSUE.—Some investigators prefer to prepare homogenates, and further subfractionate hepatic microsomal enzymes, only after removing as much blood as possible from the liver. There are several possible ways to perfuse the liver to remove blood. What seems to be more important than which method is used is, rather, how quickly after death of the animal these procedures can be effected. Other important factors besides speed (to prevent blood clotting) include nature of the perfusing solution, duration of perfusion, and perfusion pressure. A systematic study of what constitutes the best system to use has not been made, as far as this author knows. Thus, I can only mention what has been done, and caution the reader that he may find better methods himself by trial and error. The following technique has been used in our laboratory.

PROCEDURE. The animal is killed by a blow on the head. The thorax and peritoneal cavity are opened as soon thereafter as possible. The perfusion fluid is forced through the superior vena cava, and the portal vein is cut to allow escape of perfusion fluid. The liver is gently kneaded with the fingers in areas that do not blanch quickly (e.g., at edges of liver lobe). The perfusion fluid we use is isotonic KCl, though isotonic and hypertonic solutions of sucrose have also been used. The entire operation is carried out in a cold room, and should be completed in less than five minutes with most species. Such perfusion of liver is used when one wishes to study the microsomal cytochromes (especially cytochrome b_5), or when one has reason to believe hemoglobin or other blood proteins may interfere with the enzymes to be assayed. For the usual drug-metabolizing enzyme systems, such as those involved in hexobarbital, aminopyrine, codeine, or aniline metabolism, such a preliminary perfusion process is not without a price. It has been our experience that the enzyme activity of homogenates, 9,000 × *g* supernatant fractions, or microsomes isolated from perfused livers is less than in liver not perfused. This is true regardless of how enzyme activity is expressed (per gram liver, per gram protein, or per gram nitrogen of the fractions isolated).

Either perfused or not, the liver should be quickly excised and minced with scissors as soon as possible after the animal's death. The liver can be weighed before or after mincing, but again, all operations should be carried out in the cold. Gallbladders should be removed from all species having them, prior to mincing and further homogenizing. Bile constituents (both bile acids and bile pigments) are potent inhibitors of most microsomal drug-metabolizing enzymes (McLuen and Fouts, 1961). Fine mincing of liver tissue, or even forcing the liver through a tissue press of some sort, may be necessary to facilitate adequate homogenizations when abnormal livers are being studied. Thus, livers from animals that are either very old or have been exposed to hepatotoxic materials for some time are often full of fibrous tissue. Such fibers make homogenization with Potter-type homogenizers difficult, if not impossible. This is less true if the Waring Blendor or Virtis-type homogenizer is used. At the very least, such fibers contribute only inert protein to the mixture; at worst, they may interfere with subcellular fractionation or make cell membrane breakdown less complete than if they are removed prior to homogenizing.

Occasionally in some species, small areas of liver appear to be abnormal. These areas are, in our laboratory, excised before the remainder of the liver is homogenized. Thus, in winter, we often find some encysted areas in rabbit livers, in animals who are otherwise apparently quite healthy. Our veterinarian tells us these areas contain coccidia and sometimes tapeworm. Such liver has not in our experience been abnormal, with respect to drug-metabolizing enzyme activity, as long as the number of such encysted areas is not large. We recommend that liver without such inclusions be used whenever possible, but in some cases this is not practical—particularly with rabbits and dogs, and particularly in winter.

HOMOGENIZING.—The purpose in homogenizing is to prepare a uniform suspension of liver constituents, without excessive damage to the enzymes of interest, e.g., the microsomal drug-metabolizing enzymes. Compared with some other enzyme systems, these hepatic drug-metabolizing enzymes appear to be fairly rugged in most species. Several studies have been made of the homogenizing apparatuses likely to be used in such studies (see Leadbeater and Davies, 1964; and von Jagow et al., 1965). Much attention has been paid to the speed of homogenizing, the duration of homogenizing, and the clearance between pestle and container walls in Potter-type homogenizers. What seems to have resulted from all this is the predictable fact that enzyme activity, either per gram liver or per gram protein of isolated microsomes, can be affected by the homogenization technique used. One major source of variation seems to be that the more strenuous modes of homogenizing do not improve the yield of microsomal enzymes, but do increase the yield of inert protein, even when isolated microsomes are used in the enzyme assays. Within reasonable limits of homogenizing technique, there does not seem to be much microsomal drug-metabolizing enzyme destruction during homogenization, though we have found that prolonged homogenizing with any apparatus can cause some losses of enzyme activity. Most liver, if minced at all well prior to homogenizing, can be made into an acceptably smooth suspension within 30 seconds of homogenizing. With any liver we have yet used, with any homogenizing apparatus commonly available, such a short homogenization will not cause significant losses of enzyme activity for most of the drug-metabolizing enzymes in liver microsomes.

Some of our results comparing drug-metabolizing enzyme activities after Potter vs. Waring blendor homogenizing, with rat versus rabbit liver, are shown in Table 1. These data indicate that either method is satisfactory for preparing

TABLE 1

Drug-Metabolizing Enzyme Activity in 9000 X g Supernatant Fractions from Liver Homogenates Prepared by Potter versus Waring Blendor Homogenizers.

Animal*	Substrate† or Component Measured	Enzyme activity‡ or nitrogen content in fractions prepared from homogenates made with:	
		POTTER HOMOGENIZER	*WARING BLENDOR*
Rat	Hexobarbital	1,020	1,090
	Zoxazolamine	230	250
	Aniline	190	190
	p-Nitrobenzoic acid	60	90
	9,000 X *g* nitrogen	17.9 ± 0.7	17.7 ± 0.7
	Microsomal nitrogen	4.1 ± 0.4	4.1 ± 0.7
Rabbit	Hexobarbital	1,280	1,350
	Zoxazolamine	395	455
	Aniline	320	360
	p-Nitrobenzoic acid	260	270
	9,000 X *g* nitrogen	18.4 ± 1.1	18.9 ± 1.3
	Microsomal nitrogen	3.9 ± 0.7	4.1 ± 0.6

*Rats were Long-Evans, male, 200 to 300 g, and rabbits were Dutch, male, 1 to 2 kg. No pretreatment.

†Metabolic pathways: Hexobarbital and zoxazolamine by substrate disappearance. Aniline by *p*-aminophenol formation; *p*-nitrobenzoic acid by *p*-aminobenzoic acid formation. Substrate concentrations, cofactor, 9,000 X *g* supernatant fraction and buffer additions as described in text. Phosphate buffer, pH 7.4, 0.1 M, was used. Nitrogen was assayed by a micro-Kjeldahl technique. Microsomes were washed once with KCl prior to Kjeldahl analysis.

‡Enzyme activity expressed as μmoles drug metabolized or product formed in 30 minutes (for rat) or 60 minutes (for rabbit) per gram of microsomal nitrogen in the 9,000 X *g* supernatant fraction. Values are from single experiments (in triplicate) in which the animal's liver was minced and divided into two samples of approximately equal size. One of these samples was homogenized with the Potter, the other with the Waring blendor homogenizer. KCl was used to homogenize both samples. Nitrogen is expressed as mean (±SD) mg nitrogen per gram (wet weight) liver with N = 6 to 9 animals. Homogenization time was varied between 15 sec and 60 sec with similar results. Values in the table were obtained using 20 sec homogenizing time. Excessively long homogenization with Waring blendor (> 1 minute) caused marked increases in 9,000 X *g* supernatant fraction and microsomal nitrogen content (the latter increased almost 30 percent). Decreases in oxidative drug metabolisms after prolonged homogenizing with the Waring blendor were more marked with rat than with rabbit liver.

homogenates. For purposes of minimizing variability between individual liver samples and between different treatment groups, the same homogenizer should be used for the same time, and under the same conditions (speed, chilling, etc.) for all samples. This is the most important point as far as this author is concerned: *Standardize the technique used, and use it for all samples.*

As far as media in which to homogenize the liver, and the ratio of liver tissue to media to use, we once more enter a realm of subjective preference. No one has made a systematic or exhaustive study of these questions to this author's knowledge. Two reports should, however, be mentioned. Roth and Bukovsky (1961) homogenized rat liver in a variety of buffers, including sodium phosphate, potassium phosphate, and tris buffers. The microsomal *N*–demethylase system they were studying was affected by the buffer used in homogenization. For this enzyme system, sodium phosphate buffer, at 0.3 M, was optimal as far as they were concerned. Sucrose (0.25 M) definitely gave a less active preparation than did phosphate buffer, when used for making the homogenate.

Kato et al. (1964) compared the activity of the hexobarbital oxidizing enzyme in 9,000 × *g* supernatant prepared from rat liver homogenates, when these homogenates were made using Krebs phosphate bufter, sodium phosphate buffer (0.1 M and 0.2 M), potassium phosphate buffer (0.1 M and 0.2 M), sucrose (0.25 M), or KCl (1.15 percent). Of these various media used, isotonic KCl was the best. Kato et al. (1964) also compared homogenates made with KCl, wherein the tissue to media ratio was varied from 1:2 to 1:4, but found no striking differences in hexobarbital metabolizing activity between these ratios.

Our own experience would agree with that of Kato et al. (1964). For most of the enzyme systems we have studied, either in 9,000 × *g* supernatant fractions or in isolated microsomes, *the preliminary homogenization is done in KCl (isotonic) rather than sucrose or a buffer,* since these latter (sucrose or buffers) do not give us as much activity as when we use KCl. Isotonic KCl can, however, be rather acid, depending on where you get your distilled water. We commonly add a small amount of tris buffer (0.05 M) to all KCl solutions used for perfusion or homogenization of liver, in order to assure a pH of about 7.5. At pH below 6, microsomes behave as heavier particles, and can be sedimented more rapidly than expected (see Karler et al., 1967). This would have undesirable effects if one is going to use a homogenate for isolation of microsomes in any quantitative or reproducible fashion. The ratio of liver tissue to media has varied between 1 gram liver plus 2 ml solvent, up to 1 gram liver plus 9 ml solvent. Which ratio one uses may depend on what is to be done with the homogenate. The better separations of particulates from a homogenate seem to be made when the tissue:solvent ratio is about 1:5 or even 1:10—"better" separation, in this sense, meaning less cross-contamination of one fraction with another. If the homogenate is to be used directly for enzyme assay, then the "thickness" of the homogenate is less important (see Kato et al., 1964, as already mentioned).

PREPARATION OF 9,000 × *g* SUPERNATANT.—There are a number of reasons why one may not wish to use homogenates of liver for his enzyme source in a study of microsomal drug metabolism. The enzymes involved are in the microsomes, and nuclei and mitochondria can complicate the study of microsomal enzymes in several ways: (a) The drug substrate added can be bound extensively to nuclei and mitochondria, making it difficult to supply the microsomal enzymes with sufficient substrate to make the activity measured reflect the amount of enzyme present. (b) Nuclei and mitochondria may have systems capable of destroying cofactors, etc., needed by the microsomal enzyme systems.

For a discussion of these problems with homogenates, the reader is referred to the review by Gillette (1963b, especially pages 53 to 57). As mentioned in that review, it is not uncommon to find that homogenates metabolize a drug more slowly than do 9,000 × *g* supernatant fractions from the same liver. This seems to be true particularly with rats and mice. The view that 9,000 × *g* supernatant fractions, or microsomal fractions prepared therefrom, may give better enzyme activity and provide less chance for complicating factors interfering with the assays than when homogenates are used has been challenged by Kinoshita et al. (1966). These authors state that

> Conclusions concerning alterations in drug-metabolizing ability of animals that are drawn on the basis of assays performed on cell fractions may be misleading if the particular reaction under investigation is not confined to the cell fraction assayed. An example of this practical consideration was seen in the present investigation in connection with reductase activity. Neither DDT nor toxaphene produced any elevation of nitro reductase activity of whole liver homogenates in contrast to the increase in activity observed by Hart and Fouts (1950) in a cell fraction (9,000 × *g* supernatant) from the livers of rats fed DDT.

This allegation should not go unchallenged, since it raises some serious questions– are homogenates superior to 9,000 × *g* supernatants, and if so, why use 9,000 × *g* supernatants? The arguments accepted by most workers in the field suggest the opposite; homogenates can give misleading results, yet Kinoshita et al. (1966) argue the reverse. Since publication of the article by Kinoshita et al. (1966), we have made some studies of the problem, but first a few disclaimers: (a) Kinoshita et al. (1966) found qualitative discrepancies between homogenate and 9,000 × *g* supernatant enzyme activity only for one enzyme activity (nitro reductase), though they studied several enzymes; and they worked only with rats. (b) It is my opinion that one is always on tenuous ground when he seeks to extrapolate from one microsomal enzyme to the complex of microsomal drug-metabolizing enzymes found in the liver, especially if the study is confined to only one animal species. Nevertheless, we have repeated our experiments using homogenates, instead of 9,000 × *g* supernatant fractions, from control versus DDT-treated rats.

Using our incubation conditions, we have established stimulation of nitro reductase activity in both homogenates and 9,000 × *g* supernatant fractions. We believe the discrepancy between our results and those of Kinoshita et al. (1966) can be resolved on the basis of differences in incubation mixtures: we use much higher concentrations of TPN and substrate than they did, and we use more enzyme per incubation mixture.

I have spent so much time on this one issue because I think it is an important one. *To my knowledge, homogenates have never given answers about microsomal drug-metabolizing enzymes that cannot be obtained with 9,000 ×* g *supernatant or isolated microsomes, and these latter are, in this author's opinion, usually superior for quantitative studies.*

Although the term "9,000 × *g* supernatant fraction" is often seen in the literature of microsomal drug metabolism, it is not a well-defined preparation in terms of its contents. With adult rodents–mice, rats, or rabbits–the "9,000 × *g* supernatant" of liver is a fairly reproducible fraction. This 9,000 × *g* supernatant contains most of the microsomes of a liver homogenate, not many mitochondria, and most of the enzymes found in the soluble fraction of the cell. It may be important to realize that some of the microsomes of the homogenate are lost when the homogenate is spun at 9,000 × *g*, and that mitochondria can be found in the 9,000 × *g* supernatant. The degree of contamination of 9,000 × *g* supernatant fraction with mitochondria may depend on species; it is our "clinical impression" that this happens more often with rats than with rabbits.

So far we have talked only about adults and only about liver. The composition of 9,000 × *g* supernatant fractions in other tissues than liver is unknown to this author, but there are reports that age can markedly affect hepatic 9,000 × *g* supernatant fraction composition in the rat. Thus, Chatterjee et al. (1965) report that liver microsomes, from the embryonic rat, sediment at much lower *g* forces than liver microsomes from young or adult rats. The fraction, sedimenting between 200 × *g* and 8,000 × *g* in fetal liver homogenates, was composed 95 percent of microsomes, and the rest of the sediment was mitochondria and other particles. In the 14-day-old or adult rat liver, this sediment (8,000 × *g* sediment) was almost pure mitochondria (Chatterjee, et al., 1965).

The composition of 9,000 × *g* supernatant fractions may also be affected by the suspending media, its metal composition, and its pH. In concentrated sucrose solutions (e.g., 0.88 M and higher), the rate of sedimentation of mitochondria can be slow, leading to increased contamination of 9,000 × *g* supernatant fractions with mitochondria. Microsomes are capable of reacting with monovalent and divalent cations, and in so doing, their sedimentation velocity can be markedly increased. Thus, cesium causes a four- to nine-fold increase in sedimentation velocity of rough-surfaced microsomes (Dallner and Nilsson, 1966). Finally, low pH (< pH 6) favors sedimentation of microsomes at low *g* forces (Karler et al., 1967). The point of this rather extensive discussion is that each laboratory should establish for itself the composition of the 9,000 × *g* supernatant fractions used for drug metabolism, particularly if any new species, different ages, nonhepatic tissue, or unusual suspending media are being employed. The only acceptable criterion of composition of subcellular fractions, in my opinion, is examination with the electron microscope of the particulates prepared. This should be done on several different preparations of the 9,000 × *g* supernatant fraction versus 9,000 × *g* sediment, so that one can obtain some idea of the reproducibility of the technique being used to prepare this 9,000 × *g* supernatant fraction.

PROCEDURE. In our laboratory, the 9,000 × *g* supernatant fraction is prepared in the following way:

Liver is homogenized in isotonic KCl (containing 0.05 M tris buffer), having a pH of 7.5. Each gram of liver is homogenized with 3 ml of KCl. The homogenate is centrifuged for 20 minutes at 9,000 × *g* in a refrigerated centrifuge. The supernatant fraction is aspirated off carefully with a large syringe, leaving in the centrifuge tube the last volumes of 9,000 × *g* supernatant (about 0.5 cm) above the sediment. If the species used was the rabbit, this 9,000 × *g* supernatant fraction can be used immediately for enzyme assay or preparation of microsomes. If the species being studied was rat or mouse, a second spin at 9,000 × *g* for 15 minutes is used on the 9,000 × *g* supernatant from the first spin. This second spin removes all detectable mitochondrial contamination of the second 9,000 × *g* supernatant fraction. Again the 9,000 × *g* supernatant fraction is aspirated off carefully with a syringe, leaving in the centrifuge tube the last volumes of 9,000 × *g* supernatant above the sediment. If instead of aspirating, one merely decants the 9,000 × *g* supernatant fraction from the centrifuge tube, one will find this supernatant fraction heavily contaminated with mitochondria and lipid.

With rats, mice, and rabbits, these same procedures give equivalent (morphologically) preparations of 9,000 × *g* supernatant from liver if 0.25 M or 0.4 M sucrose, instead of KCl, is used in homogenizing.

PREPARATION OF MICROSOMES.—Microsomes can be isolated from 9,000 × *g* supernatant fractions by centrifugation in an ultracentrifuge for some 70,000 to 200,000 *g*-hours. What has yet to be determined, in any systematic fashion, is whether the many varieties of time and *g* force used make significant differences in recoveries of microsomes from 9,000 × supernatant fractions. The rate at which microsomes sediment will be affected by pH, concentration, and metal ion composition of the suspending medium has already been discussed.

One other factor may also make a difference in the isolation procedure chosen, and that is the amount of glycogen in the liver. Glycogen can trap certain elements of the endoplasmic reticulum (particularly smooth-surfaced microsomes) and sediment more quickly than the bulk of microsomes. Thus, the 9,000 × *g* *sediment* from a liver rich in glycogen may contain an appreciable amount of microsomes (Dallner et al., 1965). Glycogen in the 9,000 × *g* supernatant fraction may also affect the rate of sedimentation of microsomes from this 9,000 × *g* supernatant and the firmness of packing of the microsomal pellet obtained by centrifugation. It is our "clinical impression" that 9,000 × *g* supernatant fractions from livers rich in glycogen require longer centrifugation times for complete harvesting of their microsomes, and that the microsomes obtained therefrom are loosely packed. It is, therefore, recommended that animals be starved at least 12 hours, prior to sacrifice when microsomes are to be prepared from their livers; this period of starvation will reduce glycogen stores to levels where microsomal isolation will be much more reproducible, and quicker, than if animals are not so starved. Before this technique of preliminary food deprivation is embarked on too enthusiastically, the investigator must ascertain whether such starvation affects the enzyme activity he wishes to study. In our experience, no appreciable effects of 12-hour starvation on microsomal drug-metabolizing enzyme activity is seen in rats or rabbits, but we are not sure about the mouse.

In our laboratory, the microsomes are harvested from 9,000 × *g* supernatant fraction in the following ways:

a. Using the Spinco type 30 rotor—centrifugation at 72,000 × *g* for 60 to 75 minutes; all *g* forces are to center of centrifuge tube.
b. Using the Spinco type 40 rotor—centrifugation at 105,000 × *g* for 45 to 60 minutes.
c. Using the IEC rotor A 321—centrifugation at 220,000 × *g* for 30 minutes.

The microsomes so sedimented are freed of soluble fraction by aspiration of the latter to within 0.5 cm of the pellet surface, using a large syringe. The pellet is resuspended in KCl and resedimented as many times as necessary for the purpose of the experiment. We do not know whether extensive "washing" of microsomes is deleterious to their drug-metabolizing enzymes and whether species might differ in the susceptibility of their microsomes to loss by washing. Generally in our laboratory we wash microsomes only once. It is our "clinical impression" that rat liver microsomes are particularly prone to lose enzyme activity with repeated washing. It is also our "clinical impression" that microsomes sediment much more rapidly the second time than from the 9,000 × *g* supernatant fraction. In our experience, the times of centrifugation do not seem to need changing if 0.25 M or 0.4 M sucrose are used as the suspending medium, rather than KCl.

After washing, the microsomal pellet can be resuspended in KCl, sucrose, or the buffer to be used in the incubation mixture. The final resuspension is made so that each ml of the suspension contains 1 to 4 mg of microsomal protein (as determined by Kjeldahl, biuret, or Lowry protein assays). Such resuspension is performed when the microsomes are to be used for enzyme assays immediately; if such is not contemplated, storage of microsomes is probably best done in the pellet form, as will be described.

SUBFRACTIONATION OF MICROSOMES.—The microsomal pellet, as prepared above, can be further subfractionated into rough-surfaced versus smooth-surfaced types of microsomes. The procedures used for this further subfractionation are varied, but all depend on the fact that the rough-surfaced microsome behaves as though it were heavier than the smooth-surfaced microsome. We have recently completed a study comparing two methods of microsomal subfractionation in two species of animal—the rat versus the rabbit (Gram et al., 1967). The purpose of this study was to see if the microsomal drug-metabolizing enzymes might be relatively concentrated in one kind of microsome, and how the methods of preparing microsomal subfractions would affect such intramicrosomal enzyme distribution. It was our conclusion that, with either rat or rabbit liver microsomes, the best method for subfractionation was a slight modification of that originally published by Dallner (1963). This procedure will now be described.

PROCEDURE. Liver homogenates are made in 0.25 M sucrose, and the 9,000 × *g* supernatant fraction is isolated from the homogenate. This supernatant fraction is respun at 9,000 × *g* if the species being studied is the rat. The 9,000 × *g* supernatant fraction is then treated with CsCl solution (0.15 M in 0.25 M sucrose) to give a final concentration of CsCl of 15 mM; i.e., add 1 ml of 0.15 M CsCl in 0.25 M sucrose to each 9 ml of 9,000 × *g* supernatant fraction. Ten ml of this CsCl-containing 9,000 × *g* supernatant fraction is placed in the 3- × 5/8-inch tube, fitting the type 40 Spinco rotor. The remaining volume of this centrifuge tube (3.5 ml) is made up by a second phase of 1.3 M sucrose, containing 15 mM CsCl. This heavy sucrose phase is introduced into the bottom of the tube, and under the 9,000 × *g* supernatant fraction, through a long needle attached to a syringe. Thus two phases are set up in the centrifuge tube—the upper phase, consisting of 9,000 × *g* supernatant fraction in 0.25 M sucrose, and a bottom phase of 1.3 M sucrose. The two-phase system is spun at 105,000 × *g* for 2 hours and 25 minutes. At the end of this centrifugation, the smooth-surfaced microsomes are at the interface between the two layers, and the rough-surfaced microsomes are pelleted at the bottom of the centrifuge tube. The smooth-surfaced microsomes are removed, by aspiration with a syringe and needle, and sedimented at 105,000 × *g* for 30 minutes. The rough-surfaced and smooth-surfaced microsomal pellets can be resuspended in buffer, KCl, or sucrose, for enzyme assay, or washed once before assay. Final suspensions are made such that each ml of microsomal subfraction contains 1 to 4 mg of microsomal protein.

The purity of the subfractions was assessed by electron microscopy (Gram et al., 1967), and each investigator should do the same if he uses this technique, and if he uses it for any other species, any other tissue, or modifies it in *any way*. For example, we have recently been using the International B-60 ultracentrifuge and the A-321 rotor, instead of the Spinco system just described. In terms of equivalent *g*-minutes, we should have to spin only 68 minutes at 60,000 rpm to get equivalent separation of rough- from smooth-surfaced liver microsomes, from rat or rabbit. We have, however, not been able to do this apparently because the higher *g* force, used in the B-60 centrifuge, results in fractions of different purity and amounts of cross-contamination. This has manifested itself in different ratios of drug-metabolizing enzyme activity in smooth- versus rough-surfaced microsomes, and in changes in morphology of these fractions as examined with the electron microscope. Even grossly, we have observed marked differences in the tube contents of subfractionated microsomes using the type 40 rotor as opposed to the A-321 rotor. After the centrifugation with the Spinco ultracentrifuge, the area in the centrifuge tube between the smooth-surfaced microsome band and the pellet of rough-surfaced microsomes was usually clear. With the B-60 ultracentrifuge, the area between the smooth-surfaced microsome band and the pellet of rough-surfaced microsomes was often cloudy. The pellet of rough-surfaced microsomes often has a fluffy layer on top of it. This fluffy layer has the same enzyme activity and morphology as smooth-surfaced microsomes and should not be included in the rough-surfaced microsomal subfraction. The amount of fluffy layer on top of the rough-surfaced microsomal pellet differs when one uses the Spinco type 40 rotor spun at 40,000 rpm for 2 hours 25 minutes as opposed to the IEC A-321 rotor spun at 60,000 rpm for 68 minutes.

I have spent so much time on these problems for two reasons: (a) *the subfractionation of microsomes may become quite important in trying to correlate hepatic cell ultrastructure and the function of drug metabolism,* and (b) *there are quite conflicting reports in the literature about the relative distributions of drug-metabolizing enzymes in smooth- versus rough-surfaced microsomes* (see Orrenius and Ernster, 1964). From our studies, it seems apparent that the technique used to separate smooth-from rough-surfaced microsomes is crucial to the results obtained, and the experimeter who wishes to make such separations must be extremely careful to validate the method he uses, both in terms of chemical (or enzyme) methods and in terms of morphology.

One other point should be mentioned. All of the techniques for subfractionating cell particulates take time, and the further one takes the isolation of enzymes, the longer it will be between time of animal sacrifice and time of enzyme assay. The relative stability of the various microsomal drug-metabolizing enzymes is almost unknown. What little information we do have suggests that some pathways are much more labile than others, and that microsomal enzymes from different species differ in their lability. We also know that rough- and smoth-surfaced microsomes may have enzymes catalyzing the same drug metabolic pathway, but having different stability. Thus, we have shown that in rats (but not in rabbits) the enzyme systems oxidizing hexobarbital and zoxazolamine are unstable in smooth-surfaced microsomes, but not in rough-surfaced microsomes (Gram et al., 1967). Such information should be considered in designing experiments seeking to establish where in any given cell, or species, a particular drug-metabolizing enzyme may be located.

STORAGE OF ENZYMES.—Many and varied techniques have been tried, and many and different results obtained, with the storage of microsomal drug-metabolizing enzymes. What we do seem to agree on is relatively little, but perhaps can be summarized as follows: (a) No one method of storing enzymes will preserve all microsomal drug-metabolizing enzyme activity—the different enzyme activities appear to have different labilities, and this may differ from one species to another. (b) *The best methods of storage seem to be either as lyophilized and frozen powders or as frozen, concentrated suspensions or pastes of microsomes, containing small amounts of soluble fraction.* (c) The colder the storage temperature, the better.

One of the more recent studies of this problem is by Leadbeater and Davies (1964), and although their findings agree with most of the foregoing statements, it must be pointed out that they followed only four microsomal enzyme activities.

In our laboratory, we try to keep to a minimum the time between animal sacrifice and enzyme assay, and never rely on any enzyme activity obtained from a microsomal preparation that has had to be stored for any period exceeding a few hours. In our experience, the major problem in storing microsomes and preserving enzyme activity has been variability. Hepatic microsomes from one animal may be quite stable to storage for long periods of time, while another preparation (from the same animal or a different one), made the same way (sometimes on the same day), and stored in the same way (even in the same freezer), can be quite labile—at least for some of the enzymes studied. In my opinion, anyone who can devise a method for storing liver microsomes in a way that consistently preserves most drug-metabolizing enzyme activities unchanged for even relatively short times (e.g., one week), and which method can be used for several animal species, will have made a large contribution to the field.

The Assay of Hepatic Drug-Metabolizing Enzyme Activities In Vitro

There are a large variety of procedures used in assays for liver microsomal drug-metabolizing enzyme activity. The methods used vary to some extent, depending on whether homogenates, 9,000 × *g* supernatant fractions, or microsomes are used as the enzyme source. Factors that are most commonly varied are (1) amount of tissue preparation used, (2) amount of cofactor or cofactor-generating system used, (3) amount of substrate used, and (4) time of incubation. Other factors that I feel should be more intensively studied, are (1) the type of cofactor-generating system used, (2) the type of buffer used, and (3) the temperature used. I also feel that these studies should be carried out anew whenever a different source of enzyme is used (e.g., homogenate vs. 9,000 × *g* vs. microsomes, or liver vs. kidney), or whenever a new species, or strain, or sex, of animal is investigated.

The goals that one usually tries to attain in in vitro assays are (1) direct proportionality between enzyme concentration and measured enzyme activity and (2) maximal enzyme activity for any given amount of enzyme. The first of these goals is usually approached by providing excess cofactor and substrate concentrations, using relatively small amounts of enzyme and keeping the incubation time short. The second goal is approximated by studies on pH optima, temperature optima, effects of buffers on activity, and studies on the nature of the enzyme and the reaction being catalyzed (thereby hoping to find unsuspected activators of the enzyme). Although the two goals mentioned are related, they are not necessarily attained at the same time. One can often obtain the first goal without reaching the second. Indeed one wonders if such is not sometimes desirable, since the in vivo situation is very likely not that which allows maximal enzyme activity for any of the hepatic microsomal drug-metabolizing enzymes with which I am familiar. In my opinion, the following are the most important criteria to satisfy in assays of drug-metabolizing enzyme activity: (1) linear relationships between enzyme activity and time, and (2) linear relationships between enzyme activity and amount of tissue preparation used. If these conditions are met, it is my opinion that the results obtained can be valid, even if optimal or superoptimal substrate and cofactor concentrations, or optimal conditions of pH and temperature, are not used. Indeed the results obtained under suboptimal conditions may be of more practical importance, if optimal conditions for the enzyme necessitate obviously unphysiologic environment. The conclusion of this introduction, then, is that we should try to meet the ideal and work under conditions where the enzyme is maximally active *and* where this activity is directly proportional to the enzyme concentration. If, however, we cannot do both of these things, we can at least continue working, if we can satisfy the last requirement—activity proportional to enzyme concentration.

STUDY OF DRUG-METABOLIZING ENZYME ACTIVITY USING LIVER HOMOGENATES.—The major problems in using homogenates as the enzyme source are that (a) there are large amounts of inert protein, capable of binding added substrate and/or cofactors, and preventing their access to the drug-metabolizing enzymes; (b) there are several systems present, which compete with the drug-metabolizing enzymes in microsomes for cofactors or which destroy cofactors; and (c) there may be inhibitors of drug metabolism present, which act other than by limiting cofactor, or substrate concentrations. As a general rule, then, we find that the amount of drug metabolized is proportional to the amount of homogenate added only over a narrow range, and that we need much larger amounts of NADP for maximal enzyme activity than if either 9,000 × *g* supernatant or isolated microsomes are used. Usually the substrate concentration needed is not much different than with 9,000 × *g* supernatant, but if the substrate is highly bound to tissue protein, this may not be true, and a substrate concentration versus enzyme activity curve should be established.

The following represents a consensus of our experience with homogenates as enzyme source, and a variety of drugs as substrates (e.g., hexobarbital, zoxazolamine, aminopyrine, codeine, aniline, neoprontosil, and *p*-nitrobenzoic acid):

a. Enzyme activity (drug metabolized) is fairly proportional to amount of homogenate added, if this is kept between 10 and 40 mg equivalents of liver/ml. A milligram equivalent is the amount of homogenate resulting from homogenizing that amount of liver with suspending medium (e.g., KCl). Thus, in a 5-ml incubation volume, activity and amount of homogenate added are proportional within the limits of 50 mg and 200 mg of wet-weight liver tissue.
b. This is true only if incubation times are kept short (no more than 20 minutes for the rat, or less than 60 minutes for rabbit and mouse).
c. This is true only if large amounts of NADP are added—1.0 to 2.0 × 10^{-3} M final concentration.
d. We usually add 5 × 10^{-3} M glucose-6-phosphate and 2 to 4 × 10^{-3} M nicotinamide to all incubation mixtures. High concentrations of nicotinamide can inhibit some microsomal drug-metabolizing enzyme systems, particularly when enzyme or substrate concentration is low (see Schenkman, Ball, and Estabrook, 1967). Thus, the effect of nicotinamide should be checked by each investigator; if it is not needed (i.e., does not increase enzyme activity), it should be left out.
e. Substrate additions for some common drug metabolic pathways are as follows (in terms of final concentration): hexobarbital (1.2 to 2.4 × 10^{-3} M); zoxazolamine (1.2 to 2.4 × 10^{-3} M); aminopyrine (2 × 10^{-3} M for rats and 8 × 10^{-3} M for rabbits); codeine (2 to 4 × 10^{-3} M); aniline (2 to 4 × 10^{-3} M); neoprontosil (2 to 4 × 10^{-3} M); and *p*-nitrobenzoic acid (1.5 × 10^{-3} M).

We use glucose-6-phosphate and its dehydrogenase to generate NADPH in all experiments on NADPH-requiring, drug-metabolizing enzymes. However, NADPH can be produced by a variety of systems, and some of these may be preferable to the glucose-6-phosphate dehydrogenase system, if there is any doubt about the ability of this system to generate NADPH. Such doubts may arise after certain drug treatments, which may either inhibit the dehydrogenase or increase the activity of phosphatases (which would limit NADPH production by destroying glucose-6-phosphate more rapidly than normal). A widely used alternative to the glucose-6-phosphate dehydrogenase system is the isocitric acid dehydrogenase system. In our experience, the isocitric acid dehydrogenase system works well, and can be added to the homogenate as follows: isocitrate (as the sodium salt, 4 to 5 × 10^{-3} M) and $MnCl_2$ (1 × 10^{-5} M).

Normally, homogenates of liver contain large excesses of both glucose-6-phosphate and isocitrate dehydrogenases. However, if you have reason to suspect either enzyme is deficient (because of drug treatment, etc.), these enzymes are available commercially, and can be added to the homogenate. We have never found this to be necessary unless we are using very small quantities of NADP (as when studying the K_m for NADP in a reaction.

Finally, certain buffer systems are incompatible with the Mn^{++} requirement of isocitrate dehydrogenase. If this system is used for NADPH generation, phosphate buffer would not be a logical choice for the incubation medium. Tris buffer is usually used instead.

STUDY OF DRUG-METABOLIZING ENZYME ACTIVITY USING HEPATIC 9,000 × *g* SUPERNATANT FRACTIONS. There are several advantages in using 9,000 × *g* supernatant fractions rather than liver homogenates. (a) NADP additions usually are lower, (b) saturation of enzyme with substrate or inhibitor usually occurs at lower concentrations of substrate, etc., (c) activity is often greater than in homogenates (Gillette, 1963a), even when expressed in terms of microsomal protein.

The following are conditions that we use in studies on drug-metabolizing enzymes in 9,000 × *g* supernatant fractions:

a. Enzyme activity is relatively proportional to amount of 9,000 × fraction added, if this is kept between the limits of 10- and 50-mg equivalents of liver per ml of incubation mixture. Thus in a 5-ml incubation mixture, 9,000 × *g* fraction derived from 50 to 250 mg of wet-weight liver can be used.
b. Incubation times are kept as short as possible, e.g., no more than 20 minutes with rat liver fractions, and less than 60 minutes with rabbit or mouse liver fractions. We have made a study of the time course of several drug-metabolizing systems in 9,000 × *g* fractions from rats, vs. rabbits, vs. mice. This study indicated that linearity obtained for different times with different species, and that, in general, rat liver preparations seemed more labile than those from rabbits or mice (Gram and Fouts, 1966).
c. Cofactor concentrations are the same as with homogenates, except we have found that NADP concentrations can be as low as 1.2×10^{-4} M. These concentrations of NADP still give linear relationships between 9,000 × *g* fraction added and drug metabolized, as well as the same activity per unit time and tissue, as with higher NADP concentrations. We routinely use 2×10^{-4}M NADP with rabbit liver fractions and 5×10^{-4} M NADP with rat and mouse liver 9,000 × *g* supernatant fractions.
d. Substrate additions are the same as for homogenates, except that in cases where a range was given, we use the lower figure with 9,000 × *g* supernatant fractions (e.g., 1.2×10^{-3} M hexobarbital with 9,000 × *g* fractions, and 2.4×10^{-3} with homogenates).
e. Again we use the glucose-6-phosphate dehydrogenase system to generate NADPH, and again, we have shown that isocitric dehydrogenase will usually work just as well, if you have reason to suspect a limitation in NADPH generation due to the use of the glucose-6-phosphate-dependent system. The 9,000 × *g* supernatant fraction usually contains plenty of endogenous glucose-6-phosphate dehydrogenase, or isocitric dehydrogenase, but these can also be added if you suspect they are deficient for any reason (due to previous drug treatment, etc.).

STUDY OF DRUG-METABOLIZING ENZYME ACTIVITY USING HEPATIC MICROSOMAL FRACTIONS.—To the "purists" among biochemists, studies on drug metabolism should always be made using isolated microsomes, rather than homogenates or 9,000 × *g* supernatants. However compelling such arguments may be, there are some problems. With most drug-metabolizing enzyme systems that we have used, we have been unable to obtain anywhere near the enzyme activity in microsomes that one can obtain in the 9,000 × *g* supernatant fraction (in terms of drug metabolized per unit time per mg of microsomal protein). Sometimes the discrepancy is only about 30 percent, but often the microsomes have one third or less of the enzyme activity of the 9,000 × *g* fraction from which they were isolated. To my knowledge, no one has yet come up with a satisfactory reason for these differences, but private conversations, and cryptic notes in the literature, refer to some factor(s) in the soluble fraction of liver which protect the microsomal enzymes. We have been unable to restore microsomal activity to that found in the 9,000 × *g* supernatant by any such maneuver as adding excess NADPH. We do believe the phenomena are real, and I look forward to some definitive study that will help us resolve this question.

When one uses microsomes, rather than 9,000 × *g* fractions or homogenates, one must add an NADPH-generating system (usually found endogenously in homogenates, etc., as glucose-6-phosphate or isocitric dehydrogenase) or NADPH itself. As I have stated previously, we always use glucose-6-phosphate plus its dehydrogenase.

The following are conditions we have used in studies on drug-metabolizing enzymes in hepatic microsomal fractions:

a. Enzyme activity is proportional to amount of microsomes added, if this is kept between 1 and 2 mg of microsomal protein per ml of incubation mixture. We have obtained linearity at even higher concentrations of microsomal protein, but these limits (1 to 2 mg/ml) will be accepted by nearly everyone.
b. Incubation times, cofactor concentrations (NADP, glucose-6-phosphate), and substrate concentrations are the same as with 9,000 × *g* supernatant fraction. One is more likely to see inhibitory effects of nicotinamide with microsomes than with either 9,000 × *g* or homogenate fractions, at least in our experience. I would recommend therefore that, when microsomes are used, the effect of nicotinamide be checked carefully and that nicotinamide be used only when you have shown it to have a beneficial effect.
c. Glucose-6-phosphate dehydrogenase, isocitric dehydrogenase, or already-reduced NADPH must be added to complete the system. How much glucose-6-phosphate dehydrogenase or isocitric dehydrogenase to add should be determined empirically by the investigator. We normally use 1 to 2 units of either enzyme in a 5-ml incubation mixture, but I have seen experiments by several laboratories where up to 10 units of these enzymes is added per ml of the incubation mixture. The empirical approach is suggested, since batches of these enzymes do lose activity with time, and pathways do vary in their requirements for NADPH. If already reduced NADP is to be added to the incubation, this is again where the investigator must determine for himself

what is needed. It has been our experience that you might as well add all the NADPH at once (at the start of the incubation), rather than dribble it in every 5 to 15 minutes. We have used 1 to 2 $\times 10^{-3}$ M final concentration of added NADPH in most of our studies with isolated microsomes.

It is perhaps pertinent here to note that there may be differences between generating NADPH (with glucose-6-phosphate or isocitric dehydrogenases) and adding it already reduced. This is in terms of drug metabolized per unit time per mg microsomal protein. We have shown that NADPH generated by either isocitrate or glucose-6-phosphate dehydrogenase allows differentiation of enzyme activity in smooth- versus rough-surfaced microsomes, whereas added NADPH does not (Gram and Fouts, 1967). In this paper, we also showed that the amount of enzyme activity per unit of microsomal protein used was highest when the NADPH-generating system was that found in soluble fraction; less when glucose-6-phosphate dehydrogenase was used; and least when NADPH itself was added (without an NADPH-generating system). Until reasons for these differences are explored more fully, the investigator can merely be cautioned that his choice of NADPH generator may affect the results he obtains.

FACTORS THAT CAN AFFECT DRUG-METABOLIZING ENZYME ACTIVITY.—We have already discussed the major factors that everyone agrees are most likely to cause variability in the enzyme activity one can obtain with any given liver preparation. There are some other things about which we have some information, and these should at least be mentioned. They include (a) the buffer systems used in the incubation mixture and (b) the temperature of incubation.

The Buffer Systems Used in Incubation. Most people working with liver preparations in studies of drug metabolism have used either phosphate buffer or tris buffer in the final incubation mixture. In a paper by Good et al. (1966) it is pointed out that both of these buffers (phosphate and tris) have definite drawbacks in most biologic work with enzymes. In this paper by Good et al. (1966), a number of buffers capable of being used in the range of physiologic pH (6 to 8) and in the presence of what we believe are physiologic quantities of cations (Mg^{++}, Ca^{++}, Mn^{++}, etc.) are described. We have been making studies of some of these "new" buffers in incubation mixtures used for studying drug metabolism by liver from rats and rabbits. We have found that tris and phosphate buffers are not the best buffers for several microsomal drugs-metabolizing enzymes, and that the best buffer for one pathway is not the best for all. We hope to finish these studies soon, but for the time being we recommend that anyone who wishes to obtain the maximum enzyme activity possible with any given liver preparation make a systematic study of buffers other than tris or phosphate for use in this incubation mixture. In addition to the type of buffer used, some attention should be directed to the final concentration of buffer. One may find that high concentrations (>0.1 M) of buffer will inhibit the enzymes being studied.

Temperature of Incubation. When animals whose normal body temperature is not that of mammals are studied, it would be wise to investigate the rate of metabolism of drugs at temperatures other than 37°C. Thus, Adamson et al. (1965) showed that the hepatic nitro reductase enzyme in the turtle was 20 times as active at 21°C as at 37°C. The nitro reductase activity of turtle liver at 37°C would be missed by most investigators, whereas that at 21°C is easily detectable.

ASSAYS FOR THE DRUG BEING METABOLIZED BY DRUG-METABOLIZING ENZYMES.

Extraction of Drug (with Organic Solvents) from Incubation Mixtures. Several drug metabolic pathways of interest are followed by disappearance of the parent drug when it is incubated with liver preparations. Other pathways are quantified by measuring appearance of a given metabolite. Of these two procedures, the best is obviously the latter, particularly if one is studying the effects of various inducers or inhibitors on the drug-metabolizing systems. One of the major gaps in our knowledge of drug-metabolizing enzymes is that dealing with the possibility that the pathway by which a given drug disappears (e.g., hexobarbital) may be altered by induction or inhibition, so that a normally minor route of metabolism becomes more important.

In any event, after incubation of drug with enzyme, it is common to extract an aliquot of the incubation mixture with some organic solvent. This process removes drug or metabolite into the organic phase and leaves much interfering material in the aqueous phase. The drug or metabolite can then be assayed in the organic phase, or can be returned to an aqueous phase, if assays are best conducted in such a phase.

Much of the older literature, describing such extraction procedures for drugs, prescribes long periods of shaking of incubation mixtures or tissues with organic solvents. Thus, Brodie et al. (1953) describe a method for estimating pentobarbital in biologic materials, which calls for shaking the aqueous phase (tissue homogenate, urine or plasma) with the organic phase (petroleum ether and 1.5 percent isoamyl alcohol) for 45 minutes. This particular method of extraction is also prescribed for other barbiturates such as secobarbital and hexobarbital. As far as I have been able to determine, this procedure is still widely used, and in most cases the 45-minute shaking time is still observed. One publication dealing with barbiturate metabolism (Kamm and Van Loon, 1966) describes a method wherein urine is shaken for 20 minutes with the organic solvent.

There is really no theoretical justification for such prolonged periods of shaking. Unless the apparatus used to mix organic and aqueous phases is incredibly inefficient, equilibration between phases should be extremely rapid. If extraction is inefficient, it could be improved more markedly by increasing the number of times extraction is performed than by increasing the duration of mixing organic phase and aqueous phase for any given extraction. Therefore, we have recently reexamined some of our methodology of extraction to see if prolonged shaking together of organic and aqueous phases is really needed. The methods we have restudied include those for hexobarbital, zoxazolamine, amphetamine, and morphine. In all of these, the previously-called-for periods of shaking organic and aqueous phase together have been a minimum of 20 minutes. Our recent results indicate that in no case is a shaking time in excess of 5 minutes needed. We use the IEC Cat. #6306 size 2 bottle shakers for all extractions. These shakers provide a rotary and up-and-down movement which, in our experience, is one of the best for quick equilibration of two immiscible solvents.

It is my opinion, then, that any extraction procedure, used to estimate drugs, that calls for a shaking time of more than 5 minutes should be reevaluated. Longer shaking times markedly increase the problems of emulsification, and should be avoided if at all possible. If extraction is inefficient (less than 70 percent of drug extracted from aqueous phase), I would suggest using two extractions instead of one, and combining the extracts for further assay. No more than two extractions should be necessary for any usable method. Before going to more than two extractions, a wiser approach might be the use of a more polar organic solvent (e.g., instead of heptane, use chloroform or diethyl ether).

Finally, if emulsions are produced, these can be broken by cold temperatures (dry ice-acetone bath) and/or centrifugation, in nearly all cases.

Precipitation of Protein and Use of Clarified Supernatant. Several drug metabolic pathways can be followed by measuring a metabolite in a supernatant resulting after protein precipitation. One of the most common adaptations of this principle is used in estimating the amount of formaldehyde produced by microsomal enzymes removing methyl groups from various portions of a drug molecule. Indeed the method is so simple and quick that microsomal demethylases are perhaps the most widely studied of the drug-metabolizing enzyme systems. It is because of this that I wish to call attention to a publication by Stitzel et al. (1966) in which it has demonstrated that the protein precipitant used can affect the assay for formaldehyde by the NASH reagent. The principle is, I think, a very important one, and perhaps applies to more than the determination of formaldehyde. It would be my suggestion that anyone using a method for drug-metabolizing enzyme activity that requires a protein precipitant should determine for himself whether the method of precipitating protein can affect the amount of metabolite that he is measuring.

EXPRESSING ACTIVITY OF THE DRUG-METABOLIZING ENZYMES.— The activity of the drug-metabolizing enzymes has been expressed in terms of drug metabolized per gram tissue (wet-weight liver) or per mg nitrogen, protein, or phospholipid in the fraction being studied. Many workers in this field would argue that any expression of enzyme activity, other than that based on a microsomal component (e.g., per mg microsomal protein), is open to criticism, since the composition of the liver can vary so widely with diet, etc. Since the enzymes are in microsomes, their activity should be expressed in those (microsomal composition) terms. Though this point can be debated (since microsomal composition can also vary), it is perhaps more germane to at least ask on which microsomal component should we base enzyme activity? Convention would dictate protein, but perhaps phospholipid would serve better. Thus, we could have enzyme activity as μ moles drug metabolized per unit time, per mg protein, or per mg phospholipid (measured as phosphorous). The hepatic microsomal enzymes are apparently enclosed in phospholipid membranes, and their activity is dependent, in most cases, on the integrity of this membrane, since they have resisted nearly all attempts at solubilization.

If we remain conventional, however, we come to a final question—what method should one use to measure microsomal protein so that he may express enzyme activity on this basis? We have recently completed a study of several methods that might be used to measure protein content of liver homogenate subfractions, and were surprised at the marked variation in the answers we got (Juchau and Fouts, 1967). Our experience might seem to indicate that the micro-Kjeldahl and Lowry protein (or nitrogen) assays should be the ones used to quantify microsomal protein. Whatever method is used, it is important to specify in detail what was done.

Thus, regardless of the enzyme source (whether homogenate, 9,000 × *g* supernatant fraction, or microsomes), drug-metabolizing enzyme activity should be expressed in terms of a microsomal component (probably per mg protein to satisfy the referees most quickly). This requires that unless microsomes are used, one must isolate these from the tissue fraction employed (homogenate or 9,000 × *g* supernatant), at least for protein assay. It is perhaps not out of place to remind the investigator that such microsomes (for protein or nitrogen assay) should be resuspended, for that assay, in a buffer that will not interfere with the protein assay. Thus, do not use tris buffer or glycylglycine buffer for this preparation, if you are going to use the biuret or micro-Kjeldahl techniques.

The Assay of Hepatic Microsomal Drug-Metabolizing Enzyme Activity After Induction or Inhibition

ENZYME ACTIVITY AFTER INDUCTION.

Problems of Cofactor Concentration, Substrate Concentration, etc. Occasionally we have found it necessary to increase the amount of NADP added to liver fractions prepared from animals treated with inducers of microsomal drug-metabolizing enzyme systems. We do not know why this should be so, unless systems destroying NADP are also induced by the stimulators of the microsomal drug-metabolizing enzymes. I would therefore suggest that this point be investigated by anyone who is studying microsomal drug-metabolizing enzyme activity in control versus treated animals. Maximum enzyme activity after induction may require two to five times as much NADP as in the control animal.

Naturally, with more enzyme present, one will probably also have to either increase substrate concentration (to keep the enzyme saturated during the incubation) or decrease incubation time, as compared with the preparations from control animals.

Problems Due to Residual Inducer. Many compounds that induce hepatic microsomal drug-metabolizing enzymes can themselves react with these enzymes. An

TABLE 2

Effect of Incubator on Enzyme Activity in Hepatic 9,000 × g Supernatant Fractions from Control versus Phenobarbital-Pretreated Rabbits.

Type of Incubator	Substrate*	Drug Metabolism† by Hepatic 9,000 × *g* Supernatant Fraction from: CONTROL μMOLES/g LIVER/30 MIN	PHENOBARBITAL-TREATED‡ μMOLES/g LIVER/30 MIN	Ratio** Stim. : Control
Small Capacity††	Hexobarbital	2.40 ± 0.05	8.57 ± 0.23	3.6
	Aminopyrine	0.54 ± 0.03	1.19 ± 0.05	2.2
Large Capacity††	Hexobarbital	2.31 ± 0.51	3.50 ± 0.36	1.5
	Aminopyrine	0.56 ± 0.02	0.70 ± 0.05	1.3

*Final concentration of substrate in incubation mixture = 1.2×10^{-3} M for hexobarbital and 8.0×10^{-3} M for aminopyrine. NADPH concentration = 2.5×10^{-4} M, glucose-6-phosphate concentration = 5×10^{-3} M. Final volume of incubation mixture = 5 ml made to volume with 0.1 M phosphate buffer, pH 7.4. The final mixture contained 9,000 × *g* fraction from 1/3 g liver.

†Metabolism expressed as μmoles drug metabolized (hexobarbital) or metabolite formed (4-aminoantipyrine) in 30 minutes by 9,000 × *g* fraction from 1.00 g (wet weight) liver. Samples were incubated under oxygen at 37° C with shaking rate in each incubator at 100 oscillations per minute. The same 9,000 × *g* fractions were used to obtain all values in any given vertical column (e.g., control or phenobarbital-treated). Thus, the same 9,000 × *g* fraction from control rabbits was used in beakers incubated in the large or the small incubator and with either hexobarbital or aminopyrine as substrate. The values are mean ± SD with three animals. Hexobarbital and aminopyrine metabolisms by 9,000 × *g* supernatant fractions from control rabbits are the same in small vs. large incubator. Hexobarbital and aminopyrine metabolisms by 9,000 × *g* supernatant fractions from phenobarbital-treated rabbits are significantly ($P < .05$) different in small versus large incubator.

‡Male, Dutch rabbits, weighing 1 to 2 kg, were treated with phenobarbital sodium, 15 mg/kg intraperitoneally, once a day for four days. Assays were run 24 hours after the last dose of phenobarbital.

**Ratio of enzyme activity in 9,000 × *g* fraction from phenobarbital-treated rabbits to enzyme activity in 9,000 × *g* fraction from control rabbits.

††Small-capacity incubator holds 30 to 36 of the 20-ml capacity beakers we use in incubations. The large-capacity incubator holds 72 of these beakers. Oxygen flow rate in both incubators = 1,800 ml/min.

enzyme partially tied up with inducer may not be available to react with the drug used as substrate in the assay of enzyme activity. This is one reason why enzyme assays for enzyme induction are made several hours to several days after the last dose of inducer. By this delay, we hope to (1) get rid of most of the residual inducer in liver and (2) allow maximal response of the enzymes to the inducer. One can check for possible interference by inducer with the enzyme assay by determining the levels of inducer present in the liver at the time of assay. Adding these levels of inducer to the control preparation of enzymes will give you some idea of whether enzyme inhibition by the inducer will occur at the time you assay for enzyme induction. Generally speaking, the times (suggested in Section I) between last dose of inducer to the animal and sacrifice of the animal are those that have been found to allow disappearance of inducer, but still be within the time of maximal induction. With new inducers, this point should be checked.

Comparison of Effects in Homogenates versus 9,000 × g Supernatant Fraction versus Microsomes. As already mentioned, reports have appeared in the literature claiming stimulation of drug metabolism could be obtained in one cell fraction and not another. The problem already cited (homogenate versus 9,000 × *g*—see

Kinoshita et al., 1966) is, we believe, typical. A little more enzyme (homogenate) and a lot more cofactor seem to resolve the problem, so that induction can be demonstrated in both homogenates and 9,000 × *g* fractions.

Failure to Show Enzyme Induction In Vitro When It Has Been Demonstrated In Vivo. We have sometimes obtained 9,000 × *g* supernatant fractions from animals (rats or rabbits) known to have been treated with drug-metabolizing enzyme inducers (e.g., phenobarbital), which did not show or showed only slightly increased enzyme activity, compared with controls. We have finally discovered that this is due to the type of incubator that we use. Most shaking incubators used for in vitro studies provide quite adequate mixing and gassing conditions for our studies. However, some of the larger-capacity incubators are so deep, and provide such smooth shaking motions, that optimal conditions for assay of drug-metabolizing enzymes do not seem to be met. The problem seems to come down to the difference in vigor of shaking—the small-capacity incubators providing more vigorous mixing at any given shaking rate than the large-capacity incubators. The difference in enzyme activity between incubators is only great when preparations containing a lot of enzyme are used. Thus, enzyme activity in control preparations is often comparable when large versus small incubators are used, but enzyme activity in preparations from phenobarbital-treated animals is quite different. A typical experiment is shown in Table 2.

ENZYME ACTIVITY AFTER INHIBITORS.

Determination of Mechanism of Inhibition. Microsomal drug-metabolizing enzymes can be inhibited by any of several mechanisms, and at any of several sites along the chain between NADPH and the final stage of oxidation of the drug molecule. Between NADPH and this final oxidative stage are probably at least two links—a flavoprotein and at least one cytochrome (P450). Thus, when we study inhibitors of the microsomal enzymes, such studies should try to pin down the locus of action and the type of action of these inhibitors, if such is possible. At the very least, the following questions should be answered:

(1) Is the inhibition reversible or irreversible—can the inhibitor be removed by dialysis or similar treatment (e.g., dilution)?
(2) Is the inhibitor competitive with substrate or cofactor of the enzyme system (what is the effect of changing substrate concentration and/or NADPH concentration on the inhibition)?
(3) Does the inhibitor form a complex with P450 of microsomes? This can be followed by adding inhibitor, at various concentrations, to a suspension of microsomes (about 1 to 2 mg protein/ml cuvette contents) in buffer, and scanning the absorption spectrum (against a blank of microsomes plus buffer) between 350 mμ and 500 mμ. The troughs or peaks one may obtain in such spectra should be proportional in extent to the amount of inhibitor added. From such studies, one can calculate a dissociation constant of the P450 and

inhibitor (K_s), and compare this with the K_I (inhibitor constant) for the inhibition of the drug metabolism being studied. If K_s and K_I are about the same, then we have presumptive evidence that the inhibitor may act via its effect on P450. (See Schenkman et al., 1967, for a fuller discussion of this approach.) The microsomes used in this study of inhibitor-microsome interaction should either be prepared from a perfused liver or be extensively (two to three times) washed with isotonic KCl to remove hemoglobin which can interfere with the absorption spectrum.

If these questions were answered for all presently known and newfound inhibitors of the drug-metabolizing enzymes, we would be much further along in our understanding not only of the enzymes and inhibitors but also of the mechanisms by which therapeutically useful manipulations of these enzymes might be made.

Some Assay Problems. Occasionally one will find an inhibitor of microsomal enzymes in vivo (e.g., by prolongation of sleeping times, biologic half-lives, etc.) which, when added to liver fractions, is inactive. Several possible reasons exist for this, but one that should be suspected is that the added "inhibitor" is really not the active moiety. Thus, the inhibitor may be altered in some tissue other than liver, and act in the form of this metabolite on the hepatic microsomal enzymes. One other possibility that might be considered is that the drug-metabolizing enzymes in vivo are operating under suboptimal conditions–e.g., low substrate concentrations and low NADPH concentrations. The in vitro assay systems previously described would provide most of these enzymes with much more substrate and cofactor than available in vivo. The in vitro effects of the inhibitor may not, therefore, become measureable, unless the substrate and/or cofactor concentrations are lowered.

Other points to remember: (1) It will probably take a different concentration of inhibitor to effect the same degree of inhibition in homogenate versus 9,000 × *g* supernatant fraction versus microsomes. More inhibitor may be needed in homogenates because of nonmicrosomal binding of the inhibitor. Less inhibitor may be needed for microsomes, not only because of less inert protein to bind inhibitor (inert protein is present in homogenates as nuclei, mitochondria, and soluble fraction, and in 9,000 × *g* fractions as soluble fraction), but also because soluble fraction may have factors that stabilize the drug-metabolizing enzymes in microsomes, and these stabilizers are lost when isolated microsomes are used. (2) The solvent used to dissolve the inhibitor may itself affect the microsomal enzymes. Some inhibitors of microsomal enzymes are virtually water-insoluble. They can be added in vitro as solutions in alcohol, or acetone, or suspended in something like carboxymethyl cellulose. All of these (alcohol, acetone, CMC) can inhibit the microsomal enzymes, so that controls must always be run (liver fractions plus substrate and cofactors, to which solvent alone, in the same volume, is added). We have found that as long as the volume of alcohol or acetone added is less than 0.2 ml (in a total incubation volume of 5 ml), and is immediately mixed with the incubation mixture, there are minimal effects on most drug-metabolizing enzymes. We usually add the acetone or alcohol solution before the liver fraction (e.g., microsomes) is added to the incubation mixture.

CONCLUSIONS

In this discussion of methods in drug metabolism, I have tried to present a few of the practical aspects involved in an approach to this field. Many things have been left out because of the space limitations imposed. The study of glucuronidating enzymes in hepatic microsomes has not been described at all, primarily because I have had little practical experience with these systems. The purpose of what has been written can be summed up best as a description of what some of us do, and why we do it, when we study hepatic microsomal drug-metabolizing enzymes. In a sense, I have written these chapters for a very selfish reason: I have tried to gather together in one place much of what I would like my technicians and graduate students to know, and I hope such a compilation will also be of value to others.

REFERENCES

Adamson, R. H., Dixon, R. L., Francis, F. L., and Rall, D. P. 1965. Comparative biochemistry of drug metabolism by azo and nitro reductase. Proc. Nat. Acad. Sci. U.S.A., 54:1386-1391.

Aggeler, P. M., O'Reilly, R. A., Leong, L., and Kowitz, P. E. 1967. Potentiation of anticoagulant effect of warfarin by phenylbutazone. New Eng. J. Med., 276:496-501.

Booth, J., and Gillette, J. R. 1962. The effect of anabolic steroids on drug metabolism by microsomal enzymes in rat liver. J. Pharmacol. Exp. Ther., 137:374-379.

Brodie, B. B., and Axelrod, J. 1950. The fate of aminopyrine (pyramidon) in man and methods for the estimation of aminopyrine and its metabolites in biological material. J. Pharmacol. Exp. Ther., 99:171-179.

—Burns, J. J., Mark, L. C., Lief, P. A., Bernstein, E. and Papper, E. M. 1953. The fate of pentobarbital in man and dog and a method for its estimation in biological material. J. Pharmacol. Exp. Ther., 109:26-34.

Brown, R. R., Miller, J. A., and Miller, E. C. 1954. The metabolism of methylated aminoazo dyes. IV. Dietary factors enhancing demethylation in vitro. J. Biol. Chem., 209:211-222.

Burns, J. J., Cucinell, S. A., Koster, R., and Conney, A. H. 1965. Application of drug metabolism to drug toxicity studies. Ann. N. Y. Acad. Sci., 123:273-286.

Chatterjee, I. B., Price, Z. H., and McKee, R. W., 1965. Biosynthesis of L-ascorbic acid in different sub-cellular fractions of prenatal and postnatal rat livers. Nature (London), 207:1168-1170.

Chiesara, E., Clementi, F., Conti, F., and Meldolesi, J. 1967. The induction of drug metabolizing enzymes in rat liver during growth and regeneration: A biochemical and ultrastructural study. Lab. Invest., 16:254-267.

Conney, A. H., and Garren, L. 1961. Contrasting effects of thyroxin on zoxazolamine and hexobarbital metabolism. Biochem. Pharmacol., 6:257-262.

—Miller, E. C., and Miller, J. A. 1956. The metabolism of methylated aminoazo dyes. V. Evidence for induction of enzyme synthesis in the rat by 3—methylcholanthrene. Cancer Res., 16:450-459.

—Davison, C., Gastel, R., and Burns, J. J. 1960. Adaptive increases in drug metabolizing enzymes induced by phenobarbital and other drugs. J. Pharmacol. Exp. Ther., 130:1-8.

Cram, R. L., and Fouts, J. R. 1967. The influence of DDT and γ-chlordane on the metabolism of hexobarbital and zoxazolamine in two mouse strains. Biochem. Pharmacol., 16:1001-1006.

—Juchau, M. R., and Fouts, J. R. 1965. Differences in hepatic drug metabolism in various rabbit strains before and after pretreatment with phenobarbital. Proc. Soc. Exp. Biol. Med., 118:872-875.

Dallner, G. 1963. Studies on the structural and enzymic organization of the membranous elements of liver microsomes. Acta Path. Microbiol. Scand. (Suppl. 166).

—and Nilsson, R. 1966. Mechanism of the cation effect in subfractionation of microsomes. J. Cell Biol., 31:181-193.

—Siekevitz, P., and Palade, G. E. 1965. Synthesis of microsomal membranes and their enzymic constituents in developing rat liver. Biochem. Biophys. Res. Commun., 20:135-141.

Driever, C. W., and Bousquet, W. F. 1965. Stress-drug interactions; evidence for rapid enzyme induction. Life Sci., 4:1449-1454.

Ferguson, H. C. 1966. Effect of red cedar chip bedding on hexobarbital and pentobarbital sleep time. J. Pharm. Sci., 55:1142-43.

Fine, B. C., and Molloy, J. O. 1964. Effects of insecticide synergists on duration of sleep induced in mice by barbiturates. Nature (London), 204:789-790

Fujimoto, J. M. 1965. Effect of gum tragacanth, urethan, and phenobarbital on hexobarbital narcosis in mice. Toxic. Appl. Pharmacol., 7:287-290.

Gelboin, H. V., and Blackburn, N. R. 1964. The stimulatory effect of 3-methylcholanthrene on benzpyrene hydroxylase activity in several rat tissues: Inhibition by actinomycin D and puromycin. Cancer Res., 24:356-360.

Gillette, J. R. 1963a. Factors that affect the stimulation of the microsomal drug enzymes induced by foreign compounds. Advances Enzym. Regulat., 1:215-223.

—1963b. Metabolism of drugs and other foreign compounds by enzymatic mechanisms. *In* Progress in Drug Research., Jucker, E., ed. Birkhauser Verlag, Basel, Vol. 6, pp. 13-73.

Good, N. E., Winget, G. D., Winter, W., Connolly, T. N., Izawa, S., and Singh, R. M. M. 1966. Hydrogen ion buffers for biological research. Biochemistry, 5:467-477.

Gram, T. E., and Fouts, J. R. 1966. Time course differences in the metabolism of drugs by hepatic microsomes from rats, rabbits and mice. J. Pharmacol. Exp. Ther., 152:363-371.

—and Fouts, J. R. 1967. Further studies on the metabolism of drugs by subfractions of hepatic microsomes. III. Effects of the NADPH-generating system. J. Pharmacol. Exp. Ther., 158:317-322.

—Rogers, L. A. and Fouts, J. R. 1967. Further studies on the metabolism of drugs by subfractions of hepatic microsomes. J. Pharmacol. Exp. Ther., 155:479-493.

Hart, L. G., and Fouts, J. R. 1965a. Studies on the possible mechanisms by which chlordane stimulates hepatic microsomal drug metabolism in the rat. Biochem. Pharmacol., 14:263-272.

—and Fouts, J. R. 1965b. Further studies on the stimulation of hepatic microsomal drug metabolizing enzymes by DDT and its analogs. Naunyn Schmiedeberg Arch. Pharm. Exp. Path., 249:486-500.

Juchau, M. R., and Fouts, J. R. 1967. A comparison of assays for the analysis of protein content of liver homogenate subfractions. Biochem. Pharmacol., 16:155-161.

Kamm, J. J., and Van Loon, E. J. 1966. Amobarbital metabolism in man: A gas chromatographic method for the estimation of hydroxyamobarbital in human urine. Clin. Chem., 12:789-796.

Karler, R., Turkanis, S. A., and Steinman, S. P. 1967. Acid precipitation of liver microsomes for the study of drug metabolism. Fed. Proc., 26:354.

Kato, R., and Takayanaghi, M. 1966. Differences among the action of phenobarbital, methylcholanthrene and male sex hormone on microsomal drug metabolizing enzyme systems of rat liver. Jap. J. Pharmacol, 16:380-390.

—Chiesara, E., and Vassanelli, P. 1962. Factors influencing induction of hepatic microsomal drug metabolizing enzymes. Biochem. Pharmacol., 11:211-220.
—Vassanelli, P., Frontino, G., and Chiesara, E. 1964. Variation in the activity of liver microsomal drug metabolizing enzymes in rats in relation to the age. Biochem. Pharmacol., 13:1037-1051.
Kinoshita, F. K., Frawley, J. P., and DuBois, K. P. 1966. Quantitative measurement of induction of hepatic microsomal enzymes by various dietary levels of DDT and toxaphene in rats. Toxic. Appl. Pharmacol., 9:505-513.
LaDu, B. N., Gaudette, L., Trousof, N. and Brodie, B. B. 1955. Enzymatic dealkylation of aminopyrine (Pyramidon) and other alkylamines. J. Biol. Chem., 214:741-752.
Leadbeater, L., and Davies, D. R., 1964, The stability of the drug metabolizing enzymes of liver microsomal preparations. Biochem. Pharmacol., 13:1607-1617.
Lindsay, H. A., and Kullman, V. S. 1966. Pentobarbital sodium: Variation in toxicity. Science, 151:576-577.
Lutsch, E. F., and Morris, R. W. 1967. Circadian periodicity in susceptibility to lidocaine hydrochloride. Science, 156:100-102.
McLuen, E. F., and Fouts, J. R. 1961. The effect of obstructive jaundice on drug metabolism in rabbits. J. Pharmacol. Exp. Ther., 131:7-11.
Mullen, J. O., Juchau, M. R., and Fouts, J. R. 1966. Studies on interactions of 3,4-benzpyrene, 3-methylcholanthrene, chlordane, and methyltestosterone as stimulators of hepatic microsomal enzyme systems in the rat. Biochem. Pharmacol., 15:137-144.
Neubert, D. 1962. Hemmung der Oxydativen N-Demethylierung in Lebermikrosomen durch Alkylphosphate in vitro. Naunyn Schmiedeberg Arch. Pharm. Exp. Path., 243:302-3.
Novick, W. J., Stohler, C. M., and Swagzdis, J. 1966. The influence of steroids on drug metabolism in the mouse. J. Pharmacol. Exp. Ther., 151:139-142.
Orrenius, S., and Ernster, L. 1964. Phenobarbital-induced synthesis of the oxidative demethylating enzymes of rat liver microsomes. Biochem. Biophys. Res. Commun., 16:60-65.
Philleo, W. W., Schonbrod, R. D., and Terriere, L. C. 1965. Methylenedioxyphenyl compounds as inhibitors of the hydroxylation of naphthalane in houseflies. Agric. and Food Chem., 13:113-115.
Remmer, H. 1962. Drug tolerance. *In* Ciba Foundation Symposium on Enzymes and Drug action. Monger, and de Reuck, eds. Boston, Little, Brown and Company, pp. 276-298.
Rogers, L. A., Alcantara, G. A., and Fouts, J. R. 1963. p—Aminosalicyclic acid-induced prolongation of hexobarbital sleeping time. J. Pharmacol. Exp. Ther., 142:242-247.
Roth, J. S., and Bukovsky, J. 1961. Studies on an n-demethylating system in rat liver microsomes. J. Pharmacol. Exp. Ther., 131:275-281.
Rümke, C. L., Van Strik, R., deJonge, H., and Delver, A. 1963. Experiments on the duration of hexobarbital narcosis in mice. Arch. Int. Pharmacodyn., 146:10-26.
Schenkman, J. B., Ball, J. A., and Estabrook, R. W. 1967. On the use of nicotinamide in assays for microsomal mixed-function oxidase activity. Biochem. Pharmacol., 16:1071-1081.
Schenkman, J. B., Remmer, H., and Estabrook, R. W. 1967. Spectral studies of drug interaction with hepatic microsomal cytochrome. Molec. Pharmacol., 3:113-123.
Stitzel, R. E., Greene, F. E., Furner, R., and Conaway, H. 1966. Factors affecting the measurement of formaldehyde produced by enzymatic demethylation. Biochem. Pharmacol., 15:1001-1003.
von Jagow, R., Kampffmeyer, H., and Kiese, M. 1965. The preparation of microsomes. Naunyn Schmiedeberg Arch. Pharm. Exp. Path., 251:73-87.
Wattenberg, L. W., and Leong, J. L. 1965. Effects of phenothiazines on protective systems against polycyclic hydrocarbons. Cancer Res., 25:365-370.
Winne, D. 1964. Experimentelle und biometrische Untersuchungen über den Zusammenhang von Gehirnkonzentration, Eliminationsgeschwindigkeit, Schlafzeit und Körpertemperatur bei der Hexobarbitalnarkose der Maus. Naunyn Schmiedeberg Arch. Pharm. Exp. Path., 247:278-294.

CHAPTER 10

Sarcoplasmic Reticulum: Calcium Uptake and Release Systems in Muscle

Y. Ogawa, S. Harigaya, S. Ebashi

Department of Pharmacology, Faculty of Medicine
University of Tokyo, Tokyo, Japan

and K. S. Lee

Department of Pharmacology, State University of New York
Downstate Medical Center, Brooklyn, New York

INTRODUCTION

Early electron microscopic study indicated that the sarcoplasmic matrix surrounding the myofibrils contained small vesicular or tubular structures which subsequently were found to consist of longitudinally disposed tubules or cisternae forming a loose network. This network was interrupted at intervals to accommodate transversely oriented tubules (T-system). In general, the term *sarcoplasmic reticulum* is used to designate these longitudinally disposed tubules. Recognition of the existence of transversely and longitudinally oriented membrane-limited channels in the sarcoplasm stimulated conjecture on the possible role of these structures in the internal conduction of a signal from the fiber surface to the contractile system throughout the muscle cell. The sarcoplasmic reticulum is currently assigned an important role in the excitation-contraction coupling process of muscle contraction. According to the generally accepted view, the spread of the electrical excitation wave along the muscle membrane releases Ca^{++} from the sarcoplasmic reticulum which, in turn, initiates contraction of the myofibrils; after termination of excitation, relaxation is presumably brought about by the reuptake of Ca^{++} by the sarcoplasmic reticulum (Ebashi, 1965; Ebashi and Endo, 1968; Hasselbach, 1964; Weber, 1966; Lee et al., 1966; Smith, 1966).

The so-called relaxing factor,* which appears to be the main constituent of the heavy "microsomal" fraction of muscle, is derived from the sarcoplasmic reticulum. The preparation induces relaxation of contractile systems, by its ATP-dependent Ca^{++}-binding capacity (Ebashi, 1961; Ebashi and Endo, 1968; Hasselbach, 1964; Weber, 1966). Therefore, the evaluation of preparations of "relaxing factor" can be made by its Ca^{++}-binding capacity (Table 1). This section will be confined to the preparative method for "relaxing factor" from white and red skeletal muscle of rabbit, and assays for same. A detailed description for the isolation of a similar system from cardiac muscle is presented on pp. 335-336, in Inesi et al., 1964, and in Harigaya and Schwartz, 1969.

The preparation of "relaxing factor" from smooth muscle has not as yet been successful.

PREPARATION

White Skeletal Muscle of Rabbit

All the procedures described should be carried out below 4°C.

STEP 1. A young and healthy rabbit weighing 2.0 to 2.5 kg is anesthetized by ether and then exsanguinated through the carotid arteries. After removal of connective tissue, tendons, fatty tissue, nerves, vessels and red muscle, the hind leg muscle is chopped into small pieces on a glass plate using stainless-steel scissors and a knife.

STEP 2. One hundred grams of these chopped small pieces are put into 100 ml of 0.01 N NaOH in a silicone-coated stainless-steel cup of a Waring blendor and immediately homogenized. The homogenization for 20 sec is repeated every 3 minutes. During this process the pH of the homogenate should be kept at about 6.8 (use bromthymol blue indicator paper) by adding 0.01 N NaOH, up to a total volume of 300 ml; use N NaOH, if required. Changes in pH become most pronounced about 40 min after the beginning of homogenization. When the pH of the homogenate becomes constant at pH 6.8, homogenization is stopped. Usually, one hour is necessary for this step, and 2 to 3 ml of N NaOH are consumed.

*This factor owes its name to historical background. It is now called, in various ways, microsomes, fragmented or isolated sarcoplasmic reticulum, or reticulum fragments; some of these are also used in this text.

Scheme 1
Summary

chopped pieces of hind leg muscle 100 g + 0.01 N NaOH 400 ml

homogenized in Waring blendor. The medium is added in aliquots keeping the pH constant at 6.8 to 7.0. When more alkalinity is required, N NaOH is added.

centrifugation

9,000 × *g* 20 min

sup — ppt discarded

centrifugation

9,000 × *g* 20 min

sup — ppt discarded

filtration (Toyo Roshi No. 5A)

filtrate — residue discarded

centrifugation

Spinco No. 30 rotor

25,000 rpm 30 min

sup — ppt + (20 mM tris-maleate pH 6.80, 50 mM KCl) ~ 40 ml

pellet is uniformly suspended

centrifugation

6,000 × *g* 10 min

sup — ppt discarded

centrifugation

Spinco No. 30 rotor

25,000 rpm 30 min

sup — ppt + (20 mM tris-maleate pH 6.80, 50 mM KCl) ~ 3 ml

protein concentration ~ 40 mg/ml

4-5 ml

TABLE 1

*Some Properties of the Ca^{++}-Binding Activity of Rabbit White Muscle Microsomes**

STEADY-STATE FILLING	
1. Capacity	
in the absence of oxalate	0.12-0.16μmole/mg protein
in the presence of 5 mM oxalate (effective minimum concentration of oxalate: 0.3-0.5 mM)	2-3 μmoles/mg protein [30-40 μmoles/mg N (Hasselbach and Makinose, 1963)]
2. Apparent binding constant	$8 \times 10^{6}\ M^{-1}$ †
3. Temperature dependence	independent above 15°C; dependent below 15°C (cf. Inesi and Watanabe, 1967; Martonosi and Feretos, 1964)
4. ATP dependence	$K_m = 2 \times 10^{-7}$ M (reaches plateau at 10^{-6} M; secondary rise at 10^{-4} to 10^{-3} M was reported by some workers) (Inesi et al., 1967; Weber et al., 1966)
5. Mg^{++} dependence	maximum at 10 mM (cf. Carvalho and Leo, 1967; Weber et al., 1966)
6. pH dependence	optimum 6.0-6.5 (cf. Carvalho and Leo, 1967; Hasselbach, 1964)
7. Coupling with extra-ATPase (Ca-dependent ATPase)	confirmative: Ca/Pi = 1 (Hasselbach and Makinose, 1961); Ca/Pi = 2 (Hasselbach and Makinose, 1963; Weber et al., 1966) negative: (Ebashi and Yamanouchi, 1964)
RATE	
1. Rate constant	$4{,}000\ M^{-1}\ sec^{-1}$ at room temperature (proportional to concentration of free Ca^{++} and remaining available binding sites) (cf. Ohnishi and Ebashi, 1964; Weber et al., 1966)

2. Temperature dependence	$Q_{10} = 3.5$
3. Mg^{++} dependence	maximum at 4 mM (cf. Weber et al., 1966)
4. pH dependence	optimum: 5.6-6.4 (cf. Hasselbach, 1964)

INHIBITORS AND ACTIVATORS

1. Inhibitors	ADP (Ebashi and Lipmann, 1962), detergents (Ebashi and Endo, 1964; Ebashi and Lipmann, 1962; Martonosi, 1964), phospholipase C (Martonosi, 1963, 1964), trypsin (Nagai et al., 1960), Salyrgan (Hasselbach and Makinose, 1961), PCMB (Carsten and Mommaerts, 1964), inorganic anions (Ebashi, 1965), amytal (Carsten and Mommaerts, 1964), reserpine (Balzer et al., 1968)
2. Activators	None (agents that increase Ca uptake by the formation of insoluble Ca salt: oxalate (Hasselbach and Makinose, 1961), phosphate (Ebashi and Endo, 1964; Lorand and Molnar, 1962), pyrophosphate (Ebashi and Endo, 1964; Lorand and Molnar, 1962),
3. Releaser	caffeine (Weber, 1966)
4. Effect of metabolic inhibitors	no effect was observed with DNP (Harigaya et al., 1968), dicoumarol, cyanide (Weber et al., 1966), oligomycin (Weber et al., 1966; Harigaya et al., 1968), and azide (Harigaya et al., 1968).

---

*Original and unpublished data were obtained in the authors' laboratory (Ebashi et al.) during the past two years. The references cited "cf," are those that have shown inconsistencies with the preceding data.

†This value is obtained by using $5 \times 10^5\ M^{-1}$, instead of $2 \times 10^6\ M^{-1}$, as "apparent binding constant" for GEDTA for Ca^{++} at pH 6.80 (Ogawa, 1968). The former is measured directly in the presence of 20 mM tris-maleate buffer. Twenty millimolar histidine or imidazole buffer gives fairly similar value to that obtained with tris-maleate buffer, whereas the phosphate buffer gives a value similar to the latter which was calculated from Schwarzenbach's results (Ogawa, 1968; Portzehl et al., 1964; Schwarzenbach et al., 1957).

TABLE 2

Effect of Various Homogenizing Media on Ca-Binding Activity of Isolated Sarcoplasmic Reticulum from Rabbit White Skeletal Muscle. *

Medium	Activity (percent)
distilled water	(100)
0.1-0.15 M KCl	100
0.25 M sucrose with or without 0.1 mM $CaCl_2$	50
0.25 M sucrose treated with Dowex A-1	60
0.88 M sucrose	35
5 mM oxalate	65
5 mM GEDTA	60

*Reaction mixture, 10 ml in total, contains 100 mM KCl, 20 mM tris-maleate (pH 6.80), 10 mM $MgCl_2$, 0.01 mM ($CaCl_2$ + $^{45}CaCl_2$), 0.1 mg protein/ml "relaxing factor," and 2 mM ATP. Immediately after the addition of ATP, the tubes are centrifuged at 40,000 rpm for 15 min at No. 40 rotor of Spinco ultracentrifuge. Ca^{++} content in the sediment was calculated from the radioactivity in the supernatant and in the sediment, also from the total amount of Ca^{++} in the reaction mixture. All the above procedures are carried out below 4°C.

STEP 3. The homogenate is centrifuged at 9,000 × *g* for 20 min and the supernatant is again centrifuged at 9,000 × *g* for 20 min. The resulting supernatant is then passed through a filter paper (Toyo Roshi No. 5A or Whatman No. 41 or 43) to remove fat.

STEP 4. The filtrate is centrifuged at 25,000 rpm for 30 min in the No. 30 rotor of the Spinco ultracentrifuge. The pellet is suspended in about 40 ml of solution containing 50 mM KCl and 20 mM tris-maleate (pH 6.80) using a Teflon pestle of the Potter-Elvehjem type.*

STEP 5. The suspension is centrifuged at 6,000 × *g* for 10 min and the sediment is discarded. The resulting supernatant is again centrifuged at 25,000 rpm for 30 min in the No. 30 rotor of the Spinco ultracentrifuge. The pellet is thoroughly suspended in about 3 ml of the solution in the manner previously described. The protein concentration of the suspension is usually about 40 mg/ml (according to the biuret method and standardized by the Kjeldahl procedure). The total volume of the suspension amounts to 4 to 5 ml. See Scheme 1 for a summary of the preparation.

Some properties of fragmented sarcoplasmic reticulum thus obtained are shown in Table 1.

DISCUSSION AND WARNINGS

1. Animals: Back muscle should not be used. The use of aged rabbits should be avoided.

*A "Komagome" type of pipette is very useful for making a uniform suspension.

2. Water: Deionized water by resin should not be used. Only carefully prepared glass-distilled water, preferably twice-distilled, should be employed.
3. Homogenizing medium: Water, at the appropriate pH, is best. Using 0.1 to 0.15 M KCl, we can obtain a preparation as good in its quality as that by water. In this case, however, it is very troublesome to remove contaminated actomyosin. In Table 2, Ca^{++} binding activities of microsomes prepared by using various kinds of media are compared. (In this case, Ca^{++} accumulation was examined in the *absence of oxalate* by using fresh microsomes—*only a few hours old.*) However, Ca^{++} *uptake* activity in the presence of 5 mM oxalate is almost the same for all samples irrespective of the kind of medium used. Thus Ca^{++} accumulating activity in the presence of oxalate cannot define the *quality* of preparations. Microsomes prepared in a solution containing 5 mM GEDTA* lose their activity very rapidly and show no Ca^{++} binding activity 24 hours after preparation.
4. Tubes for centrifugation: The best tubes for centrifugation are of hard glass or stainless-steel coated with silicone resin. Among tubes made of synthetic resins, the polypropylene or cellulose tube will do in the case of white muscle, but polyallomer tubes should not be used. Synthetic resin tubes must be avoided in the case of red muscle (to be discussed next).

Red Skeletal Muscle of Rabbit

Since the microsomal preparation of red muscle is extremely labile compared with the microsomes of white muscle, it is impossible to obtain an active preparation from red muscle by the usual procedure (just described). Therefore, in preliminary investigations, the participation of the sarcoplasmic reticulum in the relaxation of red muscle was questionable (Gergely et al., 1965; Sreter and Gergely, 1964).

All the procedures to be described should be carried out as quickly as possible, below 4°C, exerting the greatest of care, particularly with respect to water, reagents, and equipment.

STEP 1: A young rabbit weighing about 2 kg is suitable. *d*-Tubocurarine, 3 mg/kg, is intravenously administrated and artificial respiration is performed for 15 min before exsanguination. Soleus and semitendinosus muscle should be used. Other muscles that appear red in color contain white muscle fibers. Usually, about 7 to 10 g of soleus and semitendinosus muscle can be obtained from one rabbit.

STEP 2: Ten grams of red muscle are cut into small pieces with scissors and homogenized in 50 ml of 0.15 M KCl†, containing 5 mM sodium bicarbonate, in

*GEDTA: glycoletherdiaminetetraacetic acid, or ethylene glycol bis(β-aminoethylether)-N,N′-tetraacetic acid (EGTA).

†Using water instead of 0.15 M KCl as with white muscle, or 0.1 M KCl containing 5 mM bicarbonate, the homogenates have a tendency to separate before centrifugation into debris and liquid, and an active preparation cannot be obtained.

Scheme 2
Summary

chopped pieces of red muscle 10 g

+ 50 ml $\begin{pmatrix} 0.15\ M\ KCl \\ 5mM\ NaHCO_3 \end{pmatrix}$ + 2 ml of 20 mM ATP

homogenized in Waring blendor

centrifugation

9,000 X *g* 20 min (stainless-steel tube coated with silicone resin)

sup — ppt discarded

sup: centrifugation

9,000 X *g* 20 min (stainless-steel tube coated with silicone resin)

sup — ppt discarded

sup: filtration (Toyo Roshi No. 5A)

filtrate — residue discarded

filtrate: + KCl (final concentration 0.6 M)

centrifugation

Spinco No. 40 rotor

40,000 rpm 15 min (stainless-steel tube coated with silicone resin)

sup — ppt + (5 mM $NaHCO_3$ 1 ml)

pellet is uniformly suspended

centrifugation

9,000 X *g* 10 min (glass tube)

sup — ppt discarded

sup: protein concentration 7-9 mg/ml

a Waring blendor coated with silicone resin, ten times for 30 seconds, each time with intervals of 30-sec rest. During this time 2 ml of 20 mM ATP (4μmoles ATP per gram of muscle) are added to the homogenate.

STEP 3: The homogenate is then centrifuged at 9,000 × *g* for 20 min, using stainless-steel tubes coated with silicone resin. The supernatant is again centrifuged at 9,000 × *g* for 20 min. The resulting supernatant is then passed through filter paper. Potassium chloride (0.355 g) is added to 10 ml of filtrate to give a final concentration of 0.6 M KCl, to solubilize contaminating actomyosin.

STEP 4: The filtrate is centrifuged at 40,000 rpm for 15 min in a No. 40 rotor in a Spinco ultracentrifuge using stainless-steel tubes coated with silicone resin. The pellet is thoroughly suspended in 1 ml of 5 mM sodium bicarbonate solution in the manner previously described.

STEP 5: The suspension is centrifuged at 9,000 × *g* for 10 min using glass tubes, and the resulting supernatant is used as the microsomal fraction. The protein concentration of this suspension is usually about 7 to 9 mg/ml, and the amount of contaminated Ca^{++} in the preparation is about 0.017 to 0.02 μmoles per mg protein. The capacity of Ca^{++} binding of the microsomal fraction of a rabbit red muscle prepared by this method is about 50 to 60 mμmoles (picomoles) per mg protein (in the absence of oxalate), which corresponds to about one third that of white muscle. The microsomal fraction of red muscle is extremely labile. The Ca^{++} binding capacity of this fraction decreases to almost half of the initial capacity in one day. See Scheme 2 for a summary of the preparation.

Cardiac Muscle (by K. S. Lee)

The preparation of reticulum fragments from cardiac muscle is similiar to the procedure for skeletal muscle except that α-tocopherol, 0.2 mM, is added in the extraction medium, since it was found that the presence of this agent in the medium preserves the stability of Ca^{++} uptake function in the cardiac reticulum fragments (Inesi et al., 1964); the last precipitate is resuspended in 20 mM tris-maleate buffer, pH 6.5, instead of KCl-histidine solution. It is important to know that the Ca^{++} uptake function of cardiac sarcoplasmic reticulum deteriorates very rapidly, and only the freshly prepared reticulum fragments should be used.

It should also be mentioned that the Ca^{++} uptake capacity of cardiac reticulum fragments is about one half to one third of the skeletal counterpart under the same conditions of incubation.

Solution used for the extraction:

120 mM KCl + 5 mM histidine buffer (pH 6.5)
+ 0.2 mM α-tocopherol

PROCEDURE.

PREPARATION OF TISSUE . All operations are performed at preferably 4°C in a cold room. When a cold room is not available, solutions can be kept in ice buckets. Cardiac tissue is obtained, as fresh as possible, from rabbit (dog, guinea pig, and other small animals may also be used).

Animals are killed by an intravenous injection of sodium pentobarbital, or by a blow on the head, and the heart is excised as rapidly as possible and chilled in ice. One volume of chilled muscle is homogenized with 4 volumes of cold extraction solution, at 0°C in a Waring blendor for a total of 40 seconds with pauses of 20 seconds after each 10 seconds of homogenization. The homogenates are centrifuged for 30 min each at 5,000 and 10,000 $\times$ *g* in a Lourdes centrifuge or other appropriate refrigerated centrifuges for the removal of myofibrils and mitochondria, respectively. The supernatant is passed through three layers of cheesecloth to remove the lipid layer and is then centrifuged at 38,000 $\times$ *g* for one hour in a Spinco centrifuge Model L. The resulting precipitate is washed twice with an approximately fortyfold volume of the extraction solution, followed by centrifugation at 56,000 $\times$ *g*. During the washing procedure, the bottom layer of the precipitate, which has a darker color, is discarded. The final precipitate is then suspended in the extraction solution, in a volume ratio to the original muscle of approximately 1:10. Usually, the final suspension of sarcoplasmic reticulum should contain approximately 7 to 10 mg of protein per ml.

METHODS FOR INVESTIGATION OF THE "RELAXING SYSTEM"

The experiments should be carried out on the same day of preparation in the cases of cardiac and red muscle "microsomes," and within a few days in the case of white skeletal muscle microsomes.* There are numerous methods of study. Only a few selected ones are included in this chapter, although a complete list of published procedures is given in the reference section.

A. Experiments using the "relaxing factor" (fragmented sarcoplasmic reticulum)
 1. Ca^{++}-binding activity
  a. centrifugation method
   (1) by counting radioactivity of ^{45}Ca (Ebashi, 1961; Ebashi and Lipmann, 1962; Hasselbach and Makinose, 1961; Weber et al., 1963)

*It is important to mention that the presence of inorganic phosphate (3 to 5 mM) or oxalate (1 to 5 mM) markedly increases the Ca^{++} uptake of reticulum fragments. This increased amount of Ca^{++} uptake can be obtained even with fairly aged samples. The characteristics of Ca^{++} uptake in the presence of oxalate are, however, quite different than in the absence of oxalate or phosphate, and may not represent physiologic properties of the reticulum.

(2) direct measurement of Ca^{++}
colorimetric (Ebashi and Yamanouchi, 1964)
atomic absorption (Carvalho and Leo, 1967; Weber et al., 1966; Willis, 1963)
titration with metal indicators (Weber et al., 1966).

b. millipore filter method (Martonosi and Feretos, 1964; Seidel, 1967; Weber et al., 1966)
by using ^{45}Ca

c. double-beam spectrophotometry (Ohnishi and Ebashi, 1963, 1964)

2. Relaxing activity
This is expressed by the extent to which one of the following processes is inhibited (or reversed in the case of "a").
a. contraction of glycerinated muscle (Bendall, 1953; Ebashi et al., 1960)
b. syneresis of myofibrils (Ebashi and Endo, 1964; Harigaya et al., 1968; Weber and Herz, 1963; Weber et al., 1963)
c. superprecipitation of myosin B (natural actomyosin) (Ebashi, 1961; Ebashi and Endo, 1964; Harigaya et al., 1968)
d. actomyosin-type ATPase of myofibrils or myosin B (Ebashi, 1961; Nagai et al., 1960; Weber and Herz, 1963; Weber et al., 1963)
Concerning "b" and "c", measuring the change in absorbance at 660 mμ is most convenient (Ebashi, 1961; Ebashi and Endo, 1964).
3. Mg^{++}-activated microsomal ATPase with special reference to Ca^{++} uptake and Ca^{++}-dependent ATPase (Ebashi and Yamanouchi, 1964; Ebashi and Lipmann, 1962; Hasselbach and Makinose, 1961, 1963; Makinose and Hasselbach, 1965; Weber et al., 1966)
4. Reconstitution of the membrane structure (Martonosi, 1963, 1964)

B. Experiments on the sarcoplasmic reticulum in situ
1. Determination of the localization of Ca-binding sites by radioautography (Winegrad, 1968)
2. Time course of Ca^{++} release from the sarcoplasmic reticulum on stimulation visualized by using special indicators (Jöbsis and O'Connor, 1966; Ridgway and Ashley, 1967)
3. Effects of the Ca^{++} on Natori's fiber in oil (Natori, 1954; Podolsky and Constantin, 1964) and in a relaxing solution (Endo, 1967; Hellam and Podolsky, 1966)

SOME SELECTED PROCEDURES

Centrifugation Method. The reaction mixture, 10 ml in total, consists of 0.1 M KCl, 20 mM tris-maleate (pH 6.80), 10 mM (or 4 mM) $MgCl_2$, 0.1 mg protein/ml of relaxing factor, 0.01 mM ($CaCl_2$ + $^{45}CaCl_2$), 2 mM ATP, and various additions as desired. This mixture is put into a 12-ml cellulose Spinco ultracentrifuge tube. The reaction is started by adding ATP. Immediately after the addition of ATP, the tubes are centrifuged at 40,000 rpm for 15 min in No. 40 rotor of Spinco ultracentrifuge. All procedures up to this point are usually carried out below 4°C. Both the precipitate and supernatant are analyzed for ^{45}Ca radioactivity using a gas-flow counter or liquid scintillation counter. The following procedure employs a gas-flow counter. The precipitate is uniformly suspended* in 0.3 ml of distilled water with the aid of a glass rod, and poured onto a planchette. The tube is washed once with 0.1 ml of 0.1 N NaOH and twice with 0.3 ml of water. The washings are added to the planchette. An aliquot of the supernatant (usually 1 ml) is put onto a planchette. After the planchettes are once dried by an infrared lamp, the sediment is dissolved in water, and again thoroughly dried.† The amount of Ca^{++} bound to the "relaxing factor" is calculated according to the following equation:

Amount of Ca^{++} bound to the relaxing factor (A) =

$$\frac{\text{radioactivity of precipitate (cpm)}^{\ddagger}}{\text{total radioactivity (cpm)}^{\ddagger}} \times (\text{total } Ca^{++} \text{ in reaction mixture}^{\S})$$

ATP-dependent Ca^{++} binding = (A) with ATP − (A) without ATP

Double-Beam Spectrophotometry. Murexide is the only metal indicator that reacts with free Ca^{++} at neutral pH (its apparent binding constant at neutral pH is $4 \times 10^2\ M^{-1}$). The absorption spectrum of murexide shifts to the blue side if the dye is complexed with Ca^{++}.

The difference spectrum is zero at 507 mμ, maximum at 470 mμ, and minimum at 542 mμ. By measuring the optical density difference at two different wavelengths, 507 mμ and 542 mμ, in the same light path, artifacts resulting from the dispersion are practically negligible. The optical density differences between 507 mμ and 542 mμ changes linearly with the concentration of free Ca^{++}. Therefore, this method can determine with accuracy changes in the concentration of free Ca^{++} in the medium.

REACTION MIXTURE: 3 ml in total, consists of 0.1 M KCl, 20 mM tris-maleate (pH 6.80), 10 mM (or 4 mM) $MgCl_2$, 0.4 to 0.6 mg/ml of the relaxing factor, 0.5 mM murexide, and additions as desired. The temperature is adjusted by a circulating water bath. First, 30 microliters of 10 mM $CaCl_2$ and then 30 microliters of 40 mM ATP are added. The medium should be vigorously stirred after each addition. These procedures must be done as quickly as possible. Convenient instruments are the Hitachi Two-Wavelength/Double-Beam Spectrophotometer (Model 356) and the Aminco-Chance Dual Wavelength Spectrophotometer. A sample tracing is presented in Figures 1 and 2.

*Before this procedure, it is recommended that the wall of the centrifuge tube be wiped with filter paper carefully to remove any attached supernatant.

†This procedure is recommended to obtain constant and reproducible results.

‡These are values corrected to infinite thinness. In the case of Ca^{++}, this correction is necessary because of the low energy level of radiation (0.25 MeV).

§Total Ca = added Ca^{++} + contaminated Ca^{++} which should be determined by other methods (atomic absorption spectrophotometry or colorimetric measurements).

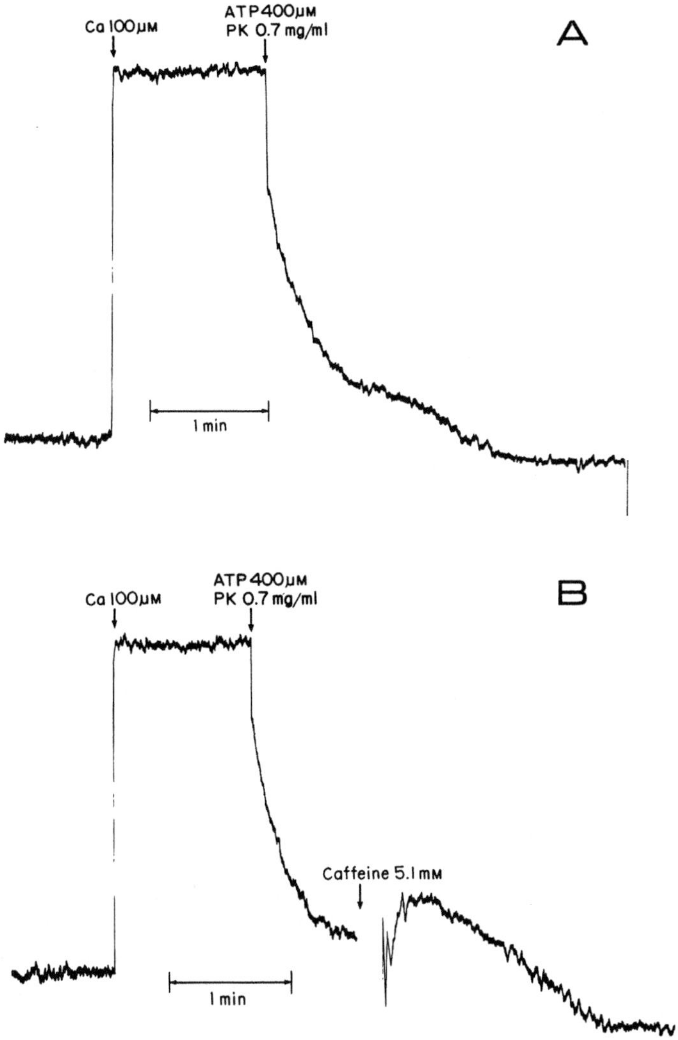

FIG. 1. The use of a dual wave length spectrophotometer for rapid measurement of "relaxing factor activity." (A) The reaction mixture consisted of 0.1 M KCl, 4 mM $MgCl_2$, 20 mM tris-maleate (pH 6.80), 2 mM phosphoenolpyruvate, 0.4 mg protein/ml of frog "relaxing factor" (9,000 — 54,500 × *g*), 0.5 mM murexide, 0.1 mM CaCl, 0.4 mM ATP, and 0.7 mg/ml of pyruvate kinase. Temperature, 15 °C. (B) The Ca-releasing effect of caffeine. Experimental conditions were the same as those in (A).

Millipore Filter Method. This method, introduced by Martonosi, is quite valuable for the measurement of Ca^{++} uptake by "relaxing factor" preparation. Usually, an appropriate funnel assembly (millipore-type, connected to a vacuum line) should be available. Ca^{++} uptake is terminated by filtration through the millipore filter (0.3 to 0.45 micron pore size). Since the diameter of the vesicles is about 0.1μ,

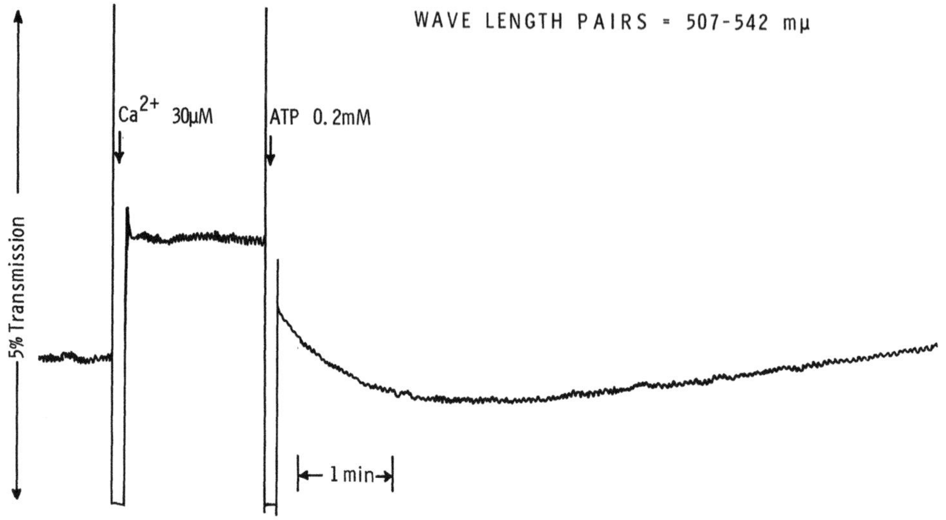

FIG. 2. The use of a dual wavelength spectrophotomer for rapid measurement of "relaxing factor activity." The reaction mixture consisted of 0.1M KCl, 10 mM $MgCl_2$, 20 mM tris-maleate buffer (pH 6.8), 0.3 mM murexide (Ammonium purpurate, Matheson Co., East Rutherford, New Jersey) and 1.3 mg/ml of cardiac "relaxing factor" from rabbit muscle; (Extraction medium contained 10 mM $NaHCO_3$ and 5mM Na azide, pH 7.0) the total volume was 3 ml. Thirty μl of 3 mM Ca solution (final concentration 30 μM), and 15 μl of 40 mM ATP (final conc. 0.2 mM) were added to the reaction mixture as indicated in the Figure. The first sharp peak after addition of ATP is an artifact. The reaction was carried out at room temperature (about 23 °C).

absorption of vesicles at the filter surface might be an important factor in separation of vesicles from the incubation mixture. The ingredients of the reaction medium have a great influence on the absorption, so one must check the extent of removal of the "relaxing factor" by the millipore filter, whenever the ingredients are changed. For example, Seidel (1967) reported that the bovine serum albumin makes the filter "leaky" to the "relaxing factor." Since the millipore filter has some detergent action which might damage the vesicles, contact of the mixture with the filter must be as short as possible.

PROCEDURE. After incubation for the selected time interval and at a specific temperature, 0.5 to 1.0 ml aliquot of the incubation mixture (the same as for the centrifugation method) is withdrawn with a pipette and immediately placed on the millipore suction apparatus connected to a vacuum line. 0.1 ml of the filtrate is added to scintillation vials containing appropriate fluid for liquid scintillation counting. The amount of Ca^{++} binding by the "relaxing factor" is calculated from the residual radioactivity in the filtrate compared with a control which is incubated in absence of ATP. As with the other calculation methods, the filter-entrapped sediment is dissolved in the fluid for liquid scintillation counting.*

*This fluid contains 10% naphthalene, 0.6% 2-5-diphenyl-oxazole (PPO) and 2% Methylcellosolve (ethylene glycol monoethylether) in dioxane. The radioactivity of the filter and the filtrate is counted, and the calcium content is calculated as described in the centrifuge method.

Superprecipitation of Actomyosin. Superprecipitation may be defined as the shrinkage of actomyosin gel in the presence of ATP. As a result, a considerable amount of water must be expelled from the gel. Consequently, superprecipitated actomyosin shows a higher local concentration of protein and, therefore, an increased apparent refractive index, which gives rise to the increase in the scattered light.

Actually, the optical absorbancy of actomyosin suspension increases markedly when actomyosin gel is "shrunken" by ATP (it decreases to some extent when the "clearing response" takes place). This change in absorbancy (turbidity) can be measured by an ordinary spectrophotometer.* The value of the change in absorbancy obtained by the spectrophotometer should be accepted only as a *relative* one, since scattered light due to the gel suspension is enormous in the direction near zero degrees, and therefore the absorbance is cancelled by the scattered light to a great extent. To avoid this difficulty, a particular device must be added to the spectrophotometer. However, this kind of consideration is not necessary if the experiment is concerned only with relative values.

The method is not difficult and the results obtained are very reproducible. However, if the preparations of actomyosin are not of good quality, a fine suspension cannot be formed after the addition of ATP, and there appears a tendency toward the formation of large aggregates, which make optical determinations impossible. To avoid this, the preparation of actomyosin should be made carefully, paying particular attention to the quality of the water used during the preparation. Resin-treated water should not be used in any case.

To determine the activity of "relaxing factor" we cannot use *synthetic* actomyosin; myosin B (natural actomyosin) must be employed, since the former lacks native tropomyosin (= tropomyosin + troponin), which enables actomyosin to respond to the changes in Ca^{++} concentration

Another important point is how to mix the reaction mixtures. The most convenient way of mixing is to use a "Komagome"-type pipette. If the quality of actomyosin preparation is good, only one mixing by this pipette after the addition of ATP is enough to follow the time course of absorbancy change of actomyosin suspension for at least 20 minutes.

This method is also applicable to the determination of syneresis of myofibrils (Ebashi and Endo, 1964).

REACTION MIXTURES: The response of myosin B (actomyosin) to ATP is variable from preparation to preparation and influenced by various conditions, particularly the ionic strength and the concentration of ATP (see Fig. 3). Therefore, appropriate conditions should be determined by preliminary experiments. The following is an example: Final concentrations: 30 mM KCl, 1 mM $MgCl_2$, 20 mM tris-maleate (pH 6.8), 0.5 mM ATP, 0.5 mg myosin B/ml, and a specific amount of the "relaxing factor" (0.02 to 0.2 mg/ml).

*The turbidometer (nephelometer) which measures scattered light at 90° cannot be used for this purpose. Scattered light due to large aggregates such as actomyosin gels does not follow the principle of Rayleigh's scattering. The degree of scattered light at 90° usually decreases in spite of the increase in the total scattered light.

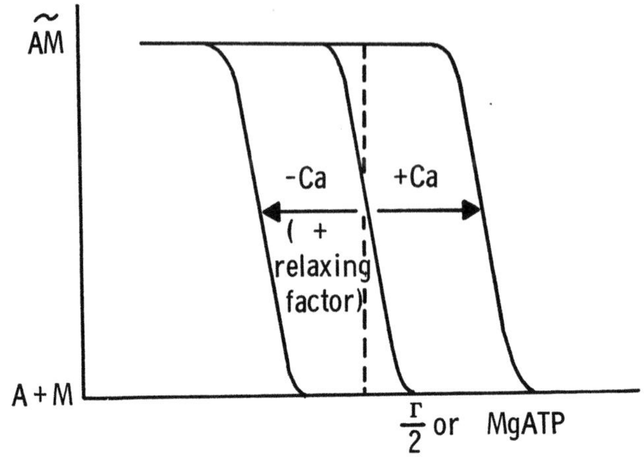

FIG. 3. Schematic presentation of the effect of ionic strength, the concentration of ATP, and Ca^{++} ions on the response of myosin B to ATP. $\widetilde{AM}$: Response of myosin B which corresponds to contraction. A+M: Response which corresponds to relaxation.

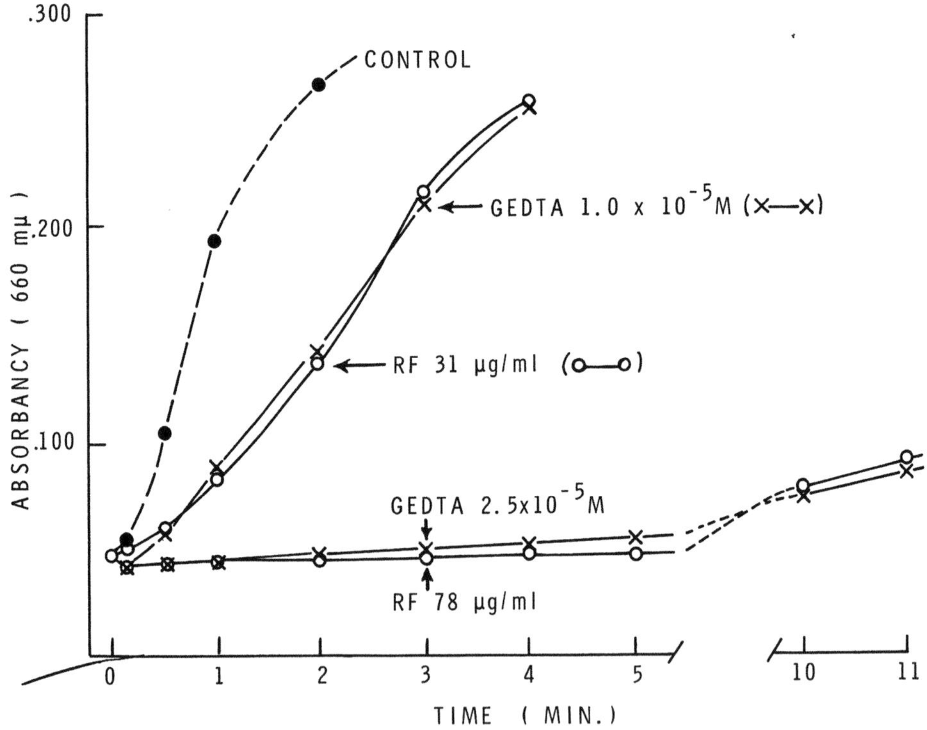

FIG. 4. Relaxing activities of GEDTA and the "relaxing factor" (RF). The reaction mixture contains 50 mM KCl, 1 mM $MgCl_2$, 20 mM tris-maleate buffer (pH 6.80), 0.50 mg of myosin B per ml, and GEDTA or "relaxing factor" as indicated. ATP, in a final concentration of 1 mM, was added at zero time. Temperature, 19°C.

PROCEDURES: A 4-ml cuvette is filled with the preceding ingredients, except ATP, up to 3.9 ml. The order of addition of these ingredients does not matter. The reaction is started by adding 0.1 ml of ATP solution and the change in optical density at 660 mμ is read at intervals of 30 sec. The delay in the time course of the turbidity development in the presence of the "relaxing factor" compared with that in the absence of the "relaxing factor" is considered due to the relaxing action of the "factor." To obtain quantitative results, the degree of inhibition should be compared with an appropriate concentration of GEDTA (Fig. 4).

In the case of the "relaxing factor" of red muscle, Ca^{++} binding is lower in quantity and slower in velocity than a similar preparation from white muscle. The development of the turbidity increase in the control experiment should be much slower than in the case of "relaxing factor" from white muscle. This can be accomplished by elevating the ionic strength of the reaction mixture or the concentration of MgATP (Harigaya et al., 1968).

Preparation of Ca^{++} Buffer. Most experiments involving relaxing systems should be carried out in a medium containing a very low concentration of Ca^{++} (about 10^{-6} M). Therefore, in order to maintain a constant concentration of Ca^{++} in the presence of Mg^{++}, we must use a Ca^{++} buffer system. GEDTA is the most preferable agent, since this substance has a high affinity for Ca^{++} and low affinity for Mg^{++} (practically negligible at neutral pH). The apparent binding constant (K′)* of GEDTA for Ca^{++} depends on pH in accordance with the following equation (around neutral pH):

$$\log K' = \log K - (pk_3 + pk_4) + 2pH \qquad (1)$$

Where K represents the binding constant ($K = 10^{11.0}$) and k_3 and k_4 the third and fourth dissociation constants ($pk_3 = 8.85$, $pk_4 = 9.43$). The following equations are obtained:

$$\left.\begin{aligned} K' &= \frac{[CaG]}{[Ca]_{free}[G]_{free}} \\ [Ca]_{total} &= [CaG] + [Ca]_{free} \\ [G]_{total} &= [CaG] + [G]_{free} \end{aligned}\right\} \qquad (2)$$

where $[Ca]_{total}$ and $[G]_{total}$ represent the total concentrations of Ca^{++} and GEDTA respectively; $[Ca]_{free}$ and $[G]_{free}$ the concentration of free Ca^{++} and GEDTA not complexed with Ca^{++} respectively; and [CaG] the concentration of Ca-GEDTA chelate. From equation (2)

$$[G]_{total} = ([Ca]_{total} - [Ca]_{free})\frac{1 + K'[Ca]_{free}}{K'[Ca]_{free}} \qquad (3)$$

$$\left(\text{if } [Ca]_{total} \gg [Ca]_{free}, \text{ then } [G]_{total} = [Ca]_{total}\frac{1 + K'[Ca]_{free}}{K'[Ca]_{free}}\right)$$

*See footnote, Table 1.

Using equation (3), the amount of Ca^{++} and GEDTA can be determined for the desired concentration of free Ca^{++} to be employed. When GEDTA chelates Ca^{++} at neutral pH, GEDTA liberates nearly two protons for one Ca^{++}. To avoid acidification of the solution due to this proton liberation, it is convenient to prepare two solutions, Ca-GEDTA (1:1) solution and GEDTA solution, the pH's of which are adjusted.
The final Ca^{++} buffer solution can be obtained by mixing both solutions in an appropriate ratio without giving rise to a marked pH change. Even with these conditions, it is preferable that the pH of the resulting solution should be checked.

EFFECTS OF DRUGS ON Ca^{++} UPTAKE

Caffeine is the only drug thus far whose effect on fragmented sarcoplasmic reticulum has been proved to be a possible mechanism underlying its pharmacologic action on living muscle. The primary effect of caffeine on the "relaxing factor" or fragmented sarcoplasmic reticulum is to release Ca^{++} which has been accumulated in the reticulum (Weber, 1966). This releasing effect is completely blocked by procaine.

Ca^{++}, once released by caffeine, is eventually taken up by the reticulum even in the presence of caffeine, and the amount of accumulated Ca^{++} in the final stage is not so much different from that of control experiments (Fig. 1). The rate of Ca^{++} uptake is moderately depressed by caffeine. The sarcoplasmic reticulum has an inherent property to release Ca^{++} which has been accumulated. Caffeine is considered to be a promotor of this releasing mechanism, rather than to be an inhibitor of Ca^{++} accumulating processes.

Other drugs or agents that affect the Ca^{++} uptake of the sarcoplasmic reticulum are listed in Table 1. Although the action of some of them is very pronounced, their action does not seem to have pharmacologic significance.

Addendum in Proof

(i) An improved method for the preparation of red muscle microsomes has been reported (Harigaya, S., and Schwartz, A., 1969. Circ. Res., 25:781). The crucial point of the method was the use of Polytron instead of Waring Blendor. It was applicable to the preparation of heart muscle microsomes or brain microsomes. (ii) Although further conclusive evidence is required, the sarcoplasmic reticulum seems to be involved in the mechanism of action of ryanodine ($C_{25}H_{35}NO_9$, an alkaloid from the ground stem wood and root of *Ryania speciosa;* cf. Jenden, D.J., and Fairhurst, A.S., 1969. Pharmacol. Rev., 21:1-26).

REFERENCES

Balzer, H., Makinose, M., and Hasselbach, W. 1968. The inhibition of the sarcoplasmic calcium pump by prenylamine, reserpine, chlorpromazine and imipramine. Naunyn-Schmiedebergs Arch. Pharm. Exp. Path., 260:444-455.

Bendall, J. R. 1953. Further observation on a factor (the 'Marsh' factor) effecting relaxation of ATP-shortened muscle-fibre models, and the effect of Ca and Mg ions upon it. J. Physiol. (London), 121:232-254.

Carsten, M. E., and Mommaerts, W. F. H. M. 1964. The accumulation of calcium ions by sarcotubular vesicles. J. Gen. Physiol., 48:183-197.

Carvalho, A. P., and Leo, B. 1967. Effects of ATP on the interaction of Ca^{++}, Mg^{++} and K^{+} with fragmented sarcoplasmic reticulum isolated from rabbit skeletal muscle. J. Gen. Physiol., 50:1327-1352.

Ebashi, F. and Yamanouchi, I. 1964. Calcium accumulation and adenosine triphosphatase of the relaxing factor. J. Biochem., 55:504-509.

Ebashi, S. 1961. Calcium binding activity of vesicular relaxing factor. J. Biochem., 50:236-244.

—1965. The sarcoplasmic reticulum and excitation-contraction coupling. *In* Molecular Biology of Muscular Contraction. Ebashi, S., Oosawa, F., Sekine, T., and Tonomura, Y., eds. Amsterdam, Elsevier Publishing Company, pp. 197-206.

—and Endo, M. 1964. Further Studies on the calcium binding activity of the relaxing factor. *In* Biochemistry of Muscle Contraction. Gergely, J., ed. Boston, Little, Brown and Company, pp. 199-206.

—and Endo, M. 1968. Calcium ion and muscle contraction. Progr. Biophys. Mol. Biol., 18:123-183.

—and Lipmann, F. 1962. Adenosine triphosphate-linked concentration of calcium ions in a particulate fraction of rabbit muscle. J. Cell Biol., 14:389-400.

—Ebashi, F., and Fujie, Y. 1960. The effect of EDTA and its analogues on glycerinated muscle fibers and myosin adenosinetriphosphatase. J. Biochem., 47:54-59.

Endo, M. 1967. Regulation of contraction-relaxation cycle of muscle (in Japanese). Proc. XVII Gen. Ass. Japan Med. Congr., pp. 193-197.

Gergely, J., Pragay, D., Scholz, A. F., Seidel, J. C., Sreter, F. A., and Tompson, M. M. 1965. Comparative studies on white and red muscle. *In* Molecular Biology of Muscular Contraction. Ebashi, S., Oosawa, T., Sekine, T., and Tonomura, Y., eds. Amsterdam, Elsevier Publishing Company, pp. 145-159.

Harigaya, S., and Schwartz, A. 1969. The rate of calcium binding and uptake in animal and human cardiac muscle: Membrane vesicles ("relaxing system") and mitochondria. Circ. Res., 25:781-794.

—Ogawa, Y., and Sugita, H. 1968. Calcium binding activity of microsomal fraction of rabbit red muscle. J. Biochem., 63:324-331.

Hasselbach, W. 1964. Relaxing factor and the relaxation of muscle. Progr. Biophys. Biophys. Chem., 14:167-222.

—and Makinose, M. 1961. Die Calciumpumpe der "Erschlaffungsgrana" des Muskels und ihre Abhängigkeit von der ATP-spaltung. Biochem. Z., 333:518-528.

—and Makinose, M. 1963. Über der Mechanismus des Calciumtransportes durch die Membranen des sarkoplasmatischen Reticulums. Biochem. Z., 339:94-111.

Hellam, D. C., and Podolsky, R. J. 1966. The relation between calcium concentration and isometric force in skinned frog muscle fibers. Fed. Proc., 25:466.

Inesi, G. and Watanabe, S. 1967. Temperature dependence of ATP hydrolysis and calcium uptake by fragmented sarcoplasmic reticulum. Arch. Biochem. Biophys., 121:665-671.

—Ebashi, S., and Watanabe, S. 1964. Preparation of vesicular relaxing factor from bovine heart tissue. Amer. J. Physiol., 207:1339-1344.

—Goodman, J. J., and Watanabe, S. 1967. Effects of diethylether on the adenosine triphosphatase activity and the calcium uptake of fragmented sarcoplasmic reticulum of rabbit skeletal muscle. J. Biol. Chem., 242:4637–4643.

Jöbsis, F. F., and O'Connor, M. J. 1966. Calcium release and reabsorption in the sartorius muscle of the toad. Biochem. Biophys. Res. Commun., 25:246-252.

Lee, K. S. 1965. Present status of cardiac relaxing factor. Fed. Proc., 24:1432.

—Ladinsky, H., Choi, S. J., and Kasuya, Y. 1966. Studies on the in vitro interaction of electrical stimulation and Ca^{++} movement in sarcoplasmic reticulum. J. Gen. Physiol., 49:689.

Lorand, L., and Molnar, J. 1962. Biochemical control of relaxation in muscle systems. *In* Muscle as a Tissue. Rodahl, K., and Horvath, S. M., eds. New York, McGraw-Hill Book Company, pp. 97-127.
Makinose, M., and Hasselbach, W. 1965. Der Einfluss von Oxalat auf den Calciumtransport isolierter Vesikel des sarkoplasmatischen Reticulum. Biochem. Z., 343:360-382.
Martonosi, A. 1963. The activating effect of phospholipids on the ATPase activity and Ca^{++} transport of fragmented sarcoplasmic reticulum. Biochem. Biophys. Res. Commun., 13:273-278.
—1964. Role of phospholipids in ATPase activity and Ca transport of fragmented sarcoplasmic reticulum. Fed. Proc., 23:913-921.
—and Feretos, R. 1964. Sarcoplasmic reticulum: I. The uptake of Ca^{++} by sarcoplasmic reticulum fragments. J. Biol. Chem., 239:648-658.
Nagai, T., Makinose, M., and Hasselbach, W. 1960. Der physiologische Erschlaffungsfaktor und die Muskelgrana. Biochim. Biophys. Acta, 43:223-238.
Natori, R. 1954. The property and contraction process of isolated myofibrils. Jikeikai Med. J., 1:119-126.
Ohnishi, T., and Ebashi, S. 1963. Spectrophotometrical measurement of instantaneous calcium binding of the relaxing factor of muscle. J. Biochem., 54:506-511.
—and Ebashi, S. 1964. The velocity of calcium binding of isolated sarcoplasmic reticulum. J. Biochem., 55:599-603.
Ogawa, Y. 1968. The apparent binding constant of glycoletherdiaminetetraacetic acid for calcium at neutral pH. J. Biochem. (In press.)
Podolsky, R. J., and Costantin, L. L. 1964. Regulation by calcium of the contraction and relaxation of muscle fibers. Fed. Proc., 23:933-939.
Portzehl, M., Caldwell, P. C., and Rüegg, J. C. 1964. The dependence of contraction and relaxation of muscle fibres from the crab *Maia squinado* on the internal concentration of free calcium ions. Biochim. Biophys. Acta, 79:581-591.
Ridgway, E. B., and Ashley, C. C. 1967. Calcium transients in single muscle fibers. Biochem. Biophys. Res. Commun., 29:229-234.
Schwarzenbach, G., Senn, H., and Anderegg, B. 1957. Komplexone XXIX Ein grosser Chelateffekt besonderer Art. Helv. Chim. Acta, 40:1886-1900.
Seidel, J. C., 1967. The effect of soluble proteins on the fragmented sarcoplasmic reticulum. Biochim. Biophys. Acta, 131:213-217.
Smith, D. S. 1966. The organization and function of the sarcoplasmic reticulum and T-system of muscle cells. *In* Progress in Biophysics and Molecular Biology. New York, Pergamon Press, Vol. 16, pp. 107-142.
Sreter, F. A., and Gergely, J. 1964. Comparative studies of the Mg activated ATPase activity and Ca uptake of fractions of white and red muscle homogenates. Biochem. Biophys. Res. Commun., 16:438-443.
Takauji, M., Yamamoto, T., and Nagai, T. 1967. On the relaxing factor system in rabbit red muscle. Jap. J. Physiol., 17:111-121.
Weber, A. 1966. Energized calcium transport and relaxing factors. *In* Current Topics in Bionergetics. Sanadi, D. R., ed. New York, Academic Press, Inc., Vol. 1, pp. 203-254.
—and Herz, R. 1963. The binding of calcium to actomyosin systems in relation to their biological activity. J. Biol. Chem., 238:599-605.
—Herz, R., and Reiss, I. 1963. On the mechanism of the relaxing effect of fragmented sarcoplasmic reticulum. J. Gen. Physiol., 46:679-702.
—Herz, R., and Reiss, I. 1966. Study of the kinetics of calcium transport by isolated fragmented sarcoplasmic reticulum. Biochem. Z., 345:329-369.
Willis, J. B. 1963. Analysis of biological materials by atomic absorption spectroscopy. *In* Methods of Biochemical Analysis. Glick, D., ed. London, Interscience Publishers, Vol. 2, pp. 1-67.
Winegrad, S. 1968. Intracellular calcium movements of frog skeletal muscle during recovery from tetanus. J. Gen. Physiol., 51:65-83.

CHAPTER **11**

The Erythrocyte Ghost

A Model for the Study of Drug Effects on the Two Related Processes of Ion Transport and Cell Metabolism

Amir Askari

Department of Pharmacology, Cornell University Medical College
New York, New York

INTRODUCTION

> I have been told that I tend to speak of the red cell as if it were a microcosm, and as if an understanding of its nature and properties would include an understanding of nearly everything else in the cellular world. To some extent this is true, for there is scarcely a fundamental problem in General Physiology which does not have a relation, of one kind or another, to the problems which have arisen in connection with the erythrocyte.
>
> E. Ponder (1948).

In the complex and delicate world of biology, general concepts and theories are often evolved from the interpretation of observed properties of an experimen-

The investigations of the author referred to or described in this chapter were supported by the U.S. Public Health Service grant HE 10884 from the National Heart Institute and by a grant-in-aid from the New York Heart Association.

tal model system. Judgment about the value of any such model should be based neither on its obvious limitations nor on its esthetic qualities, but rather on the utility (not correctness!) of concepts that have evolved from it. From this viewpoint, the red cell has been an invaluable model in the development of our present knowledge of the physiology and biophysics of the cell membrane.

The use of the red cell for the study of cellular transport phenomena began in the latter part of the nineteenth century. It was assumed then that this cell was nearly dead and, therefore, a good model at a level of complexity somewhere between inanimate systems and living cells. Although subsequent events proved the red cell to be quite alive, the enthusiasm of the biologist for it as a model was in no way dampened. In fact, the recognition of the control of membrane permeability to ions by cellular metabolism, and the development of the concept of active transport, were based largely on studies with the red cell. The complete history of these investigations may be found in several excellent monographs (Ponder, 1934, 1948; Prankerd, 1961; Whittam, 1964).

Early in this century it was realized that from the hemolysates of erythrocytes a precipitate or sediment could be separated which consists not of disrupted cells, but of cell-like bodies or "ghosts." The ghost has approximately the same size as the intact erythrocyte, and under the microscope appears as a vacuole with a surrounding wall. Thus, it was quite natural to suspect that the ghost is the membrane of the erythrocyte. This led a number of investigators to direct their attention to determinations of the chemical composition, structure, and a variety of physical properties of the ghosts. An exhaustive review of these studies up to 1961 has been published (Ponder, 1961).

A few contradictory observations on the alkali cation permeability of ghosts appeared in the older literature. The first detailed study showing that the ghost, like the intact erythrocyte, could maintain appreciable concentration differences of Na^+ and K^+ across its membrane was that of Teorell (1952). However, he stated in this report that "whether this phenomenon is due simply to very low cation permeability or to active transport processes cannot be decided, although the first assumption appears more probable." A stimulus to the further development of the ghost systems for the study of alkali cation transport mechanisms came from the work of Gardos (1954). He demonstrated that active transport of K^+ occurs in ghosts that are obtained by the hemolysis of erythrocytes in a hypotonic solution containing ATP. Since then, the ability of ghosts to transport both Na^+ and K^+ actively has been demonstrated in several different preparations of ghosts (Hoffman et al., 1960; Hoffman, 1962; Garrahan and Glynn, 1967a).

Some of these ghosts are particularly suitable for studies on the mechanism of coupling between cellular chemical reactions and the transport of ions because (a) they are deficient in metabolic substrates and intermediates; (b) most, if not all, of the glycolytic enzymes are present in them and therefore metabolism and active transport may be initiated with the addition of appropriate substrates; and (c) it is possible to introduce various substrates and large molecules, such as foreign proteins and enzymes, into them at the time of preparation. These interesting properties have already enabled investigators to provide answers to several previously unsettled questions. For example, the role of ATP as an energy source for the active transport of alkali cations has been demonstrated in the ghosts (Hoffman, 1960; Gardos, 1964; Garrahan and Glynn, 1967b). Prior to this work, the role of ATP was strictly inferred from studies of intact cells and isolated enzyme systems.

It is quite evident from the current literature that the most popular view is that "the ghost of the mammalian red cell, when prepared by osmotic and even most lytic means, represents as closely as possible a plasma membrane" (Parpart and Ballentine, 1952). It should be pointed out, however, that after a critical review of the available evidence, Ponder (1961) stated: "Nothing proves that the ghost represents a membrane of preexisting nature situated at the surface of the intact red cell." Since this statement was made, no additional evidence that is sufficiently compelling to settle this controversy has appeared. Whether the ghost is an intact saclike membrane or a solid structured body derived from the cell is usually decided on the basis of preexisting opinions rather than adequate evidence.

Whatever else the ghost may be, it is certain that at this time it is the simplest known model system in which transport of alkali cations and the biochemical energetics of the transport can be studied *simultaneously*. It is this feature that makes the ghost an attractive model to the cellular pharmacologist. Drugs whose actions are suspected to relate to their influence on the biochemical mechanisms controlling Na^+ and K^+ transport can be studied in ghosts with the hope that what is found in this model system will shed light on the molecular mechanism of drug action at the site of pharmacologic interest (e.g., Rao and Askari, 1968).

In this chapter two different preparations of ghosts that have been used extensively in the author's laboratory are described. Both are modifications of methods first used by others. It is hoped that these detailed descriptions will remove the aura of mystery that has surrounded the preparation of ghosts and has made it useful in the hands of only a few.

Some final words of caution about the ghosts are appropriate. There are perhaps as many different ghost preparations as the number of people who have worked with them. The investigator who begins to work with ghosts should not be surprised if by simple modifications of techniques he obtains a preparation that behaves differently from those described by others. One could argue endlessly as to which preparation is more "real," in respect either to the intact cell or to the "pure membrane." Instead, it would be more profitable to search for different preparations and to exploit them much in the same way that the biochemist has used the various preparations of submitochondrial particles and fractions.

PREPARATION OF ^{22}Na-LABELED GHOSTS (TYPE I)

SOLUTIONS

1. Wash Solution: 12 mM $MgCl_2$, 1.7 mM tris-HCl (pH 7.4). The solution must be cold (4° to 6°C) when used.
2. ^{22}Na solution: A convenient stock solution, sufficient for approximately thirty ghost preparations as described here, is made as follows: One millicurie of ^{22}Na, which is usually supplied in a small volume of hydrochloric acid

solution, is diluted to about 8 ml in a small plastic container. A few drops of concentrated tris solution (1 M) is added to raise the pH to a range of 6 to 8. The use of small strips of pH test paper is suggested for this purpose. The final volume is adjusted to 10 ml, and the container is stored behind a lead shield.

PROCEDURE. Forty milliliters of blood are withdrawn from a healthy adult using a 50-ml plastic syringe and an 18-gauge needle. After taking the needle off the syringe, blood is delivered with gentle mixing into a 50-ml polycarbonate centrifuge tube containing 150 mg of trisodium citrate. The tube is capped and centrifuged at 6,000 × *g* (5,000 rpm, Lourdes 9 RA rotor) for 10 minutes at 4°C. The plasma, buffy coat, and the top layer of the red cells are removed with a Pasteur pipette. Packed cells (about 14 ml) are transferred to a breaker. Then 150 ml of deionized water at room temperature are poured over the cells with rapid mixing. The mixture (hemolysate) is allowed to stand at room temperature for 10 minutes and is then thoroughly mixed with 0.3 ml of the stock solution of ^{22}Na. The vessel containing the mixture is now placed in a water bath at 37°C and shaken for 40 minutes. The incubated hemolysate is divided into four equal parts and each part is placed in a 50-ml polycarbonate centrifuge tube. The tubes are capped and centrifuged at 4°C for 30 minutes at 20,000 × *g* (12,500 rpm Lourdes 9 RA rotor). After centrifugation, if each tube is held against a bright light, the presence of a sediment under the dark red supernatant becomes evident.* The supernatant solution is decanted carefully and discarded.† Each tube is filled to a volume of 40 ml with the cold wash solution. The mixture is gently stirred with a plastic rod before being placed in the cold centrifuge rotor. After standing for 3 minutes, the hemolysates are centrifuged at 20,000 × *g* for 10 minutes. This is sufficient to sediment the ghosts at this stage of the preparation. The red supernatant solution is again discarded, and the washing is repeated as before. After four washings, the colorless (or slightly pink) supernatant is discarded and the loosely packed ghosts are pooled and mixed. The volume of the ghost suspension at this point is about 18 to 20 ml.

STORAGE: It is best to plan the experiments so that the ghosts are used immediately after preparation. If they must be stored, they may be kept at 4° to 6°C for no more than 4 hours. Longer storage periods increase the possibility of failure of experiments (see pp. 356-357). After overnight storage the ghosts are completely deteriorated.

*It is important to ascertain the proper packing of the ghosts at this point. Occasionally, for unknown reasons, complete sedimentation does not occur. In these cases centrifugation for another 20 minutes at the same speed should be repeated. The routine centrifugation of every preparation for longer periods, or at higher speeds, is not recommended. While such procedures result in better and more consistent packing, they also make the subsequent resuspension and washing of the ghosts more difficult.

†Since the largest portion of Na is discarded in this supernatant, it is appropriate to point out that throughout these experiments the local regulations concerning the disposal of radioactive materials should be followed.

PREPARATION OF ATP-FILLED AND ^{22}NA-LABELED GHOSTS (TYPE II)

SOLUTIONS

1. Hemolysis solution: 12 mM NaCl; 2 mM Na_2ATP, 3 mM MgCl. This solution (150 ml) is made freshly for each ghost preparation.

2. Wash solution: 30 mM $MgCl_2$, 3.5 mM tris-HCl (pH 7.4). This solution must be cold (4° to 6°C) when used.

3. ^{22}Na solution: This is the same solution that is described above (pp. 349-350).

PROCEDURE. This procedure is the same as that previously described (p. 350) with the following exceptions:

1. Packed cells are hemolyzed in the ATP-containing hemolysis solution instead of water.
2. After hemolysis, the mixture is allowed to stand at room temperature for 50 minutes before it is centrifuged and washed.
3. A different wash solution (see 2, above) is used. The final volume of the Type II ghost suspension is about 22 to 26 ml.

STORAGE. The remarks made about the stability of Type I ghosts (p. 350, Storage) also apply to Type II ghosts.

DEMONSTRATION OF ACTIVE TRANSPORT OF Na^+ IN TYPE I AND TYPE II GHOSTS

The design of experiments for the determination of ^{22}Na release from either of the foregoing ghost preparations depends on the purpose of the experiments, parameters other than ^{22}Na release which are to be measured, and the available equipment in the laboratory. The procedures described in this section are intended to serve as examples of the type of experiments that could be performed with these ghosts. The aims of the described experiments are to show (a) that a fairly accurate determination of the time course of ^{22}Na release from the ghosts may be made with the aid of relatively simple equipment; (b) that in Type I ghosts active transport of Na^+ occurs, and is coupled to the metabolism of a substrate; and (c) that in Type II ghosts, the Na^+ pump may be driven by ATP in the absence of substrate metabolism.

SOLUTIONS.

1. NaCl stock solution: 160 mM NaCl, 10 mM tris-HCl (pH 7.45). Appropriate amounts of NaCl and tris base are dissolved in water, and the pH is adjusted by addition of HCl. After final volume adjustment, the solution is stored at cold temperature (4° to 6°C).

2. KCl stock solution: 160 mM KCl, 10 mM tris-HCl (pH 7.45). This is prepared and stored as above.

3. NaCl-inosine stock solution: 155 mM NaCl, 5 mM inosine, 10 mM tris-HCl (pH 7.45). Inosine is added prior to pH adjustment. This solution should not be stored for more than a week.

4. NaCl-iodoacetate solution: This is similar to solution 1. Sodium iodoacetate (1 mM, 0.2 mg/ml) is added prior to pH adjustment.

5. NaCl-inosine-iodoacetate solution: This is similar to solution 3. Sodium iodoacetate (1 mM) is added prior to pH adjustment. The stability is the same as that of solution 3.

6. Ouabain stock solution: 5 mM ouabain (36 mg/10 ml of water). This solution is stable in cold for several months.

7. Phosphate stock solution: 120 mM phosphate (pH 7.45). Appropriate amounts of disodium phosphate are dissolved in water and the pH is adjusted with the addition of HCl.

EXPERIMENTS WITH TYPE I GHOSTS.

Incubation media:

1. 43 ml of NaCl-inosine solution
   2 ml of KCl solution
   5 ml of phosphate solution

2. 43 ml of NaCl-inosine solution
   2 ml of KCl solution
   5 ml of NaCl solution

3. 45 ml of NaCl-inosine solution
   5 ml of phosphate solution

4. 43 ml of NaCl solution
   2 ml of KCl solution
   5 ml of phosphate solution

5. 43 ml of NaCl-inosine-iodoacetate solution

2 ml of KCl solution
5 ml of phosphate solution

6. 43 ml of NaCl-inosine solution
   2 ml of KCl solution
   5 ml of phosphate solution
   0.1 ml of ouabain solution

Two ml of Type I ghosts are added to each of the above media. The release of ^{22}Na into each medium is measured at five different time intervals according to the method described below (pp. 353-354).

EXPERIMENTS WITH TYPE II GHOSTS.

Incubation media:
1. 50 ml of NaCl solution

2. 48 ml of NaCl solution
   2 ml of KCl solution

3. 48 ml of NaCl-iodoacetate solution
   2 ml of KCl solution

4. 48 ml of NaCl solution
   2 ml of KCl solution
   0.1 ml ouabain solution

Two ml of Type II ghosts are added to each of the above media, and the ^{22}Na released into each medium is measured according to the following method.

DETERMINATION OF TIME COURSE OF ^{22}Na RELEASE. Fifty milliliters of the incubation medium (as in the two previous experiments) are placed in a 250-ml flask and incubated for 10 minutes in a shaking water bath at 37°C. Two milliliters of the ghost suspension are mixed with the solution. Immediately after mixing, approximately 8 ml of the mixture are rapidly withdrawn and delivered into a plastic centrifuge tube placed in an ice bath. The remainder of the mixture is shaken in the water bath. Using a volumetric pipette, 3 ml of the withdrawn sample are transferred to a counting tube ($S^0{}_1$). The tube containing the remainder of the sample is placed in the refrigerated centrifuge. The centrifuge is started, its speed raised to 20,000 × *g*, and then immediately turned off. This is sufficient to separate the ghosts from the medium. Without disturbing the sedimented button of ghosts, 3 ml of the clear supernatant solution are withdrawn and transferred to a counting tube ($S^0{}_2$). Both samples ($S^0{}_1$ and $S^0{}_2$) may be saved for counting at a later time (see, however, p. 356, B). At suitable time intervals, 8-ml portions of the incubation mixture are withdrawn and treated as above. At the end of the experiment all samples ($S^0{}_1$, $S^{t_1}{}_1$, $S^{t_2}{}_1$. . .; and $S^0{}_2$, $S^{t_1}{}_2$, $S^{t_2}{}_2$ . . .) are counted in

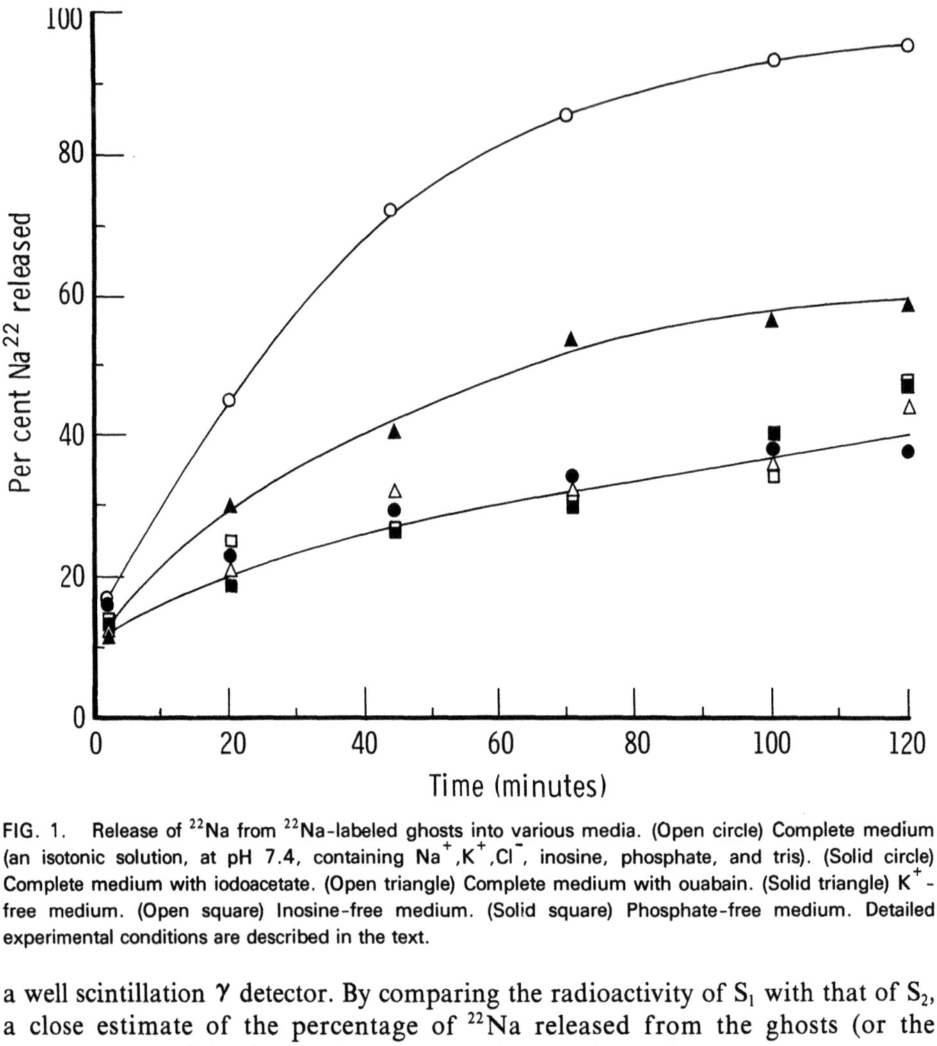

FIG. 1. Release of ^{22}Na from ^{22}Na-labeled ghosts into various media. (Open circle) Complete medium (an isotonic solution, at pH 7.4, containing Na^+,K^+,Cl^-, inosine, phosphate, and tris). (Solid circle) Complete medium with iodoacetate. (Open triangle) Complete medium with ouabain. (Solid triangle) K^+-free medium. (Open square) Inosine-free medium. (Solid square) Phosphate-free medium. Detailed experimental conditions are described in the text.

a well scintillation γ detector. By comparing the radioactivity of S_1 with that of S_2, a close estimate of the percentage of ^{22}Na released from the ghosts (or the percentage remaining in the ghosts) at any time can be made.*

RESULTS. The results of experiments described on pp. 352 and 353 are shown in Figues 1 and 2. As evident from the data of Figure 1, in Type I ghosts there is a component of ^{22}Na release which is dependent on the simultaneous

*It should be realized that the measured ^{22}Na of the ghost-free supernatant in this procedure does not, in fact, indicate the exact value of the release of ^{22}Na at the time of sample withdrawal from the incubation mixture. This is due to the fact that a few minutes elapse between the moment of withdrawal and the time that ghosts are cooled and finally separated from the mixture in the centrifuge. Another source of error introduced at the beginning of the experiment is the time lapse between the moment of addition of the ghosts to the medium and the time of withdrawal of the first sample. It is evident that the errors due to both of the foregoing factors are increased when two or more experiments are performed simultaneously, as in the experiments described on pp. 352 and 353. However, in such experiments of long duration, the preceding errors do not affect the results significantly. When more accurate measurements of ^{22}Na release within a short period of time after incubation are desired, these errors, which are inherent in the technique, must be considered seriously. In such cases, it is advisable to use a rapid filtration technique, rather than cooling and centrifugation.

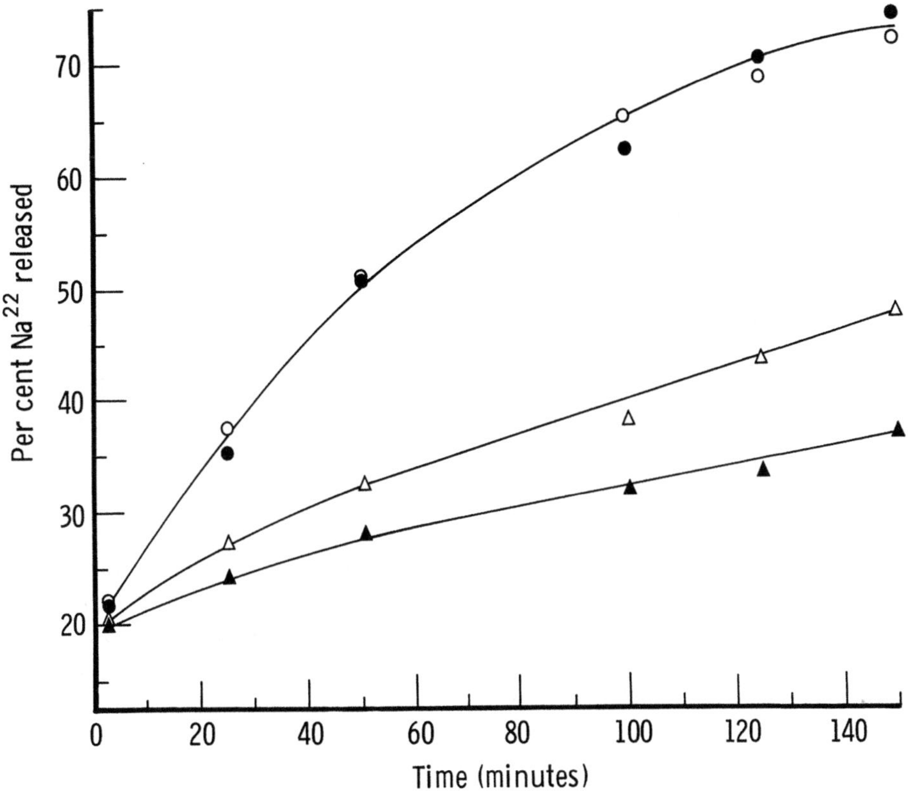

FIG. 2 Release of ^{22}Na from ATP-filled and ^{22}Na-labeled ghosts into various media. (Open circle) Complete medium (an isotonic solution, at pH 7.4, containing Na^+,K^+,Cl^-, and tris). (Solid circle) Complete medium with iodoacetate. (Solid triangle) Complete medium with ouabain. (Open triangle) K^--free medium. Detailed experimental conditions are described in the text.

presence of inosine, phosphate, and K^+ in the outside medium. Ribose of inosine and some endogenous substrates supply the triosephosphate for substrate level phosphorylation (Askari and Rao, 1968). The requirement of this component of Na^+ efflux for external K^+ and its sensitivity to ouabain characterize it as the classical coupled Na^+-K^+ pump. In these ghosts, the absolute dependence of the pump on substrate-level phosphorylation is evident by the immediate and complete inhibition of the pump by iodoacetate. The date of Figure 2 show that in Type II ghosts, without supplying the ghosts with an external substrate, there is a component of ^{22}Na release which is dependent on external K^+ and is ouabainsensitive. These facts again characterize this component as the coupled Na^+-K^+ pump. It is also evident that iodoacetate has no effect on the pump in Type II ghosts, thus indicating that here the pump is not dependent on metabolism and is being driven by ATP.

SOME OTHER POSSIBLE EXPERIMENTS. A correlation between the pump and metabolism in Type I ghosts, or a relationship between ATP hydrolysis and the operation of the pump in Type II ghosts, may be demonstrated more directly by modifying the experiments of pp. 352-353 to obtain higher ghost/medium values. In the first case, lactate is determined by standard methods in the course of the experiment, and in the second case either the increase in inorganic phosphate or the decrease in "easily hydrolyzable" phosphate is determined.

"BAD" GHOSTS

Even with strict adherence to the previous procedures, some of the ghost preparations are not suitable for the type of experiments described here. In the course of a year approximately 10 percent of 110 preparations made in our laboratory were considered failures. The different kinds of failures, their possible causes, and methods for detecting them with the minimum amount of wasted effort follow:

A. It should be evident that if experiments described in previous sections are to be successful, sufficient ^{22}Na should be retained by the ghosts after the repeated washings described on pp. 349-350 and 351. For unknown reasons the variation in the amount of retained ^{22}Na in different preparations (especially in Type I ghosts) is quite large. We have adapted the following arbitrary procedure for determining the adequacy of retained ^{22}Na. After each preparation is completed, 0.1 ml of the ghost suspension is diluted with 3 ml of water, and the radioactivity of the sample is determined with a γ counter (Nuclear Chicago DS-202 detector and 186 Scaler). If the activity is less than 5,000 cpm over the background (300 to 500 cpm), the preparation is considered a failure. Only about 4 percent of the preparations are rejected on this basis. In the rest of the preparations the average activity is about 13,000 cpm. Of course, it is possible to eliminate the "low count" failures by increasing the amount of ^{22}Na added to the hemolysis mixture. This is desirable when the number of preparations to be made is relatively small. However, when a great number of routine experiments are to be done, it is more economical to use the minimum required amounts of ^{22}Na and accept the possibility of a small number of "low-count" failures.

B. In those preparations that contain sufficient ^{22}Na there is still a possibility that experiments of the type described on pp. 351-356 may not be successful. The suitability of the ghosts for such studies depends on the fact that the ghosts undergo "reversal" (regain relative impermeability) at the moment they are added to the isotonic incubation medium (Hoffman, 1962). For unknown reasons, however, reversal does not occur in some preparations. Unfortunately, this is not found until the experiments on ^{22}Na release are performed. The following suggested procedure permits the test of the suitability of the ghosts at an early stage of the experiments. At the beginning of the experiments on p. 353, when the 3-ml aliquots of the ghost suspension and the ghost-free medium are obtained ($S^0{}_1$ and $S^0{}_2$), one-minute counts of the radioactivity of these samples are determined before proceeding with the remainder of the experiment. From these counts the approximate percentage of the ^{22}Na released from the ghosts at zero time is calculated. As evident from the results of Figures 1 and 2, even when reversal of ghosts does occur properly, about 15 percent of the ^{22}Na is released at zero time.* The cause of this relatively large amount of release at the time of reversal is not known (Hoffman, 1962). However, in the course of a great number of experiments we have found that there is a correlation between the size of the release at zero time and the process of reversal: The larger the value of this release, the greater the possibility of the failure of occurrence of reversal. Again we have established an arbitrary rule for our experiments: If the release at zero time is greater than 30 percent of the total content of the ghosts, we do not proceed with the remainder of the experiment. On this basis, about 6 percent of the preparations are rejected.

IONIC COMPOSITIONS OF TYPE I AND TYPE II GHOSTS

It is important to emphasize that the intracellular concentrations of Na^+ and K^+ in the ghost preparations described here cannot be determined accurately. Of course it is possible to measure the ionic content of the ghost phase when it is separated from the hemolysate by centrifugation either before or after the washings. For example, the Na^+ contents of the final ghost suspensions (see pp. 350 and 351) are in the ranges of 0.5 to 1 mM for Type I and 4 to 6 mM for Type II ghosts. However, the exact intracellular concentrations cannot be determined from these values since (a) ghosts shrink during the washing procedure and at the time of reversal, and (b) the exact extent of the shrinkage is difficult to estimate under experimental conditions. It should also be pointed out that, in the ghost systems described here, it is possible to distinguish several compartments of Na^+ with different properties, especially in respect to exchangeability with isotopic Na^+. Due to this heterogeneity and to the difficulty of determination of intercellular ionic concentrations, these ghost preparations are not suitable for the study of net movements of sodium. The work of Hoffman (1962) presents detailed discussions of the factors influencing the amounts of retained ions in the ghosts, and the possible causes of the heterogeniety of the ghost population.

Data of possible interest on the phosphate content of the ghosts is given in Table 1.

TABLE 1

Phosphate Content of Ghosts

	Type I	Type II
Inorganic phosphate (μmoles/ml of ghost suspension)	0.1 ± 0.03	0.5 ± 0.1
"Easily hydrolyzable phosphate" (μmoles/ml of ghost suspension)	Not detectable	2.1 ± 0.3

Aliquots of final suspensions of Types I and II ghosts (pp. 350 and 351) were added to two volumes of cold 8 percent perchloric acid. After centrifugation, inorganic phosphate contents of aliquots of the supernatants were determined before and after 15 minutes of boiling. The values given are averages of determinations on 10 different preparations.

*If efflux of Na is to be calculated from data such as those of Figures 1 and 2, the value of Na release at each time interval should be corrected for the release at zero time.

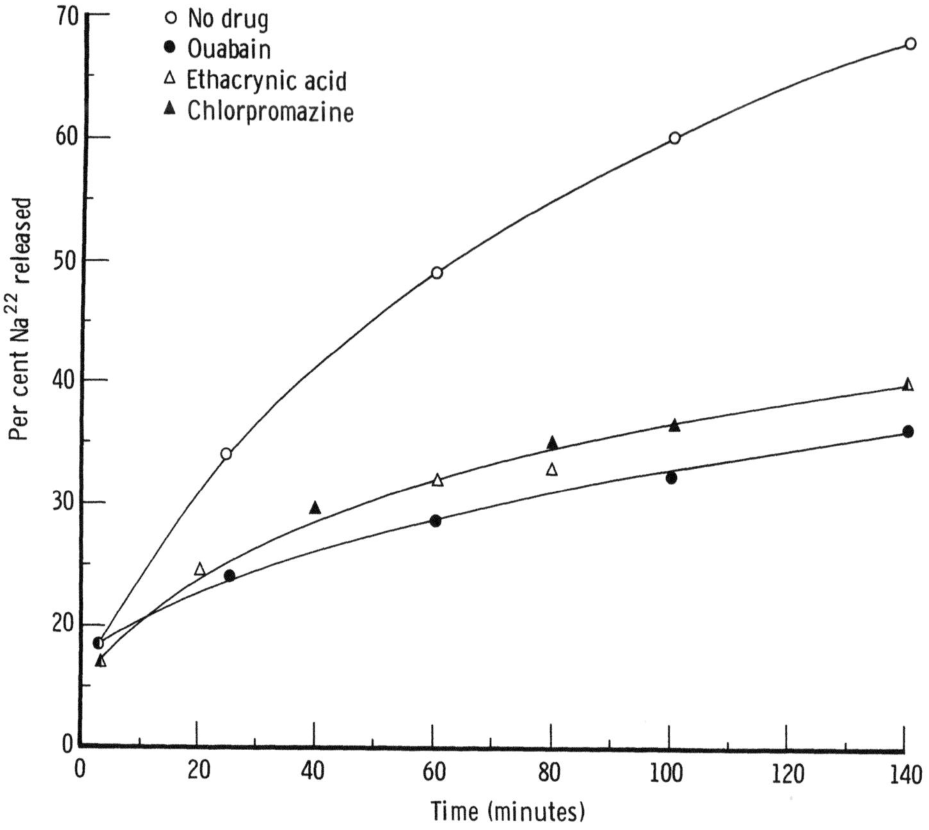

FIG. 3. Effects of ouabain (10^{-5}M), ethacrynic acid (10^{-4}M), and chlorpromazine (10^{-4}M) on the release of ^{22}Na from Type II ghosts. Experimental conditions were the same as those described on pp. 352-353.

EXAMPLES OF SOME DRUG EFFECTS ON SODIUM TRANSPORT IN GHOSTS

The ghost preparations described here have been used in the author's laboratory for the study of the effects of several classes of drugs on sodium transport (Askari and Rao, 1968, 1970; Rao and Askari, 1968). Examples of some of these drug effects are shown in Figure 3. It has been suggested that changes in cell membrane permeability induced by pharmacologically active phenothiazines may explain the various effects of these drugs (Guth and Spirtes, 1964). Substituted phenothiazines have also been shown to inhibit the Na^+, K^+-ATPase activity of membrane preparations (Davis and Brody, 1966). Duggan and Noll (1965) have shown that ethacrynic acid is another drug that inhibits the Na^+, K^+-ATPase activity, and have suggested the possibility of a relation of this action of the drug to its pharmacologic effects (contrast Nechay et al., 1967). For these reasons it was of interest to study the effects of these drugs on the erythrocyte ghost as a model. The results of Figure 3 show that ethacrynic acid and chlorpromazine, like ouabain, inhibit the ATP-supported sodium pump of the ghosts. It should be emphasized that, in addition to this common action, each of the foregoing three drugs has other effects on sodium permeability of the ghost membrane which differ from the effects of the other two. The presentation and discussion of these effects is, however, beyond the scope of this chapter.

REFERENCES

Askari, A., and Rao, S. N. 1968. The effects of purine nucleosides on sodium transport and lactate production in human erythocyte ghosts. J. Pharmacol. Exp. Ther., 163:407-416.

—and Rao, S. N. 1970. Drugs affecting sodium transport in human erythrocyte ghosts. J. Pharmacol. Exp. Ther., (in press.)

Davis, P. W., and Brody, T. M. 1966. Inhibition of Na^+ K^+-activated adenosine triphosphatase activity in rat brain by substituted phenothiazines. Biochem. Pharmacol., 15:703-710.

Duggan, D. E., and Noll, R. M. 1965. Effects of ethacrynic acid and cardiac glycosides upon a membrane adenosine triphosphatase of renal cortex. Arch. Biochem., 109:388-396.

Gardos, G. 1954. Akkumulation der Kaliumionen durch menschliche Blutkorperchen. Acta Physiol. Acad. Sc. Hung., 6:191-199.

—1964. Connection between membrane adenosinetriphosphatase activity and potassium transport in erythrocyte ghosts. Experientia, 20:387.

Garrahan, P. J., and Glynn, I. M. 1967a. Factors affecting the relative magnitudes of the sodium:potassium and sodium:sodium exchanges catalyzed by the sodium pump. J. Physiol.(London), 192:189:216.

—and Glynn, I. M. 1967b. The stoichiometry of the sodium pump. J. Physiol. (London), 192:217-235.

Guth, P. S., and Spirtes, M. A. 1964. The phenothiazine tranquilizers: biochemical and biophysical actions. Int:Rev. Neurobiol, 7:231-278.

Hoffman, J. F. 1960. The link between metabolism and the active transport of Na in human red cell ghosts. Fed. Proc., 19:127.

—1962. The active transport of sodium by ghosts of human red blood cells. J. Gen. Physiol., 45:837-859.

—Tosteson, D. C., and Whittam, R. 1960. Retention of potassium by human erythrocyte ghosts. Nature, 185:186-187.

Neehay, B. R., Palmer, R. F., Chinoy, D. A., and Posey, V. A. 1967. The problem of Na^+ and K^+ adenosine triphosphatase as the receptor for diuretic action of mercurials and ethacrynic acid. J. Pharmacol. Exp. Ther., 157:599-617.

Parpart, A. K., and Ballentine, R. Molecular anatomy of the red cell plasma membrane. *In* Modern Trends in Physiology and Biochemistry, E. S. G. Barron, ed. New York, Academic Press, Inc., p. 136.

Ponder, E. 1934. The Mammalian Red Cell and the Properties of Haemolytic Systems. Vol. 6 of Protoplasma Monographien. Berlin, Verlag Gehruder Borntraeger.

—Hemolysis and Related Phenomena. 1948. New York, Grune & Stratton, Inc., p. 1.

—1961. The cell membrane and its properties. *In* The Cell, J. Brachet and A. E. Mirsky, eds. Vol. 2. New York, Academic Press, Inc., pp. 1-84.

Prankerd, T. A. J. 1961. The Red Cell. Springfield, Illinois, Charles C Thomas, Publisher.

Rao, S. N., and Askari, A. 1968. Effects of phenothiozines and dibenzazepines on sodium transport in erythrocyte ghosts. Fed. Proc., 27:64.

Teorell, T. 1952. Permeability properties of erythrocyte ghosts. J. Gen. Physiol., 35:667-701.

Whittam, R. 1964. Transport and Diffusion in Red Blood Cells. London, Edward Arnold, Ltd.

CHAPTER 12

The Sodium- and Potassium-Activated Adenosinetriphosphatase System

A. Schwartz, K. Nagano, M. Nakao
G. E. Lindenmayer, and J. C. Allen

Department of Pharmacology, Division of Myocardial Biology
Baylor College of Medicine, Texas Medical Center
Houston, Texas

and H. Matsui

Department of Biochemistry, Tokyo Medical and
Dental University, Tokyo, Japan

INTRODUCTION

Ion regulation and active transport are known to be fundamental processes characteristic of all membranes. Membranes are biologically active, enzymatically invested structures, consisting of complex lipoproteins (Korn, 1968).

Most cells possess a process that actively maintains concentration gradients of sodium and potassium. There are essentially three general mechanisms by which differential concentrations of Na^+ (extracellular) and K^+ (intracellular) may be maintained: passive diffusion or leak, exchange diffusion, and active transport. Active transport is defined as the transfer or movement of substances across a

The original studies referred to in this paper were supported in part by U.S. Public Health Service grants HE 07906, HE 05435, P8; by National Science Foundation grant GB 6895; by the Texas and Houston Heart Association, by the Liberty Foundation, and by the National Cystic Fibrosis Foundation. A. Schwartz is a Career Research Development Awardee (K_3HE 11,875).

membrane, which requires energy derived from cellular metabolism, whether the energy is used to overcome the potential difference, a concentration difference, or a combination of both. The ouabain-sensitive transport ATPase system (Na^+,K^+-activated ATPase or Na^+,K^+-ATPase) is regarded as a structural part of the membrane and is thought by some to be the so-called sodium pump.

In 1957 Skou reported the presence of an ATP-hydrolyzing enzyme system in membranous fractions of leg nerves from the shore crab *Carcinus maenas.* This enzyme possessed the peculiar property of requiring both Na^+ and K^+ ions in addition to magnesium for optimal activity. Two sites of activity were proposed, one with preferential affinity for Na^+ and the other with high affinity for K^+. Concentrations of both ions required for optimal enzyme activity in vitro were almost identical with the intracellular and extracellular concentration of Na^+ and K^+, respectively, in the crab nerve. Furthermore, *g*-strophanthin (ouabain) specifically inhibited that ATPase activity due to Na^+ plus K^+ (Skou, 1960). This inhibition is of importance since it had previously been shown that cardiac glycosides specifically inhibit active cation transport (Schatzmann, 1953; Glynn, 1964). Only those cardiac glycosides possessing a positive inotropic action on heart muscle (an increase in the force of contraction) are effective inhibitors of this ATPase as well as active cation transport.

In attempts to explain the molecular mechanism for active transport, a number of theories have evolved, all of which suggest that some common energy source is concerned with the transport of cations. The Na^+,K^+-dependent adenosine triphosphatase (Na^+,K^+-ATPase) comes closest to fulfilling the requirements of an active transport system.

The enzyme system is of particular interest to pharmacologists in that chemical agents which purportedly have direct effects on active cation transport may interact with the Na^+,K^+-ATPase system. Furthermore, it is possible that the ouabain-sensitive ATPase may be involved in excitation-contraction-relaxation coupling in muscle (Langer and Brady, 1968) and in the control of calcium in other tissues (Alonso and Walser, 1968). The molecular mechanism of action of at least one drug, digitalis, has been ascribed to this enzyme system (Schwartz et al., 1969; Besch et al., 1970).

PURIFICATION OF Na^+,K^+-ATPASE FROM CARDIAC TISSUE

The purification of the Na^+,K^+-ATPase is quite difficult, because the Na^+,K^+-ATPase is a membrane-bound (particulate) enzyme and has not been as yet completely solubilized. Therefore, classical purification methods such as ammonium sulfate fractionation, adsorption chromatography, and cellulose ion-exchange column-chromatography, usually useful for soluble enzymes, are not applicable to this important enzyme system. At present, partial purification methods applicable to the Na^+,K^+-ATPase are classified as follows: (1) separation of membrane fragments by differential centrifugation (Skou, 1957) or by density gradient centrifugation (Emmelot and Bos, 1962); (2) treatment with sodium deoxycholate

(Skou, 1962); (3) treatment with sodium iodide (Nakao et al., 1965). The first is actually a basic method for the collection of membrane vesicles that contain specific enzyme activity greater than that found in the original tissue homogenate. The second method has been widely used, but the effectiveness is not always satisfactory except in the case of the brain and kidney ATPases. The third method seems to be the most effective for decreasing the ouabain-insensitive Mg^{++}-ATPase activity. Combination of the foregoing three methods gives the best enzyme preparation from various tissues. A detailed procedure of the enzyme preparation from heart muscle, as an example (Matsui and Schwartz, 1966), is presented in this section. This procedure is also applicable, however, to other tissues such as brain, kidney, and salivary gland with only small modifications, and yields a highly active enzyme preparation with specific activity of from 100 to 300 micromoles inorganic phosphate liberated per milligram of protein per hour.

Deoxycholate (DOC) Treatment

SOLUTIONS.

1. Sucrose stock solution:
   1 M sucrose
   4 mM EDTA · 3 tris

   It is convenient to make 3 liters of solution and to store the solution in the cold room. Dissolve 3.5 g (= 12 mmoles) of EDTA (free acid) in 18 ml of 2 M tris (= 48 mmoles) and about 100 ml of water. Add 1,027 g (=3 moles) of sucrose and water to make 3 liters of solution.

2. EDTA stock solution (0.1 M EDTA · 3 tris):
   2.9 g of ethylenediaminetetraacetic acid (EDTA, Versene) (m.w. = 292.25) is dissolved in 15 ml of 2 M tris (= 30 mmoles) and about 50 ml of water. Adjust the volume to 100 ml. The pH of the solution is neutral.

3. Medium 1
   0.25 M sucrose
   1 mM EDTA

   Mix 1 part of sucrose stock solution with 3 parts of cold water.

4. Medium 2
   0.25 M sucrose
   1 mM EDTA
   0.1 percent DOC

   Dissolve 0.1 percent (w/v) of DOC in Medium 1. DOC = sodium desoxycholate (Fisher Scientific Co.).

5. Medium 3
   0.25 M sucrose
   1 mM EDTA
   0.05 percent DOC

   Mix equal volumes of Medium 1 with Medium 2.

6. Medium 4
   1 mM EDTA
   Dilute the EDTA stock solution 100 times with water.

PROCEDURE:

STEP 1—PREPARATION OF TISSUE. Heart muscle is obtained at a nearby slaughterhouse and kept in ice during transport to the laboratory; or animals are sacrificed and the hearts quickly removed. Whenever possible the left ventricular muscle is used for this isolation, as it is relatively homogeneous and contains little connective tissue. The pericardium, endocardium, fat and connective tissues are carefully removed with scissors. The tissue is chopped into small pieces (0.5 cm^2 or smaller) or is minced by a meat grinder for large-scale preparations and put into 9 volumes (by weight) of Medium 1.

STEP 2—DISRUPTION OF TISSUE AND COLLECTION OF CELL FRAGMENTS. The above mixture is homogenized for 35 to 40 seconds at medium speed in a Macro-Waring blendor (for large-scale preparations), or at maximum speed in a Sorvall Omnimixer (for medium- and small-scale preparations). (In the case of a small animal heart, e.g., rat, it is advisable to perfuse the excised heart through the aorta with 0.9 percent NaCl to remove the blood. The tissue is then chopped and drained on eight layers of cheesecloth; the saline is removed by rinsing several times with 0.25 M sucrose. Sufficient homogenization of tissue from small animals is usually accomplished during a 7-second treatment with the Polytron PT-20* at rheostat position 1.5.) The homogenate is passed first through four and then through eight layers of cheesecloth to remove connective tissues and lipids, and then is centrifuged for 15 minutes at 10,000 × *g* (8,750 rpm Sorvall GSA rotor).

STEP 3—FIRST DOC TREATMENT. The pellet is drained and diluted with a volume of Medium 2 equivalent to eight times the original weight of tissue. The pellet is loosened from the side of the tube with a glass rod after addition of portions of the suspending medium and rinsed into the blendor. The pellet is rehomogenized at medium speed of the Macro-Waring blendor (or top speed in the Sorvall Omnimixer in the case of smaller volumes), for six 30-second periods in ice. A 15-second interval between blendings is necessary to prevent heating of the homogenizer cup. Usually large quantities of foam are produced, but can be reduced with the addition of one drop of octyl alcohol, followed by 10 to 15 minutes of standing with occasional stirring with a glass rod. A second drop is added and the mixture allowed to stand for another 15 minutes. If necessary, a third drop of octyl alcohol may be introduced. The mixture is then placed in centrifuge cups and centrifuged for 30 minutes at 10,000 × *g* (8,750 rpm Sorvall GSA Rotor). The supernate is carefully collected by decantation from the bulk of loosely packed precipitate through eight layers of cheesecloth and centrifuged at 100,000 × *g* for 45 minutes (35,000 rpm, IEC Rotor A147), or at 65,000 × *g* for one hour (30,000 rpm, Spinco

*A shearing and sonicating device; Brinkmann Instruments, Inc.

Rotor 30). The supernate is decanted and the pellet drained by inverting the centrifuge tube on a paper towel. The lipid material is wiped from the walls of the tube with a Kimwipe.

STEP 4—SECOND DOC TREATMENT. The precipitate is resuspended in approximately 1.5 times volume of Medium 3 with a glass homogenizer and Teflon pestle and centrifuged at 20,000 × *g* for 20 minutes (13,000 rpm, IEC-B35 A147 Rotor or Sorvall-RC2B, SS34 Rotor). The supernate is collected by careful decantation through eight layers of cheesecloth and centrifuged further at 100,000 × *g* for 45 minutes (35,000 rpm, IEC A147 Rotor). If desired, the pellet resulting from the 20,000 × *g* spin may be treated as in Step 3. In this case, cheesecloth cannot be used for the above decantation.

STEP 5—STORAGE OF DOC-TREATED PARTICLES. The precipitate is finally suspended in 1 mM EDTA in a volume one half to one third the original weight of tissue used (protein must be less than 5 mg/ml for NaI treatment) with a glass homogenizer and Teflon pestle. Of this fraction, 0.1 ml is diluted 20 times with 1 mM EDTA for determination of protein content (Lowry method) and specific activity. Protein may also be determined in the undiluted homogenate by a biuret method. The remaining suspension is quick-frozen in an acetone-dry ice bath and stored at −20°C. The solution is frozen in a tube or flask large enough that swirling during freezing permits uniform cooling throughout the entire volume. Protein recovery at this stage is 1 to 2 mg per gram of original wet tissue. Specific activity of Na^+, K^+-ATPase is usually 10 μmoles Pi liberated per mg protein per hour, and the activity ratio is about 1. During storage, Mg^{++}-dependent activity is gradually decreased, but Na^+, K^+-dependent activity remains unchanged for over a month.

Sodium Iodide (NaI) Treatment

SOLUTIONS:

1. Stock solution of NaI:
   - 6 M NaI
   - 15 mM EDTA · tris
   - 150 mM tris

   To prepare 200 ml of this solution, dissolve 180 g (= 1.2 moles) of NaI (m.w. = 149.92, granular NaI, analytical reagent, Mallinckrodt Chemical Works) in about 80 ml of H_2O. The solution is very slightly yellow (the use of Baker NaI gives a much more pronounced yellowish color). Add 15 ml of 2 M tris to the solution; then add 30 ml of 0.1 M EDTA · 3 tris (pH 7.0). At this point the solution is colorless. Finally, adjust the volume to 200 ml with water. Store in a brown bottle in the refrigerator. The solution should be allowed to "age" for one week under refrigeration before use. A more active preparation is obtained when an "aged" NaI solution is used: The reasons for this are unknown. After a three-fold dilution with water, the pH of the 2 M NaI solution is usually 8.5.

2. Stock solution of $MgCl_2$: 1.5 M $MgCl_2$ ($MgCl_2 \cdot 6\ H_2O$, crystal, m.w. = 203.33) is kept in a brown bottle under refrigeration.

3. Sodium iodide (NaI) solution for purification of the enzyme:
   6 M NaI
   15 mM EDTA
   7.5 mM $MgCl_2$
   150 mM tris
   Mix one part of $MgCl_2$ stock solution with 200 parts NaI stock solution.

4. Washing medium; 1mM EDTA · tris (dilute the 0.1 M EDTA stock solution 100 times).

PROCEDURE:

STEP 1—NaI TREATMENT: The DOC-treated particle suspension is thawed at room temperature and diluted, if necessary, with enough 1 mM EDTA to give a protein concentration between 2 and 5 mg/ml. The suspension is then brought to 1.5 times volume with the addition of 0.5 volume of NaI solution (Solution 3). The NaI solution is added slowly with a capillary pipette to avoid denaturing the protein with a rapid change of the medium. The mixture is kept in a flask immersed in a beaker of ice and stirred gently with a magnetic stirrer.

STEP 2—After 30 minutes the almost clear solution is diluted to 2.5 volumes by the addition of 1.5 volumes 1 mM EDTA and allowed to stand several minutes with gentle stirring. The resulting suspension is then centrifuged at 35,000 × *g* (average *g* value) for 20 minutes (21,000 rpm, IEC A147 Rotor) or at 35,000 × *g* (maximum *g* value) for 30 minutes (17,000 rpm, Sorval SS 34 Rotor).

STEP 3—WASHING OF PRECIPITATE. The precipitate is separated from the supernatant (the pH of the supernatant should be between 8.3 and 8.5). Excess liquid is removed from the walls of the tube with a Kimwipe. This precipitate is rather soft. The pellet is loosened from the centrifuge tube with a glass rod, and the tube is rinsed thoroughly with small portions of 1 mM EDTA into a glass homogenizer. The pestle and homogenizer are rinsed with about 5 ml of the same solution. It is important to wash the precipitate thoroughly each time, thus the total volume of the washing medium is about twice the volume of the original DOC-treated particle suspension. The rinse is combined with the homogenate and centrifuged at 35,000 × *g* for 10 minutes (21,000 rpm, IEC A147 Rotor). The above resuspension and washing are repeated two additional times. The pellet becomes hard after the first washing.

STEP 4—STORAGE. The final pellet is resuspended in enough 1 mM EDTA to give a protein concentration of about 1 mg/ml or between one fifth and one half of the

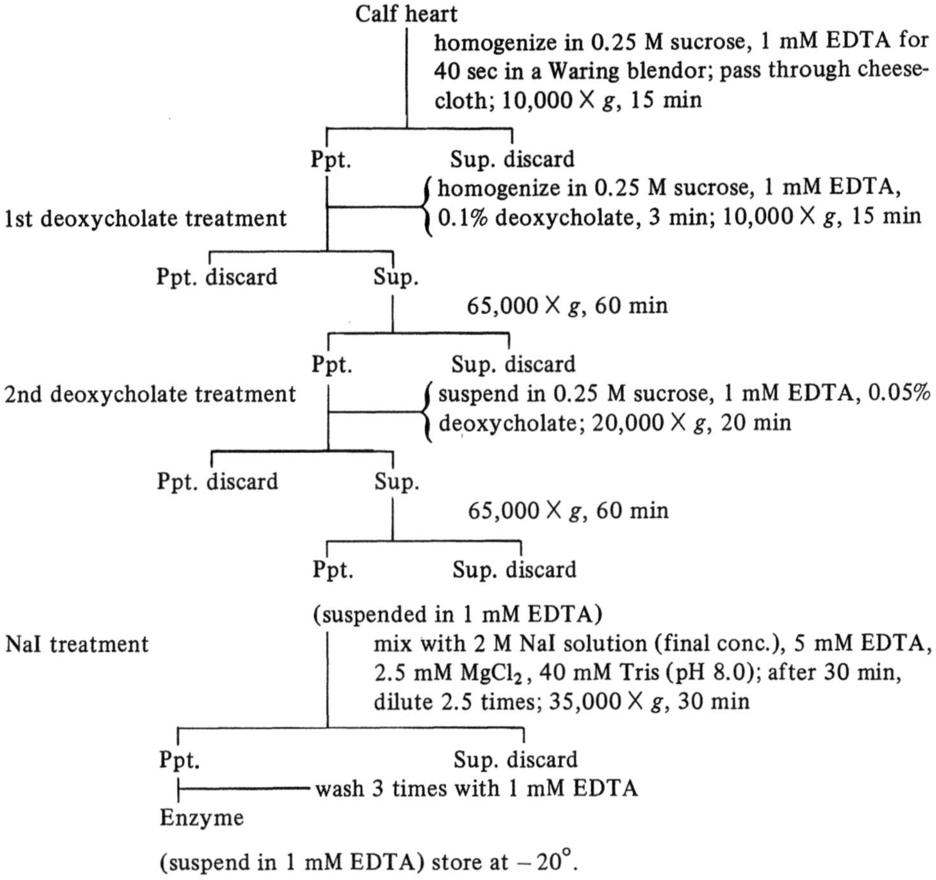

FIG. 1. Flow sheet diagram of the purification procedure for the Na^+,K^+-ATPase. (From Matsui and Schwartz. 1966. *Biochim. Biophys. Acta,* 128:380-390.)

volume of the DOC-treated suspension before the addition of NaI. The protein concentration is determined by the nature of the experiments which will be performed on the enzyme. Protein recovery by this treatment is approximately one fourth. Therefore, the one-half volume suspension will give about one half of the protein concentration of the DOC-treated particle suspension. The enzyme suspension is divided into small aliquots in culture tubes and rapidly frozen in a dry ice-acetone mixture. Quick frozen samples may be stored for more than one month without change in activity.

The flow sheet diagram of the purification procedure and the enzyme activity at each purification stage are summarized in Figure 1 and Table 1, respectively.

TABLE 1

Purification Data of Na^+, K^+-Activated ATPase from Calf Heart

Experimental Fraction	Specific activity (μmoles Pi per mg protein per hr)			Activity ratio	Recovery of	
	A + *OUABAIN*	*B* − *OUABAIN*	*B − A*	$\frac{B-A}{A}$	*PROTEIN*	*ACTIVITY* (%)
1 (a) Homogenate with deoxycholate	12.1	13.4	1.3	0.11	(100)	(100)
(b) 65,000 × *g* ppt after 1st deoxycholate treatment	9.5	19.6	10.1	1.06	3.3	24
(c) 65,000 × *g* ppt after 2nd deoxycholate treatment	13.0	24.0	11.0	0.85	1.7	14
(d) Enzyme after NaI treatment	1.7	24.9	23.2	13.7	0.47	7.8
2 (a) Homogenate with deoxycholate	10.2	12.0	1.8	0.18	(100)	(100)
(b) 65,000 × *g* ppt after 2nd deoxycholate treatment	20.2	30.5	10.3	0.50	1.2	6.6
(c) Enzyme after NaI treatment	1.1	28.1	27.0	24.6	0.26	4.0

The reaction system included 50 mM tris-HCl (pH 7.4), 1 mM EDTA, 2 mM ATP, 5 mM $MgCl_2$, 100 mM NaCl, and 20 mM KCl, in the presence or absence of 10^{-4} M ouabain, in a total volume of 1 ml. Incubation, 10 min at 37°. Deoxycholate concentration, 0.1%, 1st treatment; 0.05%, 2nd treatment.

From Matsui and Schwartz. 1966. *Biochim. Biophys. Acta, 128:380-390.*

Assays of Na^+,K^+-ATPase

Assays of the Na^+,K^+-ATPase activity are based on the increase in rate of ATP hydrolysis by Na^+ plus K^+, which is the difference between two systems in the presence of Na^+,K^+ and Mg^{++}, and Mg^{++} alone. In the case of crude enzymes, the difference between activities in the presence and absence of 10^{-4} M ouabain under the same Na^+,K^+ and Mg^{++} conditions is recommended to avoid unknown effects of ionic change on other ATPases.

ASSAY PROCEDURE A.—The reaction mixture, in a total volume of 1 ml, containing ATP, 5 mM $MgCl_2$, 1 mM EDTA-tris, 50 mM tris-HCl buffer (pH 7.4) about 50 μg enzyme protein (in the case of heart enzyme), 100 mM NaCl, and 10 mM KCl (NaCl and KCl omitted for assay of Mg^{++}-dependent ouabain-insensitive ATPase activity), is placed in a 5-ml glass test tube. The volume is brought to 1 ml with water (ouabain or other reagents may be added in appropriate concentrations, in place of a portion of the water). In addition to the experimental tubes, one tube containing the entire reaction mixture, but no enzyme, is treated simultaneously as a blank: the mixture is brought to 37°C in a shaking water bath. After 3 minutes of preincubation, the reaction is initiated by the addition of ATP. If desired, the reaction can be started by the addition of enzyme instead of ATP. The addition of ATP to each tube is made at suitable intervals (e.g., 15 seconds). After 10 minutes of incubation, the reaction is stopped by the addition of 1 ml of ice-cold 10 percent trichloroacetic acid at the same intervals. The tubes are shaken and placed in ice for 5 minutes and then centrifuged at 3,000 rpm for 3 minutes. An aliquot (1 ml) is taken for the estimation of inorganic phosphate liberated by the micromethod of Martin and Doty (see below).

ASSAY PROCEDURE B.—Na^+,K^+-ATPase activity can be conveniently determined by continuously monitoring the oxidation of NADH in a Gilford Model 2000 Recording Spectrophotometer, equipped with a constant temperature water bath (Haake), at a wavelength of 340 mμ, employing a linked enzyme system. Each cuvette should contain (in final concentration) 5 mM $MgCl_2$, 100 mM NaCl, 10 mM KCl, 25 mM tris-HCl (pH 7.4), 2.5 mM tris-ATP, 0.5 mM reduced nicotinamide adenine dinucleotide (NADH) (Sigma Chemical Co.), 2.5 mM phosphoenol pyruvic acid, and 0.02 ml of a combined pyruvate kinase-lactate dehydrogenase suspension (Sigma Chemical Co.) in a final volume of less than 2 ml.

A solution containing 100 mM $MgCl_2$, 0.5 M tris-HCl, and 50 mM phosphoenol pyruvic acid (tricyclohexylamine salt) is made, and the pH is adjusted to 7.4. The solution is then frozen in small aliquots and thawed before use, at which time NADH is added to make a final concentration of 10 mM. This solution is then used in the assay, and NaCl, KCl, and tris-ATP are added separately.

At this point the volume in each cuvette should be appropriately adjusted so that any additions of inhibitors, and the enzyme suspension, should bring the volume up to 2 ml. Ouabain is usually added in volumes not exceeding 0.1 ml. The reaction is started after an appropriate temperature equilibrium period, by the addition of the enzyme preparation, usually in a volume less than 0.1 ml, containing no more than 100 μg protein. The reaction sequence is as follows:

$$\text{ATP} \xrightarrow{Na^+ + K^+} \text{ADP} + \text{Pi}$$

$$\text{PEP} + \text{ADP} \xrightarrow[\text{kinase}]{\text{pyruvate}} \text{pyruvate} + \text{ATP}$$

$$\text{pyruvate} + \text{NADH} \xrightarrow[\text{dehydrogenase}]{\text{lactate}} \text{lactate} + \text{NAD}^+$$

A typical experiment is shown in Figure 2.

MICRODETERMINATION OF INORGANIC PHOSPHATE BY THE METHOD OF MARTIN AND DOTY.

REAGENTS:

a. 1.25 percent ammonium molybdate in 1 N H_2SO_4.
b. Isobutanol-benzene (1:1) mixture saturated with water.

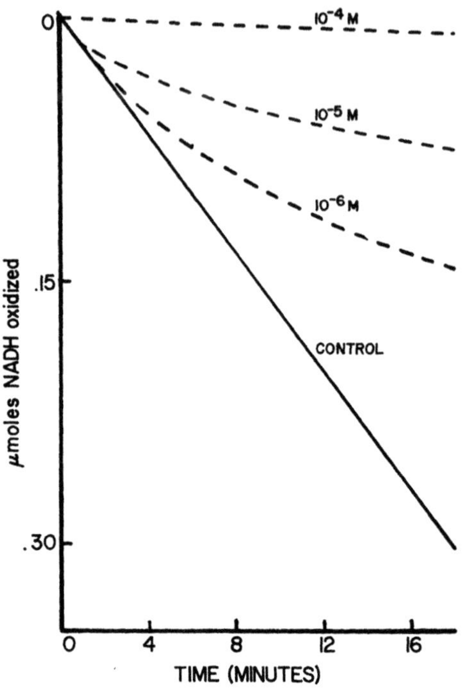

FIG. 2. Results of a typical assay carried out on the Gilford Model 2000 recording spectrophotometer. Cuvette #1 contained no added ouabain and shall be referred to as the control, cuvette #2 contained (final concentration) 10^{-6} M ouabain, cuvette #3, 10^{-5} M ouabain, and cuvette #4, 10^{-4} M ouabain. All cuvettes were allowed to equilibrate at 37°C for 5 minutes, after which time, 50 μg calf heart enzyme protein was added to each cuvette. This is designated in the graph as time 0. Since the oxidation of NADH is directly proportional to the Na^+, K^+-ATPase activity, the effect of increasing ouabain concentrations on the specific activity of the isolated enzyme system can be determined by equating the amount of NADH oxidized to the amount of inorganic phosphate formed in a certain time period, and making adjustments for the amount of protein participating in the reaction. Thus the activity of the control reaction shown in the figure would be 0.05 μmoles inorganic phosphate/30 μg protein/4 minutes. Converted to standard terms, this would be 25 μmoles inorganic phosphate/mg protein/hour. In order to determine the specific activity of the enzyme, the activity of the preparation in the presence of high concentrations of ouabain which maximally inhibit the Na^+,K^+-ATPase activity (in this case less than one) must be subtracted from the overall activity. Note the increased inhibitory effect of ouabain with increased time. The direct relationship between NADH oxidation and ATPase activity can be seen from the following sequence of reactions that occur during the linked pyruvate kinase-lactate dehydrogenase system (PK-LDH):

$$\text{ATP} \xrightarrow{Na^+,\ K^+\text{-ATPase}} \text{ADP} + \text{Pi}$$

$$\text{PEP} + \text{ADP} \xrightarrow{\text{PK}} \text{Pyruvate} + \text{ATP}$$

$$\text{Pyruvate} + \text{NADH} \xrightarrow{\text{LDH}} \text{Lactate} + \text{NAD}^+$$

c. Ethanol-H_2SO_4 (diluting solution). Mix 980 ml absolute ethanol with 20 ml concentrated H_2SO_4.

d. Stock solution of stannous chloride. 40 g stannous chloride dissolved in concentrated HCl in a total volume of 100 ml.

e. Reducing solution of stannous chloride ($SnCl_2$). $SnCl_2$ stock solution (reagent d) is diluted 200 times with 1 N H_2SO_4. Solution should be freshly diluted before each determination.

PROCEDURE: One milliliter of the sample solution is transferred to a screwcapped tube containing 1 ml molybdate solution (a) and 2.5 ml isobutanol-benzene mixture (b), and the contents are shaken vigorously for 15 seconds. The tubes are centrifuged for one minute (1,000 to 2,000 rpm) to separate the isobutanol and water layers. One milliliter of the isobutanol-benzene layer (upper layer) is transferred into another test tube containing 2 ml of ethanol-H_2SO_4 diluting solution (c). One-tenth ml of reducing solution (d) is added to the tube and the contents are mixed on a vortex mixer. The blue color, developed immediately, is stable for several hours, and the color intensity is proportional to the amount of inorganic phosphate in the sample.

Since only inorganic phosphate is extracted into iso-butanol-benzene mixture as phosphomolybdate complex, leaving ATP and other organic phosphate compounds in the water layer, the developed color is due solely to inorganic phosphate liberated. The optical density is read in a spectrophotometer at 730 (or 625) mμ. Absolute amount of phosphate is graphically obtained from a standard curve, or is calculated by standard value (0.310 OD_{730}=0.1 μmole Pi).

CALCULATION OF SPECIFIC ACTIVITY OF THE ENZYME.—Specific activity of the ATPase is conveniently expressed as μ moles of inorganic phosphate released per hour per milligram protein of the enzyme preparation. When the spectrophotometric linked-enzyme system (Assay B) is employed, specific activity may be expressed as μ moles of inorganic phosphate released per minute per milligram of enzyme protein.

MORPHOLOGIC NATURE OF THE ENZYME COMPLEX

Even in suspensions of preparations derived from homogenates, the enzyme activity appears to be associated with membranes; it is probable that the membranes maintain at least some degree of integrity, even after DOC and NaI treatment (Fig. 3). Note that the suspension consists of vesicles of minute dimensions. The NaI treatment appears to yield a preparation with smaller vesicles than the DOC treatment. Attempts to solubilize the enzyme with various detergents and lipid solvents generally result in a partial or complete loss of activity rather than a purification, although, recently a Lubrol-treated solubilized Na^+,K^+-ATPase has been reported (Medzihradsky et al., 1967; Shirachi et al., 1970). The integrity of the lipid component of the membrane is therefore essential for activity. The ATPase system itself is, in fact, probably a lipoprotein (Tanaka and Abood, 1964; Schatzmann, 1962).

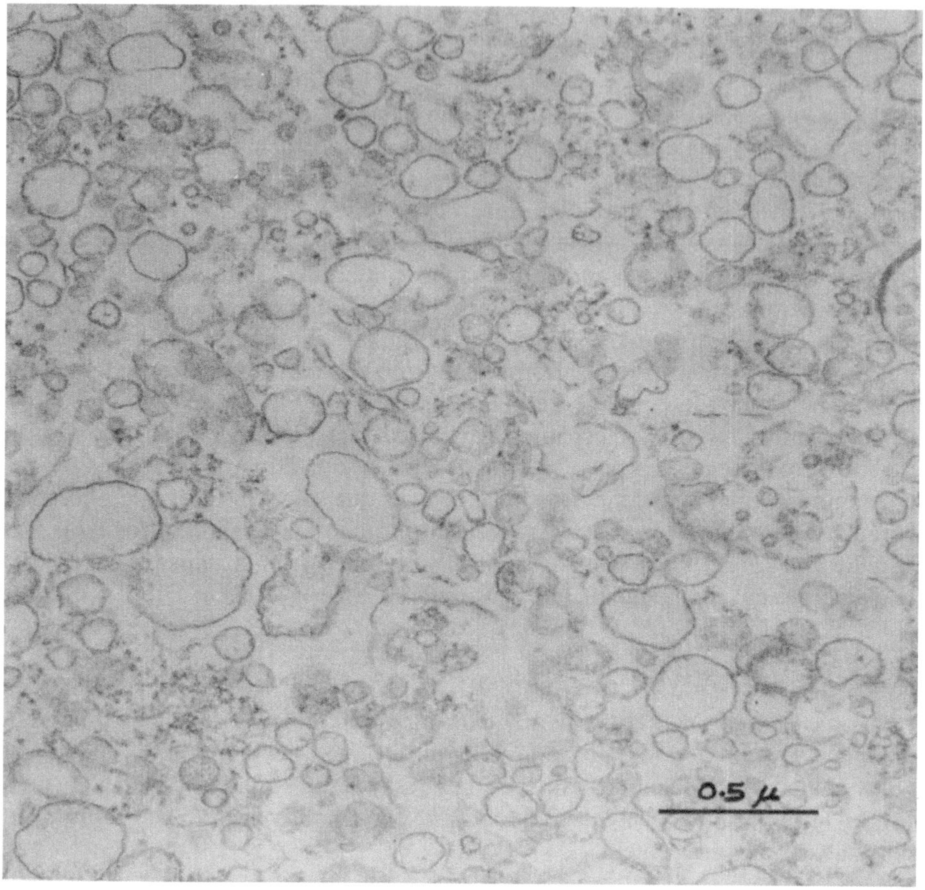

FIG. 3. An electron micrograph of a purified pellet containing Na^+, K^+-ATPase activity.

GENERAL PROPERTIES AND EFFECTS OF CHEMICAL AGENTS

In the case of the enzyme purified with NaI, the ATP hydrolysis is almost completely Na^+- and K^+-dependent and ouabain-sensitive. For example, the ouabain-insensitive basic Mg^{++}-ATPase activity is usually less than 5 percent of the total activity with the heart muscle enzyme and less than 1 percent with the brain enzyme preparations. Optimal pH of the Na^+,K^+-dependent ATP hydrolysis is around 7.5. Magnesium ion is an absolute requirement for activity. However, Mn^{++} or Co^{++} can substitute for Mg^{++} with one tenth the efficiency of Mg^{++}. Na^+ may not be replaced by any cation, while K^+ can be substituted by other monovalent cations such as Rb^+, NH^+_4, Cs^+, and Li^+. K^+ may be substituted by

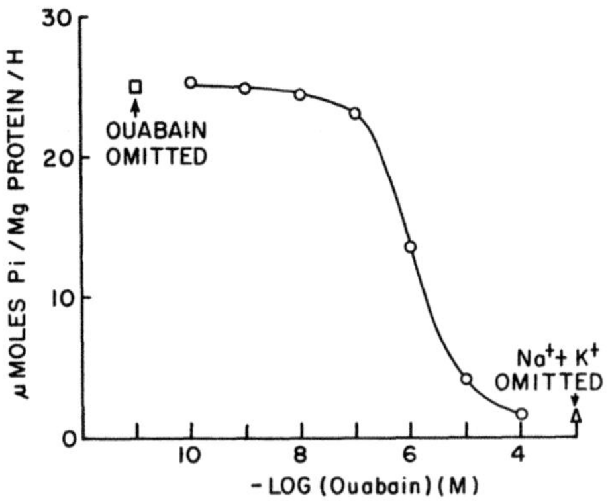

FIG. 4. Effect of ouabain on the ATPase activity. $MgCl_2$, NaCl, and KCl were employed, in 5 mM, 100 mM, and 20 mM concentrations, respectively, as indicated in the figure. The enzyme was added to the medium which contained ouabain just prior to the preincubation. (From Matsui and Schwartz. 1966. *Biochim. Biophys. Acta,* 128:380-390.)

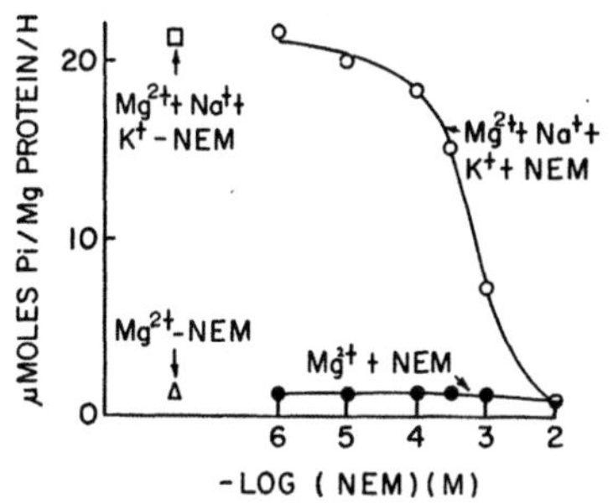

FIG. 5. Effect of N-ethylmaleimide (NEM) on the ATPase activity. Concentrations of ions and procedure are the same as in Fig. 4. (From Matsui and Schwartz. 1966. *Biochim. Biophys. Acta,* 128:380-390.)

Na^+ ($=Na^+$-ATPase), and Na^+ may only be substituted by H^+ ($=K^+$-ATPase at low pH range) (Fujita et al., 1968). CTP can substitute for ATP with less effectiveness. It is noteworthy to mention that a K^+-dependent *p*-nitrophenylphosphatase or acylphosphatase activity apparently associated with the Na^+, K^+-ATPase preparation has been observed in recent years (Fujita et al., 1966; Bader and Sen, 1966). It is generally accepted that the K^+-dependent phosphatase activity may be due to the same enzyme molecule as the Na^+, K^+-ATPase, or at least has close relationship with the ATPase activity if not due to the same enzyme molecule. The phosphatase activity may represent the partial reaction (the latter part) of the total ATP hydrolytic reaction sequence (see section on ^{32}P-labeling of the Na^+, K^+-ATPase, pp. 377-387).

Chemical agents that affect the Na^+,K^+-ATPase activity are as follows:

1. *Cardiac glycosides.* Active glycosides such as ouabain, digoxin, and scillaren are known to be specific inhibitors of the enzyme (Fig. 4). Their aglycones (e.g.,

TABLE 2

Concentration of Inhibitor Necessary to Produce Half-Maximal Inhibition of Na^+, K^+-Dependent ATPase Activity

Inhibitor	K_i(M)
Ouabain	10^{-6}
PCMB	5×10^{-6}
N-Ethylmaleimide	6×10^{-4}
Oligomycin	7×10^{-6}
Tri-*n*-butyltin	1.5×10^{-5}
Octylguanidine	3×10^{-4}

Molar concentration of oligomycin was calculated, using a molecular weight of 424.

strophanthidin) also inhibit the enzyme. Erythrophleum alkaloids, which have cardiotonic activity, are also specific inhibitors of the enzyme, and may be classified in this group in view of the similarity of their inhibitory effect to the cardiac glycosides.

2. *Mitochondrial energy transfer inhibitors: oligomycin, tri-*n*-butyltin and octylguanidine.* K_i's for Na^+,K^+-ATPase, however, are 10 to 100 times as high as those for mitochondrial ATPase (Table 2).

3. *Sulfhydryl inhibitors.* *p*-Chloromercuribenzoate, mersalyl, and *N*-ethylmaleimide (Fig. 5).

4. *Detergents.* Triton, sodium laurylsulfate, and deoxycholate (>0.1 percent) inactivate the enzyme. Organic solvents usually are inhibitory for the enzyme.

5. *Others.* The enzyme is also inhibited by Ca^{++}, Be^{++}, fluoride, and diisopropylfluorophosphate.

The list of K_i's and titration curves of the inhibitors are shown in Table 2 and Figures 4 and 5.

SPECIAL TECHNIQUES FOR THE STUDY OF THE Na^+,K^+-ATPASE SYSTEM

Binding of ^3H-Cardiac Glycoside to the Na^+,K^+-ATPase

Studies of ^3H-cardiac glycoside binding to the Na^+,K^+-ATPase published recently (Matsui and Schwartz, 1968) offer useful information for the investigation of pharmacologic actions of caridac glycosides as well as elucidation of the reaction mechanism of the Na^+,K^+-ATPase.

The principle of the determination of glycoside binding to the Na^+,K^+-ATPase is based on the measurement of radioactivity found in the enzyme-^3H-cardiac-glycoside complex which can be separated as a precipitate from the reaction mixture by ultracentrifugation. Use of millipore filter for separation of the enzyme-glycoside complex is not effective for the heart enzyme because of the clogging of enzyme particles into pores of the filter. However, millipore filtration can be readily employed in binding experiments involving Na^+,K^+-ATPase obtained from non-muscular tissues (Albers et al., 1968).

REAGENTS:

1. ^{3}H-ouabain, ^{3}H-digoxin, and ^{3}H-digitoxin are obtained from New England Nuclear Corp. If the specific radioactivity of the ^{3}H-glycoside obtained is too high, it is necessary to dilute the radioactive glycoside with unlabeled glycoside.
   a. Stock solution of 1 mM ^{3}H-ouabain (or other glycosides). 1 mM ^{3}H-ouabain water solution with specific radioactivity of 0.1-0.3 mc/μM.
   b. Diluted ^{3}H-ouabain solution. Stock solution is diluted 1,000 times with water, making 10^{-6} M ^{3}H-ouabain with the same specific radioactivity.
2. Other reagents are the same as shown in the section on ATPase assay.

PROCEDURE: The reaction mixture is pipetted directly into polycarbonate ultracentrifuge tubes (for Spinco Rotor 40 or 50). The standard reaction mixture consists of about 1 mg enzyme protein, 5 mM $MgCl_2$, 4 mM ATP-tris, 100 mM NaCl, 2×10^{-7}M ^{3}H-ouabain (or other tritiated cardiac glycoside), 1 mM EDTA-tris, and 50 mM tris-HCl pH 7.4, in a total volume of 2 ml. The reaction is initiated with addition of enzyme and allowed to proceed for 5 minutes at 37°C in a water bath. The tubes are capped and inserted into the centrifuge rotor prewarmed to 37°C, and centrifuged for 3 minutes (extra 4 minutes included for centrifuge acceleration) at $105{,}000 \times g$, Spinco Rotor 40. (Otherwise, after 10 minutes incubation the reaction is rapidly stopped by transferring the tubes into ice bath and ultracentrifuged at 0°C.) The supernates are discarded by decantation and the droplets attached to the tube wall are wiped off with a Kimwipe. The pellets are dissolved in 0.3 ml of 0.2 N NaOH by warming for 5 minutes at 100°C in a water bath. To avoid evaporation, the tubes are sealed with marbles. The entire sample solutions are transferred with capillary pipette into counting vials containing 15 ml of scintillation medium (100 g of naphthalene, 6 g of 2,5-diphenyloxazole [=PPO] in a total of 1 liter of dioxane). The walls of the tube and pipette are rinsed twice each with two drops of water. Each rinse is also transferred into the vial. The radioactivity of ^{3}H is counted in a liquid scintillation spectrometer at room temperature. The counting efficiency of ^{3}H in this system is about 50 percent. A standard ^{3}H-ouabain is also counted, and the specific radioactivity is calculated as cpm per pmole ouabain. Then, the binding of ^{3}H-ouabain is expressed as pmoles ouabain per mg enzyme protein.

PROPERTIES OF CARDIAC GLYCOSIDE BINDING TO THE Na^+,K^+-ATPase.—The specific binding level of cardiac glycoside using a heart Na^+,K^+-ATPase under "standard reaction conditions" (ATP + Mg^{++} + Na) is 20 to 30 pmoles per mg enzyme protein. The binding is Mg^{++} plus ATP-dependent and is diluted by other active cardiac glycosides to a low nonspecific level (usually 1 percent of total radioactivity used) (Figs. 6 and 7). This specific binding is almost saturation level, and the level is proportional to the enzyme unit—i.e., proportional to the specific activity of the enzyme using the same amount, as well as to the

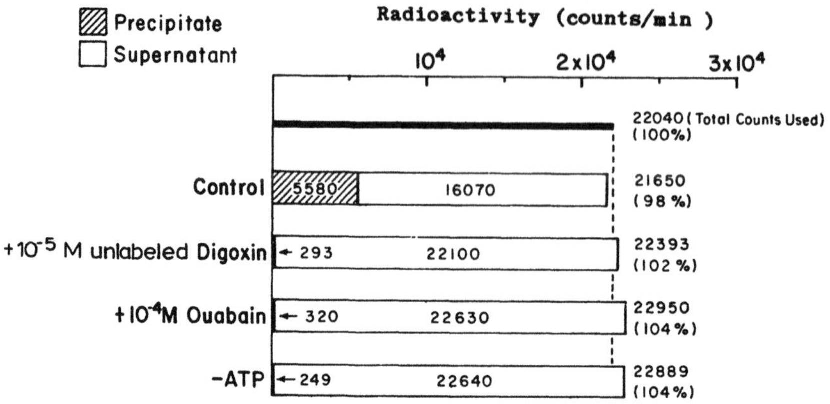

FIG. 6. Specificity of [^{3}H]digoxin binding to Na^+,K^+-ATPase and recovery of radioactivity. The standard assay conditions given in Methods were used with 10^{-7} M [^{3}H]digoxin (specific radioactivity: 140 μC/μmole) and 1 mg protein of the enzyme (specific activity: 29.3 μmoles Pi per mg per hour. Radioactivity in the supernate was also counted. Counts in precipitate and supernate were compared, after correction of quenching differences between precipitate and supernate. (From Matsui and Schwartz, 1968. *Biochim. Biophys. Acta,* 151:655-663).

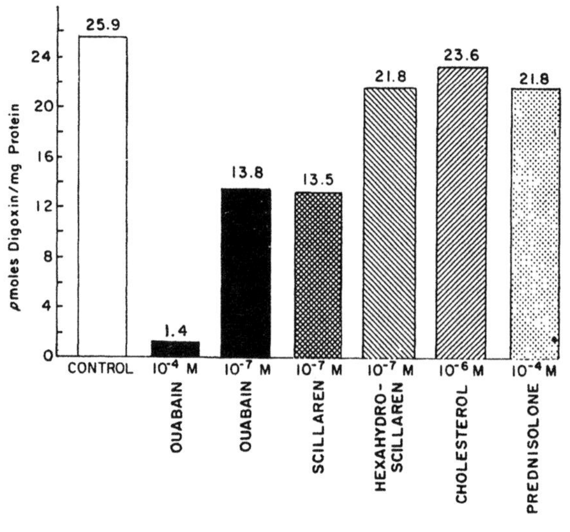

FIG. 7. Dilution of [^{3}H]digoxin binding by cardiac glycosides and steroids. Cardiac glycoside or noncardiac steroid was added in the reaction mixture containing [^{3}H]digoxin in the concentrations shown in the figure. Specific activity of the enzyme was 12.7 μmoles Pi per mg protein per hour. (From Matsui and Schwartz. 1968. *Biochim. Biophys. Acta,* 151:655-663.)

amount of the enzyme using the same preparation. The value is about 1 pmole/1 unit of enzyme (unit of enzyme activity – 1 μmole Pi released per hour). The apparent dissociation constant of enzyme-ouabain complex–i.e., concentration of ouabain that gives half maximal binding–is about 2×10^{-8}M, and this value is comparable to or less than the "K_i" for ouabain for Na^+,K^+-ATPase inhibition. Sodium is not an absolute requirement but it increases the Mg^{++} plus ATP-dependent ouabain binding, whereas potassium decreases the binding. These characteristics can explain the apparent competition between potassium and cardiac glycoside upon the ATPase activity at a molecular level. Other nucleoside triphosphates and ADP can replace ATP with somewhat less effectiveness for ouabain binding.

Acetyl phosphate and carbamyl phosphate can support the full level of ouabain binding in the presence of Mg^{++}. Na^+ does not increase this binding, while K^+ still has a significant decreasing effect. Inorganic phosphate together with Mg^{++} also supports ouabain binding. In this case, however, Na^+ as well as K^+ profoundly depresses the binding. Without monovalent cations, divalent cations such as Mg^{++} and Mn^{++} also support significant levels of ouabain binding. These requirements for the binding together with the effect of Na^+ and K^+ are summarized in Table 3.

TABLE 3

Effect of Mg^{++}, Na^+, and K^+ on ^3H-Ouabain Binding in the Presence and Absence of ATP, AcP, and Pi

System			pmoles Ouabain/mg Protein			
5 mM Mg^{++}	*100 mM Na^+*	*10 mM K^+*	*ATP*	*AcP*	*Pi*	*NONE*
+	–	–	6.4	20.7	21.9	2.1
+	+	–	21.5(0.9)	17.4	1.3	0.8
+	+	+	3.6	1.7	1.4	0.8
+	–	+	1.5	1.9	2.4	0.8
–	+	–	2.5	0.9	0.9	1.0
–	+	+	0.9	1.0	1.0	0.9
–	–	+	1.0	0.9	1.0	0.9
–	–	–	1.0	1.1	1.0	0.9

Value in parentheses represents nonspecific binding level diluted with 10^{-4} M cold ouabain.
AcP = acyl phosphate
Pi = inorganic phosphate.

^{32}P Labeling of the Na^+,K^+-ATPase from ATP (γ^{32}P) ("The Phosphorylated Intermediate")

Regardless of interpretation, Na^+,K^+-ATPase preparations (obtained by treatment with sodium iodide, urea, or sodium deoxycholate or other detergenic reagents) rapidly incorporate the terminal phosphate of ATP in the presence of Mg^{++} and Na^+ (see Albers, 1967; Post and Sen, 1967). Furthermore, the labeled protein is dephosphorylated in the presence of K^+. It has been suggested by some that phosphorylation reflects a half-step of ATP hydrolysis as indicated in the general scheme:

$$(\gamma\text{-}^{32}P)ATP + enzyme \xrightleftharpoons{Na+} (^{32}P)enzyme + ADP \qquad (1)$$

$$(^{32}P)enzyme \xrightarrow{K+} enzyme + {}^{32}Pi \qquad (2)$$

The Na^+-dependent phosphorylation is observed at lower (0° or 4°C) as well as higher (37° or 20°C) temperatures. The chemical properties of the phosphorylated protein obtained at lower and higher temperatures seem to be identical (Nagano et al., 1967). Labeling at lower temperatures is technically more convenient, since the rate of $AT^{32}P$ consumption is much slower. Moreover, the extent of possible formation of Na^+-independent labeling is more limited.

Preparation of (γ-^{32}P) ATP

Terminally labeled $AT^{32}P$ is obtained by an exchange reaction using two enzymes participating in the glycolytic phosphorylation. The following procedure is a modification of that of Glynn and Chappell (1964).

REACTION MIXTURE:

1. Carrier-free (^{32}P) inorganic phosphate (^{32}Pi), 3 mc.
2. 60 μl of 1 M tris (hydroxymethyl) aminomethane (tris). The material is recrystallized from a commercial product, in water.
3. One ml of the following mixture: 1 mM H_2Na_2EDTA; 0.1 mM NAD^+; 5 mM 3-phosphoglyceric acid (tricyclohexylammonium salt, Calbiochem Co.; and 10 mM Na_2ATP, containing about 10 percent ADP but only a trace amount of inorganic phosphate (Pi) (Pi is eliminated by column chromatography through a Dowex-1 column, eluted with 10 mM HCl, and the remaining nucleotides are eluted with 0.1 N HCl and freeze-dried).
4. 0.2 ml of 1 M tris buffer, pH 8.0.
5. 20 μM of cysteine.
6. 10 μl of 1 M $MgSO_4$.
7. 20 μl of phosphoglycerate kinase suspension (10 mg/ml, Boeringer Co.).
8. 50 μl of phosphoglyceraldehyde dehydrogenase suspension (10 mg/ml, Boeringer Co.).

PROCEDURE: To a glass vial of carrier-free ^{32}Pi, 0.5 ml of 0.1 N HCl is added through an injection needle without taking off the rubber lid of the container. The bottle is boiled in water for 30 minutes to hydrolyze pyrophosphate which might be present, the injection needle being left on the rubber lid. After cooling in air, the lid is removed and the other components (2 to 8) are added in the order listed. Before introducing the last two (7 and 8), a very small aliquot (1 μl or less) is sampled using a fine capillary on a piece of pH test paper (BTB), which should turn greenish blue. The labeling reaction is carried out in the ^{32}Pi container immersed in water at 25°C.

After 15 minutes, the extent of labeling is checked as follows: About one μl of the reaction mixture is introduced into a 10-ml centrifuge glass tube containing the following components:

1. 0.5 ml of acid-molybdate mixture. The stock solution consists of 60 ml of 10 N H_2SO_4, 60 ml of 5 percent ammonium molybdate, and enough water to make 900 ml.

2. One ml of carrier Pi solution (NaH_2PO_4, 1 mg/L). The contents are mixed, and 10 μl aliquot is plated onto a planchette, 1.5 ml of isobutanol-benzene mixture (1:1 v/v) added, and the tube is thoroughly agitated on a laboratory vibrator. The

tube is centrifuged at low speed and a 20 μl aliquot is taken from the upper layer which contains extracted inorganic ^{32}P. The degree of ^{32}P-exchange between Pi and ATP is estimated from comparison between the total and inorganic ^{32}P counts. The labeling usually comes to a constant level within an hour.

SEPARATION OF RADIOACTIVE ATP: The radioactive ATP is separated by chromatography on a column of anion exchange resin as follows: Dowex-1 × 10, 100-300 mesh, is converted to the chloride form and packed into a column of diameter 1.2 cm × 2 cm height. The column is washed with water; the radioactive sample, diluted to 50 ml, is then passed through the resin at a flow rate not exceeding 1 ml per minute. The column is eluted stepwise in the following sequence:

1. 40 ml of water
2. 40 ml of 30 mM HCl
3. 15 mM NH_4Cl in 20 mM HCl
4. 20 ml of 10 mM HCl
5. 20 ml of 0.1 N HCl

ADP is eluted in the eluent No. 3. An ultraviolet monitoring system is connected to the column, and elution with this eluant (No. 3) is continued until the level of ultraviolet absorption becomes sufficiently low. Elution No. 4 is included to eliminate any trace of NH_4^+ retained within the resin particles, since contamination of $AT^{32}P$ with this cation will disturb the labeling experiments. $AT^{32}P$ is eluted with eluant No. 5. Specific activity of $AT^{32}P$ is determined, using a small portion of this eluant, and the remainder is neutralized with 2 M tris (base) to pH 7.7 while held 0° in an ice bath. About 1.2 ml of tris is needed to neutralize 20 ml of the eluant.

The radioactive incorporation is about 30 percent, and the preparation has a specific activity of 3 to 6 × 10^7 cpm/μmole ATP (counted in a gasflow counter). The preparation is stored at –20°C. In experiments of the scale, as described in the next section, the $AT^{32}P$ preparation is usable for about two months.

Preparation of Phosphorylated Enzyme

The following procedure is a slight modification of that of Nagano et al. (1967).

REACTION MIXTURE:

1. 0.1 ml of 0.4 M tris buffer, pH 7.7
2. 0.1 ml of 50 mM $MgCl_2$.
3. 0.1 ml of 5 mM EDTA, neutralized to pH 7.7 with 1 M tris (free base).
4. 0.1 ml of 1.4 M NaCl or 0.14 M KCl.
5. 0.1 ml of Na^+, K^+-ATPase suspension containing about 1 mg of protein.
6. 0.1 ml of (γ-^{32}P) ATP preparation. The preparation is 6 × 10^{-4} M, about 10^6 cpm per 0.1 ml.

The total volume is made to 1.0 ml.

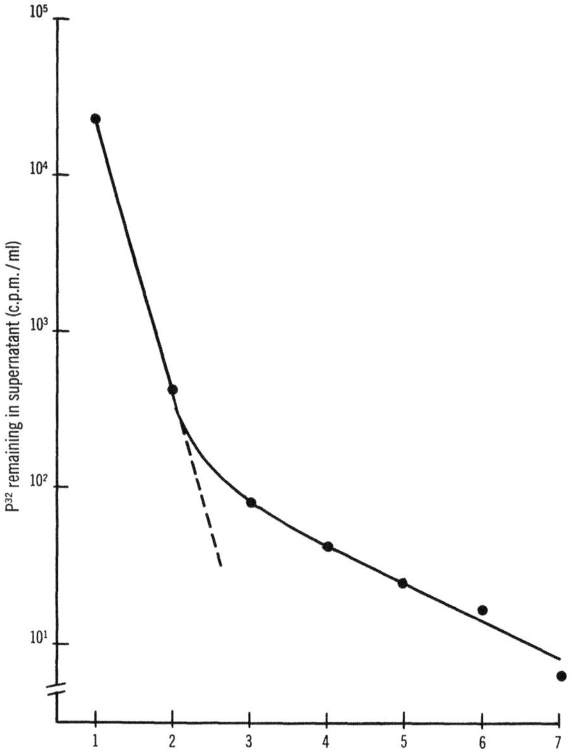

FIG. 8. Washing of the labeled protein and release of P^{32} into supernatant therefrom.

ENZYME PREPARATION: The preparation is made according to the procedure of Nakao et al. (1965) or Matsui and Schwartz (1966). It may be stored without significant loss of activity at –20°C for at least two months.

LABELING PROCEDURE: The reaction is carried out at 0°C in a polycarbonate 10-ml centrifuge tube with stirring by a small magnetic bar. The reagents are added in the sequence previously given, and the labeling is started by the addition of $AT^{32}P$. After the desired period of labeling (usually 5 to 10 seconds), the reaction is stopped by the addition of 3 ml of ice-cold 3 percent perchloric acid ($HClO_4$) containing 10 mM NaH_2PO_4 and 0.1 mM ATP as diluting carriers. Carrier ATP is added to the acid phosphate solution immediately before use. After termination of labeling, the magnetic bar is pulled up using a magnet from the outside along the wall of the tube, rinsed with an additional 3 ml of perchloric acid then taken out of the tube. The suspension of the labeled protein is precipitated in a refrigerated centrifuge at 16,000 rpm for 5 minutes. The supernatant is carefully decanted; the mouth portion of the inverted tube is washed using a squeeze bottle and wiped with a Kimwipe. The precipitate is homogenized with a glass rod (2 mm thick) on a laboratory vibrator. Some of the protein does not precipitate to the bottom but adheres to the wall of the

TABLE 4
Washing Conditions to Obtain Phosphorylated Na^+, K^+-ATPase

Monovalent cation present at the time of incubation (mM)	Carrier ATP added at the time of labeling termination (mM)	Carrier ATP concentration during washing of the precipitate (mM)	Phosphorylated protein (mμmoles ^{32}P/g protein)
(No incubation)	–	0	18, 21
(No incubation)	–	0.1	13, 11
(No incubation)	–	1	8, 6
Na^+, 140	0	1	242, 256
Na^+, 140	0.1	1	234, 240
Na^+, 140	1	1	239, 228
K^+, 14	0	1	68, 63
K^+, 14	1	1	58, 47

Enzyme (1.2 mg protein per vessel). *Labeling conditions:* 10 seconds at 0°C. *Washing:* Pi, 10 mM, was present throughout. ATP was added as indicated. *Centrifugation:* At 0°C in a refrigerated centrifuge, in 10-ml polycarbonate tubes, 12,000 × *g* for 5 minutes.

centrifugation tube, forming a thin line. Special care is paid not to wash off this precipitate when the tube is rinsed, but to rub it off with a glass rod. The homogenized suspension is diluted to 7 ml with the cold perchloric acid-carrier mixture. The cycles of centrifugation, decantation, and homogenization are repeated at least three times. By careful handling, more than one hundred times diluting of the contaminant $AT^{32}P$ (and ^{32}Pi) is achieved per one cycle of washing without any significant loss of the phosphorylated protein (Fig. 8).

The standard procedure, using an NaI-treated enzyme, yields 0.3 μM of incorporated phosphate per 1 mg of protein. It corresponds to 0.5 percent of the added radioactivity. Centrifugation at 1,500 × *g* may also be used, but the resulting pellet is more fluffy. In that case decantation may not be feasible, and the efficiency of washing is significantly lower.

To determine protein recovery, the final precipitate is solubilized in 2 percent sodium dodecylsulfate (SDS), pH 11, with NaOH. An aliquot is used for protein assay. The acid-denatured protein may not be immediately soluble in alkaline SDS, but may need mild warming and vibration and subsequent centrifugation to remove the froth formed. In a typical experiment, the protein recovery was 85 percent (average of 14 samples; the range of recovery among these samples was 83 to 90 percent).

COMMENTS: Released counts into the supernatant after each washing cycle are plotted in Figure 8. A part of the continuous leakage of weak radioactivity after repeated washes may come from occluded $AT^{32}P$ (and ^{32}Pi) possibly held in the vesicular-formed precipitate. To obtain a correct estimate of nonspecifically incorporated or occluded radioactivity, a control experiment where K^+ replaces Na^+ is required. The incorporation level at zero time, in which perchloric acid is added before $AT^{32}P$, is much lower than the potassium control (see Table 4). However, these complexities are not an important cause of error as long as full phosphorylation in an Na^+ system is present, since the phosphorylation level in an Na^+ system is one order higher than in other systems.

Possibility of partial unlabeling by carrier ATP at the moment of termination of the reaction was studied. It is seen from the result in Table 4 that essentially no decrease in labeling occurred even if ATP was present at 1 mM concentration.

In some of the experiments shown in Table 4, ATP was present at 1 mM concentration throughout all washing cycles. Routinely, however, the presence of 0.1 mM ATP during the first two cycles is sufficient.

As for the 15 percent loss of protein during washing procedure, three possibilities must be considered: (1) Loss of a part of the precipitate into supernatant. (2) Some protein component of Na^+,K^+-ATPase preparation is soluble in PCA. (3) Colorimetric efficiency becomes lower after acid denaturation. The first possibility seems remote if the tubes are carefully handled.

Properties of the Phosphorylated Protein

RATE OF PHOSPHORYLATION: The protein is phosphorylated rapidly in the presence of both Na^+ and K^+ at lower as well as higher temperatures. The rate of phosphorylation is of the same order as rate of ATP hydrolysis by the enzyme when both are compared at 0°C (Nagano et al., 1967). In the presence of Na^+ but no K^+, phosphorylation reaches saturation level more slowly.

The amount of the phosphorylated protein decreases rapidly by subsequent addition of K^+ to the Na^+ system (Gibbs et al., 1965; Post et al., 1965; Nagano et al., 1967).

NATURE OF THE PHOSPHATE BOND: The phosphate is relatively stable at acidic pH (pH 2 to 5), but very unstable and is hydrolyzed rapidly at alkaline pH (above pH 9) (Nagano et al., 1965; Hokin et al., 1965; Bader et al., 1966). Treatment of the phosphorylated protein by hydroxylamine under conditions similar to that for hydrolysis of acetylphosphate releases the phosphate. Hydrolysis is also accelerated by molybdate (Bader et al., 1966). The phosphate is transferred to methanol or ethanol in the presence of HCl (Hems and Rodnight, 1966; Bader et al., 1966). The bond is therefore proposed to be a carboxylphosphate.

UNIFORMITY: The incorporated phosphate in the presence of Na^+ is released from the protein according to first-order kinetics at pH 3.5 at 40°C, suggesting chemical uniformity of the bound phosphate (Nagano et al., 1965, 1967). The half-life of the incorporated phosphate under these conditions is about 40 minutes.

At longer incubation periods at 37°C, another type of phosphate incorporation appears and increases with incubation time as long as sufficient $AT^{32}P$ remains as ^{32}P-donor (Nagano et al., 1967). This kind of incorporation is independent of Na^+ and is not released by hydroxylamine treatment. The nature of this phosphorylated material is unknown.

THE PHOSPHORYLATED UNIT: The phosphorylated moiety seems to be a unit having an Avogadro number of about 2×10^5 (result of gel filtration using Sephadex G-200, Sepharose 4–B, or Biogel P-200; see the next section).

Incubation with acidic proteases including pepsin (Bader et al., 1966) and proctase A (Tashima et al., to be published) digests the protein and solubilizes phosphorylated peptide(s).

Digestion and analysis of the phosphorylated protein after hydroxylamine (or its derivative) treatment, where the carboxyl residue possibly has been converted to a hydroxamate, can also be performed. However, quantitative results with reasonably high recovery have not yet been reported.

Gel Filtration of the Phosphorylated Protein. By addition of sodium dodecylsulfate (SDS), the labeling reaction is terminated and the phosphorylated protein is solubilized. The protein is then separated from the remaining $AT^{32}P$ (and ^{32}Pi) by means of gel filtration through a Sephadex G-25 column using SDS solution as eluant (Nagano et al., 1965, 1967). Acid-washed phosphorylated protein (see the previous section) is also solubilized by SDS, giving similar results.

PREPARATION OF SEPHADEX G-25 COLUMN: Ten g of dry Sephadex G-25 gel is swollen and equilibrated in 2 percent solution dodecylsulfate containing 0.1 percent acetic acid at room temperature, poured into a chromatographic column equipped with a water mantle, and allowed to settle for an hour before use. The column (1.6 cm diameter × 16 cm) is maintained at 10°C by water circulation through the mantle.

PROCEDURE: One mg of Na^+,K^+-ATPase is labeled as described in the former section, but using a total volume of 0.6 ml. The reaction is stopped by addition of 0.1 ml of 20 percent SDS containing 1 percent acetic acid. The slightly turbid solution is centrifuged at 12,000 × *g* for 10 minutes at about 10°C. Usually more than 95 percent of the protein remains in the supernatant. However, high protein concentrations may give considerable precipitation. Lower temperature may cause SDS to crystallize out. One-half ml of the supernatant is carefully applied to the top of the gel column. Just when the sample has infiltrated into the gel, 0.5 ml of 2 percent SDS containing 0.1 percent acetic acid is carefully layered onto the gel surface. After three successive additions each of 0.5 ml of SDS solution, about 20 ml of the eluant is layered over the top of the column, and the column is connected to a reservoir to continue the elution. Eluting speed should not exceed about 1 ml per minute and is usually maintained at 0.6 ml per minute. Each ml is fractionated and assayed for protein and radioactivity.

Protein determination is performed according to the method of Lowry scaled down to one tenth (0.1 ml sample in a final volume of 0.65 ml), and optical density is determined at 680 mμ with a Zeiss PMQ-II spectrophotometer in microcuvettes (each 0.35 ml). SDS does not interfere with protein determination at the concentration used.

Both protein and radioactivity appeared in the void volume which was determined separately by Blue Dextran (Pharmacia Co., Uppsala, Sweden). The specific radioactivity is constant over most of the main peak (Fig. 9). It takes about 30 minutes before the peak is eluted.

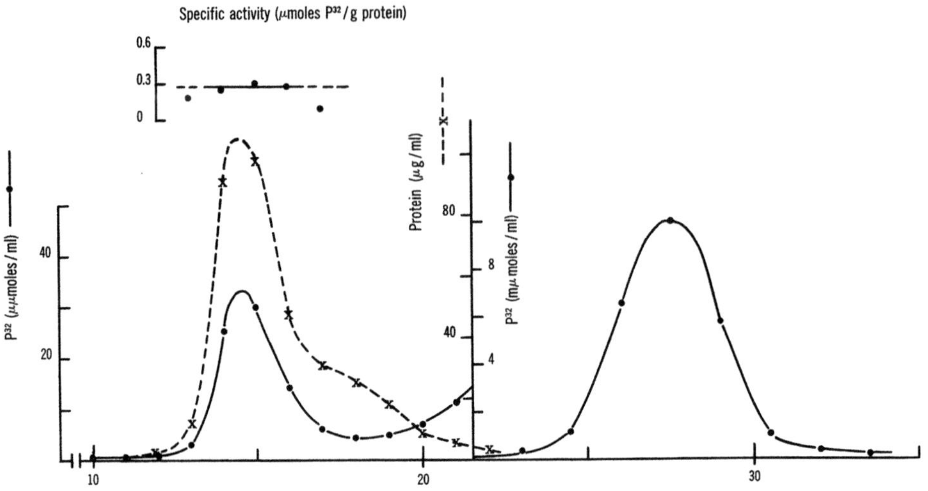

FIG. 9. Gel filtration of the phosphorylated protein through a Sephadex G-25 column.

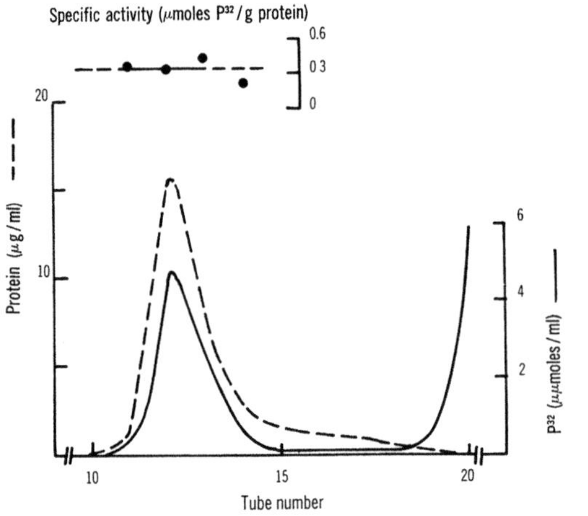

FIG. 10. Complete separation of the phosphorylated protein from ATP^{32} through a longer Sephadex G-25 column. Column size: 2.5 cm × 43 cm. Charged protein: 2.07 mg in 0.7 ml. Flow rate: 50 ml/hour. Each 5.2 ml was fractionated. Protein recovery in fractions 10 to 17 was 92 percent.

Clearer separation between the phosphorylated protein and $AT^{32}P$ (and ^{32}Pi) is obtained using a longer column (Fig. 10). Release of ^{32}P from the phosphorylated protein during its elution through the column is negligible, as is seen from the absence of any significant "tailing" of the radioactivity.

COMMENTS: The phosphorylated enzyme obtained by gel filtration has the same property as that previously described, in regard to its sensitivity to hydroxylamine as well as its rate of ^{32}P release at pH 3.5 at 40°C. The volume ratio

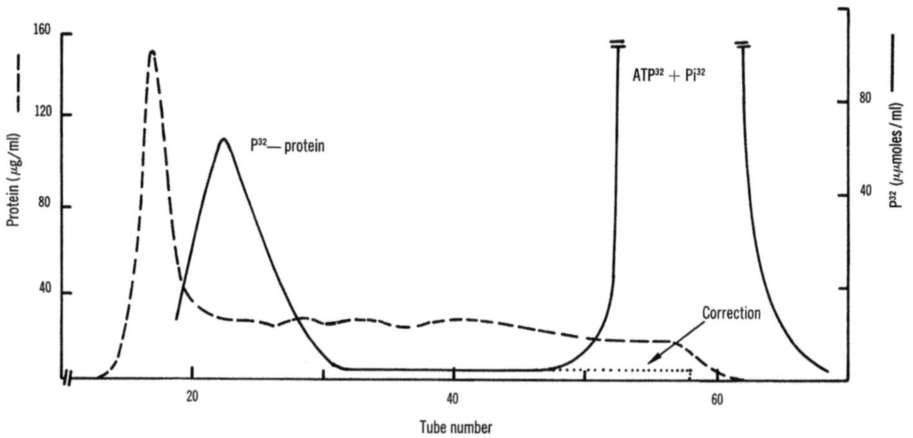

FIG. 11. Separation of the phosphorylated protein as a single radioactive peak by gel filtration through Sephadex G-200. Column size: 2.5 cm × 37 cm. Charged protein: 4.7 mg in 1.0 ml. Flow rate: 22 ml per hour. Each 3.9 ml was fractionated. Protein recovery was 102 percent. Apparent specific activity at the top of the peak (fraction #21) was 2.0 μ moles P^{32}/g protein.

of the charged sample to column size should not exceed 1:50 to avoid obscuring the weak incorporation by the overwhelming $AT^{32}P$ peak. Both protein and ^{32}P radioactivity are recovered almost quantitatively.

In order to compare levels of labeling at different labeling conditions, it is sufficient to monitor the protein peak of each sample by ultraviolet absorption and determine its specific radioactivity.

Sephadex G-15 is not suitable since $AT^{32}P$ is partially excluded by this gel and overlaps on the protein peak.

SEPARATION OF THE PHOSPHORYLATED PROTEIN THROUGH SEPHADEX G-200: Gel filtration of labeled Na^+,K^+-ATPase may also be performed through Sephadex G-200 (Nagano et al., in preparation). Particular attention must be paid to these points:

1. Too high hydrostatic pressure from the reservoir should be avoided. Otherwise, the gel particles become strongly compressed and the flow becomes too slow or may stop.
2. Suitable flow rates must be maintained, particularly when using Sephadex (10 ml per hour using a 2-cm × 30-cm column). Some tailing of the released ^{32}P may occur, making a low plateau of radioactivity after the peak. An approximate correction is made as shown in Figure 11 (dotted line).

The phosphorylated protein is retarded from the void volume and appears at the position of R = 1.35 (R, ratio of the elution volume of the peak to the void volume determined by Blue Dextran). The position corresponds to a molecular weight of about 2 × 10^5. Rechromatography of the eluted phosphorylated protein through Sephadex G-200 gives a peak at the same position of R = 1.30—1.35. When 5 mM Mg^{++} is included in the eluant, the radioactive peak is eluted earlier (R = 1.20) and is not symmetrical, suggesting some interaction between void volume protein and the phosphorylated protein under these conditions.

Similar gel filtration using Sephadex G-150, Sepharose 4-B, or Biogel P-200 also gives an eluting position which coincides with the estimate of particle size as 2 $\times 10^5$.

MEASUREMENTS OF INORGANIC ^{32}PHOSPHATE (^{32}PI) INCORPORATION INTO Na^+,K^+-ATPase PREPARATIONS. Carrier free inorganic ^{32}orthophosphate was obtained from the Union Carbide Corporation (Tuxedo, N.Y.) and immediately diluted and neutralized to pH 7.4 with tris-base. In some cases, aliquots of this solution were passed through Dowex-1 (Cl^- form) columns; in other cases the solution was boiled for 15 minutes. These procedures were used in an attempt to minimize the concentration of polyphosphates, especially pyrophosphate. Identical results were obtained, however, when the pretreated or the treated ^{32}Pi solutions were used. ^{32}Pi incorporation into calf-brain cortical Na^+,K^+-ATPase preparations was observed under specific assay conditions. Experiments may be carried out at 37°C in 50 mM tris-Cl, pH 7.4, 0.1 mM ouabain, 3 mM $MgCl_2$, 0.5 to 0.7 mg protein, and any other desired additions. The reactions are started by addition of 5 nmoles of inorganic ^{32}phosphate (final volume = 1 ml). After two minutes of incubation, the reaction is stopped by the addition of 4 ml of freshly prepared, ice-cold 5% tricholoracetic acid (TCA) which contains 1 mM phosphoric acid. The tubes are placed on ice for 5 minutes and subsequently centrifuged for 4 minutes (table top centrifuge kept at 23 to 25°C). Longer centrifugations cause tight packing of the precipitates, difficulty in redispersion of the precipitates, and loss of precision. The pellets are resuspended in 3 ml of the TCA-Pi solution (maintained at 0°C), finely dispersed with a Super Mixer (Lab-Line Instruments, Inc., Melrose Park, Ill.), and centrifuged as described above. The wash is usually repeated three times. (Preliminary experiments indicated that this number of washes is adequate for quantitative results; additional washes, in fact, lead to an increasing loss of the label.) In some cases the TCA washes can be followed by the treatments listed below:

(1) Absolute ethanol wash
(2) Two chloroform:methanol (2:1) washes
(3) Absolute ethanol wash

These washes do not alter the results in a quantitative manner, and are not routinely employed (Lindenmayer, et al., 1968). The washed pellets are suspended in 0.2 N NaOH and solubilized in a boiling water bath for 5 minutes. An aliquot of this solution is analyzed for protein by the Lowry Method (Lowry, et al., 1951); a second aliquot is placed in scintillation fluid (see Part A) and analyzed for ^{32}P content.

In this laboratory it was found that ouabain, in a dose-related manner, stimulates ^{32}P incorporation. The amounts of drug required for ^{32}Pi incorporation were similar to that for ouabain-induced inhibition of enzyme activity. Potassium inhibited the ouabain effect (Table 5).

TABLE 5

The Incorporation of Inorganic ^{32}Phosphate (^{32}Pi) into Calf-Brain Na^+, K^+-ATPase Preparations.

Conditions	^{32}Pi incorporated (pmoles/mg protein)
No additions	7.0
Ouabain	8.1
Mg^{2+}	14.2
Mg^{2+} + ouabain	38.4
Mg^{2+}, ouabain + K^+	21.6

The experiment was carried out at 37°C in the presence of 50 mM tris-Cl, pH 7.4, 0.57 mg protein, and where indicated 3 mM $MgCl_2$, 0.1 mM ouabain, 20 mM KCl. The reactions were started by the addition of 5 nmoles of tris-$^{32}PO_4$ (final volume = 1 ml) and were stopped after two minutes with cold trichloroacetic acid containing 1 mM phosphoric acid.

REFERENCES

Albers, R. W. 1967. Biochemical aspects of active transport. Ann. Rev. Biochem., 36:727-756.

—Koval, G. J., and Siegel, G. J. 1968. Studies on the interaction of ouabain and other cardioactive steroids with sodium-potassium-activated adenosine triphosphatase. Molec. Pharmacol., 4:324-336.

Alonso, G., and Walser, M. 1968. ATP-splitting and calcium binding by brain microsomes measured with a rapid perfusion method. J. Gen. Physiol., 52:111-135.

Bader, H., and Sen, A. K. 1966. (K^+)-dependent acyl phosphatase as part of the (Na^+ + K^+)-dependent ATPase of cell membrane. Biochim. Biophys. Acta, 118:116-123.

—Sen, A. K., and Post, R. L. 1966. Isolation and characterization of a phosphorylated intermediate in the (Na^+ + K^+) system-dependent ATPase. Biochim. Biophys. Acta, 118:106-115.

Besch, H. R., Jr., Allen, J. C., Glick, G., and Schwartz, A. 1970. Correlation between the inotropic action of ouabain and its effects on subcellular enzyme systems from canine myocardium. J. Pharmacol. Exp. Ther., 171:1-12.

Danielli, J. F., and Davson, H. 1935. A contribution to the theory of permeability of thin films. J. Cell. Comp. Physiol., 5:495-500.

Emmelot, P., and Bos., C. J. 1962. Adenosine triphosphatase in the cell-membrane fraction from rat liver. Biochim. Biophys. Acta, 58:374-375.

Fujita, M., Nakao, T., Yashima, Y., Mizuno, N., Nagano, K., and Nakao, M. 1966. Potassium-ion stimulated p-nitrophenylphosphatase activity occurring in a highly specific adenosine triphosphatase preparation from rabbit brain. Biochim. Biophys. Acta, 117:42-53.

—Nagano, K., Mizuno, N., Tashima, Y., Nakao, T., and Nakao, N. 1968. Comparison of some minor activities accompanying a preparation of sodium-plus-potassium ion-stimulated adenosine triphosphatase from pig brain. Biochem. J., 106:113-121.

Glynn, I. M. 1964. The action of cardiac glycosides on ion movements. Pharmacol. Rev., 16:381-407.

—and Chappell, J. B. 1964. A simple method for the preparation of P^{32}-labelled ATP of high specific activity. Biochem. J., 90:147-149.

Hems, D. A., and Rodnight, R. 1966. Properties of phosphate bound to cerebral microsomes during adenosine-triphosphatase activity. Biochem. J., 101:516-523.

Hokin, L. E., Sastry, P. S., Galsworthy, P. R., and Yoda, A. 1965. Evidence that a phosphorylated intermediate in a brain transport adenosine triphosphatase is an acyl phosphate. Proc. Nat. Acad. Sci. U. S. A., 54:177-184.
Korn, E. D. 1968. Structure and function of the plasma membrane: A biochemical perspective. J. Gen. Physiol., 52: 257s-278s.
Langer, G. A., and Brady, A. J. 1968. The effects of temperature upon contraction and ionic exchange in rabbit ventricular myocardium. J. Gen. Physiol., 52:682-713.
Lindenmayer, G. E., Laughter, A. H., and Schwartz, A. 1968. Incorporation of inorganic phosphate-32 into a Na^+,K^+-ATPase preparation: Stimulation by ouabain. Arch. Biochem. Biophys., 127:187-192.
Lowry, O. H., Rosebrough, N. J., Farr, A. L., and Randall, R. J. 1951. Protein measurement with the folin phenol reagents. J. Biol. Chem., 193:265.
Matsui, H., and Schwartz, A. 1966. Purification and properties of a highly active ouabain-sensitive Na^+,K^+-dependent adenosine-triphosphatase from cardiac tissue. Biochim. Biophys. Acta, 128:380-390.
—and Schwartz, A. 1968. Mechanism of cardiac glycoside inhibition on the (Na^+-K^+)-dependent ATPase from cardiac tissue. Biochim. Biophys. Acta, 151:655-663.
Medzihradsky, F., Kline, M. H., and Hokin, L. E. 1967. Studies on the characterization of the sodium-potassium transport adenosine triphosphatase. 1. Solubilization, stabilization and estimation of apparent molecular weight. Arch. Biochem. Biophys., 121:311-316.
Nagano, K., Kanazawa, T., Mizuno, N., Tashima, Y., Nakao, T., and Nakao, M. 1965. Some acyl phosphate-like properties of P^{32}-labeled sodium-potassium-activated adenosine triphosphatase. Biochem. Biophys. Res. Commun., 19:759-764.
—Mizuno, N., Fujita, M., Tashima, Y., Nakao, T., and Nakao, M. 1967. On the possible role of the phosphorylated intermediate in the reaction mechanism of (Na^+-K^+)-ATPase. Biochim. Biophys. Acta, 143:239-248.
Nakao, T., Tashima, Y., Nagano, K., and Nakao, M. 1965. Highly specific sodium-potassium-activated adenosine triphosphatase from various tissues of rabbit. Biochem. Biophys. Res. Commun., 19:755-758.
Post, R. L., and Sen, A. K. 1967. ^{32}P-labeling of a $(Na^+ + K^+)$-ATPase intermediate. *In* Methods in Enzymology. Estabrook, R. W., and Pullman, M. E., eds. Vol. 10, pp. 773-776.
—Sen, A. K., and Rosenthal, A. S. 1965. A phosphorylated intermediate in adenosine triphosphate-dependent sodium and potassium transport across kidney membranes. J. Biol. Chem., 240:1437-1445.
Robertson, J. D. 1959. The ultrastructure of cell membranes and their derivatives. Biochem. Soc. Sympos., 16:3-43.
Schatzmann, H. J. 1953. Herzglycoside als hemmstoffe fur den aktiven kalium uns natrium transport durch die erythrocytenmembran. Helv. Physiol. Pharmacol. Acta, 11:346-354.
—1962. Lipoprotein nature of red cell adenosine triphosphatase. Nature, 196:677.
Schwartz, A., Allen, J. C., and Harigaya, S. 1969. Possible involvement of cardiac Na^+,K^+-ATPase in the mechanism of action of cardiac glycosides. J. Pharmacol. Exp. Ther., 168:31-41.
Shirachi, D., Allard, A., and Trevor, A. 1970. Lubrol extracted Na-K-ATPase from brain and cardiac tissue. Fed. Proc., 29:806.
Skou, J. C. 1957. The influence of some cations on adenosinetriphosphatase from peripheral nerves. Biochim. Biophys. Acta., 23:394-401.
— 1960. Further investigations on a Mg^{2+} + Na^+-activated adenosinetriphosphatase, possibly related to the active linked transport of Na^+ and K^+ across the nerve membrane. Biochim. Biophys. Acta, 42:6-23.
—1962. Preparation from brain and kidney of the enzyme system involved in active transport of Na^+ and K^+. Biochim. Biophys. Acta, 58:314-325.
Tanaka, R., and Abood, L. G. 1964. Phospholipid requirement of Na^+,K^+-activated adenosine triphosphatase from rat brain. Arch. Biochem. Biophys., 108:47-52.

CHAPTER **13**

Contractile Proteins

Arnold M. Katz

Mount Sinai School of Medicine
of the City University of New York
New York, New York

INTRODUCTION

In vitro model systems, made up of various combinations of the purified myofibrillar proteins of cardiac muscle, have long been employed in the search for the molecular sites of action of drugs that modify myocardial contractility. Over the years, methods for the isolation and purification of these proteins have been refined, and procedures once thought to yield single contractile proteins are now known to have resulted in the extraction of mixtures of the myofibrillar proteins. Kühne, in 1864, isolated a viscous protein, which he called *myosin*, when muscle was extracted with neutral salts. For several decades these myosin preparations were believed to consist of a single protein. However, Banga and A. Szent-Györgyi (1941) found that the properties of the myosin obtained after prolonged extraction

Supported by research grant HE 08515 and FR 5367, U.S. Public Health Service, and grant-in-aid 65–G–61 of the American Heart Association. Much of this work was carried out while Dr. Katz was an Established Investigator of the American Heart Association. Dr. Katz is currently Philip J. and Harriet L. Goodhart Professor of Medicine (Cardiology) at the Mount Sinai School of Medicine.

The author would like to thank Miss Doris I. Repke, with whom many of these techniques were evolved, and Mrs. Margaret R. Levy, for many contributions to the preparation of this manuscript.

of the muscle mince (myosin B) differed from those of myosin A, which was obtained by short extraction.

These studies led to more detailed examinations of the composition of these myosins and culminated in the discovery of *actin* (Straub, 1942, 1943). Straub found that protracted extraction of the muscle mince with neutral salts led to the extraction of myosin that contained large amounts of actin, whereas short extraction gave myosin preparations that contained little or no actin. Subsequently, many of the properties of myosin B were found to be due to the fact that it was a complex of two proteins, myosin and actin. During the following two decades the properties of actin were actively studied in a number of laboratories throughout the world in the belief that this was a single protein.

In 1962, however, several investigators demonstrated that the actin preparations employed by most, but not all, groups contained significant quantities of *tropomyosin* (Laki et al., 1962; Drabikowsky and Gergely, 1962; Martonosi, 1962a). This third myofibrillar protein had been isolated from muscle mince several years earlier by Bailey (1948), but the ease with which tropomyosin could be incorporated into polymerized actin had not been recognized.

Shortly thereafter, analysis of tropomyosin-containing actin preparations demonstrated that, in addition to actin and tropomyosin, they contained an additional protein (Katz, 1966a). This protein appears to be *troponin,* which had been isolated from whole muscle mince by Ebashi and Kodama (1965). It is apparent, therefore, that the older myosin preparations, once regarded as being composed of a single molecular species, in fact contained at least four distinct proteins: myosin, actin, tropomyosin, and troponin. Additional evidence now indicates that this list remains incomplete. Ebashi and Ebashi (1965) have described the isolation of α-actinin from conventional actin preparations, and Maruyama (1965) isolated β-actinin, yet another protein from the actins made by some, but not all, preparative procedures. Thus, at this time, it is likely that Kuhne's "myosin" contained six different proteins, and the list may yet be extended (see Katz, 1970).

In addition to the myofibrillar proteins just described, many of which have been obtained by purification of apparently homogeneous contractile proteins, several additional proteins can be prepared from striated muscle (A. G. Szent-Györgyi, 1960; Poglazov, 1966). These include the delta protein (Amberson et al., 1957), contractin or γ-myosin (Dubuisson, 1948; Schapira et al., 1957; Kay and Pabst, 1962), Y-protein (Dubuisson, 1950), metamyosin (Raeber et al., 1955), and "extra proteins" or "X-proteins" (Villafranca, 1956). Some of these, notably delta protein (White et al., 1957) and the extra protein (Corsi, 1957; Perry and Corsi, 1958; Perry and Zydowo, 1959), appear to be heterogeneous. The possible identity between these proteins and the more recently discovered proteins previously mentioned remains to be established.

In the present chapter, consideration shall be limited to four of these proteins: *myosin, actin, tropomyosin,* and *troponin.* Although the other myofibrillar proteins may be of importance in determining the biologic properties of the intact muscle, for the most part their functional significance remains unclear. On the other hand, it is now possible to relate many features of muscular contraction to the activities of these four proteins.

PROPERTIES OF THE INDIVIDUAL PROTEINS

Myosin

The only myofibrillar protein known to possess an active ATPase is myosin, which catalyzes the hydrolysis of ATP to ADP and Pi (Engelhardt and Ljubimova, 1939; Green et al., 1953). The importance of this enzymatic activity to the performance of the intact muscle is well established, and ATP appears to be the immediate source for the chemical energy utilized in muscle contraction (Infante and Davies, 1965). In addition, there is excellent evidence that the speed of shortening in a muscle is determined by the intrinsic ATPase activity of myosin (M. Bárány et al., 1965; Gergely et al., 1965; Katz et al., 1966b; M. Bárány, 1967). This relationship between the rate of ATP hydrolysis by the contractile proteins and the speed of muscle shortening is of considerable importance in the analysis of the physiologic and pharmacologic modulation of cardiac muscle performance as changes in myocardial contractility are paralleled by prominent changes in shortening velocity (Wiggers, 1927; Abbott and Mommaerts, 1959; Sonnenblick, 1962). While it is possible that mechanisms which bring about these important changes in myocardial contractility act by increasing the ATPase activity of the heart's contractile proteins (Katz, 1967a), serious problems exist in defining this relationship (see Katz, 1970).

The extensive literature concerning the molecular weight of rabbit skeletal myosin has been reviewed by Dreizen et al. (1967). It now appears that the molecular weight of myosin prepared by conventional methods is approximately 500,000, whereas myosin prepared by ammonium sulfate fractionation appears to have the slightly higher molecular weight of 600,000, due possibly to a small degree of aggregation. In the case of cardiac myosin, the previously accepted molecular weight of approximately 225,000 (Ellenbogen et al., 1960; Olson et al., 1961) has been found to be in error (Gergely et al., 1956; Gergely, 1959; Davis et al., 1960; Brahms and Kay, 1962b, 1963; Mueller et al., 1964a; Luchi et al., 1965; Conway and Roberts, 1965). Thus, as in the case of rabbit skeletal myosin, the current best estimate for the molecular weight of cardiac myosin is approximately 500,000.

Like skeletal myosin, cardiac myosin is an elongated molecule, approximately 1,600 to 1,700 Å in length (Gergely and Kohler, 1957; Mueller et al., 1964a; Conway and Roberts, 1965). In the case of both cardiac and skeletal myosins, these hydrodynamic estimates of molecular dimensions have been confirmed by electromicroscopic examinations of individual myosin molecules (Rice, 1961; Zobel and Carlson, 1963; Mueller et al., 1964a; Carney and Brown, 1965, 1966; Rice et al., 1966). Electromicrographs show one end of the rodlike myosin molecule to be enlarged. As will be discussed, the globular end of the myosin molecule probably represents the site for both actin-binding and ATPase activity. Measurements of the optical rotatory dispersions of skeletal (C. Cohen and Szent-Györgyi, 1957; Simmons et al., 1961; C. Cohen, 1961; Tonomura et al., 1962, 1963) and cardiac (Brahms and Kay, 1963; Kay and Green, 1964) myosin give similar values. By the usual criteria for estimating α-helix content, approximately 55 to 65 percent of the peptide chain of both myosins exists in the α-helical configuration. A similar value for the α-helix content of skeletal myosin has been obtained from a study of ultraviolet circular dichroism (Mommaerts, 1966). Solvents such as ethylene glycol cause similar changes in the optical rotatory dispersions of both cardiac and skeletal myosins (Kay et al., 1964).

When monomeric skeletal myosin is allowed to form aggregates, the myosin monomers associate in a linear manner that allows the globular ends of the individual molecules to project from the filament (Huxley, 1963; Kaminer and Bell, 1966; Josephs and Harrington, 1966). The resulting aggregate closely resembles the thick filament of muscle in which the projecting cross bridges correspond to the actin-binding and ATPase sites of the myosin molecules (Huxley, 1963).

The extremely large size of the myosin molecule strongly suggests that it is composed of more than one peptide chain. Thus, several approaches have been utilized in an attempt to separate and isolate myosin subunits. One of the earliest and most valuable methods employed to degrade the myosin molecule has been exposure to the proteolytic enzyme trypsin (Gergely, 1950). Following tryptic digestion, the high viscosity of native myosin becomes reduced, whereas the myosin ATPase activity (Gergely, 1950, 1953; Mihályi, 1953) and actin-combining ability (Mihályi and Szent-Györgyi, 1953b) are preserved. Early in the course of the tryptic digestion of skeletal myosin, two components can be identified in the analytical ultracentrifuge (Mihályi and Szent-Györgyi, 1953a; A. G. Szent-Györgyi, 1953). These have been designated the meromyosins. The more rapidly sedimenting heavy meromyosin (HMM) contains both ATPase activity and the ability to bind to actin (Mihályi and Szent-Györgyi, 1953b; Lowey and Holtzer, 1959), whereas the smaller component, light meromyosin (LMM), has solubility properties similar to those of native myosin (A. G. Szent-Györgyi, 1953). The molecular weight of HMM now appears to be approximately 350,000; that of LMM is approximately 150,000 (Mueller, 1964).

Proteolytic enzymes other than trypsin can produce meromyosins from native myosin. Chymotrypsin (Gergely et al., 1955), subtilisin (Middlebrook, 1958), and snake venon esterase (Laki, 1958) all lead to formation of meromyosins that are generally similar to those released by trypsin. Because these enzymes cleave the myosin molecule at different points, the meromyosins cannot be considered to represent true subunits of myosin, if a subunit is defined as a separate polypeptide linked to other peptide chains by noncovalent bonds.

Significant differences between the actions of trypsin on cardiac and skeletal myosins have been observed. Unlike the tryptic hydrolysis of skeletal myosin, which shows an initial fast rate followed by a slower rate (Mihályi, 1953; Mihályi and Harrington, 1959; Lowey and Cohen, 1962), the digestion of cardiac myosin by low concentrations of trypsin proceeds only at a slow rate (Iyengar et al., 1961;

Brahms and Kay, 1963; Kay and Green, 1964; Theiner et al., 1963; Mueller et al., 1964b; M. Bárány et al., 1964b). Under these conditions, meromyosins can be identified (Gergely, 1959), but their isolation is extremely difficult (Iyengar et al., 1961; Brahms and Kay, 1963; Kay and Green, 1964), and digestion with high concentrations of myosin and trypsin is necessary to permit isolation of the meromyosins of cardiac muscle (Mueller et al., 1964b). However, once isolated, cardiac LMM and cardiac HMM have physicochemical properties that are indistinguishable from those of the corresponding skeletal meromyosin (Mueller et al., 1964b).

LMM has a highly ordered structure (C. Cohen and Szent-Györgyi, 1957; Lowey and Cohen, 1962; A. G. Szent-Györgyi et al., 1960) which may represent a coiled coil (two parallel chains each possessing a full α-helical structure) (A. G. Szent-Györgyi et al., 1960; Lowey and Cohen, 1962; Lowey, 1965). The hydrodynamic properties of HMM, on the other hand, indicate that it is composed of a globular region to which is attached a short, highly helical rod (C. Cohen, 1961; Lowey and Cohen, 1962). This interpretation has been confirmed by electron microscopic examination of HMM (Huxley, 1963; Rice et al., 1966). A helical fraction of HMM, which can be isolated by acid treatment, probably represents the rodlike portion of the molecule (Lowey, 1964), and the globular portion of HMM, which retains both the ATPase activity and actin-combining properties of myosin and HMM, has been obtained by brief tryptic degradation of HMM (Mueller and Perry, 1962). Subsequent exposure of this latter fraction (usually called HMM subfragment 1) to trypsin is followed by the appearance of a more heterogenous fraction, HMM subfragment 2, which lacks both ATPase activity and actin-combining ability. Estimates of the molecular weight of HMM subfragment 1 include values of 117,000 (Young et al., 1965), and 147,000 (Yagi and Yazawa, 1966). Mueller (1965), who obtained values up to 170,000 for molecular weight of HMM subfragment 1, attributed the variability of the molecular weight estimates to difference in the extent of degradation by trypsin.

Treatment of myosin with concentrated urea of guanidine causes the appearance of fragments that appear to be true subunits of myosin. Prolonged exposure of myosin to 6 to 8 M urea results in the production of smaller molecular particles (Weber and Stöver, 1933; Mommaerts, 1945; Snellman and Erdös, 1948; Tsao, 1953b; Wetlaufer and Edsall, 1960; Small et al., 1961). In 12 M urea, on the other hand, a single monodisperse component has been observed on both ultracentrifugal and electrophoretic analysis. (Small et al., 1961). The fragments produced in 6 to 8 M urea have not been extensively studied because the prolonged urea treatment (weeks to months) (Tsao, 1953b) has rendered this approach somewhat impractical.

High concentrations of guanidine have proven to be more useful in separating myosin into subunits. It was initially believed that concentrated guanidine (or urea) led to the appearance of a single species of myosin subunit (Kielley and Harrington, 1960; Small et al., 1961; Woods et al., 1963), but subsequent studies demonstrated the appearance of an additional low-molecular-weight component when myosin is treated with 5 M guanidine (Wetlaufer and Edsall, 1960; Dreizen et al., 1966, 1967). The larger subunit has a molecular weight of approximately

200,000 (Tsao, 1953b; Kielley and Harrington, 1960; Small et al., 1961; Woods et al., 1963; Dreizen et al., 1966, 1967). The molecular weight of the smaller component, originally estimated to be 46,000 (Dreizen et al., 1966), has recently been revised to approximately 21,000 (Gershman et al., 1966).

Agents other than concentrated urea and guanidine also cause myosin to dissociate into its apparent subunits. A light fragment of molecular weight 19,000 to 29,000 (Dreizen et al., 1967) has been obtained by exposure of myosin to 0.1 M sodium carbonate (Kominz et al., 1959). This light component constitutes 12 to 18 percent of the original myosin molecule (Kominz et al., 1959; Gershman et al., 1966), and Dreizen et al. (1967) have estimated the number of these light subunits to be three per myosin molecule. Further evidence indicates that the light component that is detached by alkali is identical with the small component released from myosin by 5 M guanidine (Dreizen et al., 1967). Other procedures that give rise to small myosin fragments include prolonged heat denaturation (Locker, 1956), storage at 20° to 30°C (Yasui et al., 1960; Johnson and Rowe, 1961), methylmercuric hydroxide (Kominz, 1961), copper cyanide (Kominz and Maruyama, 1960), trypsin treatment of ethanol-denatured myosin (Laki, 1957), sodium dodecylsulfate (Mihályi et al., 1957; Hartshorne and Stracher, 1966), succinylation (Oppenheimer et al., 1966, 1967), acetylation (Locker and Hagyard, 1967a, 1967b), carboxymethylation (Locker and Hagyard, 1967b), and treatment with tripolyphosphate (Locker and Hagyard, 1967a). Examination of the fragments obtained by alkali treatment or succinylation of myosin indicates that the small subunits are electrophoretically polydisperse (Gershman et al., 1966; Oppenheimer et al., 1967); and three distinct components have been found to be liberated by acetylation of myosin (Locker and Hagyard, 1967a, 1967b). At least two of these fragments can be obtained from HMM, but not from LMM (Locker and Hagyard, 1967b; Oppenheimer et al., 1967; K. Bárány and Oppenheimer, 1967).

The heavy fragment obtained by guanidine-treatment of myosin dissociates into two similar components having molecular weights of approximately 210,000. These findings led to the conclusion that myosin is composed of two subunits, and support the interpretations of Mueller (1965), who studied the dissociation of HMM, and of Lowey (1965), who studied the properties of LMM (see above), that native myosin is composed of two polypeptide chains. Thus, the evidence for the two-chain model of the myosin molecule appears to be stronger than that advanced in support of a three-chain model (Kielley and Harrington, 1960; Woods et al., 1963; Young et al., 1964, 1965; Kielley, 1965; see also Katz, 1970, for a more recent review of evidence favoring this view).

The amino acid compositions of rabbit skeletal and dog cardiac myosins are generally similar (Iyengar et al., 1961; Iyengar and Olson, 1965). A minor difference in the cysteine content has been found, however (Iyengar and Olson, 1965; M. Bárány et al., 1964b), and the amino acid compositions of the region around the SH group, which is protected by actin-binding, differ when the tryptic peptides rabbit cardiac and skeletal myosin are compared (Stracher, 1965). Furthermore, the small subunits obtained from cardiac myosin differ from those of white skeletal myosin (Locker and Hagyard, 1967c; Gaetjens and Bárány, 1967). These molecular differences appear to underlie the immunologic dissimilarities between cardiac and skeletal myosins (Ebert, 1953; Samuels, 1961; Finck, 1965a, 1965b), as well as differences in enzymatic activity to be discussed later.

Actin

Actin, the second major contractile protein to have been purified, exists in two forms: *G-actin* (G = globular), the monomer that exists in solutions of low ionic strength, and the *F-actin* (F = fibrous), the polymer that is formed upon addition of salts. The G-F transformation (polymerization) is accompanied by a marked rise in the viscosity of the actin solutions (Straub, 1942, 1943).

G-actin is a nearly symmetrical molecule of ovoid shape, having an axial ratio of approximately 3 (Rowe, 1964), in which one fourth to one third of the peptide chain exists in the form of an α-helix (Nagy and Jencks, 1962; Vazina et al., 1966). The molecular weight of G-actin is approximately 60,000 as determined by sedimentation and viscosity measurements (Kay, 1960), sedimentation equilibrium (Lewis et al., 1963), light scattering (Mommaerts, 1952a; Oosawa et al., 1959; Kay, 1960; Krans et al., 1965), amino acid analysis (Laki and Standaert, 1960), or ATP content (Straub and Feuer, 1950, Mommaerts, 1952c; Ulbrecht et al., 1960; Strohman and Samorodin, 1962; Tsuboi and Hayashi, 1963; M. Bárány et al., 1964a). More recently, several reports have appeared which indicate that the molecular weight of action is 46,000-48,000 (see Katz, 1970). The G-actin molecule appears to consist of a single polypeptide chain whose *N* terminal amino acid is *N*-acetyl aspartic acid (Gaetjens and Bárány, 1966; Alving and Laki, 1966). As usually prepared, G-actin contains one mole each of bound ATP (Straub and Feuer, 1950; Laki et al., 1950; Mommaerts, 1952c; Ulbrecht et al., 1960; Strohman and Samorodin, 1962) and bound Ca^{++} (M. Bárány et al., 1962; Maruyama and Gergely, 1961). Nucleotides other than ATP can be bound by the G-actin molecule (Martonosi and Gouvea, 1961; Grubhofer and Weber, 1961; Martonosi, 1962b; M. Bárány and Finkelman, 1963; Iyengar and Weber, 1964; Mihashi, 1964; Katz, 1964a; M. Bárány et al., 1966; Tonomura et al., 1966; Hayashi, 1967), though with less affinity than ATP; and other bivalent cations, notably Mg^{++} or Mn^{++}, can replace the tightly bound Ca^{++} (Oosawa et al., 1964; Drabikowsky and Strzelecko-Gołaszewska, 1963; Martonosi et al., 1964; Mihashi and Ooi, 1965). The nucleotide and bivalent cation both appear to be bound at or near a single site on the G-actin molecule, because removal of one is paralleled by loss of the other (M. Bárány et al., 1961, 1962; Martonosi and Gouvea, 1961; Grubhofer and Weber, 1961; Tonomura and Yoshimura, 1961; Strohman and Samorodin, 1962). Removal of either bound nucleotide or bound calcium is rapidly followed by loss of the ability of G-actin to polymerize, although polymerization of G-actin that contains neither bound nucleotide nor bound divalent cations has been observed (Kasai et al., 1965; M. Bárány et al., 1966). Thus, the bound nucleotide and cation probably serve to stabilize a "native" conformation of the G-actin molecule (Katz, 1963, 1964a, 1965; Kasai et al., 1965; M. Bárány et al., 1966), rather than acting as cofactors in the polymerization reaction.

Polymerization of G-actin-ATP (G-actin that contains bound ATP) is accompanied by dephosphorylation of the nucleotide, thereby leading to the formation of F-actin-ADP (Straub and Feuer, 1950; Mommaerts, 1952c; A. G. Szent-Györgyi, 1951; Ulbrecht et al., 1960). The nucleotide bound to G-actin is freely exchangeable, and can be easily removed, but F-actin contains a tightly bound nucleotide (Martonosi et al., 1960a; M. Bárány et al., 1961; Strohman and Samorodin, 1962). Similarly, the bound Ca^{++} of G-actin, but not of F-actin, is readily removed by chelating agents or ion exchangers (Chrambach et al., 1961, Tonomura and Yoshimura, 1961; Maruyama and Gergely, 1961; M. Bárány et al., 1962). In the course of polymerization, therefore, loosely bound ATP is converted to tightly bound ADP, and inorganic phosphate is liberated. On the other hand, actin-bound ADP appears not to be rephosphorylated during the depolymerization of F-actin. Instead, free ATP is exchanged for bound ADP during depolymerization, thereby giving rise to stable G-actin-ATP (Martonosi et al., 1960a; Ulbrecht et al., 1960; Grubhofer and Weber, 1961; M. Bárány and Finkelman, 1963). Similarly, formation of G-actin-ATP from G-actin-ADP requires exchange of actin-bound ATP for ADP, and cannot proceed through phosphorylation of ADP bound to the actin monomer (West et al., 1967a).

As usually defined, actin does not possess the ability to hydrolyze ATP. Although dephosphorylation of ATP does occur during polymerization, free ATP is not hydrolyzed by either G-actin of F-actin. In equilibrium mixtures of G- and F-actin, however, ATP is slowly dephosphorylated (Asakura and Oosawa, 1960); and when F-actin is disrupted by sonic vibration—a treatment that permits actin-bound ADP to exchange with free ATP (Asakura et al., 1963a; M. Bárány and Finkelman, 1963)—rapid liberation of Pi from ATP is seen (Asakura, 1961). Similarly, hydrolysis of free ATP is seen at high (55° to 60°C) temperatures (Asai and Tawada, 1966). In all of these reactions, this apparent actin ATPase activity appears under conditions in which the links between actin monomers are being repeatedly interrupted and reformed (Asakura et al., 1963b).

The role of salts in promoting the polymerization of actin has been recognized since the discovery of this protein (Straub, 1942). This action is nonspecific in that a large variety of salts can cause G-actin to polymerize, and the extent of polymerization is independent of the nature of the salt added to G-actin (Straub, 1943; Mommaerts and Khairallah, 1951; Mommaerts, 1952b). Thus, the action of a variety of salts appears to be to screen the electrostatic repulsions between the G-actin molecules, which are negatively charged at neutral pH (Mommaerts and Khairallah, 1951; Mommaerts, 1952b; Ooi, 1961). Immediately after addition of salt, small oligomers of actin are formed (Mommaerts, 1952b; Tsao, 1953a; Ooi, 1960, 1961). These appear to serve as nuclei for an autocatalytic growth, or condensation, of linear F-actin polymers. Thus the rapid increase in viscosity when salts are added to G-actin in concentrations above a "critical" level has been interpreted as evidence for an autocatalytic growth, or condensation, of linear F-actin (Oosawa et al., 1959; Kasai et al., 1962b), although this phenomenon may, instead, represent the transition from a single-stranded flexible polymer to a double-stranded rigid polymer (Yoshimura et al., 1963).

In addition to their nonspecific effects to screen charges that separate G-actin monomers, bivalent cations have specific effects on the rate of actin's polymerization. Of particular interest are the actions of Ca^{++} and Mg^{++}, which have opposing effects on polymerization rate. The polymerization of actin is accelerated by Mg^{++}, whereas Ca^{++}, which itself is capable of initiating polymerization, acts to slow polymerization induced by other salts (Feuer et al., 1948; Asakura et al., 1957; Kasai et al., 1962a; Oosawa et al., 1965; Mihashi and Ooi, 1965). These effects of Ca^{++} and Mg^{++} appear to reflect cation-induced changes in the conformation of the G-actin molecule (Katz, 1963).

Attempts to define conformational changes in the actin monomer following dephosphorylation of actin-bound nucleotide have given conflicting results. Dephosphorylation of this actin-bound nucleotide appears to change neither intrinsic viscosity (L. B. Cohen, 1966), optical rotatory dispersion (Nagy, 1966), nor the ultraviolet spectrum of the protein between 270 and 310 mμ (Higashi and Oosawa, 1965). Although gross changes in secondary and tertiary structure cannot be clearly identified, slight differences in the ultraviolet absorption at wavelengths below 240 mμ have been reported (Higashi and Oosawa, 1965) and different spectral shifts following removal of nucleotide from G-actin-ATP and G-actin-ADP have been seen (West et al., 1967b). A significant difference between the conformations of G-actin-ATP and G-actin-ADP is suggested by the finding that the rates of reaction of *p*-mercuribenzoate with sulfhydryl groups of G-actins containing bound ATP or ADP are comparable (Katz, 1964a). In addition, bivalent cations have different effects on the SH reactivity of G-actin ATP and G-actin-ADP (Katz, 1963, 1964a). Thus, depolymerization of actin-bound nucleotide appears to cause minor, but significant, conformational changes in the actin monomer.

Polymerization itself causes large changes in ultraviolet absorption (Higashi and Oosawa, 1965) which are due primarily to the increased scattering of light by the large F-actin polymers (Mommaerts, 1952b). Specific changes in the absorption of ultraviolet light between 270 and 310 mμ have been interpreted as evidence that tyrosine and tryptophane residues, which are exposed in the case of G-actin, become folded within the F-actin molecule (Higashi and Oosawa, 1965; Oosawa et al., 1965). Polymerization of actin is also accompanied by changes in the spectrum below 240 mμ, which suggest that parts of the peptide chains in F-actin may exist in the β structure, as well as in the α-helical conformation (Higashi and Oosawa, 1965).

The helical structure of the F-actin polymer, predicted by thermodynamic and kinetic analyses of the polymerization of actin (Oosawa and Kasai, 1962; Kasai et al., 1962b), has been observed when actins prepared from both skeletal muscle (Hanson and Lowy, 1963; Huxley, 1963) and cardiac muscle (Katz and Hall, 1963) are examined in the electron microscope. Isolated thin filaments of muscle, examined by similar methods, have a structure indistinguishable from that of F-actin (Hanson and Lowey, 1963). F-actin appears to be a right-handed helix (Depue and Rice, 1965).

Cardiac actin is identical with skeletal actin in all respects studied to date. Physicochemical properties (Katz and Hall, 1963; Jenney, 1967), amino acid compositions (Katz and Carsten, 1963; Jenney 1967), and the number and reactivities of sulfhydryl groups (Katz and Maxwell, 1964) are the same for cardiac and skeletal actins. The myosins and actins from heart and skeletal muscle are interchangeable in combining to form actomyosin (Gergely and Gouvea, 1953; Katz et al., 1966a); the stoichiometry of the interaction between cardiac actin and myosin is the same as that for skeletal actin; and the extent of activation of either cardiac or skeletal myosin is the same for both actins (M. Bárány et al., 1964b; Katz et al., 1966b; Jenney, 1967).

Tropomyosin

Tropomyosin, first purified by Bailey (1948), constitutes 10 to 12 percent of the myofibrillar proteins of skeletal muscle (Perry and Corsi, 1958). It is a highly helical protein (C. Cohen and Szent-Györgyi, 1957; C. Cohen, 1961; Lowey, 1965; Fraser et al., 1965), having a molecular weight of approximately 70,000 (Holtzer et al., 1965; Lowey, 1965; Woods, 1966). Tropomyosin, like LMM, appears to exist as a coiled-coil (Lowey, 1965). Tropomyosin preparations often contain a nucleotide contaminant, but when prepared with care, nucleotide-free tropomyosin can be obtained (Simmons et al., 1961; Katz 1964b). In solutions containing high concentrations of urea along with a sulfhydryl stabilizing reagent, tropomyosin dissociates into two subunits of approximately 34,000 molecular weight (Woods, 1965, 1966). Solutions of tropomyosin are highly viscous at low ionic strength, but additions of salt cause a marked fall in viscosity (Bailey, 1948; Ooi et al., 1962). This behavior is in marked contrast to that of actin, which exists in monomeric form at low ionic strength, and forms a thixotropic gel in the presence of salts.

The physicochemical properties of cardiac tropomyosin are indistinguishable from those of skeletal tropomyosin (Katz and Converse, 1964; McCubbin et al., 1967), and both tropomyosins form identical needlelike crystals (Bailey, 1948; Tsao et al., 1956; Kominz et al., 1957). The amino acid compositions and peptide patterns after tryptic digestion of cardiac and skeletal tropomyosins are the same (Katz and Converse, 1964) as are the electrophoretic mobilities of cardiac and skeletal tropomyosins (Tsao et al., 1956). Thus cardiac and skeletal tropomyosins, like cardiac and skeletal actins, appear to be identical with each other.

Tropomyosin itself has no known enzymatic activity, but this protein has been found to bind stoichiometrically with actin (Laki et al., 1962; Maruyama, 1964). The presence of tropomyosin in F-actin modulates the ability of the latter to activate the Mg^{++}-activated actomyosin ATPase activity (Katz, 1964, to be discussed). Thus, during the clearing phase, tropomyosin delays superprecipitation by inhibiting the ATPase activity, whereas after the onset of superprecipitation tropomyosin increases the extent of activation of myosin ATPase by F-actin (Katz, 1964b; Azuma and Watanabe, 1965a). These effects become maximal at tropomyosin concentrations at which the binding to actin is maximal, and it appears likely that these effects of tropomyosin are due to the presence of this protein in combination with F-actin (Katz, 1964b).

Tropomyosin has been found to contaminate actin preparations when the acetone-dried muscle powder is extracted at room temperature (Laki et al., 1962; Drabikowsky and Gergely, 1962; Martonosi, 1962a). The incorporation of tropomyosin into F-actin is greatly reduced when actin is polymerized in dilute $MgCl_2$. More recently a protein in addition to tropomyosin has been discovered in actin preparations extracted at room temperature (Katz, 1966). This additional protein, which in combination with tropomyosin sensitizes reconstituted actomyosin to Ca^{++}, is troponin (to be discussed).

Calcium-Sensitizing Proteins

On several occasions it has been recognized that the ATPase activity of reconstituted actomyosins made from highly purified actin and myosin often failed to be inhibited when Ca^{++} concentration was reduced by chelating agents (Perry and Grey, 1956; A. Weber and Winicur, 1961). The presence or absence of Ca^{++} sensitivity appeared to depend on the actin preparation used, rather than the myosin (A. Weber and Winicur, 1961). A. Szent-Györgyi and Kaminer (1963) found that a tropomyosin-containing fraction possessed the metachromasia that they suggested might be a property of Ca^{++}-binding anionic groups and S. Ebashi (1963) and S. Ebashi and Ebashi (1964) found that a tropomyosin-like protein conferred this Ca^{++} sensitivity on reconstituted actomyosin. Examination of actins extracted on ice and at room temperature demonstrated that a Ca^{++}-sensitizing protein complex is included with actin when the acetone-dried muscle powder is extracted at higher temperature (Katz, 1966). The protein complex, which now appears to be responsible for sensitizing actomyosin to Ca^{++}, is troponin plus tropomyosin (S. Ebashi and Kodama, 1965, 1966a, 1966b; S. Ebashi et al., 1967; Hartshorne and Mueller, 1967). Isolation of the Ca^{++}-sensitizing proteins from highly purified room-temperature extracted actins facilitates exclusion of other myofibrillar proteins (Katz, 1966), but these proteins have generally been isolated from whole muscle mince (S. Ebashi and Ebashi, 1964; A. Szent-Györgyi and Kaminer, 1963; Azuma and Watanabe, 1965a, 1965b; Mueller, 1966; Watanabe and Staprans, 1966) or natural actomyosin (Perry et al., 1966; Hartshorne and Mueller, 1967). The actual site of Ca^{++} binding appears to be upon troponin (Ebashi et al., 1967). For a more recent discussion of the properties of troponin, see Katz (1970).

The calcium affinity of the troponins prepared from cardiac and skeletal muscle (Katz et al., 1966a; S. Ebashi et al., 1966; H. H. Weber and Ruegg, 1966) appear to be similar (Katz, 1970). Thus, the level of free Ca^{++} needed to effect a given degree of activation of the cardiac contractile proteins is similar to that which causes similar activation of the contractile proteins of white skeletal muscle (Fanburg, 1964; Katz et al., 1966a). Slight differences in the Sr^{++} affinity of these proteins have been noted, however (Ebashi et al., 1968).

ADENOSINETRIPHOSPHATASE ACTIVITY

Myosin

A large number of factors influence the ATPase activity of the contractile proteins, making this subject one of the most complex aspects of muscle biochemistry. Many contradictions have arisen from studies of myosins that contained unrecognized contaminating proteins, so that discovery of additional myofibrillar proteins has often permitted conflicting findings concerning the effects of various agents upon this enzymatic activity.

In the absence of salts, myosin has little or no ATPase activity (Mommaerts and Seraidarian, 1947), and as stated by A. Szent-Györgyi (1947): "all metals that do not denature protein have an activating effect." Alkali-metal salts stimulate myosin ATPase activity when they are present in low concentrations (Banga and Szent-Györgyi, 1943; A. Szent-Györgyi, 1947; Mommaerts and Seraidarian, 1947; Mommaerts and Green, 1954; Maruyama and Ishikawa, 1963), whereas at higher concentrations they inhibit this activity. The inhibition of myosin ATPase activity by high concentrations of alkali-metal salts follows the order predicted by the nonspecific structure-disrupting effects of the cation (Warren et al., 1966). In the case of KCl, the alkali-metal salt used most commonly in studies of the contractile proteins, maximal myosin ATPase activity is seen at concentrations of 0.2 to 0.3 M (Mommaerts and Seraidarian, 1947; Banga and Szent-Györgyi, 1943; Mommaerts and Green, 1954).

Calcium salts have a marked stimulatory action upon myosin ATPase activity (Bailey, 1942; Mommaerts and Seraidarian, 1947; Mommaerts and Green, 1954). In the presence of KCl, however, the effects of calcium become biphasic, with stimulation of ATPase activity at low $CaCl_2$ concentrations and inhibition at higher concentrations (Mommaerts and Green, 1954). The optimal calcium concentration in the presence of KCl varies with pH. In the pH range around 7.0, maximal ATPase activity is seen in approximately 1 mM Ca^{++} (Mommaerts and Green, 1954). Kinetically, the activation of myosin by Ca^{++} at pH 6.4 reflects an increase in V_{max}, although K_s also is increased, whereas at pH 9.0 Ca^{++} increases V_{max} while K_s is reduced (Green and Mommaerts, 1954). The kinetic interpretation of these changes in K_s is difficult, especially that seen at pH 6.4. These findings appear to reflect an "anomaly" in the pH dependence of myosin ATPase activity, in which the Ca^{++}-activated myosin ATPase first rises, then falls at neutral pH, and then rises again as the pH becomes more alkaline. The decline in activity at neutral pH is abolished by agents such as mercurials and dinitrophenol (to be discussed).

Unlike Ca^{++}, Mg^{++} has a marked inhibitory effect on myosin ATPase activity (Banga and Szent-Györgyi, 1943; Mommaerts and Seraidarian, 1947; Braverman and Morgulis, 1948; Hasselbach, 1952). In the presence of Mg^{++} and Ca^{++} together, the effects of the former predominate, so that Mg^{++} has a strong inhibitory effect on the Ca^{++}-activated myosin ATPase (Mommaerts and Seraidarian, 1947; Mommaerts and Green, 1954).

The ATPase activity of cardiac myosin is less than that of white skeletal myosin (Bailey, 1942; Csapó, 1949; Gelotte, 1951; Gergely and Gouvea, 1953; Tenow and Snellman, 1954; Gergely et al., 1956; Gergely, 1959, Ellenbogen et al., 1960; M. Bárány et al., 1964b; Katz et al., 1966b; Seidel, 1967). However, when the ATPase activity of red skeletal myosin is compared with that of cardiac myosin, little difference is seen (Katz et al., 1966b; Seidel, 1967). Comparison of myosin ATPase activity with the constants that characterize the physiologic function of a given muscle (Hill, 1938) strongly suggests that myosin ATPase activity determines the velocity of shortening of the muscle (Katz et al., 1966b; M. Bárány, 1967; Katz, 1967a, 1967b).

The patterns of activation and inhibition of both cardiac and white skeletal myosins by various cations generally are similar (Gergely et al., 1956; Brahms and Kay, 1963; M. Bárány et al., 1964b; Mueller et al., 1964a; Katz et al., 1966b; Luchi and Kritcher, 1966). However, the KCl sensitivity of the Ca^{++}-activated cardiac myosin ATPase is less than that of white skeletal myosin, and the activation of this ATPase activity at alkaline pH is much less in the case of cardiac myosin (M. Bárány et al., 1964b). Although the extent of Mg^{++} inhibition of cardiac myosin is the same as that of white skeletal myosin, the extent of Ca^{++} activation is less in cardiac myosin (Jenney, 1965; Katz et al., 1966b).

As mentioned, treatment of myosin with a variety of agents has been found to activate the ATPase activity at neutral pH. Thus, blocking of some myosin sulfhydryl groups (Greville and Needham, 1955; Chappell and Perry, 1955; Kielly and Bradley, 1956; Morales et al., 1957; Morales and Hoffa, 1960; Blum, 1960, 1962; Levy and Ryan, 1961; Gilmour and Gellert, 1961; Tonomura et al., 1963; Martonosi and Meyer, 1964; Rainford et al., 1964; Sekine and Kielley, 1964; Blum and Sanadi, 1964a, 1964b; Gaetjens et al., 1964) or treatment with dioxane (Tonomura et al., 1961, 1963; Rainford et al., 1964), dinitrophenol (Greville and Needham, 1955; Chappell and Perry, 1955; Rainford et al., 1962; Levy and Ryan, 1961; Levy et al., 1963), hydrogen peroxide (Rainford et al., 1964), and low concentrations of urea or guanidine (Brahms and Kay, 1962a) have all been found to increase the Ca^{++}-activated ATPase of white skeletal myosin. The mechanism responsible for this activation remains uncertain, although many of these agents abolish the anomalous fall in activity around neutral pH. As the latter appears to reflect a conformational change in the myosin molecule (Gilmour and Griffith, 1957; Levy et al., 1959; Blum, 1960), these agents probably cause activation of myosin ATPase by producing a local change in the conformation around the active center of the myosin molecule (Rainford et al., 1964). These phenomena can also be demonstrated in the case of cardiac myosin (Mueller et al., 1964a; Luchi and Kritcher, 1966; Katz and Repke, unpublished results).

Actomyosin

When considering the enzymatic behavior of actomyosin,* it is important to distinguish between two types of phenomena. The first, analogous to those seen as in the case of myosin alone, are those mechanisms that cause activation or inhibition of the ATPase activity of the actomyosin complex. In addition, however, a variety of activators of actomyosin ATPase activity can, in high concentration, reduce the rate of ATP hydrolysis by promoting the dissociation of actin and

*Confusion can arise from the terminology that has been used to describe various myosin and actomyosin preparations (see A. G. Szent-Györgyi, 1960). Previous terms used to designate myosin itself include L-myosin and Myosin A, whereas Myosin B or natural actomyosin refers to the actomyosin preparations obtained by prolonged extraction of muscle with salt solutions. Reconstituted actomyosin is made by combining individually purified actin and myosin.

myosin. These phenomena are exemplified in the following consideration of the effects of cations and nucleotides in actomyosin ATPase activity.

A variety of cations have a dual effect on actomyosin ATPase activity, exhibiting activation at lower concentrations and inhibiting this activity at higher concentrations. Thus, actomyosin ATPase activity is stimulated by low concentrations of alkali metal ions, Ca^{++}, Mg^{++}, and other metal ions, whereas high concentrations of these ions inhibit this activity (Banga and Szent-Györgyi, 1943; Mommaerts and Seraidarian, 1947; Hasselbach, 1952; Watanabe et al., 1953; Maruyama and Watanabe et al., 1962). Although these phenomena bear a general resemblance to the effects of some of these ions on myosin itself, the observed effects on ATPase activity reflect, in addition, variations in the degree of association between myosin and actin. Thus, dissociation of actomyosin, by reducing activation by actin, causes ATPase activity to decrease. Similar findings have been obtained in studies of myofibrils, which when prepared from rabbit white skeletal muscle have properties generally similar to those of actomyosin (Perry, 1951). However, the amounts of salt needed to effect dissociation of actin and myosin in myofibrils are higher than those that cause dissociation of actomyosin (Perry, 1951, 1956; Hasselbach, 1952). This quantatative difference is probably due to the greater structural organization of the contractile proteins in the myofibrils, as compared to the rather loose aggregations seen in both natural and reconstituted actomyosin.

In the presence of Mg^{++}, as in its absence, the alkali metal salts have a dual effect on actomyosin ATPase activity, with stimulation of ATP hydrolysis at lower ionic strengths and inhibition at higher ionic strengths (Bowen and Gershfeld, 1957; Maruyama and Ishikawa, 1963). The optimal KCl concentration in 1 mM $MgCl_2$ is approximately 0.035 M (Maruyama and Ishikawa, 1963). Likewise, in the presence of KCl, either Mg^{++} (Maruyama and Ishikawa, 1963) or Ca^{++} (Bowen and Gershfeld, 1957) will stimulate actomyosin ATPase activity at low concentrations and inhibit this activity at high concentrations (Mommaerts and Seraidarian, 1947; Bowen and Gershfeld, 1957). The stimulation of actomyosin ATPase activity by low concentrations of Mg^{++} is in marked contrast to the inhibitory effects of this cation on myosin alone, and agents that dissociate actomyosin into actin and myosin will change the effect of Mg^{++} on ATPase activity from enhancement to inhibition (Hasselbach, 1952). Adenosinetriphosphate, like the metal ions, has a dual action on actomyosin ATPase activity (Perry, 1956). These effects will be considered further in the next section.

Evidence for the participation of actin-bound nucleotide in the ATPase activity of actomyosin has been sought in a number of studies. Neither F-actin-bound ADP (Martonosi et al., 1960a; Moos, 1964a, 1964b) nor G-actin-bound ADP (West et al., 1967a) appears to be susceptible to rephosphorylation, so that cyclic phosphorylation-dephosphorylation of actin-bound ADP would require exchange of free ATP for bound ADP in a depolymerized or disrupted (Asakura et al., 1963b) portion of the F-actin polymer. However, little incorporation of ^{32}P administered to the intact animal into the bound ADP of muscle extracts, most of which exists in association with F-actin, has been found (Martonosi et al., 1960b). During superprecipitation of actomyosin (to be discussed), little or no exchange of

F-actin-bound ADP with free ATP has been found by Martonosi et al. (1960a) and Nakamura and Tonomura (1967). However, A. G. Szent-Györgyi and Prior (1966) and Iyengar and Cain (1966) reported that up to half the F-actin bound ADP can be exchanged during superprecipitation of actomyosin. This finding would indicate that, in this in vitro analogue of contraction, actin-bound nucleotide is dephosphorylated and, subsequently, replaced by free ATP from the medium. Strong evidence against the participation of actin-bound nucleotide in the rapid hydrolysis of ATP by actomyosin has been obtained in studies of actomyosin reconstituted from nucleotide-free actin. M. Bárány et al. (1966) reported that the actomyosin type of ATPase activity can proceed in actomyosin reconstituted from myosin and nucleotide-free actin in the presence of deoxyATP, which does not bind to actin. Furthermore, M. Bárány et al. (1966) found the hydrolysis of deoxyATP by such actomyosin to proceed at the same rate as did hydrolysis of ATP, thus suggesting that binding of the nucleotide to actin is not necessary for these phenomena. On the other hand, Tonomura et al. (1966) and Tokiwa et al. (1967) found that nucleotide-free F-actin, when incorporated into reconstituted actomyosin, was much less effective than F-actin containing ADP in activating the hydrolysis of deoxyATP, and Hayashi (1967) reported that actomyosin reconstituted with nucleotide-free F-actin did not superprecipitate in the presence of deoxyATP. This important question of the role of actin-bound nucleotide in the superprecipitation of actomyosin thus remains unsettled.

PHYSICAL CHANGES IN THE ACTOMYOSIN COMPLEX: SUPERPRECIPITATION

As mentioned previously, many effects of ions, nucleotides, and other agents upon actomyosin can be interpreted in terms of a primary action upon the state of association between actin and myosin. Thus ions may promote formation of the actomyosin complex; or they may cause dissociation, with loss of the activating effect of actin, upon myosin enzymatic activity.

The manifestations of these phenomena are different at high and low ionic strength. In the presence of high concentrations of salts, the actomyosin is dissolved and exists as a sol, whereas at lower ionic strengths the proteins exist as an insoluble gel. Most studies of the physiologic properties of actomyosin are carried out on actomyosin gels. Although such preparations are inconvenient to work with, and the irregular nature of these insoluble aggregates can complicate interpretation of certain experimental findings, it must be recognized that the actomyosin in the living muscle also is not in solution, though in a more ordered structure than can be obtained with the extracted proteins. The following description of the changes that occur in the actomyosin complex will be centered around the dual effects of ATP. Similar phenomena result from the actions of a number of cations, as has already been discussed on pp. 399-402 of this chapter.

Addition of ATP to actomyosin sols at high salt concentration (0.5 to 0.6 M KCl) causes a marked fall in viscosity and flow birefringence (Needham et al., 1941; Dainty et al., 1944; A. Szent-Györgyi, 1947; H. H. Weber, 1950). This effect is due to dissociation of actomyosin into actin and myosin (H. H. Weber, 1950; Johnson and Landolt, 1950; A. Weber, 1956; Gergely, 1959; Martonosi et al., 1960c). Reduction in ATP concentration, due to hydrolysis of ATP, causes the original high viscosity to be restored. The rate of viscosity increase is accelerated by Ca^{++} and inhibited by Mg^{++}, as would be predicted from the actions of these cations on the ATPase activity of myosin alone (Mommaerts, 1948).

When similar experiments are carried out at lower ionic strengths–e.g., at KCl concentrations between 0.10 and 0.15 M–these phenomena are generally similar in nature, though they have quite different manifestations. Thus addition of high concentrations of ATP to actomyosin gels in the presence of Mg^{++} again causes a marked decrease in turbidity which is due to dissociation of actin and myosin (A. Szent-Györgyi, 1947; Spicer, 1952). Hence the term "clearing phase" is used to describe the dissociated state of actomyosin gels under the influence of high ATP concentrations. Addition of lower concentrations of ATP, on the other hand, causes a prompt increase in turbidity which is due to shrinkage and dehydration of the actomyosin gel. This process, also called syneresis, causes a reduction in the volume of the actomyosin precipitate collected by low-speed centrifugation (A. Szent-Györgyi, 1947). To describe this diminution in the volume of the actomyosin gel, Szent-Györgyi coined the term "superprecipitation," which is now commonly used to describe the syneresis of actomyosin.

The dissociation of actomyosin gels by ATP is not an "all-or-none" phenomenon, but may be more or less complete, depending on the ionic strength and the concentrations of Mg^{++} and ATP. With partial dissociation–e.g., at KCl concentrations of approximately 0.10 M in 1 mM $MgCl_2$ and 1 mM ATP at pH 6.8– the ATPase activity during the clearing phase remains higher than that of myosin alone under identical conditions (Maruyama and Gergely, 1962a; Katz, 1964b, 1966). Studies of the actin-HMM complex under these conditions indicate that a relatively stable actomyosin complex can be formed at a time when the actomyosin suspension appears to be clear (Eisenberg and Moos, 1967). Following the addition of a high concentration of ATP to actomyosin at constant ionic strength and $MgCl_2$ concentration, the ATPase activity will gradually increase. The initial ATPase activity will be low, but as ATP concentration is reduced (as a result of slow hydrolysis by dissociated actomyosin) (Maruyama and Gergely, 1962a; Katz, 1964), this activity will increase. The initial increase in ATPase activity is gradual, but when actin and myosin recombine, the ATPase will accelerate abruptly and the clearing phase will end. The time course of ATP hydrolysis under such conditions is not linear, so that the use of a single phosphate sample to determine actomyosin ATPase activity may be subject to significant quantitative misinterpretation, depending on the state of the actomyosin gel at the time of sampling.

The ATPase activity during the clearing phase is modified by a variety of agents. In general, those factors that inhibit myosin ATPase activity will prolong the clearing phase. Thus increasing concentrations of KCl, $MgCl_2$, and ATP all delay the onset of superpreciptation (Katz, 1964b). However, superprecipitation itself requires the presence of small amounts of Mg^{++}, but not Ca^{++} (Maruyama and Watanabe, 1962; Weber and Herz, 1962; Maruyama and Ishikawa, 1964; Yasui and Watanabe, 1965). Similarly, the shortening of glycerinated muscle fibers requires small amounts of Mg^{++}, but not Ca^{++} (Watanabe and Sleator, 1957). The optimal Mg^{++} concentration for superprecipitation is approximately 10 μM (Watanabe and Yasui, 1965).

It has been suggested that the rapid hydrolysis of ATP that is associated with superprecipitation occurs only during the process of superprecipitation and is not a characteristic of fully superprecipitated actomyosin (Kuschinsky et al., 1954; Yasui and Watanabe, 1965). However, Endo (1964) attributed the decline in the rate of ATP hydrolysis after superprecipitation to impaired diffusion of ATP into the contracted actomyosin gel.

Sulfhydryl reagents that, in low concentration, accelerate the ATPase activity of myosin alone (see previously) also stimulate the ATPase activity during the clearing phase of actomyosin (Maruyama and Gergely, 1962b; Katz, 1964b). When myosin preparations are allowed to age, or when glassware containing traces of heavy metal ions is used during the preparation of myosin, the properties of the myosin are altered, due probably to sulfhydryl oxidation. As a result, the actomyosins prepared from aged myosins behave like actomyosin made from myosins that have had some of their SH groups blocked. Thus, the ATPase activity during the clearing phase is accelerated, and certain interactions with tropomyosin (Katz, 1964b) and cations (Katz et al., 1966a) are altered.

The time course of superprecipitation can be followed by measuring the volume of the actomyosin precipitate at various times after addition of ATP (A. Weber and Winicur, 1961). Measurement of the protein concentration in the supernatant provides an estimate of the protein that is not superprecipitated, but this additional measurement is not essential to the interpretation of data obtained more readily by measurement of the precipitate volume. Another method used to quantify superprecipitation has been to measure the increased turbidity that develops after the clearing phase. Because the scattering of light by the actomyosin gel increases during superprecipitation, measurements of the turbidity change at wavelengths around 660 mμ have been commonly employed to follow this process (S. Ebashi, 1961; Yasui and Watanabe, 1965). This method has found wide acceptance, but several difficulties in interpretation of measurements of the turbidity change have been noted. For example Briskey et al. (1967) found that gel syneresis, measured by low-speed centrifugation, can proceed in the absence of a turbidity increase. Furthermore, not only the extent but also the direction of a turbidity change have been found to depend on the geometrical optics of the spectrophotometer used to record the turbidity changes during superprecipitation (Briskey et al., 1967). Thus, during superprecipitation an increase in turbidity is measured by a wide-beam spectrophotometer (such as the Beckman DU), in which there is considerable forward scattering of the incident light, whereas a decrease in turbidity can be recorded under identical conditions when measurements are made in a narrow beam spectrophotometer in which most of the forward-scattered light is eliminated (Briskey et al., 1967).

The rate of change in optical density measured in a wide-beam spectrophotometer does not always parallel the rate of ATP hydrolysis (Endo, 1964; Levy and Fleisher, 1965), and addition of minute amounts of previously superprecipitated actomyosin can greatly accelerate the turbidity change without modifying ATPase activity (Tada and Tonomura, 1966). Turbidity changes can be observed when deoxyATP is added to reconsituted actomyosin prepared from ADP-free F-actin (Tonomura et al., 1966), conditions under which these investigators failed to see the actomyosin type of ATPase.

Cardiac actomyosin, like cardiac myosin, is a weaker ATPase than white skeletal actomyosin (Bailey, 1942; Benson and Hallaway, 1958; Miyahara, 1962; M. Bárány et al., 1964b; Katz et al., 1966a, 1966b), but the viscosity drop on addition of ATP (Kasavina and Balyashaya, 1947; Kováts, 1949; Edman, 1950, 1951; E. H. Bárány et al., 1952; Davis et al., 1959; Inchiosa, 1964) and phenomena of superprecipitation (Miyahara, 1962; Katz et al., 1966a, 1966b) are qualitatively similar when cardiac and white skeletal actomyosins are compared.

PREPARATIVE TECHNIQUES*

General Comments

While different techniques are needed to prepare the various contractile proteins, certain general rules can be laid down. Of prime importance is the need always to keep the muscle mince and purification mixtures ice cold. All solutions and glassware must be prechilled to near 0°C, as must centrifuge rotors, tubes, caps, grinders, homogenizers, etc. Initial procedures involving large volumes of solution should be carried out in a cold room at or near 0°C.

For all of these procedures, one must use distilled water that has been deionized prior to use. Most commercial deionizers will be satisfactory, but the ion-exchange resin should be changed when any reading on a conductance meter is obtained. Redistillation of water is not essential if traces of cations have been removed. Similarly, all glassware must be free of traces of heavy metals. Reagent grade chemicals should be used, and reagents that will be used in high concentrations (e.g., ammonium sulfate) should either be deionized or obtained as a special ion-free grade. It has been the author's experience that certain lots of "Special Enzyme Grade" reagents contain sufficient contaminants to inactivate the more sensitive heart-muscle enzymes.

Dialysis tubing (one-fourth inch) should be precut, placed in distilled water, and allowed to remain at 100 °C for several hours. This can be accomplished by placing a beaker containing the dialysis tubing in a larger beaker of boiling water. Once moistened, dialysis tubing must not be allowed to dry (it may leak afterward) but be kept in distilled water in the cold room.

Various methods can be used to sacrifice the animals from which muscle tissue is obtained, and effects of the commonly used anaesthetics on the purified contractile proteins have not been noted. The use of curare has been advocated to avoid muscle twitching, which could cause hydrolysis of ATP during the removal of

*Additional details of these techniques can be obtained from most of the references at the end of the chapter. Excellent general discussions will be found in articles by A. Szent-Györgyi (1947) and Mommaerts (1950, 1958).

skeletal muscle. However, this agent is not without effect on the heart. If curare is to be used, it must *never* be given to conscious animals, but only after prior anaesthesia because the flaccid state induced by curare, in which the sensorium is clear, cannot be distinguished from true anaesthesia.

Preparation of Tropomyosin-Free Cardiac Actin

Several methods are available for purification of cardiac actin (Katz and Hall, 1963). The following method is based on Straub's original method and has been found to give excellent yields. However, this actin probably contains α-actinin, so that preparation of α-actinin-free actin would require additional steps (see Seraidarian et al., 1967). Rigorous exclusion of all traces of tropomyosin also requires an additional purification procedure (Grant et al., 1964).

The starting material in this preparation can be fresh, aged, or frozen muscle (Katz and Maxwell, 1964). If simultaneous preparation of myosin is desired, the residue from the first extraction of the muscle mince for myosin may be used (see below).

For certain procedures, notably to improve stability of G-actin-ADP, solutions of alkaline pH (Solutions 2 and 3) must be avoided, and dilute $NaHCO_3$ at pH 7.6 should be used instead (Ulbrecht et al., 1960). This modification will greatly reduce the yield of actin.

PREPARATION OF THE ACETONE-DRIED MUSCLE POWDER.

SOLUTIONS:

1. "Guba-Straub" solution: 0.3 M KCl, 0.15 M K_2HPO_4 adjusted to pH 6.5. This solution is stable in the cold for several months, though pH should be checked monthly.
2. 0.4 percent $NaHCO_3$. 4 g $NaHCO_3$ to 1 liter water. This should be made up immediately prior to use.
3. 0.05 M $NaHCO_3$, 0.05 M Na_2CO_3. This should be made up immediately prior to use.
4. 0.1 M $CaCl_2$.
5. Acetone.

PROCEDURE (for 100 g muscle):

1. Grind muscle through fine holes of a commercial meat grinder, regrind once. If residue from myosin extraction is used, regrinding at this initial stage is not essential. For very small tissue samples, use a tissue press. In our experience, muscle homogenized in the Waring blendor gives poor yields of actin.
2. Add 330 ml cold Guba-Straub solution and stir gently for 15 minutes. An overhead stirrer, rather than a magnetic stirrer, will be needed.
3. Add 1,300 ml cold water to this mixture. Immediately thereafter strain through gauze, retaining the muscle mince and discarding the liquid. The filtration through gauze, which must be done in a cold room, is easily effected by placing two to four thicknesses of gauze over a large (12-inch) plastic funnel

allowed to rest in a large flask. A flask with an open outlet at the bottom is most useful, as these and all subsequent washings will be discarded. In the early steps of this procedure the muscle residue is gelatinous, and vigorous attempts to remove the liquid associated with the muscle mince will be futile.

4. To the muscle mince add 400 ml 0.4 percent $NaHCO_3$. Stir gently for 20 minutes and again filter over gauze, retaining the muscle mince.
5. Regrind the residue in the meat grinder. This step greatly increases the yield of actin.
6. Add 100 ml of 0.05 M $NaHCO_3$, 0.05 M Na_2CO_3, and stir 10 minutes. Then add 1 L of 0.5mM $CaCl_2$ (5 ml of 0.1 M $CaCl_2$ + 995 ml H_2O) and again stir for 10 minutes.
7. Pour over gauze and discard liquid. Squeeze muscle residue as dry as possible.
8. Wash three times with 300 ml cold acetone, discarding the washing each time. (Note: *Explosion hazard* exists at this step so that, if the cold room is not explosion-proof, carry out this step in the hood. Use care in discarding the washings!) It is imperative that all portions of the muscle mince be effectively dehydrated. This is best accomplished by kneading the mince by hand while it is in acetone. Failure to dehydrate fully the muscle powder will greatly reduce the final yield of actin.
9. Spread powder over filter paper and allow to dry overnight in the hood.
10. Collect acetone-dried muscle powder and store in deep freeze. These powders can yield an active actin after several years of storage.

EXTRACTION OF ACTIN.

SOLUTIONS:

1. Acetone-dried muscle powder (see previous).
2. 0.1 mM ATP at pH 7.6. Commercial disodium ATP, when made up to this concentration, usually is at or near this pH.
3. 3 M KCl.
4. 30 mM $MgCl_2$.
5. 10 mM tris-nitrate (tris-hydroxymethylaminomethane adjusted to pH 7.6 with nitric acid).

PROCEDURE (to prepare approximately 50 mg actin):

Note: to avoid tropomyosin contamination, it is imperative that Steps 1 to 5 be carried out at or near 0°C.

1. To a chilled beaker, on ice in the cold room, add 12 g of the acetone-dried muscle powder. Then add 60 ml 0.1 mM ATP which has been chilled to 0 to 2°C. If the powder imbibes all of the ATP, add an additional 30 ml of this solution. Water may be used instead of the ATP solution, as the nucleotide will be formed from ADP present in the muscle powder (Tsuboi, 1963).
2. Stir gently (overhead stirrer) for 30 minutes, keeping the beaker on ice. Magnetic stirrers will be unsatisfactory if they warm the mixture.

3. Pour over Whatman #1 filter paper in a chilled Buchner funnel and gently filter by suction. Avoid foaming. Place filtrate on ice.
4. Reextract powder as before with 60 ml 0.1 mM ATP, again stirring gently for 30 minutes.
5. Filter as before (Step 3) and combine filtrates. This is impure G-actin.
6. Clarify filtrate by centrifugation for 30 minutes at approximately 100,000 × *g*. Discard pellet.
7. To each 30 ml of supernatant (the contents of one Spinco No. 30 rotor tube) add 0.5 ml 3M KCl (final KCl concentration: approximately 0.05 M), 0.1 ml 30 mM $MgCl_2$ (final $MgCl_2$ concentration: approximately 0.1 mM) and 0.5 ml 1 M tris-nitrate at pH 7.6. The latter is essential, as the action solution at Step 6 is quite alkaline and will polymerize poorly.
8. Allow to polymerize. This will require 1 to 12 hours, depending on temperature and actin concentration. Polymerization can be easily detected by observation of the increased viscosity, which will be manifest by trapping of air bubbles in the solution. A more sensitive means to detect polymerization is to swirl a beaker of the actin solution between crossed-polaroids. F-actin will exhibit strong flow birefringence.
9. Centrifuge two and a half hours at approximately 100,000 × *g*. Discard supernatant, allowing tube to drain completely. Rinse tube and top of pellet gently with ice-cold distilled water.
10. Depolymerize pellet in 0.1 mM ATP. For large pellets (occupying 1 to 2 ml), approximately 10 ml of this solution will be needed. Smaller volumes will be needed where yields are smaller. The F-actin can be quickly depolymerized by brief, gentle homogenization of the pellet in a hand-operated glass-Teflon Potter-Elvehjem homogenizer. (The pestle of this homogenizer provides an ideal tool with which to remove the F-actin pellet from the centrifuge tube.)
11. Centrifuge the G-actin solution for one-half to two hours at approximately 100,000 × *g* and discard the pellet. Longer centrifugation assures removal of undepolymerized F-actin, which will contain significant amounts of tropomyosin.
12. To the supernatant from Step 11, add $MgCl_2$ to a final concentration of 0.6 mM and allow to polymerize one to two hours. (If no F-actin is obtained at this point, too much ATP solution was probably added at Step 10.)
13. Centrifuge two and a half hours at approximately 100,000 × *g*.
14. Decant carefully (this pellet will be more gelatinous than that at Step 9) and discard the supernatant.
15. Depolymerize pellet in 0.1 mM ATP and 1 mM tris-nitrate at pH 7.6 as in Step 10.
16. Dialyze overnight against approximately 50 volumes of 0.1 mM ATP.

These G-actin solutions cannot be frozen, but will be stable for several days when kept on ice. Care must be taken to avoid bacterial contamination (dilute ATP solutions are an ideal medium for bacterial growth) and brief ultracentrifugation, by removing bacteria introduced during dialysis, will prolong the life of the actin preparation.

Preparation of Cardiac Myosin

General Comments: It is more difficult to prepare an actomyosin-free myosin from cardiac muscle than from white skeletal muscle. This finding may reflect the rapid hydrolysis of ATP by mitochondrial elements during the extraction procedure as the extraction of actomyosin, instead of myosin, begins when the intrinsic ATP of the muscle mince is hydrolyzed (Banga and Szent-Györgyi, 1941; Mihályi and Rowe, 1966). In addition, cardiac actomyosin is less readily dissociated than the homologous skeletal myosin (see Katz, 1970). All myosin preparations should be examined for actomyosin contamination by testing for EGTA sensitivity at low ionic strength (Katz et al., 1966b). This enzymatic method is more sensitive than the conventional test of observing a viscosity drop after addition of ATP.

Myosin readily picks up traces of heavy metals, so that all water and glassware must be free of cations. The specific ATPase activity of a myosin preparation cannot be used as an index of purity because loss of myosin SH groups may increase this enzymatic activity (see previous discussion). We have found it useful to add dithiothreitol ("Cleland's Reagent") to the distilled water used to precipitate the myosin (Katz et al., 1966a). This reagent protects SH groups and thereby stabilizes the cardiac myosin preparations, which in the absence of this reagent deteriorate within a few days. Should it be necessary to interrupt this procedure, even for an hour, the myosin should be left in a solution of high ionic strength. Precipitated myosin appears to be much less stable than dissolved myosin.

The starting material may be fresh muscle, though muscle kept on ice for long periods may be used after extensive washing (M. Bárány et al., 1964b). Frozen cardiac muscle yields poor myosins which are heavily contaminated with actomyosin (Katz et al., 1966b).

The excellent discussion by Mommaerts (1950) should be consulted for details of this, and other, methods for preparing myosin.

SOLUTIONS:

1. Guba-Straub solution (see previous).
2. 10 mg/ml dithiothreitol.
3. 0.5 M tris-acetate, pH 6.8 (tris-hydroxymethylaminomethane neutralized to pH 6.8 with acetic acid).
4. 3 M KCl.
5. 50 mM tris-nitrate, pH 8.0 (tris-hydroxymethylaminomethane neutralized to pH 8.0 with nitric acid).
6. 0.1 M MgATP (equal concentrations of disodium ATP and $MgCl_2$) adjusted to pH 7.0. The pH must be adjusted *after* addition of $MgCl_2$.

PROCEDURE (for 100 g muscle):

1. Grind muscle, once only, through coarse holes of meat grinder.
2. Extract for 15 minutes with gentle stirring in 330 ml Guba-Straub solution.

3. Add 1,287 ml cold water containing 13 ml of 10 mM dithiothreitol, as described in Step 3 of actin preparation procedure. *Retain washings*! It is important to add the 1,287 ml of water slowly while the original extract is being effectively stirred.
4. Stir the washings rapidly in a circular motion with a broad paddle and *slowly* add 2,400 ml 0.1 mM dithiothreitol (2,376 ml water and 24 ml of 10 mg/ml dithiothreitol). Failure to maintain active circular motion may result in formation of an amorphous myosin precipitate which gives a water-rich jelly that will not sediment during the centrifugation at Step 5.
5. Collect precipitate by centrifugation (e.g., in International PR-2 at 2,000 rpm for 20 minutes. If the solution at Step 4 is allowed to stand, most of the myosin precipitate will settle, so that much of the myosin-free supernatant can be poured off. However, the advantage to be gained by reducing the volume to be centrifuged must be weighed against the deleterious effects of allowing the myosin to stand at low ionic strength.
6. Suspend pellet in 0.5 mM tris-acetate, pH 6.8, and homogenize *once* gently in a loosely fitting glass-Teflon Potter-Elvehjem homogenizer. Add 0.1 volume 3 M KCl (final concentration 0.27 M) to dissolve myosin, but not actomyosin. The 3 M KCl should be added slowly with constant stirring to avoid local high concentrations of KCl which may dissolve actomyosin.
7. Centrifuge for 20 minutes at approximately 100,000 × *g*.
8. While stirring with a circular motion, add 9 volumes of cold water containing 0.1 mM dithiothreitol.
9. Collect precipitate in PR-2 as in Step 5.
10. Suspend pellet as in Step 6, omitting homogenization.
11. Centrifuge for 15 minutes at approximately 150,000 × *g*. Discard precipitate.
12. Add 9 volumes cold water containing dithiothreitol as described in Step 8.
13. Collect precipitate in PR-2 as in Step 5.
14. Suspend pellet in minimal amount of 50 mM tris-nitrate at pH 8.0. Add 0.25 volume 3 M KCl (final KCl concentration equals 0.6 M).
15. Add 0.1 volume 0.1 M MgATP (pH 7.0) and centrifuge *immediately* at 150,000 × *g* for two and a half hours. This step removes F-actin.
16. Collect upper two thirds of supernatant and dialyze against two changes of approximately 50 volumes of 0.6 M KCl and 20 mM tris-acetate at pH 6.8. The resulting myosin preparation will be stable on ice for several days, after which the sulfhydryl titer will gradually decrease.

Preparation of Cardiac Tropomyosin

This method yields troponin-poor, nucleotide-free tropomyosin. However, significant loss of tropomyosin SH groups can be expected, even with use of purified ammonium sulfate (Special Enzyme Grade, Mann Research Laboratories). Use of dithiothreitol in this procedure preserves SH groups (Mueller, 1966), but results in considerable troponin contamination. Frozen or fresh muscle may be used.

SOLUTIONS:

1. 95 percent ethanol.
2. Diethyl ether.
3. 1 M KCl.
4. Saturated ammonium sulfate (deionized, or special enzyme grade), containing 1 percent (by volume) concentrated NH_4OH.
5. Solid ammonium sulfate (deionized or special enzyme grade).

PROCEDURE (for 100 g muscle):

This method is adapted from that of Bailey (1948).

1. Grind muscle and homogenize in Waring blendor for 1 minute with 150 ml cold water. If homogenate is too thick for adequate homogenization, add an additional 20 to 50 ml water.
2. Let stand 30 minutes.
3. Add 150 ml ethanol, filter through gauze. Gently squeeze out liquid and discard washings.
4. Repeat Step 3. Be sure to break up muscle mince.
5. Add 300 ml ether (*explosion hazard*, carry out in hood), squeeze dry.
6. Repeat Step 5.
7. Allow powder to dry in hood for several hours.
8. Add powder to 700 ml 1 M KCl at room temperature. Adjust to pH 7.0 and let stand overnight in cold room.
9. Filter through gauze, collect washings.
10. Resuspend powder in 700 ml 1 M KCl; let stand two hours.
11. Repeat Step 9, combine washings and discard muscle powder.
12. Acidify to pH 4.7 with 1 N HCl to precipitate tropomyosin. Use care. If pH is made too acid (pH 4.3), the tropomyosin will dissolve.
13. Collect precipitate by centrifugation at 1,200 rpm for 20 minutes. Discard supernatant.
14. Suspend pellet in 5 volumes (or less) of water. Adjust pH to 7.0 with KOH to dissolve tropomyosin.
15. Slowly add 0.7 volume saturated ammonium sulfate (containing 1 percent NH_4OH) to precipitate contaminating protein (notably actin).
16. Centrifuge 15 minutes at 1,200 rpm. Discard pellet.
17. Add solid ammonium sulfate, 20.5 g/100 ml, to cause tropomyosin to precipitate.
18. Centrifuge 15 minutes at 35,000 × *g*. Discard supernatant.
19. Suspend pellets in *minimal* volume of water and dialyze overnight against 100 volumes of distilled water.
20. Repeat Steps 12 to 19.
21. Again, repeat Steps 12 to 19, except that the final dialysis should be extended to two to three days against several changes of 10 mM tris-acetate at pH 6.8. (The buffer is needed to avoid precipitation of tropomyosin by carbonic acid.) These tropomyosin preparations retain their ability to modify actomyosin

ATPase (Katz, 1964b) for many days, and can be lyophilized without loss of this activity.

Preparation of the Calcium-Sensitizing Tropomyosin-Troponin Complex from Cardiac Muscle

Several methods are commonly used to extract this protein complex from whole muscle mince (Ebashi and Ebashi, 1964; A. Szent-Györgyi and Kaminer, 1963; Azuma and Watanabe, 1965a, 1965b; Mueller, 1966) or actomyosin (Perry et al., 1966; Hartshorne and Mueller, 1967). The following method is based on the fact that this complex is incorporated into the F-actin polymer (Katz, 1966). The ability to purify this complex by its association with F-actin during the reversible polymerization and depolymerization of actin can be expected to increase the purity of the resulting tropomyosin-troponin complex.

Dissociation of tropomyosin and troponin can be achieved by methods described by Ebashi and Kodama (1965) and Hartshorne and Mueller (1967).

SOLUTIONS:

See methods for preparation of acetone-dried muscle powder, extraction of actin, and preparation of tropomyosin.

PROCEDURES:

Acetone-dried muscle powder is prepared in the usual manner. Extraction of actin is carried out as previously described except that both extractions (Steps 2 and 4) are prolonged to one hour and are carried out at 35 °C. Initial purification of actin is then carried out as described in Steps 6 to 13. At Step 14, however, the supernatant from the F-actin polymerized in 0.6 mM $MgCl_2$ is retained, as this contains the tropomyosin-troponin complex.

15. To each 3 volumes of this supernatant, add 2 volumes of saturated ammonium sulfate (containing 1 percent NH_4OH).
16. Centrifuge 20 minutes at 35,000 × *g*. Discard pellet.
17. Add solid ammonium sulfate to 70 percent saturation (20.5 g/100 ml).
18. Centrifuge 20 minutes at 35,000 × *g*. Discard supernatant and suspend pellet in a small amount of 5 mM tris-acetate at pH 6.8.
19. Dialyze against two changes of 50 volumes 0.1 M KCl, buffered with 5 mM tris-acetate at pH 6.8.

This protein complex when kept on ice retains its ability to sensitize actomyosin to low concentrations of Ca^{++} for over a week.

Preparation of Cardiac Actin Which Contains the Calcium-Sensitizing Tropomyosin-Troponin Complex

This shortcut is useful in preparation of calcium-sensitive reconstituted actomyosins.

PROCEDURE:

Actin is prepared by the standard method (pp. 407-409). except that the two extractions of the acetone-dried muscle powder are each carried out for one hour at 35°C (see method for preparation of tropomyosin-troponin complex). The remainder of the procedure is identical with that for preparation of tropomyosin-free actin *except* that at Step 12 polymerization is effected by addition of KCl to a final concentration of 0.05 M, instead of by adding dilute $MgCl_2$. This will cause the Ca^{++}-sensitizing proteins to be incorporated into the F-actin polymer.

Preparation of Reconstituted Cardiac Actomyosins

SOLUTIONS:

1. Tropomyosin-free cardiac actin or cardiac actin prepared to include the calcium-sensitizing tropomyosin complex. (Either G-actin or F-actin may be used.)
2. Cardiac myosin.
3. 0.1 M tris-acetate, pH 6.8.
4. 3 M KCl.

PROCEDURE:

A convenient protein concentration for superprecipitation and ATPase studies is 0.8 mg/ml. For tropomyosin-free actomyosin, the ratio of actin:myosin should be 1:4 (by weight); for actomyosin that contains the calcium-sensitizing tropomyosin complex, use a ratio of 1 g actin-tropomyosin-troponin complex per 3 g myosin.

To a small Erlenmeyer flask add undiluted actin plus 0.1 volume of 10 mM tris-acetate at pH 6.8. Add undiluted myosin (which will be in 0.6 M KCl; see myosin preparation). Allow to react at room temperature for 20 minutes, then dilute slowly with water to one third the final desired volume. (Subsequent dilution to final protein concentrations will be effected during addition of test materials, ATP, etc.) To avoid large clumps of actomyosin, the initial dilution should be carried out by adding small aliquots of cold water followed by gentle swirling of the Erlenmeyer flask. These actomyosins can be kept on ice for only a few hours, after which their properties will change.

Preparation of "Natural" Cardiac Actomyosin

In general, these preparations differ from those used to purify myosin in that finely minced muscle is extracted for prolonged periods with Guba-Straub or similar solutions, and the steps used to remove actomyosin and actin are omitted.

The author lacks extensive experience with this type of preparation, so that the reader is referred to a number of excellent papers for details of preparation

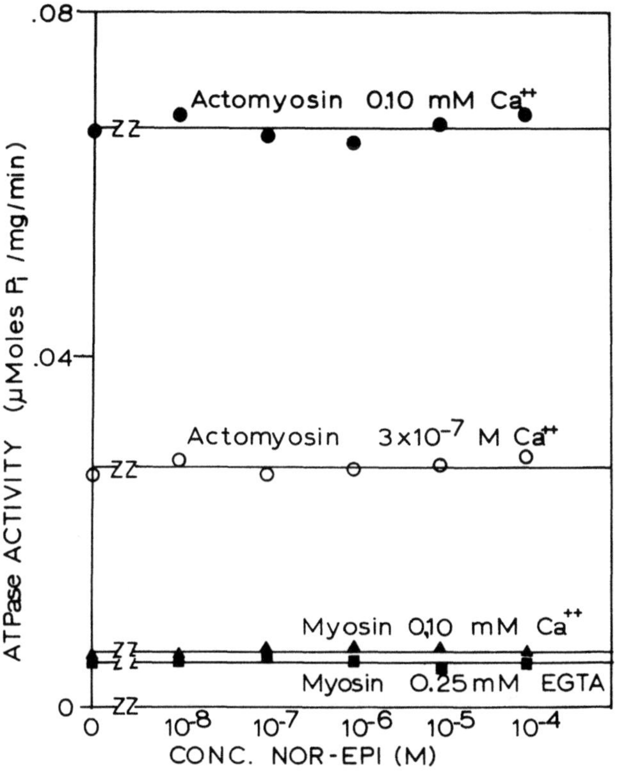

FIG. 1. Effect of norepinephrine on the initial Mg^{++}-activated ATPase activities of cardiac myosin and actomyosin. The liberation of Pi by 0.50 mg/ml cardiac myosin was examined in 0.1 mM $CaCl_2$ (solid triangle) and 0.25 mM EGTA (solid square). The ATPase activities of 0.667 mg/ml cardiac actomyosin, containing 0.50 mg/ml myosin and 0.167 mg/ml of the actin-troponin-tropomyosin complex, were measured in 0.1 mM CaCl (solid circle) and 3×10^{-7} M Ca^{++} (open circle). The total concentration of EGTA plus CaEGTA in the latter was 1.0 mM. All reactions were carried out at 25°C in 1.0 mM MgATP, 0.08 M KCl, and 20 mM histidine buffer at pH 6.8. (From Katz. 1967. *Amer. J. Physiol.*, 212:39-42.)

(Inchiosa, 1964; M. Bárány et al., 1964b; Stowring et al., 1966). As has been mentioned, such actomyosins include, in addition to actin and myosin, tropomyosin, troponin, and probably α-actinin.

Preparation of Cardiac Myofibrils

The gross contamination of cardiac myofibril preparations with mitochondrial fragments has been clearly demonstrated (Fanburg et al., 1964). In addition, one can expect the inclusion of additional ATPases derived from the Ca^{++}-transport system (sarcoplasmic reticulum) and cell surface membrane Na^+,K^+-activated ATPase enzyme system. At the present time, therefore, this type of preparation cannot be recommended for study.

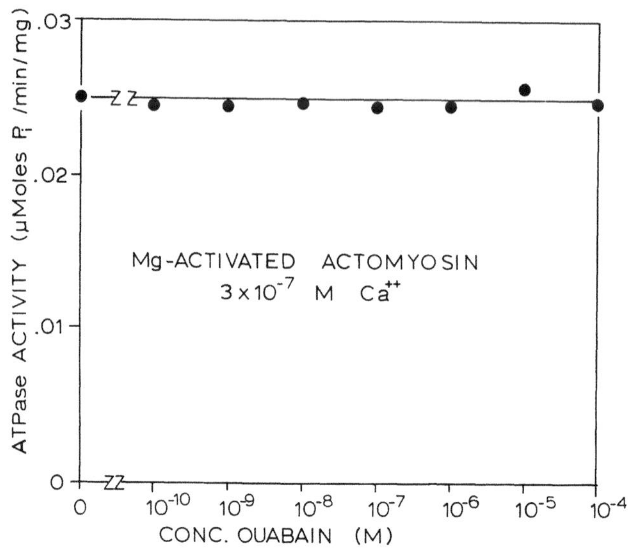

FIG. 2. Effect of ouabain on the Mg^{++}-activated ATPase activity of reconstituted cardiac actomyosin in 3 10^{-7} M Ca^{++}. The initial rates of P_i liberation by 0.667 mg/ml of cardiac actomyosin, containing 0.5 mg/ml of cardiac myosin and 0.167 mg/ml of the actin-troponin-tropomyosin complex, were measured at 25°C in 0.08 M KCl and 1.0 mM MgATP buffered with 20 mM histidine at pH 6.8. The concentration of free Ca^{++} was buffered with EGTA and CaEGTA, the total EGTA concentration being 1.0 mM. (From Katz. 1966. *J. Pharm. Exp. Ther.*, 154:558-565.)

EXPERIMENTAL PROTOCOLS AND SELECTED EXAMPLES OF DRUG EFFECTS

Some of the protocols that can be followed in studying reconstituted actomyosins are illustrated in two papers from this laboratory (Katz, 1966b, 1967c). The types of ATPase activity that can be studied are illustrated in Figure 1.

In studies of reconstituted actomyosins, the properties of the contractile proteins should be examined under conditions where the actin-myosin interaction is not complete. It has been our practice to carry out these studies in 3 × 10^{-7} M Ca^{++} (Katz, 1966b, 1967c), where cardiac actomyosin ATPase is only partially activated by Ca^{++} (Katz et al., 1966b) (Fig. 2).

For studies of ATPase activity, the following protocol has been used:

1. 0.3 ml of 0.2 M histidine buffer, pH 6.8.
2. 0.3 ml of 10 mM CaEGTA buffer (A. Weber and Winicur, 1961; Katz et al., 1966a). For a discussion of the preparation of these buffers, see Katz (1970).
3. 0.4 ml of water, solvent or drug.
4. 1.0 ml of actomyosin containing predetermined KCl concentration (see p. 414).

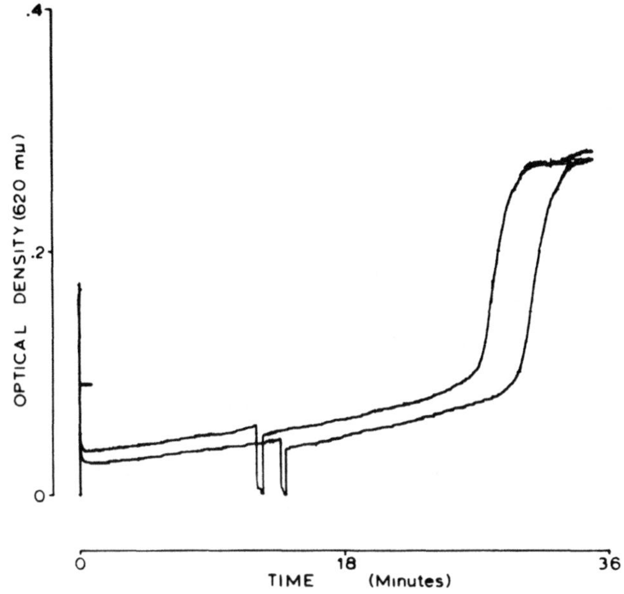

FIG. 3. Effect of ouabain on superprecipitation of a Ca^{++}-sensitive, reconstituted cardiac actomyosin. The effects of 10^{-6} M ouabain (lower curve) were compared to a control reaction (upper curve) in 0.05 M KCl and 1.0 mM MgATP buffered with 22 mM histidine at pH 6.8. The concentration of ionized Ca^{++} was buffered at 3 × 10^{-7} M by 1.0 mM EGTA plus CaEGTA buffer, and the concentration of actomyosin was 0.8 mg/ml. The abrupt downward deflections occurring between 12 and 14 min are artifacts resulting from restandardization of the photomultiplier. The initial optical density of the actomyosin gel, determined on a blank, was 0.09, and is indicated by a short horizontal line on the ordinate. (From Katz. 1966. *J. Pharm. Exp. Ther.*, 154:558-565.)

5. Allow to incubate 5 minutes at 25°C.
6. Start reaction by adding 1.0 ml of 3 mM MgATP (equal concentrations of Mg^{++} and disodium ATP) adjusted to pH 6.8.

Samples are taken for phosphate analysis when approximately 20 percent of the ATP has been hydrolyzed. Aliquots of 1.2 ml are added to 1.2 ml 20 percent TCA; the mixture is filtered through Whatman #41 filter paper and analyzed for phosphate. We have found the following adaptation of the method of Taussky and Shorr (1953) to be reliable and convenient:

To each cuvette add:

1. 1.0 ml of 2 percent ammonium molybdate in 2 N H_2SO_4.
2. 2.5 ml of water.
3. 1.0 ml of filtrate.
4. 0.5 ml ferrous sulfate* (10 g per 25 ml 1 N H_2SO_4).

Read after 5 minutes at 700 mμ.

*Mallinckrodt A. R. This solution must be prepared daily.

This reaction can also be carried out in the pH-Stat (Radiometer, Inc., see Katz, 1964b).

For studies of superprecipitation, the following protocol has been used:

1. To a 1 cm × 1 cm cuvette, arranged for stirring (Katz, 1966b, 1967c), add
   a. 0.3 ml of 0.2 M histidine buffer, pH 6.8.
   b. 0.3 ml of 10 mM CaEGTA buffer.
   c. 0.4 ml water, solvent or drug.
   d. 1.0 ml actomyosin containing predetermined KCl concentration (see p. 414).
2. Incubate 5 minutes at 25°C in water-jacketed spectrophotometer holder.
3. Add 1.0 ml 3 mM MgATP.
4. Measure change in OD at 540 to 560 mμ.

Data illustrating the clearing phase and superprecipitation are illustrated in Figure 3.

Alternatively, these suspensions can be centrifuged by the method of A. Weber and Winicur (1960) (see also Briskey et al., 1967).

REFERENCES

Abbott, B. C., and Mommaerts, W. F. H. M. 1959. A study of inotropic mechanisms in the papillary muscle preparation. J. Gen. Physiol., 42:533-551.

Alving, R. E., and Laki, K. 1966. N-terminal sequence of actin. Biochemistry, 5:2597-2601.

Amberson, W. R., White, J. I., Bensusan, H. B., Himmelfarb, S., and Blankenhorn, B. E. 1957. Δ protein, a new fibrous protein of skeletal muscle: preparation. Amer. J. Physiol., 188:205-211.

Asai, H., and Tawada, K. 1966. Enzymatic nature of F-actin at high temperature. J. Molec. Biol., 20:403-417.

Asakura, S. 1961. F-actin adenosine triphosphatase activated under sonic vibration. Biochim. Biophys. Acta, 52:65-75.

—and Oosawa, F. 1960. Dephosphorylation of adenosine triphosphate in actin solutions at low concentration of magnesium. Arch. Biochem. 87:273-280

—Taniguchi, M., and Oosawa, F. 1963a. The effect of sonic vibration on exchangeability and reactivity of the bound adenosine diphosphate of F-actin. Biochim. Biophys. Acta, 74:140-142.

—Taniguchi, M., and Oosawa, F. 1963b. Mechano-chemical behavior of F-actin. J. Molec. Biol., 7:55-69.

—Hotta, K., Imai, N., Ooi, T., and Oosawa, F. 1957. G-F transformation of actin by divalent cations. *In* Conference on the Chemistry of Muscular Contraction. Tokyo, Igaku Shoin, Ltd.

Azuma, N., and Watanabe, S. 1965a. The major component of metin from rabbit skeletal and bovine cardiac muscle. J. Biol. Chem., 240:3847-3851.

—and Watanabe, S. 1965b. The minor component of metin from rabbit skeletal muscle. J. Biol. Chem., 240:3852-3857.

Bailey, K. 1942. Myosin and adenosine triphosphatase. Biochem. J., 36:121-139.

—1948. Tropomyosin: a new asymmetric protein component of the muscle fibril. Biochem. J., 43:271-279.

Banga, I., and Szent-Györgyi, A. 1941. Preparation and properties of myosin A and B. Stud. Inst. Med. Chem., Univ. Szeged, 1:5-16.

—and Szent-Györgyi, A. 1943. The influence of salts on the phosphatase action of myosin. Stud. Inst. Med. Chem., Univ. Szeged, 3:72-75.

Bárány, E. H., Edman, K. A. P., and Palis, A. 1952. The influence of electrolytes on the rate of viscosity drop in ATP-actomyosin mixtures. Acta Physiol. Scand., 24:361-367.

Bárány, K., and Oppenheimer, H. 1967. Succinylated meromyosins. Nature, 213:626-627.

Bárány, M. 1967. ATPase activity of myosin correlated with speed of muscle shortening. J. Gen. Physiol., 50(No. 6, Pt. 2):197-216.

—and Finkelman, F. 1963. The exchange of the F-actin-bound adenosine 5′-diphosphate. Biochim. Biophys. Acta, 78:175-195.

—Finkelman, F., and Therattil-Anthony, T. 1962. Studies on the bound calcium of actin. Arch. Biochem., 98:28-45.

—Tucci, A. F., and Conover, T. E., 1966. The removal of the bound ADP of F-actin. J. Molec. Biol., 19:483-502.

—Nagy, B., Finkelman, F., and Chrambach, A. 1961. Studies on the removal of the bound nucleotide of actin. J. Biol. Chem., 236:2917-2925.

—Gaetjens, E., Bárány, K., and Karp, E. 1964b. Comparative studies of rabbit cardiac and skeletal myosins. Arch. Biochem., 106:280-293.

—Bárány, K., Reckard, T., and Volpe, A. 1965. Myosin of fast and slow muscles of the rabbit. Arch. Biochem, 109:185-191.

—Koshland, D. E., Jr., Springhorn, S. S., Finkelman, F., and Therattil-Antony, T. 1964a. Adenosine triphosphate cleavage during the G-actin to F-actin transformation and the binding of adenosine diphosphate to F-actin. J. Biol. Chem., 239:1917-1919.

Benson, E. S., and Hallaway, B. E. 1958. Interaction of actomyosin and adenosinetriphosphate as studied with glycerol-extracted cardiac muscle bundles. Amer. J. Physiol., 194:564-572.

Blum, J. J. 1960. Interaction between myosin and its substrates. Arch. Biochem., 87:104-119.

—1962. Observations on the role of sulfhydryl groups in the enzymatic activity of myosin. Arch. Biochem., 97:309-320.

—and Sanadi, D. R. 1964a. Activation of myosin adenosine triphosphatase by carbonyl cyanide p-chlorophenylhydrazone. J. Biol. Chem., 239:452-454.

—and Sanadi, D. R. 1964b. Activation of myosin adenosine triphosphatase by gamma-(p-arsenosophenyl)-n-butyrate. J. Biol. Chem., 239:455-459.

Bowen, W. J., and Gershfeld, M. 1957. The effect of monovalent salts on the acceleration of myosin B ATPase by magnesium. Biochim. Biophys. Acta, 24:315-323.

Brahms, J., and Kay, C. M. 1962a. The role of solvent-induced conformational changes on the enzymatic adenosine triphosphatase activity of cardiac myosin A. J. Biol. Chem., 237:3449-3454.

—and Kay, C. M. 1962b. Molecular and enzymatic studies of cardiac myosin. J. Molec. Biol., 5:132-137.

—and Kay, C. M. 1963. Molecular and enzymatic properties of cardiac myosin A as compared with those of skeletal myosin A. J. Biol. Chem., 238:198-205.

Braverman, I., and Morgulis, S. 1948. The inhibition of the adenosine triphosphatase activity of actomyosin by magnesium ions. J. Gen. Physiol., 31:411-415.

Briskey, E. J., Seraidarian, K., and Mommaerts, W. F. H. M. 1967. The modification of actomyosin by α-actinin. II. The effect of α-actinin upon contractility. Biochim. Biophys. Acta, 133:412-423.

Carney, J. A., and Brown, A. L., Jr. 1965. Human cardiac myosin: electron microscopic observations. Circ. Res., 17:336-339.

—and Brown, A. L., Jr. 1966. An electron microscope study of canine cardiac myosin and some of its aggregates. J. Cell Biol., 28:375-389.

Chappel, B. J., and Perry, S. V. 1955. The stimulation of the adenosine triphosphatase activities of myofibrils and L-myosin by 2:4-dinitrophenol. Biochim. Biophys. Acta, 16:285-287.

Chrambach, A., Bárány, M., and Finkelman, F. 1961. The bound calcium of actin. Arch. Biochem., 93:456-457.

Cohen, C. 1961. Discussion of paper by Schellman and Schellman. J. Polymer. Sci., 49:144-145.
—and Szent-Györgyi, A. G. 1957. Optical rotation and helical polypeptide chain configuration in α-proteins. J. Amer. Chem. Soc., 79:248.
Cohen, L. B. 1966. Viscosity of G-ADP and G-ATP actin. Arch. Biochem., 117:289-295.
Conway, G. F., and Roberts, J. L. 1965. Comparison of molecular weight of myosin from normal and failing dog hearts. Amer. J. Physiol., 208:243-249.
Corsi, A. 1957. Some observations on the extra-protein of cross-striated muscle. Biochim. Biophys. Acta, 25:640-641.
Csapó, A. 1949. Studies on the adenosine-triphosphatase activity of uterine muscle. Acta Physiol. Scand., 19:100-114.
Dainty, M., Kleinzeller, A., Lawrence, A. S. C., Miall, M., Needham, J., Needham, D. M., and Shen, S.-C. 1944. Studies on the anomalous viscosity and flow-birefringence of protein solutions. III. Changes in these properties of myosin solutions in relation to adenosine triphosphate and muscular contraction. J. Gen. Physiol., 27:355-399.
Davis, J. O., Trapasso, M., and Yankopoulos, N. A. 1959. Studies of actomyosin from cardiac muscle of dogs with experimental congestive heart failure. Circ. Res., 7:957-968.
—Carroll, W. R., Trapasso, M., and Yankopoulos, N. A. 1960. Chemical characterization of cardiac myosin from normal dogs and from dogs with chronic congestive heart failure. J. Clin. Invest., 39:1463-1471.
Depue, R. H., and Rice, R. V. 1965. F-actin is a right-handed helix. J. Molec. Biol., 12:302-303.
Drabikowski, W., and Gergely, J. 1962. The effect of the temperature of extraction on the tropomyosin content in actin. J. Biol. Chem., 237:3412-3417.
—and Strzelecko-Gołaszewska, H. 1963. The exchange of actin-bound calcium with various bivalent cations. Biochim. Biophys. Acta, 71:486-487.
Dreizen, P., Hartshorne, D. J., and Stracher, A. 1966. The subunit structure of myosin. J. Biol. Chem., 241:443-448.
—Gershman, L. C., Trotta, P. P., and Stracher, A. 1967. Myosin. Subunits and their interactions. J. Gen. Physiol., 50(No. 6, Pt. 2):85-113.
Dubuisson, M. 1948. Apparition d'une protéine nouvelle, la contractine, dans les extraits de muscles contractés. Experientia, 4:437-440.
—1950. "Y-Protein": a new component of the muscle machine. Nature, 166:1116.
Ebashi, S. 1961. Calcium binding activity of vesicular relaxing factor. J. Biochem. (Tokyo), 50:236-244.
—1963. Third component participating in the superprecipitation of "natural actomyosin." Nature, 200:1010.
—and Ebashi, F. 1964. A new protein component participating in the superprecipitation of myosin B. J. Biochem., 55:604-613.
—and Ebashi, F. 1965. α-Actinin, a new structural protein from striated muscle. I. Preparation and action on actomyosin-ATP interaction. J. Biochem., 58:7-12.
—and Kodama, A. 1965. A new protein factor promoting aggregation of tropomyosin. J. Biochem., 58:107-108.
—and Kodama. A. 1966a. Interaction of troponin with F-actin in the presence of tropomyosin. J. Biochem., 59:425-426.
—and Kodama, A. 1966b. Native tropomyosin-like action of troponin on trypsin treated myosin B. J. Biochem., 60:733-734.
—Ebashi, F., and Kodama, A. 1967. Troponin as the Ca^{++}-receptive protein in the contractile system. J. Biochem., 62:137-138.
—Kodama, A., and Ebashi, F. 1968 Troponin. I. Preparation and physiological function. J. Biochem. (Tokyo), 64:465-477.
—Iwakura, H., Nakajima, H., Nakamura, R., and Ooi, Y. 1966. New structural proteins from dog heart and chicken gizzard. Biochem. Z., 345:201-211.
Ebert, J. D., 1953. An analysis of the synthesis and distribution of the contractile protein, myosin, in the development of the heart. Proc. Nat. Acad. Sci. U.S.A., 39:333-344.

Edman, K. A. P. 1950. The action of ouabain on heart actomyosin. Acta Physiol. Scand., 21:230-237.
—1951. Wirkung des ouabains auf das Aktomyosin der Herzmuskulatur. Experientia, 7:71-72.
Eisenberg, E., and Moos, C. 1967. The interaction of actin with myosin and heavy meromyosin in solution at low ionic strength. J. Biol. Chem., 242:2945-2951.
Ellenbogen, E., Iyengar, R., Stern, H., and Olson, R. E. 1960. Characterization of myosin from normal dog heart. J. Biol. Chem., 235:2642-2648.
Endo, M. 1964. The superprecipitation of actomyosin and its ATPase activity in low concentration of ATP. J. Biochem. (Tokyo), 55:614-622.
Engelhardt, W. A., and Ljubimova, M. N. 1939. Myosin and adenosine triphosphatase. Nature, 144:668-669.
Fanburg, B. 1964. Calcium in the regulation of heart muscle contraction and relaxation. Fed. Proc., 23:922-925.
—Finkel, R. M., and Martonosi, A. 1964. The role of calcium in the mechanism of relaxation of cardiac muscle. J. Biol. Chem., 239:2298-2306.
Feuer, G. Molnár, F., Pettko, E., and Straub, F. B. 1948. Studies on the composition and polymerization of actin. Acta Physiol. Acad. Sci. Hung., 1:150-163.
Finck, H. 1965a. Immunochemical studies on myosin. II. Cardiac myosin. Biochim. Biophys. Acta, 111:221-230.
—1965b. Immunochemical studies on myosin. III. Immunochemical comparison of myosins from chicken skeletal, heart and smooth muscles. Biochim. Biophys. Acta, 111:231-238.
Fraser, R. D. B., MacRae, T. P., and Miller, A. 1965. X-ray diffraction patterns of α-fibrous proteins. J. Molec. Biol., 14:432-442.
Gaetjens, E., and Bárány, M. 1966. N-acetylaspartic acid in G-actin. Biochim. Biophys. Acta, 117:176-183.
—and Bárány, M. 1967. Discussion of paper by Dreizen et al., 1967. J. Gen. Physiol., 50(No. 6, Pt. 2):113-115.
—Therattil-Antony, T., and Bárány, M. 1964. Modification of L-myosin by disulfide-sulfydryl interchange reaction. Biochim. Biophys. Acta, 86:554-566.
Gelotte, B. 1951. Myosin from cardiac muscle. Biochim. Biophys. Acta, 7:378-386.
Gergely, J. 1950. Relationship of ATPase and myosin. Fed. Proc. 9:176.
—1953. Studies on myosin-adenosinetriphosphatase. J. Biol. Chem., 200:543-550.
—1959. Muscle proteins and energy utilization. Ann. N. Y. Acad. Sci., 72:538-554.
—and Gouvea, M. A. 1953. Combining ratio of cardiac myosin and actin. Fed. Proc., 12:207.
—and Kohler, H. 1957. Molecular parameters of cardiac myosin. Fed. Proc., 16:185.
—Gouvea, M. A., and Karibian, P. 1955. Fragmentation of myosin by chymotrypsin. J. Biol. Chem., 212;165-177.
—Gouvea, M. A. and Kohler, H. 1956. Cardiac myosin. Circulation, 14:940-941.
—Pragay, D., Scholz, A. F., Seidel, J. C., Sreter, F. A., and Thompson, M. M. 1965. Comparative studies on white and red muscle. *In* Molecular Biology of Muscular Contraction. Ebashi, S., F. Oosawa, T. Sekine, and Y. Tonomura, eds. Amsterdam, Elsevier. pp. 145-159.
Gershman, L. C., Dreizen, P., and Stracher, A. 1966. Subunit structure of myosin. II. Heavy and light alkali components. Proc. Nat. Acad. Sci. U.S.A., 56:966-973.
Gilmour, D., and Gellert, M. 1961. The binding of p-chloromercuribenzoate by myosin. Arch. Biochem., 93:605-616.
—and Griffiths, M. 1957. The action of 2,4-dinitrophenol on myosin. Arch. Biochem., 72:302-315.
Grant, R. J., Cohen, L. B., Clark, E. E., and Hayashi, T. 1964. A low viscosity G-actin preparation. Biochem. Biophys. Res. Comm., 16:314-318.
Green, I., and Mommaerts, W. F. H. M. 1954. Adenosinetriphosphatase systems of muscle. IV. Kinetics of myosin adenosinetriphosphatase. J. Biol. Chem., 210:695-702.
—Brown, J. R., and Mommaerts, W. F. H. M. 1953. Adenosinetriphosphatase systems of

muscle. II. Identification of the reaction products. J. Biol. Chem., 205:493-501.
Greville, G. D., and Needham, D. 1955. Effect of 2:4-dinitrophenol and phenylmercuric acetate on enzymic activity of myosin. Biochim. Biophys. Acta, 16:284-285.
Grubhofer, N., and Weber, H. H. 1961. Über actin-nucleotide und die Funktion und Bindung der Nucleotidphosphatase im G- und F-actin. Z. Naturforsch., 16b:435-444.
Hanson, J., and Lowy, J. 1963. The structure of F-actin and of actin filaments isolated from muscle. J. Molec. Biol., 6:46-60.
Hartshorne, D. J., and Mueller, H. 1967. Separation and recombination of the ethylene glycol bis (β-aminoethyl ether)-N, N′-tetraacetic acid-sensitizing factor obtained from a low ionic strength extract of natural actomyosin. J. Biol. Chem., 242:3089-3092.
—and Stracher, A. 1966. Effect of detergents on muscle proteins. Biochem. Z., 345:70-79.
Hasselbach, W. 1952. Die Umwandlung von Aktomyosin-ATPase in L-Myosin-ATPase durch Aktivatoren und die resultierenden Aktivierungseffekte. Z. Naturforsch., 7b:163-174.
Hayashi, T. 1967. Reactivities of actin as a contractile protein. J. Gen. Physiol., 50(No. 6, Pt. 2):119-132.
Higashi, S., and Oosawa, F., 1965. Conformational changes associated with polymerization and nucleotide binding in actin molecules. J. Molec. Biol., 12:843-865.
Hill, A. V. 1938. The heat of shortening and the dynamic constants of muscle. Proc. Roy. Soc.[Biol.], B126:136-195.
Holtzer, A., Clark, R., and Lowey, S. 1965. The conformation of native and denatured tropomyosin B. Biochemistry (Wash.), 4:2401-2411.
Huxley, H. E. 1963. Electron microscope studies on the structure of natural and synthetic protein filaments from striated muscle. J. Molec. Biol., 7:281-308.
Inchiosa, M. A., Jr. 1964. Actomyosin content of rabbit heart ventricle. Amer. J. Physiol., 206:541-546.
Infante, A. A., and Davies, R. E. 1965. The effect of 2,4-dinitrofluorobenzene on the activity of striated muscle. J. Biol. Chem., 240:3996-4001.
Iyengar, M. R., and Cain, D. F. 1966. Exchange of the actin-bound nucleotide during the superprecipitation of actomyosin in the presence of magnesium and calcium. Life. Sci., 5:227-235.
—and Olson, R. E. 1965. The amino acid composition of dog-heart myosin. Biochim. Biophys. Acta, 97:371-373.
—and Weber, H. H. 1964. The relative affinities of nucleotides to G-actin and their effects. Biochim. Biophys. Acta, 86:543-553.
—Theiner, M. R., and Olson, R. E. 1961. The chemical nature of cardiac myosin. Abstr. 5th Int. Cong. Biochem., 9:259.
Jenny, E. 1965. Physikalisch-chemische und enzymatische Untersuchungen von Kalbsherzmyosin. Helv. Physiol. Pharmacol. Acta, 23:357-373.
—1967. Actin aus Kalbsherzmuskel. Experientia, 23:106-109.
Johnson P., and Landolt, R., 1950. Muscle proteins and their interaction with adenosine triphosphate. Nature, 165:430-432.
—and Rowe, A. J. 1961. The spontaneous transformation reactions of myosin. Biochim. Biophys. Acta, 53:343-360.
Josephs, R., and Harrington, W. F. 1966. Studies on the formation and physical chemical properties of synthetic myosin filaments. Biochemistry (Wash.), 5:3474-3487.
Kaminer, B., and Bell, A. L. 1966. Myosin filamentogenesis: effects of pH and ionic concentration. J. Molec. Biol., 20:391-401.
Kasai, M., Asakura, S., and Oosawa, F. 1962a. The G-F equilibrium in actin solutions under various conditions. Biochim. Biophys. Acta, 57:13-21.
—Asakura, S., and Oosawa, F. 1962b. The cooperative nature of G-F transformation of actin. Biochim. Biophys. Acta, 57:22-31.
—Nakamo, E., and Oosawa, F. 1965. Polymerization of actin free from nucleotides and divalent cations. Biochim. Biophys. Acta, 94:494-503.

Kasavina, B. S., and Balyashaya, A. J. 1947. Actomyosin from heart muscle. Byull. Eksp. Biol. Med., 24:146-149.
Katz, A. M. 1963. The influence of cations on the reactivity of the sulfhydryl groups of actin. Biochim. Biophys. Acta, 71:397-407.
—1964a. The sulfhydryl reactivity of G-actin-ADP. J. Molec. Biol., 8:776-779.
—1964b. Influence of tropomyosin upon the reactions of actomyosin at low ionic strength. J. Biol. Chem., 239:3304-3311.
—1965. Stabilizing actions of free nucleotides on the sulfhydryl groups of G-actin. Biochemistry (Wash.), 4:987-991.
—1966a. Purification and properties of a tropomyosin-containing protein fraction that sensitizes reconstituted actomyosin to calcium-binding agents. J. Biol. Chem., 421:1522-1529.
—1966b. Absence of effects of cardiac glycosides on cardiac myosin and a Ca^{++}-sensitive reconstituted cardiac actomyosin. J. Pharmacol. Exp. Ther. 154:558-565.
—1967a. Regulation of cardiac muscle contractility. J. Gen. Physiol., 50(No. 6, Pt. 2):185-196.
—1967b. Patterns of energy production and energy utilization in cardiac and skeletal muscle. *In* Factors Influencing Myocardial Contractility. Tanz, R. D., Kavaler, F. and Roberts, J., eds. New York, Academic Press, Inc. pp. 401-415.
—1967c. Absence of direct actions of norepinephrine on cardiac myosin and actomyosin. Amer. J. Physiol., 212:39-42.
—1970. The contractile proteins of the heart. Physiol. Rev., 50:63-158.
—and Carsten, M. E. 1963. Actin from heart muscle: Studies on amino acid composition. Circ. Res., 13:474-477.
—and Converse, R. P. 1964. Comparison of tropomyosins from cardiac and skeletal muscle. Circ. Res., 15:194-198.
—and Hall, E. J. 1963. Actin from heart muscle: isolation, purification and physicochemical properties. Circ. Res., 13:187-198.
—and Maxwell, J. B. 1964. Actin from heart muscle: sulfhydryl groups. Circ. Res., 14:345-350.
—Repke, D. I., and Cohen, B. R. 1966a. Control of the activity of highly purified cardiac actomyosin by Ca^{2+}, Na^{+} and K^{+}. Circ. Res., 19:1062-1070.
—Repke, D. I., and Rubin, B. B. 1966b. The adenosinetriphosphatase activity of cardiac myosin. Comparison of the enzymatic activities and activation by actin of dog cardiac, rabbit cardiac, rabbit white skeletal and rabbit red skeletal myosins. Circ. Res., 19:611-621.
—Repke, D. I., Upshaw, J. E., and Polascik, M. A. 1970. Characterization of dog cardiac microsomes. Use of zonal centrifugation to fractionate fragmented sarcoplasmic reticulum, (Na^{+} + K^{+})-activated ATPase and mitochondrial fragments. Biochim. Biophys. Acta. In press.
Kay, C. M. 1960. A re-examination of the molecular characteristics of G-actin. Biochim. Biophys. Acta, 43:259-267.
—and Green, W. A. 1964. Physicochemical and enzymatic studies on cardiac myosin A. Circ. Res. 15: Suppl., 2:38-51.
—and Pabst, H. F. 1962. Physicochemical properties of α-myosin from dystrophic muscle. J. Biol. Chem., 237:727-732.
—Green, W. A., and Oikawa, K. 1964. Influence of solvent composition on cardiac and skeletal myosin A as determined by optical rotatory dispersion measurements. Arch. Biochem., 108:89-98.
Kielley, W. W. 1965. Studies on the structure of myosin. *In* Molecular Biology of Muscular Contraction. Ebashi, S., Oosawa, F., Sekine, T. and Tonomura, Y. Tokyo, Igaku Shoin. pp. 24-32.
—and Bradley, L. B. 1956. The relationship between sulfhydryl groups and the activation of myosin adenosinetriphosphatase. J. Biol. Chem., 218:653-659.

—and Harrington, W. F. 1960. A model for the myosin molecule. Biochim. Biophys. Acta, 41:401-421.
Kominz, D. R. 1961. Molecular changes in myosin caused by methylmercuric hydroxide. Biochim. Biophys. Acta, 51:456-463.
—and Maruyama, K. 1960. The 3 S fragments of rabbit and crayfish myosin obtained by copper cyanide treatment. Arch. Biochem., 90:52-56.
—Saad, F., Gladner, J. A., and Laki, K. 1957. Mammalian tropomyosins. Arch. Biochem., 70:16-28.
—Carroll, W. R., Smith, E. N., and Mitchell, E. R., 1959. A subunit of myosin. Arch. Biochem., 79:191-199.
Kováts, J. 1949. Myosin and actomyosin content of the heart-muscle. Nature, 163:606-607.
Krans, H. M. J., von Eijk, H. G., and Westenbrink, H. G. K. 1965. A study of G-actin. Biochim. Biophys. Acta, 100:193-201.
Kühne, W. 1864. Üntersuchungen über das Protoplasma und die contractilität. Leipzig.
Kuschinsky, G., Lange, G., and Turba, F. 1954. Über die Dephosphorylierung von Adenosintriphosphat (ATP) zu Adenosindiphosphat (ADP) bei der Synärese von Aktomyosin-Gel, der Kontraktion glycerinextrahierter und frischer Muskelfibrillen. Biochem. Z., 325:321-328.
Laki, K. 1957. A tropomyosin-like fragment of denatured myosin. *In* Conference on the Chemistry of Muscular Contraction. Tokyo, Igaku Shoin. pp. 77-79.
—1958. Personal communication cited by A. G. Szent-Györgyi. 1960.
—and Standaert, J. 1960. The minimal molecular weight of actin estimated with the use of carboxypeptidase A. Arch. Biochem., 86:16-18.
—Bowen, W. J., and Clark, A. 1950. The polymerization of proteins. Adenosine triphosphate and the polymerization of actin. J. Gen. Physiol., 33:437-443.
—Maruyama, K., and Kominz, D. R. 1962. Evidence for the interaction between tropomyosin and actin. Arch. Biochem., 98:323-330.
Levy, H. M., and Fleisher, M. 1965. Studies on the superprecipitation of actomyosin suspensions as measured by the change in turbidity. II. The relationship to hydrolysis of adenosine and inosine triphosphate. Biochim. Biophys. Acta, 100:491-502.
—and Ryan, E. M. 1961. Comparative effects of 2,4-dinitrophenol and *p*-chloromercuribenzoate on the magnesium-moderated nucleotide triphosphatase activity of L-myosin. Biochim. Biophys. Acta, 46:193-194.
—Sharon, N., and Koshland, D. E. 1959. A mechanism of dinitrophenol action on myosin. Fed. Proc., 18:273.
—Leber, P. D., and Ryan, E. M. 1963. Inactivation of myosin by 2,4-dinitrophenol and protection by adenosine triphosphate and other phosphate compounds. J. Biol. Chem., 238:3654-3659.
Lewis, M. S., Maruyama, K., Carroll, W. R., Kominz, D. R., and Laki, K. 1963. Physical properties and polymerization reactions of native and inactivated G-actin. Biochemistry (Wash.), 2:34-39.
Locker, R. H. 1956. The dissociation of myosin by heat coagulation. Biochim. Biophys. Acta, 20:514-521.
—and Hagyard, C. J. 1967a. A correlation of various small subunits of myosin. Arch. Biochem., 120:241-244.
—and Hagyard, C. J. 1967b. Small subunits in myosin. Arch. Biochem., 120:454-461.
—and Hagyard, C. J. 1967c. Variations in the small subunits of different myosin. Arch. Biochem., 122:521-522.
Lowey, S. 1964. Myosin substructure: isolation of a helical subunit from heavy meromyosin. Science, 145:597-599.
—1965. Comparative study of the α-helical muscle proteins. J. Biol. Chem., 240:2421-2427.
—and Cohen, C. 1962. Studies on the structure of myosin. J. Molec. Biol., 4:293-308.
—and Holtzer, A. 1959. The homogeneity and molecular weights of the meromyosins and their relative proportions in myosin. Biochim. Biophys. Acta, 34:470-484.

Luchi, R. J., and Kritcher, E. M. 1966. Cardiac myosin adenosinetriphosphatase activity. Modifying factors and comparison with skeletal muscle myosin adenosinetriphosphatase activity. Circ. Res., 19:283-294.
—Kritcher, E. M., and Conn, H. L. Jr., 1965. Molecular characteristics of canine cardiac myosin. Circ. Res., 16:74-82.
Martonosi, A. 1962a. Studies on actin. VII. Ultracentrifugal analysis of partially polymerized actin solutions. J. Biol. Chem., 237:2795-2803.
—1962b. The specificity of the interaction of adenosine triphosphate with G-actin. Biochim. Biophys. Acta, 57:163-165.
—and Gouvea, M. A. 1961. Studies on actin. VI. The interaction of nucleoside triphosphates with actin. J. Biol. Chem., 236:1345-1352.
—and Meyer, H. 1964. The binding of pyrophosphate and adenosine triphosphate to myosin. J. Biol. Chem., 239:640-647.
—Gouvea, M. A., and Gergely, J. 1960a. Studies on actin. I. The interaction of C^{14}-labeled adenine nucleotides with actin. J. Biol. Chem., 235:1700-1703.
—Gouvea, M. A., and Gergely, J. 1960b. Studies on actin. III. G-F transformation of actin and muscular contraction (experiments in vivo). J. Biol. Chem., 235:1707-1710.
—Gouvea, M. A., and Gergely, J. 1960c. Studies on actin. IV. Actin as a component of myosin-B. J. Biol. Chem., 235:3169-3173.
—Molino, C. M., and Gergely, J. 1964. The binding of divalent cations to actin. J. Biol. Chem., 239:1057-1064.
Maruyama, K. 1964. Interaction of tropomyosin with actin. A flow birefringence study. Arch. Biochem., 105:142-150.
—1965. A new protein-factor hindering network formation of F-actin in solution. Biochim. Biophys. Acta, 94:208-225.
—and Gergely, J. 1961. Removal of the bound calcium of G-actin by ethylenediaminetraacetate (EDTA). Biochem. Biophys. Res. Comm., 6:245-249.
—and Gergely, J. 1962a. Interaction of actomyosin with adenosine triphosphate at low ionic strength. I. Dissociation of actomyosin during the clear phase. J. Biol. Chem., 238:1095-1099.
—and Gergely, J. 1962b. Interaction of actomyosin with adenosine triphosphate at low ionic strength. II. Factors influencing clearing and superprecipitation: adenosine triphosphatase and birefringence of flow studies. J. Biol. Chem., 237:1100-1106.
—and Ishikawa, Y. 1963. Effect of magnesium and calcium on the ATPase activity of actomyosin at low ionic strength. Biochim. Biophys. Acta, 77:682-685.
—and Ishikawa, Y. 1964. A further study on the requirement of magnesium for the superprecipitation of myosin B. Enzymologia, 15:341-348.
—and Watanabe, S. 1962. The role of magnesium in the superprecipitation of myosin B. J. Biol. Chem., 237:3437-3442.
McCubbin, W. D., Kouba, R. F., and Kay, C. M. 1967. Physiochemical studies on bovine cardiac tropomyosin. Biochemistry (Wash.), 6:2417-2425.
Middlebrook, W. R. 1958. The subunit structure of myosin. Abstr. Proc. 4th. Int. Congr. Biochem., 17:84.
Mihályi, E. 1953. Trypsin digestion of muscle proteins. II. The kinetics of the digestion. J. Biol. Chem., 201:197-209.
—and Harrington, W. F. 1959. Studies on the tryptic digestion of myosin. Biochim. Biophys. Acta, 36:447-466.
—and Rowe, A. J. 1966. Studies on the extraction of actomyosin from rabbit muscle. Biochem. Z., 345:267-285.
—and Szent-Györgyi, A. G. 1953a. Trypsin digestion of muscle proteins. I. Ultracentrifugal analysis of the process. J. Biol. Chem., 201:189-196.
—and Szent-Györgyi, A. G. 1953b. Trypsin digestion of muscle proteins. III. Adenosintriphosphatase activity and actin-binding capacity of the digested myosin. J. Biol. Chem., 201:211-219.

—Bradley, D. F., and Knoller, M. I. 1957. Some physical and chemical properties of the ribonucleic acid contaminant of rabbit muscle myosin preparations. J. Amer. Chem. Soc., 79:6387-6393.
Mihashi, K. 1964. Molecular characteristics of G-ADP actin. Arch. Biochem., 107:441-448.
—and Ooi, T. 1965. Effects of divalent cations and ethanol on actin. *In* Molecular Biology of Muscular Contraction. Ebashi, S., Oosawa, F., Sekine, T., and Y. Tonomura, eds. Amsterdam, Elsevier. pp. 77-89.
Miyahara, M. 1962. Studies of actomyosin of heart muscle. Jap. Circ. J., 26:8-14.
Mommaerts, W. F. H. M. 1945. On the nature of forces acting between the components of the muscle-fibrillum. I. The disaggregation of actomyosin by adenosinetriphosphoric acid and some other reagents. Archiv Kemi, Mineral. Geol., 19:No. 18, pp. 1-11.
—1948. The reaction between actomyosin and adenosine triphosphate. J. Gen. Physiol., 31:361-375.
—1950. Muscular Contraction, New York, Interscience.
—1952a. The molecular transformations of actin. I. Globular actin. J. Biol. Chem., 198:445-457.
—1952b. The molecular transformations of actin. II. The polymerization process. J. Biol. Chem., 198:459-467.
—1952c. The molecular transformations of actin. III. The participation of nucleotides. J. Biol. Chem., 198:469-475.
—1958. Chemical investigation of muscular tissues. *In* Methods in Medical Research, Vol. 7. Warren, J. V. ed. Chicago, Year Book Medical Publishers, Inc. pp. 1-59.
—1966. Ultraviolet circular dichroism of myosin. J. Molec. Biol., 15:377-380.
—and Green, I. 1954. Adenosinetriphosphatase systems of muscle. III. A survey of the adenosinetriphosphatase activity of myosin. J. Biol. Chem., 208:833-843.
—and Khairallah, P. A. 1951. Preliminary investigations of the role of salts in the polymerization of actin. Arch. Biochem., 33:483-484.
—and Seraidarian, K. 1947. A study of the adenosine triphosphatase activity of myosin and actomyosin. J. Gen. Physiol., 30:401-422.
Moos, C. 1964a. Delayed enzyme inactivation: a source of error in analyses of myofibril-bound nucleotides. Nature, 202:1177-1179.
—1964b. Can creatine kinase phosphorylate the myofibril-bound nucleotide of muscle? Biochim. Biophys. Acta, 93:85-97.
Morales, M. F., and Hotta, K. 1960. The adenosine triphosphatase activity of myosin B treated with S-β-aminoethylisothiuronium. J. Biol. Chem., 235:1979-1986.
—Osbahr, A. J., Martin, H. L., and Chambers, R. W., 1957. The effect of certain sulphur compounds on the myosin B-ATP system. Arch. Biochem. 72:54-65.
Mueller, H. 1964. Molecular weight of myosin and meromyosins by Archibald experiments performed with increasing speed of rotations. J. Biol. Chem., 239:797-804.
—1965. Characterization of the molecular region containing the active sites of myosin. J. Biol. Chem., 240:3816-3828.
—1966. EGTA-sensitizing activity and molecular properties of topomyosin prepared in the presence of a sulfhydryl protecting agent. Biochem. Z., 345:300-321.
—and Perry, S. V. 1962. The degradation of heavy meromyosin by trypsin. Biochem. J., 85:431-439.
—Franzen, J., Rice, R., and Olson, R. E. 1964a. Characterization of cardiac myosin from the dog. J. Biol. Chem., 239:1447-1456.
—Theiner, M., and Olson, R. E. 1964b. Macromolecular fragments of canine cardiac myosin obtained by tryptic digestion. J. Biol. Chem., 239:2153-2159.
Nagy, B. 1966. Optical rotatory dispersion of G-actin-adenosine-5′-diphosphate. Biochim. Biophys. Acta, 115:498-500.
—and Jencks. W. P. 1962. Optical rotatory dispersion of G-actin. Biochemistry (Wash)., 1:987-996.
Nakamura, H., and Tonomura, Y. 1967. Superprecipitation and enzymatic activity of

actomyosin as affected by the mode of polymerization and nucleotide of actin. J. Biochem., 61:242-250.
Needham, J., Shen, S.-C., Needham, D. M., and Lawrence, A. S. C. 1941. Myosin birefringence and adenylpyrophosphate. Nature, 147:766-768.
Olson, R. E., Ellenbogen, E., and Iyengar, R. 1961. Cardiac myosin and congestive heart failure in the dog. Circulation, 24:471-482.
Ooi, T. 1960. Light-scattering studies on G-F transformation of actin. J. Phys. Chem., 64:984-987.
—1961. On the initial stage of the G-F transformation of actin. J. Biochem., 50:128-134.
—Mihashi, K., and Kobayashi, H. 1962. On the polymerization of tropomyosin. Arch. Biochem. 98:1-11.
Oosawa, F., and Kasai, M. 1962. A theory of linear and helical aggregations of macromolecules. J. Molec. Biol., 4:10-21.
—Asakura, S., Hotta, K., Imai, N., and Ooi, T. 1959. G-F transformation of actin as a fibrous condensation. J. Polymer. Sci. [A1], 37:323-336.
—Asakura, S., Asai, H., Kasai, M., Kobayashi, S., Mihashi, K., Ooi, T., Taniguchi, M., and Nakano, E. 1964. Structure and function of actin polymers. *In* Biochemistry of Muscle Contraction. Gergely, J., ed. Boston, Little, Brown and Company. pp. 158-172.
Asakura, S., Higashi, S., Kasai, M., Kobayashi, S., Nakano, E., Ohnishi, T., and Taniguchi, M. 1965. Morphogenesis and motility of actin polymers. *In* Molecular Biology of Muscular Contraction. Ebashi, S., Oosawa, F., Sekine, T., and Tonomura, Y., eds. Amsterdam, Elsevier. pp. 56-76.
Oppenheimer, H., Bárány, M., Hamoir, G., and Fenton, J. 1966. Polydispersity of succinylated myosin. Arch. Biochem., 115:233-234.
—Bárány, K., Hamoir, G., and Fenton, J. 1967. Succinylation of myosin. Arch. Biochem., 120:108-118.
Perry S. V. 1951. The adenosinetriphosphatase activity of myofibrils isolated from skeletal muscle. Biochem. J., 48:257-265.
—1956. Relation between chemical and contractile function and structure of skeletal muscle cell. Physiol. Rev., 36:1-76.
—and Corsi, A. 1958. Extraction of proteins other than myosin from the isolated rabbit myofibril. Biochem. J., 68:5-12.
—and Grey, T. C. 1956. Ethylenediaminetetra-acetate and the adenosinetriphosphatase activity of actomyosin systems. Biochem. J., 64:5.
—and Zydowo, M. 1959. The nature of the extra protein fraction from myofibrils of striated muscle. Biochem. J., 71:220-228.
—Davies, V., and Hayter, D. 1966. "Natural" tropomyosin and the factor sensitizing actomyosin adenosine triphosphatase to ethylenedioxybis (ethyleneamino) tetra-acetic acid. Biochem. J., 99:1c-2c.
Poglazov, B. F. 1966. Structure and Functions of Contractile Proteins. New York, Academic Press, Inc.
Raeber, L., Schapira, G., Dreyfus, J. C. 1955. Sur une nouvelle protéine musculaire, la "metamyosine." C. R. Acad. Sci. (Paris), 241:1000-1003.
Rainford, P., Hotta, K., and Morales, M. 1964. Experiments on the modification of myosin nucleosidetriphosphatase. Biochemistry (Wash.), 3:1213-1220.
Rice, R. V. 1961. Conformation of individual macromolecular particles from myosin solutions. Biochim. Biophys. Acta, 52:602-604.
—Brady, C., Depue, R. H., and Kelly, R. E. 1966. Morphology of individual macromolecules and their ordered aggregates by electron microscopy. Biochem. Z., 345:370-394.
Rowe, A. J. 1964. The contractile proteins of skeletal muscle. Proc. Roy. Soc. [Biol.,] 160:437-441.
Samuels, A. 1961. The immuno-enzymology of muscle proteins. I. General features of myosin and 5′-adenylic acid deaminase. Arch. Biochem., 92:497-506.

Schapira, G., Marcaud-Raeber, L., and Dreyfus, J. C. 1957. Sur l'isolement et quelques propriétés de la contractine. Bull. Soc. Chim. Biol. (Paris), 39:1059-1065.
Seidel, J. C. 1967. Studies on myosin from red and white skeletal muscles of the rabbit. II. Inactivation of myosin from red muscles under mild alkaline conditions. J. Biol. Chem., 242:5623-5629.
Sekine, T., and Kielley, W. W. 1964. The enzymatic properties of *N*-ethyl maleimide-modified myosin. Biochim. Biophys. Acta, 81:336-345.
Seraydarian, K., Briskey, E. J., and Mommaerts, W. F. H. M. 1967. The modification of actomyosin by α-actinin. I. A survey of experimental conditions. Biochim. Biophys. Acta, 133:399-411.
Simmons, N. S., Cohen, C., Szent-Györgyi, A. G., Wetlaufer, D. B. and Blout, E. R. 1961. A conformation-dependent cotton effect in α-helical polypeptides and proteins. J. Amer. Chem. Soc., 83:4766-4769.
Small, P. A., Harrington, W. F., and Kielley, W. W. 1961. The electrophoretic homogeneity of the myosin subunits. Biochim. Biophys. Acta, 49:462-470.
Snellman, O., and Erdős, T. 1948. Ultracentrifugal analysis of crystallized myosin. Biochim. Biophys. Acta, 2:650-659.
Sonnenblick, E. H. 1962. Implications of muscle mechanics in the heart. Fed. Proc., 21:975-990.
Spicer, S. S. 1952. The clearing response of actomyosin to adenosinetriphosphate. J. Biol. Chem., 199:289-300.
Stowring, L., Bowen, W. J., Mattingly, P., and Morales, M. 1966. On the mechanism of cardiac glycoside action. Stimulation of myosin B superprecipitation by ouabain and digoxin. Circ. Res., 19:496-506.
Stracher, A. 1965. Characterization of the sulfhydryl residues involved in the binding of ATP and actin to myosin A. *In* Muscle. Paul, W. M., Daniel, E. E., Kay, C. M., and Monckton, G., eds. Oxford, Pergamon Press, Inc. pp. 85-92.
Straub, F. B. 1942. Actin. Stud. Inst. Med. Chem., Univ. Szeged, 2:3-16.
—1943. Actin. II. Stud. Inst. Med. Chem., Univ. Szeged, 3:23-37.
—and Feuer, G. 1950. Adenosinetriphosphate. The functional group of actin. Biochim. Biophys. Acta, 4:455-470.
Strohman, R. C., and Samorodin, A. J. 1962. The requirements for adenosine triphosphate binding to globular actin. J. Biol. Chem., 237:363-370.
Szent-Györgyi, A. 1947. Chemistry of Muscular Contraction. New York, Academic Press, Inc.
Szent-Györgyi, A., and Kaminer, B. 1963. Metin and metactomyosin. Proc. Nat. Acad. Sci. U.S.A., 50:1033-1036.
Szent-Györgyi, A. G. 1951. The reversible depolymerization of actin by potassium iodide. Arch. Biochem., 31:97-103.
—1953. Meromyosins, the subunits of myosin. Arch. Biochem., 42:305-320.
—1960. Proteins of the myofibril. *In* The Structure and Function of Muscle, Vol. 2, Biochemistry and Physiology. Bourne, G. H., ed. New York, Academic Press, Inc. pp. 1-54.
—and Prior, G. 1966. Exchange of adenosine diphosphate bound to actin in superprecipitated actomyosin and contracted myofibrils. J. Molec. Biol., 15:515-538.
—Cohen, C., and Philpott, D. E. 1960. Light meromyosin fraction I: A helical molecule from myosin. J. Molec. Biol., 2:133-142.
Tada, M., and Tonomura, Y. 1966. Superprecipitation of myosin B caused by ATP as a nucleated growth process. J. Biochem. (Tokyo), 60:480-483.
Taussky, H. H., and Shorr, E. 1953. A microcolorimetric method for the determination of inorganic phosphorus. J. Biol., Chem., 202:675-685.
Tenow, M., and Snellman, O. 1954. Salting-out curves of crystallized myosin. Biochim. Biophys. Acta, 15:395-398.
Theiner, M., Mueller, H., and Olson, R. E. 1963. Tryptic digestion of cardiac myosin. Fed. Proc., 22:350.

Tokiwa, T., Shimada, T., and Tonomura, Y. 1967. Role of ADP of F-actin in superprecipitation and enzymatic activity of actomyosin. J. Biochem. (Tokyo), 61:108-122.
Tonomura, Y., and Yoshimura, J. 1961. Removal of bound nucleotide and calcium of G-actin by treatment with EDTA. J. Biochem. (Tokyo), 50:79-80.
—Sekiya, K., and Imamura, K. 1962. The optical rotatory dispersion of myosin A. I. Effect of inorganic salt. J. Biol. Chem., 237:3110-3115.
—Sekiya, K., and Imamura, K. 1963. The optical rotatory dispersion of myosin A. II. Effect of dioxane and p-chloromercuribenzoate. Biochim. Biophys. Acta, 69:296-305.
—Tokura, S., Sekiya, K., and Imamura, K. 1961. Influence of solvent composition on the molecular shape and the enzymatic activity of myosin A. Arch. Biochem., 95:229-236.
—Tokiwa, Y., and Shimada, T. 1966. Role of ADP bound to F-actin in superprecipitation and enzymatic activity of actomyosin. J. Biochem. (Tokyo), 59:322-324.
Tsao, T.-C. 1953a. The molecular dimensions and the monomer-dimer transformation of actin. Biochim. Biophys. Acta, 11:227-235.
—1953b. Fragmentation of the myosin molecule. Biochim. Biophys. Acta, 11:368-382.
—Tan, P.-H., and Peng., C.-M. 1956. A comparative, physicochemical study of tropomyosins from different sources. Sci. Sinica., 5:91-111.
Tsuboi, K. K. 1963. The origin of native G-actin-bound adenosine triphosphate. Biochim. Biophys. Acta, 74:359-364.
—and Hayashi, T. 1963. Reaction involving the bound nucleotide component of muscle actin. Arch. Biochem., 100:312-322.
Ulbrecht, M., Grubhofer, N., Jaisle, F., and Walter, S. 1960. Die Erschöpfende Reinigung von Aktin-Präparaten Zahl und Art der phosphathaltigen prosthetischen Gruppen von G- und F- aktin. Biochim. Biophys. Acta, 45:443-459.
Vazina, A. A., Bolotina, I. A., Vol'kenshtein, Lyasotskaya, I., and Frank, G. M. 1966. Configuration of polypeptide chain in G- and F-actin. Fed. Proc., 27:T476-T478, (original in Biofizia, 10:547, 1965).
Villafranca, G. W. de. 1956. A study of the nature of the A band of cross-striated muscle. Arch. Biochem., 61:378-383.
Warren, J. C., Stowring, L., and Morales, M. F. 1966. The effect of structure-disrupting ions on the activity of myosin and other enzymes. J. Biol. Chem., 241:309-316.
Watanabe, S., and Sleator, W., Jr. 1957. EDTA relaxation of glycerol-treated muscle fibers, and the effects of magnesium, calcium and manganese ions. Arch. Biochem., 68:81-101.
—and Staprans, I. 1966. Purification of the relaxing protein of rabbit skeletal muscle. Proc. Nat. Acad. Sci., U.S.A. 56:572-577.
—and Yasui, T. 1965. Effects of magnesium and calcium on the superprecipitation of myosin B. J. Biol. Chem., 240:105-111.
—Tonomura, Y., and Shoikawa, H. 1953. Mechanism of muscular contraction. II. Kinetic studies on muscle ATP-ase. J. Biochem., 40:387-402.
Weber, A. 1956. The ultracentrifugal separation of L-myosin and actin in an actomyosin sol under the influence of ATP. Biochim. Biophys. Acta, 19:345-351.
—and Herz, R. 1962. Requirement for calcium in the synaeresis of myofibrils. Biochem. Biophys. Res. Comm., 6:364-368.
—and Winicur, S. 1961. The role of calcium in the superprecipitation of actomyosin. J. Biol. Chem., 236:3198-3202.
Weber, H. H. 1950. Muskelproteine. Biochim. Biophys. Acta, 4:12-23.
—and Rüegg, J. C. 1966. The contractile fine structure of vertebrate smooth muscle. Med. Coll. Virginia Quarterly, 2:72-77.
—and Stöver, R. 1933. Das Kolloidale Verhalten der Muskeleiweisskörper. IV. Über Teilchengewichte von Muskeleiwesskörpern und das van der Waalssche Wirkungsvolumen der myogenteilchen. Biochem. Z. 259:269-284.
West, J. J., Nagy, B., and Gergely, J. 1967a. Free adenosine diphosphate as an intermediary in the phosphorylation by creatine phosphate of adenosine diphosphate bound to actin. J. Biol. Chem., 242:1140-1145.

—Nagy, B., and Gergely, J. 1967b. The effect of EDTA on the spectral properties of ATP-, ADP-and ITP-G-actin. Biochem. Biophys. Res. Comm., 29:611-616.
Wetlaufer, D. B., and Edsall, J. T. 1960. Sedimentation of myosin in urea solutions. Biochim. Biophys. Acta, 43:132-134.
White, J. I., Bensusan, H. D., Himmelfarb, S., Blankenhorn, B. E., and Amberson, W. R. 1957. Δ-protein, a new fibrous protein of skeletal muscle: properties. Amer. J. Physiol., 188:212-218.
Wiggers, C. J., and Stimson, B. 1927. Studies on the cardiodynamic actions of drugs: application of optical methods of pressure registration in study of cardiac stimulants and depressants. J. Pharmacol. Exp. Ther., 30:217-231.
Woods, E. F. 1965. Peptide chains of tropomyosin. Nature, 207:82-83.
—1966. The dissociation of tropomyosin by urea. J. Molec. Biol., 16:581-584.
—Himmelfarb, S., and Harrington, W. F. 1963. Studies on the structure of myosin in solution. J. Biol. Chem., 238:2374-2385.
Yagi, K., and Yazawa, Y. 1966. Isolation and characterization of a subfragment of myosin A. J. Biochem. (Tokyo), 60:450-458.
Yasui, T. and Watanabe, S. 1965. A study of "superprecipitation" of myosin B by the change in turbidity. J. Biol. Chem., 240:98-104.
—Hashimoto, Y., and Tonomura, Y. 1960. Physicochemical studies on denaturation of myosin-adenosinetriphosphatase. Arch. Biochem., 87:55-62.
Yoshimura, J., Matsumiya, H., and Tonomura, Y. 1963. Studies on the G-F transformation of actin. Ann. Rep. Sci. Works, Fac. Sci., Osaka Univ., 11:51-66.
Young, D. M., Himmelfarb, S., and Harrington, W. F. 1964. The relationship of the meromyosins to the molecular structure of myosin. J. Biol. Chem., 239:2822-2829.
—Himmelfarb, S., and Harrington, W. F. 1965. On the structural assembly of the polypeptide chains of heavy meromyosin. J. Biol. Chem., 240:2428-2436.
Zobel, C. R., and Carlson, F. D. 1963. An electron microscopic investigation of myosin and some of its aggregates. J. Molec. Biol., 7:78-89.

CHAPTER **14**

Nuclear Magnetic Resonance as Applied to Pharmacology

James J. Fischer

Department of Radiology, Yale University School of Medicine
New Haven, Connecticut

INTRODUCTION

It is one of the basic axioms of pharmacodynamic theory, explicitly stated or implied in almost all quantitative descriptions of drug action, that the observed pharmacologic effects come about as a result of a chain of events initiated by the interaction of the drug molecules and cellular structures called receptor sites. The similarity of the physical-chemical mechanisms involved in the drug-receptor interaction and those of antigen-antibody, enzyme-substrate, and drug-plasma protein interactions has frequently been noted. Each is characterized by narrow specificity, easy reversibility, and relatively small free-energy changes, generally arising from van der Waal's forces, ionic, hydrophobic, charge transfer, and hydrogen bonds. Clearly the possibility of rational design or alteration of drug structures will be enhanced when detailed knowledge of these interactions becomes available. Hopefully such knowledge will include the identity of all chemical groups that contribute to the binding interaction and the relative strengths of these individual contributions.

This chapter describes a method that makes use of the relaxation phenomenon of nuclear magnetic resonance (NMR) spectroscopy, which has been developed specifically to study weak binding interactions of this type. There are a number of advantages inherent in the characteristics of NMR spectroscopy that make it particularly suitable for the study of biologic material. Foremost, of course, is the nature of the information to be obtained. Often there exist no other physical-chemical techniques that can provide such detailed knowledge of molecular structure and motion, regardless of how the experimental system may be simplified. The technique itself is nondestructive and in fact does not perturb the chemical degrees of freedom of the sample to any measurable extent. Not only does this permit repeated study of valuable material in short supply, but in principle it should permit one to study living systems without producing undesirable effects upon the cellular metabolism or structure.

The radio-frequency (R-F) radiation used in NMR studies does not show excessive background absorption in biologic materials. Thus the author has been able to obtain spectra from a variety of small molecules in a suspension of isolated rat liver cells, some of which, including the penicillins, showed no effect from the cells whatsoever. This is in marked contrast to most spectroscopic techniques to which cells are essentially "opaque" and thus not suitable for study. It should be possible, in a properly chosen system, actually to observe the changes in the NMR spectrum of a drug while simultaneously monitoring the pharmacologic effect. By appropriate experimental design, making use of specific competitive inhibitors, it should be further possible to establish the exact spectral change due to the interaction with the "receptor site" as distinguished from the many other nonspecific interactions that undoubtedly occur in such a complex system. The pattern of these changes will provide information concerning the nature of the drug-receptor interaction, but furthermore it will serve as a physical-chemical "fingerprint" of the interaction which can be used as an assay technique in attempts to isolate the receptor site itself. Past attempts to isolate such structures have often failed for want of just such a specific assay procedure which could differentiate the pharmacologically meaningful interaction from other nonspecific binding.

The biggest single obstacle to the application of NMR spectroscopy to the study of biologic material has been the relative lack of sensitivity of the available spectrometers. However, continued improvement has been the rule in the past, and "raw" spectra from 10^{-3} M solutions are now possible under optimal conditions. The relatively new Fourier transform technique (Ernst and Anderson, 1966) promises to improve sensitivity by at least one order of magnitude, and when this is combined with the time-averaging procedures now available, it should permit detection of spectra from concentrations as low as 10^{-5} M. With the "amplifier effect" seen in binding studies of the type to be described, interactions with binding sites available or preparable in concentrations of 10^{-7} M should be observable. Clearly this begins to approach the range actually encountered in biologic material.

The number of published studies using NMR relaxation measurements to study binding interactions is still quite small. The serum albumin binding experiments of the author and O. Jardetzky have been the prototype for subsequent applications and therefore will be discussed in some detail. Other applications will be summarized briefly.

Before actual examples of the use of this technique are presented, however, its theoretical basis will be developed in sufficient detail both to justify the interpretation of the experimental results and to indicate possible future applications. It will be necessary to assume that the reader has some familiarity with NMR spectroscopy; fortunately there now exist a number of texts and review articles at all levels of detail and sophistication which may be consulted for background information (Abragam, 1961; Kowalsky and Cohn, 1964; Pople et al., 1959; Roberts, 1959). To be at all adequate a discussion of relaxation theory must rely heavily on quantum mechanical concepts (Bloembergen, 1961; Bloch, 1957). For those unfamiliar with this jargon, the mathematical formulations are generally followed by examples that illustrate the underlying physical nature of the phenomenon being described. An attempt has been made to use symbols and terminology consistent with the original publications and/or with the text by Abragam.

BASIC THEORY

The general Hamiltonian for a system of magnetic nuclei in an external magnetic field is given, in frequency units, by:

$$\mathcal{H} = \frac{H}{2\pi} \sum_{i} \gamma_i(1 - \sigma_i)I_z(i) + \sum_{i>j} J_{ij}I(i)I(j) + E(t) \tag{1}$$

Here H is the value of the external magnetic field, γ_i is the gyromagnetic ratio, and σ_i the shielding constant for the *i*th nucleus, $I_z(i)$ and I (*i*) are the operators for the Z component (colinear with the applied field) and the total angular momentum respectively of the *i*th nucleus; J_{ij} is the indirect spin-spin coupling constant for the indicated nuclei, and E(t) is a Hamiltonian which depends on both the nuclear spin system and the lattice, the other degrees of freedom of the system.

The first term on the right side of equation 1 corresponds to the Zeeman energy of noninteracting nuclei in a magnetic field. The shielding constants, σ_i, describe the reduction of the applied field strength actually experienced by the nuclei as a result of their local chemical environment. It is this factor that is responsible for the "chemical shift" and thus the existence of an actual spectrum with nuclei in different chemical structures absorbing different frequencies of applied radiation. The second term describes the indirect spin-spin coupling interaction between pairs of nuclei which is responsible for much of the fine structure in the NMR spectrum. In contrast to the direct dipolar interactions which are of importance in the mechanism of relaxation, indirect coupling occurs by way of the orbital electrons and thus depends on the particular chemical relationship—i.e., number and nature of intervening chemical bonds between the nuclei, rather than just on the spatial relationship.

It is often a good approximation to consider small groups of nuclei with identical values of σ and γ as if they were isolated. A typical example is a methyl group with three protons having identical chemical shifts and no significant indirect spin-spin coupling to nuclei outside of the group. It can then be shown that the only effect of indirect spin-spin coupling within the group is to shift all the energy levels by a constant amount, producing no observed change in the spectrum (Pople et al., 1959; p. 117). For this special case the second term of equation 1 can be ignored and the Hamiltonian can be rewritten:

$$\mathcal{H} = C \sum_i I_z(i) + E(t) \qquad (2)$$

with C as a new constant.

E(t) is a time-dependent Hamiltonian that couples the nuclear spin system with the chemical thermodynamic degrees of freedom of the molecules–i.e., the intramolecular vibrations and rotations, Brownian motion, etc. E(t) is usually small and may be treated as a perturbation on the energy levels established by the Zeeman Hamiltonian. The eigenstates of the Zeeman Hamiltonian occur in the direct product vector space of the eigenvectors of the individual $I_z(i)$'s. For protons, the only nuclei to be considered here, the eigenvector of the ith nucleus can be represented simply as α (i) or β (i), depending on which of the two possible orientations its Z component of angular momentum occupies with respect to the applied magnetic field. The coupling Hamiltonian, E(t), may produce transitions of the spin system between the different eigenstates with corresponding gain or loss of energy by the lattice. The result is the establishment of a "thermal" equilibrium between the spin system and the lattice in which the distribution of nuclei among the various Zeeman energy levels is Boltzman in nature, with characteristically more nuclei in the lower levels.

During a resonance experiment the nuclei are flipped from one orientation to the other under the influence of an applied radio-frequency field in such a way that the population in each of the two states, α and β, tends to be equalized. The result is a net gain in the total energy of the spin system and a resulting disruption in the thermal equilibrium established by E(t). When the resonance condition no longer exists, this equilibrium is reestablished, a process called spin-lattice relaxation and characterized by the spin-lattice relaxation time, T_1. This process is also called longitudinal relaxation since it is responsible for the reestablishment of the equilibrium value of the bulk magnetization of the sample in the direction of the externally applied field after it has been reduced in magnitude by the equalization of the energy level populations.

It should also be noted that the ability of the sample to absorb the R-F radiation and thus produce a signal in the spectrometer is related directly to the difference in the populations in the various energy levels; when the populations are equalized, the sample is said to be saturated and the absorption does not occur. The rate of recovery of the ability to absorb is frequently used to measure T_1.

The actual calculation of the relaxation rates is a quantum mechanical exercise (Abragam, 1961, Chapter 8). A time-dependent perturbation of the

Zeeman energy levels is carried out using E(t) as the perturbation. The problem thus consists of enumerating all possible coupling Hamiltonians, calculating the matrix elements of these Hamiltonians with the Zeeman eigenstates, and determining the time dependence of the operators of these Hamiltonians, assumed to arise only from changes in the lattice parameters. Since the equation of motion of the spins is dominated by the Zeeman Hamiltonian, only perturbations at the Larmor frequency will be secular, and the others may be ignored. It is then necessary to consider the Fourier spectrum of the time dependence of the operators to evaluate the intensity at the frequency of interest.

An example will help to clarify this procedure. There exists a variety of possible mechanisms that could couple the spin system with the lattice. The most important of these for our purposes is the direct dipole-dipole interaction originally described in the classic work of Bloembergen, Purcell, and Pound (BPP), which was the first successful attempt to explain the mechanism of nuclear relaxation. The magnetic dipole moments of any two nuclei interact directly with an energy that depends on both the internuclear distance and on the orientation of the internuclear vector with respect to the applied magnetic field. The interaction energy varies in time as the random Brownian motion of the molecules containing the nuclei changes these parameters. The exact expression for the dipole-dipole Hamiltonian is of the form:

$$E(t) = \sum_q F^{(q)}(t)A^{(q)} \tag{3}$$

where the A's are the operators that act in the spin space and the F's are functions of the lattice parameters, length and orientation of the internuclear vector. (The complete forms of these expressions are given in Abragam, 1961, p. 289.)

It is characteristic of the dipole-dipole interaction that energy variations of only certain frequencies—namely, the basic resonance frequency, ω_0, and $2\,\omega_0$—permit exchange of energy between the spin system and the lattice. It is thus necessary to formulate a model of the random Brownian motion and, by a Fourier analysis, evaluate the components at these frequencies. When the motion is isotropic its frequency spectrum can be obtained by a method of Wang and Uhlenbeck (1945). A correlation function is defined for each F by:

$$G(\tau) = \overline{F(t)F^*(t+\tau)} \tag{4}$$

where the bar means ensemble average taken over all the nuclei of the sample, and the * signifies complex conjugate. The Fourier transform of G gives the desired spectral density according to the Wiener-Khinchin theorem.

For a pair of identical protons it can easily be shown that the return to thermal equilibrium following a resonance experiment can be described by a single exponential process with the characteristic time given by:

$$\frac{1}{T_1} = \frac{9}{8}\gamma^4\hbar^2\,[J^{(1)}(\omega_0) + J^{(2)}(2\omega_0)] \tag{5}$$

Here the J's are the Fourier transforms of the G's appropriate for the dipole-dipole interaction and ω_0, as previously mentioned, is the Larmor or resonance frequency. In order to actually evaluate the J's it is necessary to use some particular model to describe the random motion. This has been done for some simple cases. Often it is assumed that $G(\tau)$ has the form:

$$G(\tau) = G(0)e^{-\frac{\tau}{\tau_c}} \tag{6}$$

where τ_c is a constant characteristic of the motion and is called the correlation time. This result is obtained exactly from some rigorous treatments of rotational and translation diffusion as Markov processes; and in those cases, values for τ_c can be derived from parameters of the model used. The correlation time is a measure of the length of time after which the system is unlikely to be in the same state as when originally observed. Slow random processes will have long correlation times; i.e., the parameters, such as the position or orientation of a molecule, are likely to remain unchanged for a relatively long period before randomly assuming other values.

The Fourier transform of a G of the form given in Equation 6 produces a factor

$$\frac{\tau_c}{1 + (\omega\tau_c)^2} \tag{7}$$

in the expressions for the $J(\omega)$'s. With the relatively short correlation times found in liquids, the denominator reduces to one, and $1/T_1$ depends directly on τ_c. When the latter is large, as for slow random processes, the relaxation rate will be relatively rapid.

Equation 5 can be generalized to the case of two or more identical nuclei, provided that the motion of these nuclei relative to one another is not correlated, by simply adding the contribution of each of the additional nuclei to $1/T_1$.

Before going on to discuss spin-lattice relaxation in more detail, the related phenomenon of spin-spin relaxation will be described. In addition to selectively supplying energy to the spin system, a resonance experiment also destroys the random phasing of the individual nuclear moments as they precess at the Larmor frequency, and thereby produces a nonzero component of the bulk magnetization at right angles to the applied magnetic field, H. The reestablishment of the original random condition and the decay of the transverse magnetization is called spin-spin or transverse relaxation and is characterized by a time constant, T_2. Processes that contribute to spin-lattice relaxation will also cause spin-spin relaxation–i.e., the act of flipping a spin to a different Zeeman level causes dephasing. However, dephasing also results from the near-zero frequency components in the Fourier spectrum of the dipole-dipole interaction. These are essentially inhomogeneities in the magnetic field applied to the various nuclei which arise from the presence of other nearby nuclei and do not vary in time sufficiently to be averaged out. They cause a spread in the actual Larmor frequencies and subsequent dephasing. For the case previously discussed, uncorrelated motion of identical nuclei with short τ_c's, it can be shown that T_1 equals T_2. Furthermore, when inhomogeneity of the applied magnetic field and other experimental artifacts are not limiting, the spin-spin relaxation time determines the width of the observed spectral line.

$$\Delta\nu = \frac{1}{\pi T_2} \tag{8}$$

where $\Delta\nu$ is the line width measured at half maximum height. Under certain restricted conditions which must be carefully established for each particular case, it is possible to determine $1/T_1$ values by direct measurement of line widths. Conveniently it is just when the relaxation rates are so rapid, i.e., small T_1 and T_2, and the more precise methods of measurement such as spin echo or progressive saturation are not possible, that the observed line widths are sufficiently great so that instrumental artifacts are insignificant by comparison.

So far the emphasis has been on the dipole-dipole mechanism of relaxation, which is indeed the most important for the applications of interest here. However, it is necessary to recognize that other mechanisms exist, both because at times they may be deliberately exploited to study molecular interactions and also because they may, if unsuspected, lead to erroneous interpretation of experimental results.

In situations when it is not possible to disregard the indirect spin-spin coupling terms of the general Hamiltonian (Equation 1), so-called scalar relaxation mechanisms may exist. One such involves coupling of the nucleus of interest to another nucleus which is itself undergoing rapid transitions between its Zeeman levels. In proton spectroscopy with biologic materials, the most common example of this is coupling to a nitrogen nucleus which, because of its electric quadrupole moment, can be rapidly relaxed by a time-dependent electric field gradient. Interpretation of relaxation data, particularly with regard to the causes of changes in the relaxation rates associated with molecular events, is hazardous. It is possible to remove this effect by spin decoupling, simultaneously irradiating at the nitrogen resonance frequency while observing the proton spectrum with a separate R-F source.

Another scalar mechanism requires a time dependence of the J_{ij}'s. Since coupling constants are known to vary with changes in molecular conformation, it is not inconceivable that this term in the Hamiltonian could be modulated at the Larmor frequency and thus cause transitions between Zeeman states. More often than not, the molecules of interest contain groups of nuclei suitable for relaxation studies for which the conditions for either kind of scalar relaxation mechanism clearly are not met.

Another relaxation mechanism depends on the existence of anisotropic chemical shifts. The applied magnetic field then produces a component of magnetization that can be modulated by molecular motion and thus may couple the spin system and the lattice. It is characteristic of this mechanism that the relaxation rate is directly proportional to the applied field strength. If there is reason to suspect that it is of importance in a particular case, the resonance experiment may be carried out and the relaxation rates measured at several different field strengths.

A direct spin-rotation relaxation mechanism has been described but is not usually of importance for protons (Hubbard, 1963). Electric quadrupole relaxation is not possible for the proton itself, and can play a role only indirectly as previously described.

Henceforth, discussion will be limited to dipole-dipole relaxation. Using the general approach previously outlined, detailed theoretical treatments of a number of specific examples of nuclear configurations and molecular motions have been carried out. Several of these that will be of particular usefulness in binding studies will be briefly described.

It is important to note that the dipole-dipole interaction energy varies as b^{-3}, where b is the internuclear distance; and therefore the effect of one nucleus on the relaxation rate of another varies as b^{-6}. It is because of this fact that near-neighbor nuclei are of predominant importance for relaxation, and it is possible to consider small groups of nuclei as if they were completely isolated. Methyl, methoxy, methylene, and phenyl groups are typical examples for which this assumption is valid. Furthermore, within these groups the internuclear distances are constant in time, and the dipole-dipole interaction is modulated only by reorientation of the internuclear vectors.

The simplest such case is that of two identical nuclei whose relative orientation is described by the diffusion equation on the unit sphere. The correlation function then has the exponential form previously mentioned, Equation 6, and the relaxation rate is given by:

$$\frac{1}{T_1} = \frac{3}{10}\frac{\gamma^4\hbar^2}{b^6}\left[\frac{\tau_c}{1+\omega_0^2\tau_c^2} + \frac{4\tau_c}{1+4\omega_0^2\tau_c^2}\right] \tag{9}$$

where all the symbols have their previously defined meanings. For the extreme narrowing condition $\tau_c \ll \frac{1}{\omega_0}$, this reduces to:

$$\frac{1}{T_1} = \frac{3}{2}\frac{\gamma^4\hbar^2}{b^6}\tau_c \tag{10}$$

For this particular case, T_1 equals T_2.

This result can be extended to cases with more than two nuclei, provided that the relative motion of the internuclear vectors is not correlated. In general, this condition will not be met for these rigid structures. However, it has been explicitly demonstrated by Hubbard (1958) that the required modification of the foregoing result for the case of a three-spin system with the nuclei at the corners of an equilateral triangle was indeed negligible. Using the same general approach a similar result was obtained by Richards (1963) for arbitrarily large groups of identical nuclei.

Complications arise when one considers dipole relaxation in groups of nonidentical nuclei. Using the density matrix formulation of Redfield (1957), it is possible to treat theoretically simple examples of even the most general case: nonidentical nuclei with indirect spin-spin coupling. When the conditions of extreme narrowing prevail, the relaxation of two nonidentical but noncoupled, J=0, nuclei is:

$$\frac{1}{T_2} = \frac{\gamma^4 \hbar^2}{b^6} \tau_c \tag{11}$$

The line width is two thirds of that observed for like spins. When the two nuclei are relatively strongly coupled, the resulting four spectral peaks will have unequal widths; however, the widths will still depend linearly on a correlation time which characterizes the motion of the system.

The specific examples described have demonstrated that under certain restrictions—namely,

1. Direct dipole-dipole interaction as the only mechanism of relaxation
2. Negligible contributions to 1 from nuclei other than those within the "relaxing" group, either within the same molecule or on other molecules
3. Relatively fixed geometry of the nuclei within the group
4. Isotropic motion, and
5. Extreme narrowing,

the relaxation rates and line widths of signals arising from a group of nuclei, even when the nuclei are nonidentical and are indirectly spin-spin coupled, are directly proportional to a correlation time which describes the reorientation of the group.

RELAXATION THEORY APPLIED TO BINDING STUDIES

The strategy of using relaxation rates to study the binding of small molecules to macromolecules or cell structures is based on the anticipation that such an interaction would alter the motion of the small molecule, thus changing the correlation times and the relaxation rates. Furthermore, to the extent that small chemical groups on the molecule can be considered as isolated relaxing units, it is possible to determine the extent to which the motions of these individual parts of the molecule are altered by the interaction. When attempting to identify the portions of the molecule most strongly involved in binding, it is important to compare the changes in relaxation rates observed for the various groups when binding occurs, rather than the actual values of the rates themselves, since the latter will reflect the chemical nature of the groups as well as any preferential stabilization. Under the previously listed conditions, the ratio of the relaxation times of the free and bound forms will be inversely related to their correlation times, and can be used to define a stabilization ratio, R, such that

$$(T_1)\ \text{free}/(T_1)\ \text{bound} = (\tau_c)\ \text{bound}/(\tau_c)\ \text{free} = R \tag{12}$$

When a small molecule binds to a larger and more slowly moving molecule, the description of its random motion becomes much more complicated. While it is to be expected that the linear diffusion of the small molecule will become, for the time it is attached, essentially the same as that of the large molecule, certain internal motions, such as the rotation of methyl groups about the C—C bond, might be relatively unaffected. It is important to appreciate the net effect on the relaxation processes of random motions that are the resultant of both rapid and relatively slow variations in the molecular coordinates. While the exact results of theoretical treatments are complex and applicable only to limited situations, it is possible to make the general statement that, when the motion is described by more than one correlation time, all of which differ greatly in magnitude, the shortest correlation time is most important in determining the relaxation rate (Woessner, 1962; Ullman, 1966). Thus it is not expected that the relaxation rate will be significantly increased by binding if any single degree of freedom describing the motion of the particular group is unaffected and continues to vary relatively rapidly. It is possible therefore that a molecule may be bound predominantly by an interaction at a localized site, thereby greatly increasing the relaxation rates of peaks arising from protons in that region, while those from other parts of the same molecule could be relatively unaffected. It is this specificity that permits identification of the particular portions of the small molecule that are directly involved in the binding. Furthermore the pattern of the different changes in the relaxation rates for the various peaks serves as a fingerprint to identify a particular binding interaction which may be used for example as an assay during attempts to purify the binding site from biologic material.

In order to be able to attribute changes in relaxation rates to complex formation, it is necessary to exclude nonspecific intermolecular dipole-dipole interactions as a possible cause. Specific experiments designed to do this will be described in detail subsequently; however, some approximate theoretical arguments will serve to anticipate these results. In BPP's original treatment of relaxation in liquid water the intermolecular contribution to the relaxation rate was found to be approximately 0.1 sec^{-1}. This figure, a not inconsiderable amount, will serve as a guide for the evaluation of the intermolecular contributions in the experimental situations used for binding studies. While most of these studies are carried out in aqueous solution, D_2O usually replaces over 90 percent of the water. The smaller magnetic moment of the deuterium markedly reduces the dipole-dipole interaction (Anderson and Arnold, 1956), and the expected contribution of the solvent to the relaxation rate of dissolved small molecules should be less than 0.01 sec^{-1}. The contribution from other small solute molecules, buffer substances, etc., usually present only in relatively low concentration, less than 0.1 M, should be of the same order of magnitude.

The presence of macromolecules and cell structures adds a large number of hydrogen nuclei to the sample. While it is difficult to know the exact concentrations reached, particularly for the latter, 1 to 10 M equivalent would seem to be a reasonable maximum. Relaxation rates of 0.1 sec^{-1} could result.

These contributions to the relaxation rates are relatively small compared with those seen to result from binding interactions. Moreover, they are nonspecific and will be observed for the peaks of the solvent and the other small molecules present in the solution as well as for the drug. Thus, it is usually easy to recognize these effects and appropriately control for them.

The presence of paramagnetic ions, either free in solution or bound to large molecules, can produce large relaxation effects. Again, however, in the absence of specific complex formation involving these compounds, the effects will be nonspecific. Often they can be completely removed by addition of a small amount of a chelating agent such as EDTA. Alternatively, a dialysate of the complete solution can be tested for its effect on the NMR spectrum as a control for the presence of free paramagnetic ions. A variation of this approach using the molecular sieve, Sephadex, will be described subsequently. If a paramagnetic ion is attached to the macromolecule near the binding site, the small molecule may experience significant changes in its relaxation rates by this mechanism as well as from changes in the intramolecular dipole-dipole interactions due to increases in the τ_c's. Such an effect can produce useful information concerning the nature of the interaction.

The simplest experimental system for the study of binding interactions consists of the solvent, the small molecule, and the macromolecule. In order to obtain meaningful NMR spectra, the small molecule must be present in concentrations usually greater than 10^{-3} M. It will rarely be possible to obtain solutions of the binding sites in nearly this high a concentration. In fact the ratio of the numbers of small and large molecules will usually be greater than 100:1. Because of its low concentration and because of the relatively great widths of its spectral lines, the macromolecule will generally not contribute to the total NMR spectrum. At most it may produce small, very broad peaks upon which are superimposed the spectrum of the small molecule.

It is convenient to consider the small molecule as existing in one of only two possible states, bound or free, and to ignore any transition states. In the most general case both the chemical shifts and the relaxation rates of the two forms might differ. In this case, the observed spectrum will depend on the exchange rate, $1/T_e$, of molecules between the two states. It can easily be shown that regardless of the magnitude of the exchange rate, the existence of changes in the chemical shifts upon binding cannot, under the experimental conditions previously described, alter the observed spectrum. The maximum effect upon chemical shifts, due to interactions other than actual breaking of covalent bonds, can be estimated at 200 cps caused by placing a proton into the diamagnetic region of an unsaturated ring structure (Johnson and Bovey, 1958). More commonly the effects would be an order of magnitude less. In the rapid exchange limit, $1/T_e$ much greater than 200 sec^{-1}, one peak would be observed with a shift that was the weighted average of the two. Since only approximately 1 percent of the molecules could be in the bound form, the change would be at most 2 cps, which would be difficult to detect for very broad peaks. For slow exchange rates–slow compared to the difference in the chemical shifts–two separate peaks would result; however, since one would arise from such a low concentration, it would be virtually undetectable.

On the same basis, it is possible to rule out exchange broadening as a possible mechanism for the observed changes in line widths (Pople et al., 1959). Even if the exchange rate were in the correct range, approximately 10 to 200 cps, the small fraction in the one state would make the effect negligible. In fact it will be shown later that one of the conditions for observing the dipolar broadening will require an exchange rate well in excess of that required to average the largest possible change in chemical shifts.

To explain the effects of the increased relaxation rates of the bound form of the small molecule on the observed spectrum, three different cases must be considered with respect to the exchange rate:*

$$\text{Case I} \quad 1/T_e < (1/T_2)\text{ free} < (1/T_2)\text{ bound}$$

In this case, two superimposed lines will be seen, one narrow and one broad. In general, the broad line will not actually be detectable because of its extreme width and because it arises from such a low concentration of molecules. The narrow peak will be reduced in amplitude in proportion to the number of molecules bound, but since this is small, in fact there will be no effect seen when the macromolecule is added. Binding due to covalent bond formation will usually be sufficiently strong to fall into this category, and thus interactions of this type cannot be studied by this method.

$$\text{Case II} \quad (1/T_2)\text{ free} < 1/T_e < (1/T_2)\text{ bound}$$

Here the nuclei of the bound form will relax essentially as if exchange did not occur; but the relaxation of the free molecules will depend on the exchange rate and in fact will be approximately equal to it. Frequently the widths of all the peaks will be almost the same, in contrast to the relaxation rates of the free form, and this will enable the situation to be easily recognized.

$$\text{Case III} \quad (1/T_2)\text{ free} < (1/T_2)\text{ bound} < 1/T_e$$

This is the fast exchange limit. The relaxation rates of the two forms will be averaged with the result:

$$(1/T_2)\text{ observed} = (1/T_2)\text{ free} + B[(1/T_2)\text{ bound} - (1/T_2)\text{ free}] \tag{13}$$

*For a detailed discussion of the effect of exchange rates on relaxation processes, see Zimmerman and Brittin (1957) and Woessner and Zimmerman (1963).

where B is the fraction of the total small molecules that is bound. Most biologically interesting interactions fall into this group. In general, $(1/T_2)$ bound values range from 10^2 to 10^4 sec^{-1}, and the exchange rate must be rapid compared to this in order to produce averaging. Activation energies for breakdown of the complex of less than 10 kcal/mole would meet this requirement.

The phenomenon of averaging has important practical results. Because of the very rapid relaxation rate of the bound form, detectable spectra will result only when the molecule exists mainly in the free form, approximately 500:1, so that the average line width is in the range 2 to 20 sec^{-1}. The averaging thus produces an amplifier effect in terms of sensitivity, permitting a limited number of binding sites to influence the spectrum from a large enough concentration of small molecules to actually produce a detectable spectrum, while at the same time reducing the broadening to a level that does not itself interfere with signal detection. If a signal can be obtained from a 10^{-3} M solution of the small molecule, the effect of the presence of 10^{-5} to 10^{-6} M binding sites should be observable. Since it is the concentration of the latter that usually limits application of NMR methods to biologic systems, the importance of this "increased sensitivity" is readily apparent.

EXPERIMENTAL

The author and O. Jardetzky first attempted to apply NMR spectroscopy to the study of binding interactions in biologic systems in 1959. The initial choice of experimental systems included several of the hapten-antibody interactions described in the classic work of Landsteiner, since it was felt that these interactions were already reasonably well understood and would show the specificity and reversibility characteristic of a large group of interesting interactions. These early attempts were unsuccessful largely because it proved impractical to obtain antibody concentrations sufficient to affect the relatively highly concentrated, 0.2 to 0.5 M, solutions of hapten that were required with the early spectrometers.

The next attempt was to study the various binding interactions of penicillin, which seemed particularly suitable for a number of reasons. The drug was readily soluble. Its structure was such that considerable intramolecular motion was possible; and there existed a number of chemical groups that could form hydrogen, ionic, and hydrophobic bonds with macromolecules. It produced an NMR spectrum that was interpretable and which contained, among others, three unsplit peaks, each of which arose from a group of nuclei of identical chemical shifts and which therefore would have relatively simple relaxation mechanisms. Several known binding interactions were available for study, including the weak, reversible binding to serum albumin, a macromolecule that could be prepared in solution in concentrations greater than 1 mM (Scholtan and Schmid, 1962; Chow and McKee, 1945); a binding to red cell membranes, which later was shown to be due to covalent bond formation and thus not suitable for study by this technique (Fischer and DeSimone, 1963); the interaction with a globulin antibody (Josephson, 1960); and possibly some binding phenomenon associated with its bactericidal action.

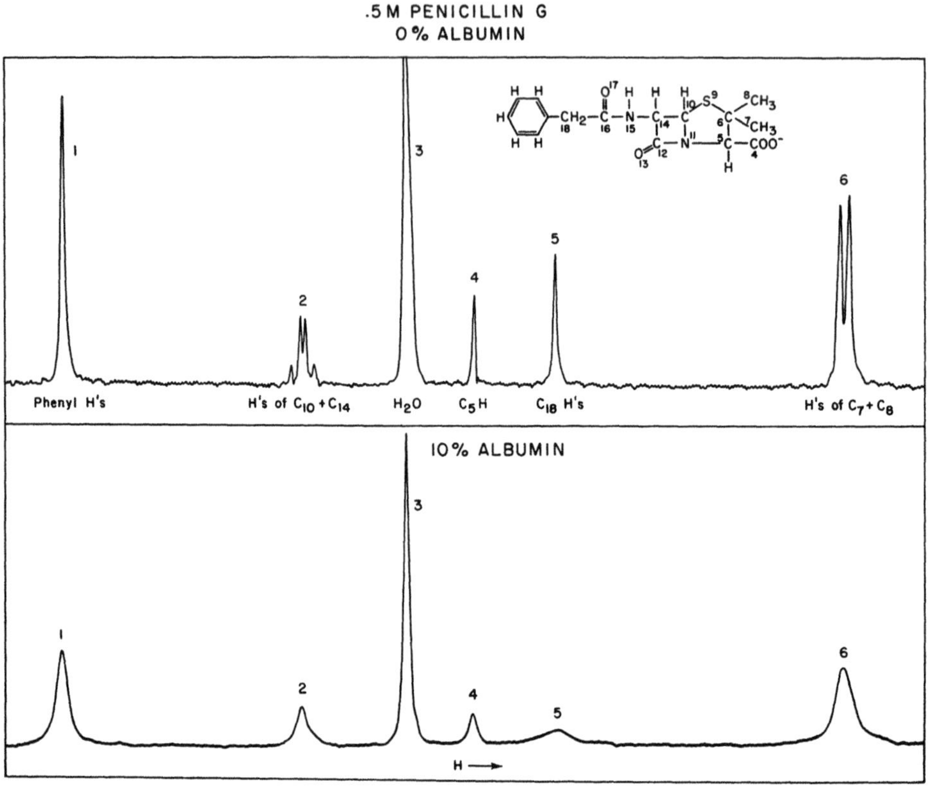

FIG. 1. The structures and the NMR spectra of penicillin G in D_2O alone and with albumin. The peak assignments are indicated. Addition of albumin broadens the peaks, particularly those arising from the phenyl and methylene groups.

The serum albumin binding experiments will be described in some detail because they have been the prototype for all of the later applications and because the results illustrate and justify the theoretical arguments previously presented. The experimental details and results of this work are available (Fischer, 1961, 1964; Fischer and Jardetzky, 1965), and only the more pertinent results together with some unpublished experiments will be given. Figure 1a shows a 60 Mc proton magnetic resonance spectrum of penicillin G; the structure and the peak assignments are also shown. The interpretation is unambiguous because of the presence of the AB system labeled #2. The effects of added albumin are shown in Figure 1b. With reference to the preceding theoretical discussion it should be noted that:

1. There are no significant changes in the chemical shifts of the penicillin peaks
2. The albumin spectrum is not seen
3. The penicillin peaks are broadened to varying degrees, which is noteworthy in order to rule out exchange Case II
4. The peak from the water impurity broadens to a much lesser extent, which

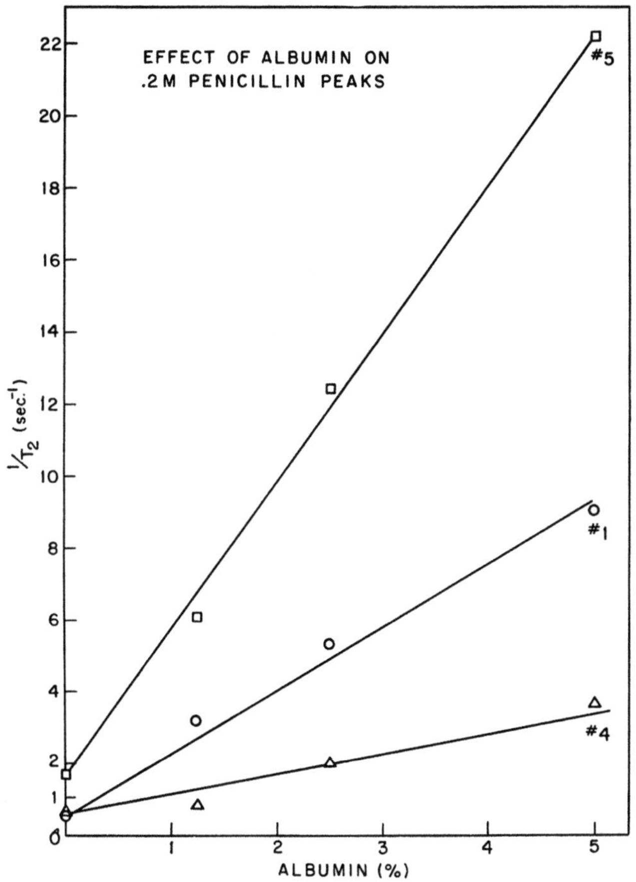

FIG. 2 The line widths (expressed as $1/T_2$) of three penicillin peaks as a function of increasing albumin concentration. Peaks are numbered as in Figure 1.

serves as a control for the anticipated broadening due to viscosity changes and eliminates the possibility of the presence of significant concentrations of paramagnetic impurities

The line widths for the three unsplit peaks, Nos. 1, 4, and 5 arising from the phenyl, methyne, and methylene groups respectively, were measured for an array of penicillin (0.01 to 0.5 M) and albumin (0 to 10 percent) concentrations. A typical result using 0.2 M penicillin G and increasing albumin concentrations is shown in Figure 2. For each peak the width was found to be directly proportional to the ratio of the albumin to penicillin concentrations for all of the absolute concentrations studied. It must be remembered that the penicillin is always present in large excess; thus the albumin binding sites are essentially completely saturated and the fraction of the total penicillin molecules that are bound depends only on the ratio of the albumin to penicillin concentrations. When this ratio becomes greater than 1:50, the penicillin peaks become too broad to detect.

For the purpose of ruling out other possible mechanisms of line broadening, it is worthwhile to point out explicitly that the addition of more pencillin to a given penicillin-albumin solution decreases the line widths. However, more penicillin increases solution viscosity, increases the possibility of nonspecific drug-drug interactions, increases the intermolecular dipole relaxation, and increases the possibility of adding paramagnetic contaminants; in fact it should increase the contribution of almost any conceivable nonspecific broadening mechanism. The only feasible alternative is to attribute the observed effect to a specific and saturable interaction with the albumin.

Using the rapid exchange model and the resulting Equation 13, it is possible to calculate from these data the values of the relaxation rates for the three peaks arising from the bound penicillin, given in Table 1.

TABLE 1

	$(1/T_2)$ bound	R
Peak #1	3,400 sec^{-1}	5,200
Peak #4	1,430 sec^{-1}	1,700
Peak #5	5,975 sec^{-1}	2,060

The methylene peak has the fastest relaxation rate; however, the stabilization ratios, Equation 12, are more meaningful in terms of the effect of binding on molecular motion. With this criterion, the phenyl peak is the one preferentially stabilized (Table 1), suggesting that the binding is hydrophobic in nature, and that the remainder of the penicillin molecule is to some extent free to move about while the ring structure is attached to the albumin.

Similar experiments with gamma globulin, which does not bind penicillin, show only very slight effects consistent with measured viscosity changes. Solutions of methyl cellulose which have extremely high bulk viscosities show essentially no effect on the penicillin spectrum. These findings support the contention that large (on a molecular scale) cells of free solvent exist within the methyl cellulose matrix which are able to dissolve the drug in the usual fashion without reflecting the measured bulk viscosity. More important here is the fact that this is another example of a nonbinding largė molecule that does not alter line width.

Penicillin V (phenoxy) also binds to serum albumin and shows similar changes in its line widths. Since not all of the spectral peaks of G and V overlap, it is possible to observe them simultaneously, alone, and with albumin, and thus to carry out an "inhibition experiment." Table 2 shows the results of $1/T_2$ measurements of the methylene peaks of the G and V in various mixtures. A fivefold excess of V reduces the line width of the 0.1 M penicillin G-2.5 percent albumin solution by approximately one half. This suggests that the two penicillins compete for a common binding site and provides more evidence that the broadening is not due to a nonspecific intermolecular interaction.

Similar studies show that 6-aminopenicillanic acid, the penicillin nucleus, and acetyl penicillin, a synthetic complete penicillin with only a methyl group on the side chain, do not bind or inhibit penicillin G binding (Table 2). In contrast

TABLE 2
Inhibition Studies: $1/T_2$ Values (sec^{-1})

	CH_{2_G}	CH_{2_V}
0.1 M Peni G	5.2	–
0.5 M Peni V	–	8.98
0.1 M Peni G 0.5 M Peni V	6.75	9.12
0.1 M Peni G 2.5% Alb	22.0	–
0.5 M Peni V 2.5% Alb	–	17.9
0.1 M Peni G 0.5 M Peni V 2.5% Alb	11.73	16.8
0.1 M Peni G 0.5 M 6-APA 2.5% Alb	26.1	–
0.1 M Peni G 0.5 M Acetyl Peni 2.5% Alb	22.3	–

phenoxyacetic acid and phenoxyacetamide specifically inhibit the effects of albumin on the penicillin G spectrum. This provides an independent verification that the phenyl group is of crucial importance for the binding interaction.

The molecular sieve compounds offer a unique tool for the study of exchange effects and the importance of intimate contact between drug and protein for broadening. Solutions of penicillin (0.05 M) alone and with albumin (1.25 percent) were examined in the presence of two types of Sephadex: G-50, which excludes albumin, and G-200, which allows free entry of the albumin as well as the penicillin.

Figure 3 shows the spectrum of penicillin with the G-200 type Sephadex (1.9 percent by dry weight). The familiar peaks of a high resolution penicillin spectrum can easily be distinguished; only the methylene peak is partially hidden by the Sephadex spectrum. Under the conditions used here, only about 1/20 of the volume of the NMR cell within the coils is occupied by extragranular solvent. The observed signals must then arise from penicillin actually inside the Sephadex; their sharpness indicates that the drug does not interact with the Sephadex itself. Furthermore the drug finds within the granules an environment very similar to that in free solution. When albumin is added, the spectrum of Figure 3b results. The extent of broadening is about what one would expect in the absence of Sephadex, showing that the protein has access to the same volume as does the drug.

When G-50 Sephadex is used, the result is quite different. The albumin is excluded from the inside of the granule, and narrow peaks are seen from the intragranular penicillin; on the other hand, the penicillin outside the granules is in contact with the protein and produces the expected broad lines. By changing the

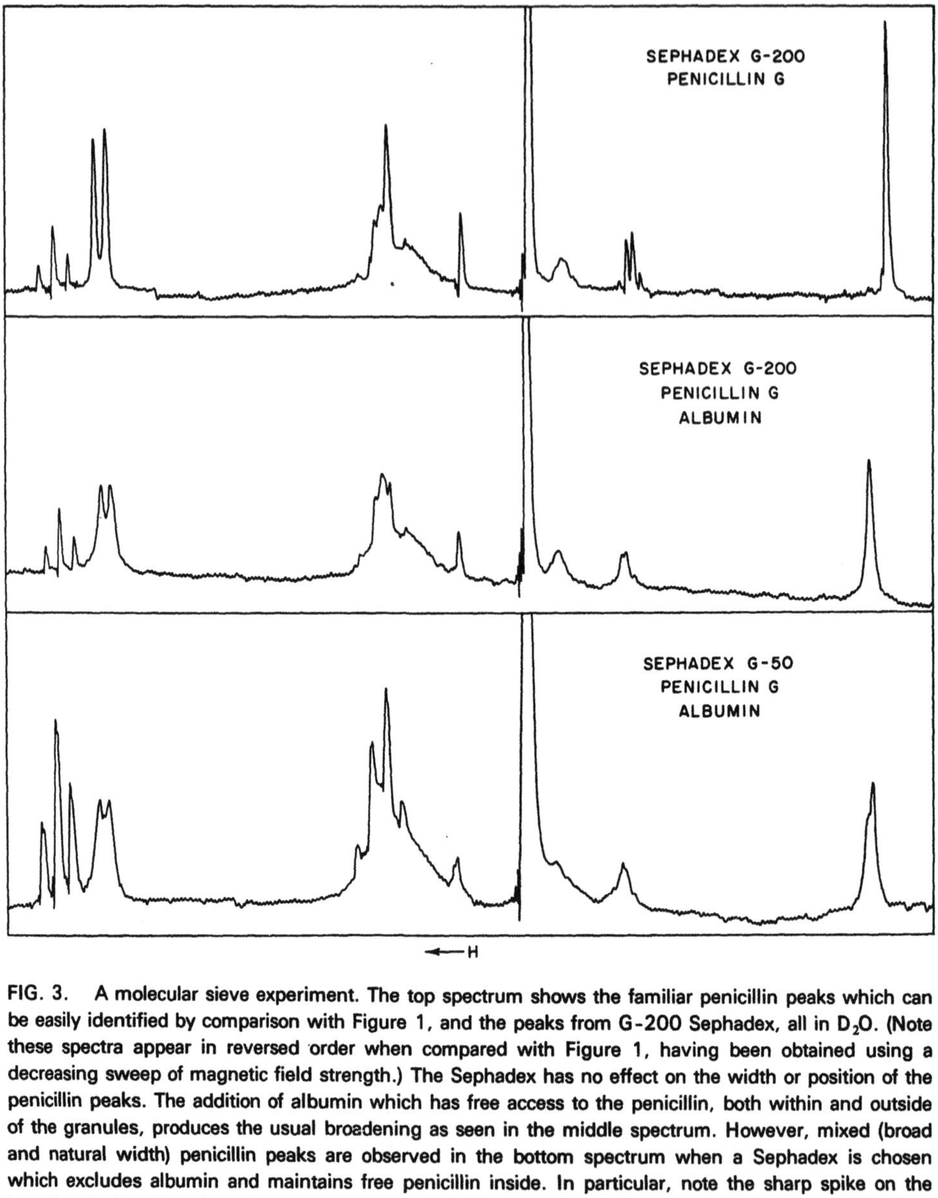

FIG. 3. A molecular sieve experiment. The top spectrum shows the familiar penicillin peaks which can be easily identified by comparison with Figure 1, and the peaks from G-200 Sephadex, all in D_2O. (Note these spectra appear in reversed order when compared with Figure 1, having been obtained using a decreasing sweep of magnetic field strength.) The Sephadex has no effect on the width or position of the penicillin peaks. The addition of albumin which has free access to the penicillin, both within and outside of the granules, produces the usual broadening as seen in the middle spectrum. However, mixed (broad and natural width) penicillin peaks are observed in the bottom spectrum when a Sephadex is chosen which excludes albumin and maintains free penicillin inside. In particular, note the sharp spike on the broadened phenyl peak at the extreme right.

proportion of granules to extragranular solution, the superposition of the broad and narrow peaks can be seen quite easily for the phenyl peak.

The potential usefulness of this kind of experiment is considerable. For purposes of interest here, it demonstrates three important points: Sephadex is another example of a large molecular structure that does not interact with penicillin; intimate contact is required between the drug and protein for broadening to occur; and rapid exchange must occur between the bound and unbound forms to produce a single broad line rather than the superposition of two lines (Fischer and Jost, 1969a).

OTHER EXPERIMENTAL RESULTS

As mentioned in the introduction, the number of published binding studies using NMR relaxation measurements is still quite small. A preliminary investigation of the interaction of diphosphopyridine nucleotide (DPN) to the enzyme yeast alcohol dehydrogenase (ADH) (Jardetzky et al., 1963) was carried out, making use for the first time of signal averaging techniques for sensitivity enhancement. Subsequently, a more detailed investigation was conducted by Hollis (1967), using more advanced equipment. It was possible to show that the addition of ADH to a solution of ethanol produced no change in the ethanol NMR spectrum under conditions such that approximately 6 percent of the substrate should have been bound to the enzyme. The author concludes that either there is no rapid exchange between free and bound forms of the ethanol (Case I or slow Case II exchange), or the binding of the substrate does not significantly restrict the motion of its methyl hydrogens to alter their relaxation rate. Further studies will be necessary to distinguish between these two possibilities, but obviously the result will be useful in understanding the mechanism of action of the enzyme.

A study of the binding of sulfonamides to serum albumin has been carried out using essentially the same experimental protocol as outlined above (Jardetzky and Wade-Jardetzky, 1965). For several of the simpler sulfonamides, binding resulted in preferential stabilization of the *p*-amino ring structure. Interestingly, sulfaphenazole seemed to bind to at least two different binding sites by two different mechanisms involving either the *p*-amino ring or the phenyl group of the specific side chain. The former mechanism could be competitively inhibited by phenylpropanol, as could the binding of the other simple sulfonamides. A variety of other compounds, including penicillin G, did not inhibit binding.

Thomas (1966) attempted to study the binding of various inhibitors to lysozyme by measuring changes in the chemical shifts of the NMR peaks of the inhibitors. The spectrum of one of the inhibitors, *N*, *N*1-diacetyl chitobiose, showed two methyl peaks, one of which broadened upon addition of the enzyme. Insufficient details are presented to interpret this observation adequately, but it certainly could be an example of a selective change in relaxation rates and clearly warrants further investigation.

Recently the results of a study of a hapten-antibody complex using a technique essentially identical with that described above have been published (Burgen et al., 1967). The antibody is directed toward the choline moiety and the line width of the *N*-methyl hydrogen nuclei increases when binding takes place. Similarly prepared gamma globulin from nonimmunized rabbits served as a control and did not alter the line width. Following a procedure that has had some

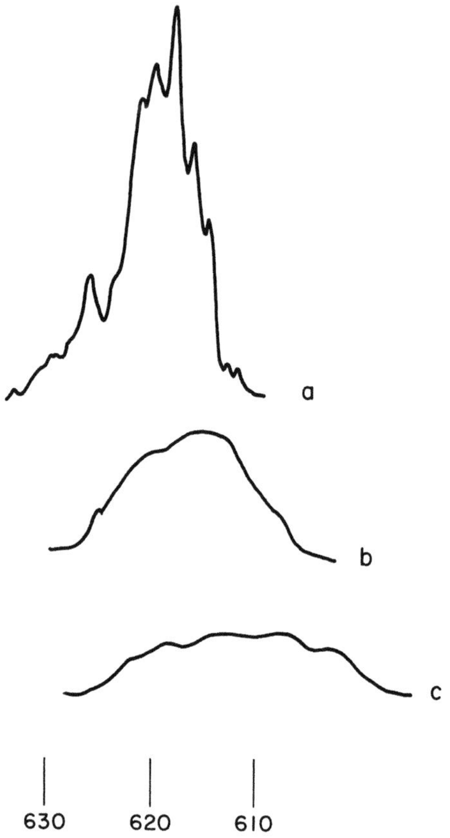

FIG. 4. 90 mHz NMR spectra of the phenyl protons of epinephrine. Scale: Chemical shift in Hz relative to internal DSS. (a) Epinephrine. (b) 0.01 M epinephrine with liver cells. (c) 0.005 M epinephrine with liver cells.

success in solid-state work,* an attempt was made to calculate an "energy barrier" to rotation of the methyl groups in the bound form from the temperature dependence of the line widths. Considering the complexity of the experimental system, it remains to be seen if the available data indeed warrant such a simple interpretation.

A very interesting study of the binding of tryptophan to chymotrypsin has been reported by Gerig (1968). D-Tryptophan shows a greater signal broadening upon addition of the enzyme that does the L isomer, a finding in agreement with the fact that the former is known to be a stronger inhibitor.

Alteration of the enzyme by phosphorylation or by substitution at the 192 methionine residue markedly reduces the line broadening. The correlation times for the bound tryptophan calculated from the relaxation rates are in excellent

*See Woessner and Snowden (1967) for a discussion of this technique and references to earlier applications.

agreement with what one would predict for tumbling of the enzyme itself (based on its known molecular dimensions) and indicate that binding constrains the tryptophan molecule to move with the enzyme as a unit.

DRUG-RECEPTOR INTERACTIONS

The first successful application of this technique to the study of a drug-receptor interaction has recently been described (Fischer and Jost, 1969b). The binding of epinephrine to liver cells, a mixed alpha and beta adrenergic interaction which leads via the adenyl cyclase system ultimately to the release of glucose, was chosen for the prototype studies for the following reasons: It is representative of an important class of pharmacologic effects; the system had been extensively studied by the indirect classical methods, including structure-activity and inhibition studies; and the dose-response curve for this effect seemed to extend to relatively high concentrations, approximately 10^{-5} M, thus perhaps indicating that the concentration of receptor sites would also be relatively great.

A suspension of isolated, intact, and viable mouse liver parenchymal cells was prepared using a method described by Rappaport and Howze (1966). Prior to use for NMR spectroscopy, the cells were incubated for approximately 24 hours in a deuterated buffer. This procedure substantially reduced the water signal from the cells, but apparently did not affect their morphology or viability. An example of the effect of these cells on the NMR spectrum of epinephrine is shown in Figure 4. The complex peak from the phenyl protons of epinephrine is shown in Figure 4a. Substantial broadening and a small upfield shift occur when the cells are present (Fig. 4b and c).

Analysis of the spectral changes indicates that the epinephrine is attached to the cells both at the ring structure and most probably at the nitrogen atom. The epinephrine ring is bound in such a way that it is in the diamagnetic region of a ring structure which is part of the binding site. The methyl group, on the other hand, seems relatively less influenced by the binding process. Dichloroisoproterenol, a beta adrenergic blocking agent, inhibits the changes in the epinephrine spectrum, while itself showing spectral changes characteristic of binding.

These conclusions concerning the nature of this drug-receptor complex confirm many of the features of models that have been developed from the classical structure-activity studies. Most important, however, this work explicitly demonstrates the feasibility of carrying out NMR binding studies with drug-receptors in intact, viable cells, and makes available for the first time a direct physical-chemical technique for the detection and investigation of these important interactions.

SUMMARY

An experimental method for the study of the weak, reversible binding of small molecules to biologic macromolecules and cellular structures based on the relaxation phenomenon of NMR spectroscopy has been described. Changes in the relaxation rates in the spectrum of the small molecule are used to identify portions of the molecule that take part in the binding interaction and to estimate the extent to which their internal motion is restricted by the binding interaction.

Although still relatively new, the method has been successfully applied to such problems as enzyme interactions with substrates, inhibitors, and coenzymes, to hapten-antibody interactions, and to the serum binding of small molecules. More recently an actual example of a drug binding to its receptor site in an intact viable cell has been investigated. Clearly there exist a large number of biologically important binding interactions for which detailed knowledge concerning molecular mechanisms is desirable. With the rapidly improving NMR instrumentation, and with the application of sufficient experimental ingenuity, an increasing number of them will be found suitable for investigation using this technique.

REFERENCES

Abragam, A. 1961. The Principles of Nuclear Magnetism. London, Oxford University Press, Inc.

Anderson, W. A., and Arnold, J. T. 1956. Proton relaxation times in H_2O-D_2O mixtures. Physiol. Rev., 101:511-512.

Bloch, F. 1957. Generalized theory of relaxation. Physiol. Rev., 105:1206-1220.

Bloembergen, N. 1961. Nuclear Magnetic Relaxation. New York, W. A. Benjamin, Inc.

Burgen, A., Jardetzky, O., Metcalfe, J. C., and Wade-Jardetzky, N. 1967. Investigation of a haptene-antibody complex by nuclear magnetic resonance. Proc. Nat. Acad. Sci., U.S.A. 58:447-453.

Chow, B. F., and McKee, C. M. 1945. Interaction between crystalline penicillin and human plasma proteins. Science, 101:67-68.

Ernst, R. R., and Anderson, W. A. 1966. Application of Fourier transform spectroscopy to magnetic resonance. Rev. Sci. Instrum., 37:93-102.

Fischer, J. J. 1961. A study of the protein binding of penicillin by nuclear magnetic resonance. Fed. Proc., 20:170.

—1964. The mechanism of the binding of penicillins to serum albumin studied by nuclear magnetic resonance spectroscopy. Ph.D. Thesis, Harvard University, Cambridge, Mass.

—and DeSimone, C. M. 1963. The role of D-benzyl-penicillenic acid in the sensitization of erythrocytes. Biochim. Biophys. Acta, 69:412-414.

—and Jardetzky, O. 1965. Nuclear magnetic relaxation study of intermolecular complexes. The mechanism of penicillin binding to serum albumin. J. Amer. Chem. Soc., 87:3237-3244.

—and Jost., M. C. 1969a. The use of molecular sieves in the study of intermolecular binding by NMR spectroscopy. Biochim. Biophys. Acta, 177:346-348.

—and Jost, M. C. 1969b. NMR studies of drug-receptor interactions. The binding of epinephrine to isolated mouse liver cells. Molec. Pharmacol., 5:420-423.

Gerig, J. T. 1968. Nuclear magnetic resonance studies of the interaction of tryptophan with α-chymotrypsin. J. Amer. Chem. Soc., 90:2681-2686.

Hollis, D. P. 1967. A nuclear magnetic resonance study of substrate binding to alcohol dehydrogenases. Biochemistry, 6:2080-2087.

Hubbard, P. S. 1958. Nuclear and magnetic relaxation of three and four spin molecules in a liquid. Physiol. Rev., 109:1153-1158.

—1963. Theory of nuclear magnetic relaxation by spin-rotational interactions in liquids. Physiol. Rev., 131:1155-1165.

Jardetzky, O., and Wade-Jardetzky, N. G. 1965. On the mechanism of the binding of sulfonamides to bovine serum albumin. Molec. Pharm., 1:214-230.
—Wade, N. G. and Fischer, J. J. 1963. Proton magnetic resonance investigation of enzyme-coenzyme complexes. Nature (London), 197:183-184.
Johnson, C. E., and Bovey, F. A. 1958. Calculation of nuclear magnetic resonance spectra of aromatic hydrocarbons. J. Chem. Phys., 29:1012-1014.
Josephson, A. S. 1960. The development of antibodies to penicillin in rabbits. J. Exp. Med., 111:611-620.
Kowalsky, A., and Cohn, M. 1964. Application of nuclear magnetic resonance in biochemistry. Ann. Rev. Biochem., 33:481-518.
Pople, J. A., Schneider, W. G., and Bernstein, J. H. 1959. High Resolution Nuclear Magnetic Resonance. New York, McGraw-Hill Book Company.
Powles, J. G., and Gutowsky, H. S. 1953. Proton magnetic resonance of the CH_3 group. I. Investigation of six tetrasubstituted methanes. J. Chem. Phys., 21:1695-1703.
Rappaport, C., and Howze, G. B. 1966. Dissociation of adult mouse liver by sodium tetraphenylboron. A potassium complexing agent. Proc. Soc. Exp. Biol. Med., 121:1010-1016.
Redfield, A. G. 1957. On the theory of relaxation processes. IBM J., 1:19-31.
Richards, P. M. 1963. Relaxation of longitudinal and transverse components of nuclear magnetization in liquids. Physiol. Rev., 132:27-32.
Roberts, J. D. 1959. Nuclear Magnetic Resonance. New York, McGraw-Hill Book Company.
Scholtan, W., and Schmid, J. 1962. Die Bindung der Penicilline and die Eiweiszkorper des Serum un des Gewebes. Arzneimittel-forschung, 12:741-750.
Thomas, E. W. 1966. Interaction between lysozyme and acetamido sugars as detected by proton magnetic resonance spectroscopy. Biochem. and Biophys. Res. Commun. 24:611-615.
Ullman, R. 1966. Nuclear magnetic relaxation of polymer solutions. Side-chain motion. J. Chem. Phys., 44:1558-1566.
Wang, M. C. and Uhlenbeck, G. E. 1945. On the theory of the brownian motion II. Rev. Mod. Phys., 17:323-342.
Woessner, D. E. 1962. Spin relaxation processes in a two-proton system undergoing anisotropic reorientation. J. Chem. Phys., 36:1-4.
—and Zimmerman, J. R. 1963. Nuclear transfer and anisotropic motional spin phenomena: Relaxation time temperature dependence studies of water adsorbed on silica gel IV. J. Phys. Chem., 67:1590-1600.
—and Snowden, B. S. Jr. 1967. Proton spin-lattice relaxation temperature dependence in ammonium bromide. J. Chem. Phys., 47:378-381.
Zimmerman, J. R., and Brittin, W. E. 1957. Nuclear magnetic resonance studies in multiple phase systems: Lifetime of a water molecule in an adsorbing phase on silica gel. J. Phys. Chem., 61:1328-1333.

CHAPTER 15

The Effect of Hormones on Nucleic Acid and Protein Synthesis

Edward Bresnick

Department of Pharmacology, Baylor College of Medicine
Texas Medical Center, Houston, Texas

INTRODUCTION

Hormones may be defined concisely as *chemical messengers* or *transmitters.* They are elaborated in specialized cells located in cell groups called glands and are transported via the circulation to a target tissue. The manner by which a specific hormone selects its target site is not known. However, the fact that hormones do localize, are concentrated, and are retained in target organs is indicative of the presence of "receptor" substances in these organs which can identify a particular hormone.

We may picture the initial events that occur after administration or elaboration of a hormone as (a) transport of the hormone across the target cell membrane, and (b) the interaction of the hormone with a specific receptor. Following the hormone-receptor interaction, a specific physiologic cellular response is elicited.

The original work of the author mentioned in this chapter was supported by grants from the National Institute of Health, CA 10290, and from the American Cancer Society, ACS–E373.

$$\text{Hormone} + \text{Receptor} \rightleftharpoons \text{Hormone-Receptor} \quad (1)$$

$$\text{Hormone-Receptor} \longrightarrow \text{Effects} \quad (2)$$

The hormone-receptor interaction would be defined in terms of Equation 1, while the hormonal action at a cellular level is represented by Equation 2. The nature of the receptor substance responsible for its recognition of a specific hormone will be briefly discussed in the ensuing paragraphs.

The exact nature of the receptor module has not been definitively established, although the latter has been conceived as a specific enzyme or enzyme complex, a system intimately involved in permeability or transport, or an "amplifier" molecule.

Both the enzyme or enzyme complex and the transport mechanism may contain fixed or flexible sites, distinct from the catalytic or transfer action, which bind the specific hormone. The subsequent complexation may lead to an augmentation in the ability of enzyme to react with its substrate or in the rate of transport. This is the definition of an allosteric interaction. Thus, Yielding and Tompkins (1962) have demonstrated the alteration in substrate specificity of glutamate dehydrogenase in the presence of estrogens. Ordinarily, the enzyme utilizes glutamate as substrate, but in the presence of estradiol or diethylstilbestrol, a conformational alteration in the enzyme molecule occurs which allows acceptance of alanine as substrate. The interplay between hormones, enzymes, and membranes has been nicely documented by Sutherland and Rall (1960). They have demonstrated the localization of the enzyme responsible for the synthesis of cyclic AMP, adenyl cyclase, within membranes. Cyclic AMP, a chemical transmitter, is known to affect several enzyme systems within the mammalian organism, in particular, the formation of the active form of phosphorylase, which governs the breakdown of glycogen and indirectly the formation of NADPH. The rate of formation of cyclic AMP, itself, is under hormonal control. Epinephrine is a potent activator of the adrenal system; ACTH a marked stimulator of the liver system.

The interactions of ligands with receptors have been explored by Changeux and his co-workers (Changeux et al., 1967; Changeux and Podleski, 1968), who have pointed out the similarities in properties between regulatory enzymes and excitable membranes. Both are excitable in that they respond to the interaction with specific substances by a defined alteration in their biologic activity. With the former, the affinity of the substrate for the enzyme is either augmented or reduced; with the latter, the permeability of ions is affected. Both also exhibit complex cooperative phenomena, i.e., dose-response curves are sigmoidal rather than linear. Consequently, the biologic activities of regulatory enzymes and excitable membranes are exquisitely sensitive to threshold concentrations of regulatory ligands.

The properties of excitable membranes are attributed to the presence within these structures of repeating globular lipoprotein units, i.e., protomers, which possess stereospecific recognition sites for excitatory ligands. The macromolecular protomers are associated in a highly ordered lattice or membrane structure. The

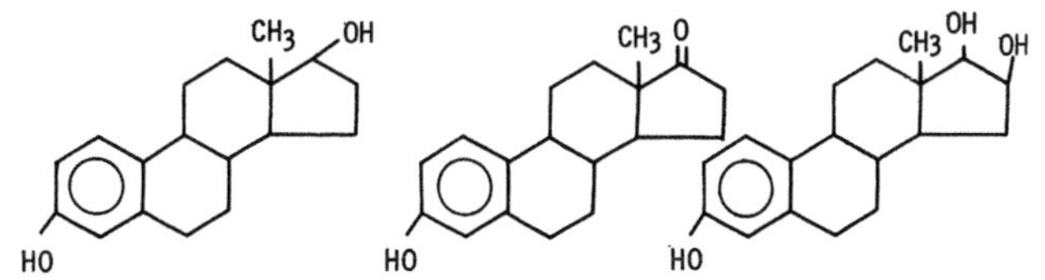

FIG. 1. Estrogens.

membrane structures are able to undergo reversible conformational changes which trigger off a biologic response. Changeux (Changeux and Podleski, 1968) has studied the binding of cholinesterase activators and inhibitors to the synaptic membranes of the isolated electroplax. He has suggested that in the resting membrane, a polarized state or conformation (P state) is maintained whereas a triggering of membrane depolarization is accomplished by a shift of the acetylcholinesterase protomer to another conformation, i.e., D conformation. The ability of drugs or of a neurohormone to induce the depolarization is related to the preferential affinity of the latter for the D state; antagonism is seen where drugs are able to differentially stabilize the P state. Consequently, the relative change in membrane potential is a reflection of the relative numbers of protomers which undergo the transition to the D state.

In the last category of receptor-like molecules, one might include the hormone-gene interactions. Thus, the complexation of a hormone with a receptor would lead to the elaboration of a substance that could activate a region or regions of the mammalian genome from which additional directions for information macromolecules would flow.

$$\text{DNA} \longrightarrow \text{RNA} \longrightarrow \text{Protein}$$

Such a mechanism was first suggested for the sex hormones by Karlson (1961).

In this chapter, we will consider only the latter mechanism, i.e., hormone-gene interaction, and we will restrict our discussion to the mechanism of action of a single class of hormones, the estrogens. The discussion will be divided essentially into two parts. The first part will be concerned with the events that occur in the uterus of ovariectomized rats following the administration of estrogens (see Fig. 1) with the emphasis placed upon interaction of the latter with a "receptor" and upon alterations in nucleic acid and protein biosynthesis. The second part will be more directly concerned with the experimental details involved in establishing the conclusions presented in the first part.

REGULATION OF UTERINE METABOLISM BY ESTROGENS

A considerable amount of effort has been expended in attempting to ascertain the initial change that takes place in the immature uterus which has just been

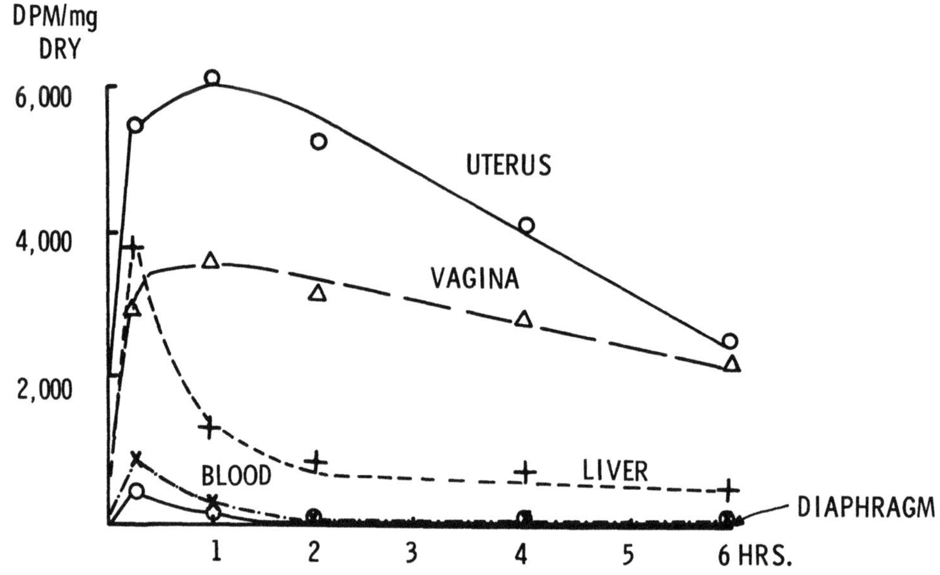

FIG. 2. Concentration of radioactivity in dried tissues of 23-day-old rats after single subcutaneous injection of 0.042 μg (8.65 μc) estradiol-6, 7-^{3}H in 0.2 ml saline. Liver and blood points are mean values of 3 aliquots portions of pooled samples; other points are median values of 5 individual animals. In this or in analogous experiments, radioactivity incorporation patterns paralleling that of blood are shown by kidney, adrenal, lung, ovary, skeletal muscle, bone, hypothalamus, and cerebrum, whereas anterior pituitary shows practically the same curve as vagina. (From Jensen et al. 1967. *Arch. Anat. Micr. Morph. Exp.*, 56:547-569.)

stimulated by estrogen administration. No clear-cut demonstration of such a change has been forthcoming. Some of the earliest effects that take place after stimulation with 17-β-estradiol are concerned with transport of water and small molecules. Markee (1932) reported the occurrence of hyperemia in the uterus occurring within 30 minutes of estrogen administration to rats. A number of other substances accumulate in the uterus within hours of administration of estradiol to rats. These events, which have been reviewed by Segal and Scher (1967), include accumulation of serum albumin and other proteins, oxygen, urea, sucrose, sodium, iron, glucose, and lactate.

Estradiol influences the metabolism of some amino acids and amino acid precursors within the uterine cell. However, neither the quantity nor the activity of free transfer RNA or the amino acid activating enzymes was increased by its action. The effect of estradiol upon the synthesis of nucleic acid precursors has been investigated by several authors (Gorski and Mueller, 1963; Jervell et al., 1958; Volfin et al., 1957, 1961). These investigators have demonstrated that the rat uterine acid-soluble adenine and uridine monophosphate pools are increased after estradiol injection; the total concentration of uridine triphosphate, as well as adenosine triphosphate, was also augmented. The effects of hormone administration upon uterine nucleic acid metabolism may be summarized as follows: Little change occurs in DNA synthesis while the synthesis of RNA increases up to 40 hours. The latter effect is observable as early as 10 to 20 minutes after administration of the hormone. The effects of the hormone upon RNA synthesis will be discussed in greater detail later.

BINDING OF ESTROGEN TO UTERINE RECEPTOR

Estradiol is very rapidly taken up by the uterus, as noted by Jensen and coworkers (reviewed in Jensen et al., 1967). Their results are presented in Figure 2. In these experiments, Jensen et al. (1967) injected tritiated estradiol of high specific activity into immature female rats and noted a rapid incorporation into the liver, vagina, and uterus. This was particularly apparent when the radioactivity was expressed on a dry weight basis. The estrogen was apparently preferentially bound in the uterus and vagina of the immature female rat. This effect was observed only when low concentrations, i.e., 0.1 mg or less of the estrogen, were injected.

The fate of the tritiated estradiol in the rat uterus was examined by Talwar et al. (1964), who demonstrated the localization of the tritiated material principally in two subcellular fractions, a nuclear myofibrillar and a supernatant fraction; approximately 58 percent of the radioactivity was associated with the latter. Noteboom and Gorski (1965) demonstrated the specificity of this binding reaction in the nuclear myofibrillar fraction. They were able to show that the binding could be prevented by pretreatment of the immature rats only with diethylstilbestrol, the synthetic "estrogen," and with unlabeled 17-β-estradiol. Of interest, the inactive isomer, 17-γ-estradiol, did not prevent the binding reaction. Furthermore, the estradiol-binding factor present in the nuclear fraction was sensitive to trypsin, suggesting protein as a major component.

Gorski and his colleagues (Toft and Gorski, 1966; Toft et al., 1967), concentrating their attention on the receptor-like material present in the supernatant fraction of uterus, have found that the receptor is a macromolecule, present only in the uterus, with a sedimentation coefficient of 9.5 S. When the amount of estrogen administered is within the physiologic range, the hormone is bound exclusively with the 9.5 S component; at higher amounts, the hormone becomes associated with other components present in the soluble fraction. The binding of estradiol to the 9.5 S component is also inhibited by diethylstilbestrol but not by any of the nonestrogenic steroids. Gorski has calculated the concentration of estrogen binding sites in the soluble fraction of uterus to be 10×10^{-13} moles per mg protein or approximately 9×10^{-13} moles per uterus. Although the relationship between the action of the estrogens and the receptor-like substance found in these soluble fractions has not been clearly established, the suggestion is that the protein acts like an activating substance for the hormone; the hormone-protein complex would be responsible for the sequence of events that ensue.

The interaction of 17-β-estradiol with uterine protein has also been examined by Jensen and his colleagues (see Jensen et al., 1967). They confirmed the presence of a "receptor" protein in a rat uterus high-speed supernatant fraction and, in addition, demonstrated the complexation of the estrogen to a protein component

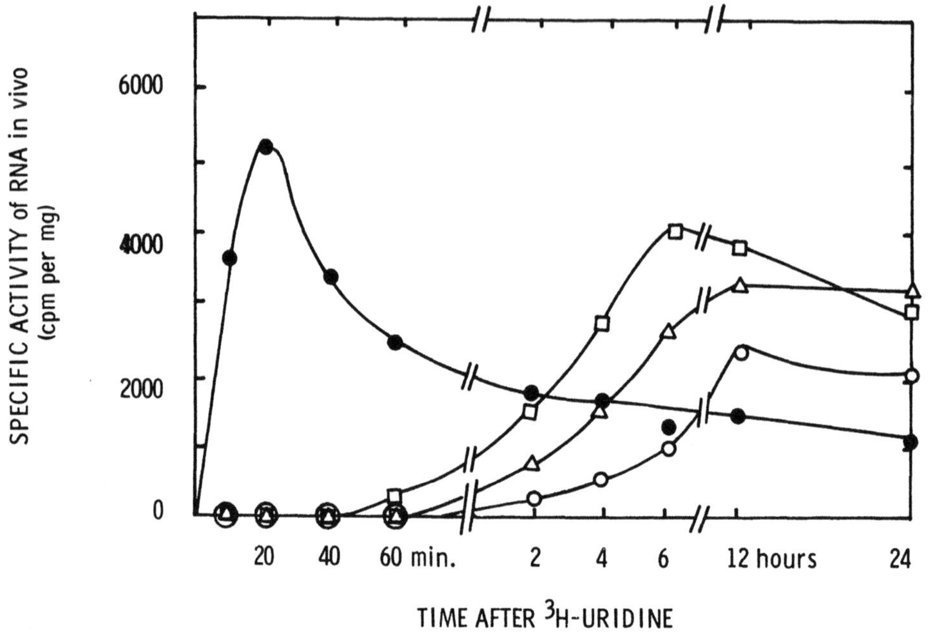

FIG. 3. Time course of incorporations of ^{3}H-uridine into uterine RNA in the intact adult rat. All animals received intraperitoneally 100 μc of ^{3}H-uridine at time zero. Animals were killed (three to five per group) at the times indicated, and the uteri were excised, weighed, and pooled. The whole tissue homogenate was prepared, the subcellular fractions were isolated, and the RNA was extracted for determination and for measurement of radioactivity. Specific activity of RNA was expressed as counts per min of ^{3}H-uridine (1.0 c per mmole) incorporated per mg of RNA. The remaining experimental details were as described in the text. Solid circles: nuclear RNA; Open circles: mitochondrial RNA; Open squares: microsomal RNA; Open triangles: cell sap RNA. (From Hamilton et al. 1968. *J. Biol. Chem.*, 243:408-417.)

in uterine nuclei. The "soluble" receptor sedimented at 9.5 S, the nuclear-bound material at 5 S. Although both proteins showed similar properties, they were not identical, i.e., the 9.5 S material was not a dimer of the 5 S. The binding of estradiol to either receptor was abolished by sulfhydryl reagents, i.e., *p*-hydroxymercuribenzoate, suggesting either the involvement of protein sulfhydryls in the complexation or the contribution of the latter to the conformation of the receptor structure.

EFFECTS OF ESTROGENS UPON RNA BIOSYNTHESIS

Within the first 24 hours after the administration of 17-β-estradiol to ovariectomized rats, an accumulation of protein occurs which is preceded by a marked augmentation in RNA biosynthesis (Mueller et al., 1958). That the inhibitor of RNA synthesis, actinomycin D, can block various aspects of the early estrogen response confirmed the necessity for RNA synthesis (reviewed in Segal

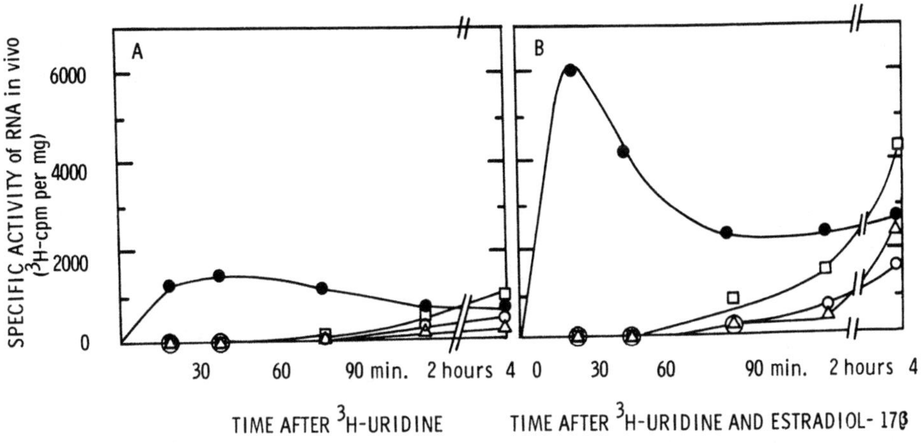

FIG. 4. Effect of a single dose of estradiol-17β on the incorporation of ^{3}H-uridine into RNA in the uterus of the ovariectomized adult rat. All animals were given 100 μc of ^{3}H-uridine (*A*) or 100 μc of the radioisotope and 10 μg of estradiol-17β (*B*) at time zero. At the times indicated, animals were killed (three to five per group), the uteri were excised and pooled, and the subcellular fractions were isolated. Solid circles: nuclear RNA; Open circles: mitochondrial RNA; Open squares: microsomal RNA; Open triangles: cell sap RNA. (From Hamilton et al. 1968. *J. Biol. Chem.*, 243:408-417.

and Scher) in the subsequent hormonal events. The question arises, what is the nature of the ribonucleic acid whose synthesis is augmented by estrogen treatment? Ui and Mueller (1963) and Gorski and Nicolette (1963) have indicated that the administration of the hormone does not result in the synthesis of any specific type of RNA. The quantitative increases in RNA synthesis are due to enhanced formation of messenger, transfer, and ribosomal RNA.

A detailed study of the synthesis of RNA in the rat uterus during early estrogen action has been conducted by Hamilton et al., (1968). The temporal relationships of the incorporation of tritiated uridine into cytoplasmic and nuclear RNA of the uterus in the intact adult rat are indicated in Figure 3. It is apparent that nuclear RNA is very rapidly labeled, reaching a maximum at approximately 20 minutes after injection of the precursor. As the specific activity of the latter RNA is reduced, concomitantly, the specific activity of cytoplasmic RNA is increased; maximal labeling is achieved in the latter by 6 to 12 hours. Such a relationship is strongly suggestive of parent-progeny interplay, with nuclear RNA being emitted from the nucleus into the cytoplasm.

The effects of ovariectomy upon the isotopic incorporation into uterine RNA are depicted in Figure 4A. The procedure is accompanied by a marked reduction of the incorporation into both nuclear and cytoplasmic RNA which is restored upon administration of 17-β-estradiol (Fig. 4B). The pattern of incorporation is identical in the uterus from estradiol-treated ovariectomized and intact rats.

One of the major activities of the nucleus (more definitely, the nucleolus) is in the elaboration of ribosomal RNA. That nuclear RNA synthesis is markedly enhanced in the uterus after the administration of 17-β-estradiol to ovariecto-

TABLE 1

Effect of Ovariectomy, Hormone Treatment, and Phase of Estrous Cycle on the Ratio of RNA to DNA and the Ratio of Protein to DNA in the Uterus or the Nuclei of Its Individual Cells.

Interval after hormone treatment (hr)	DNA in uterus (mg)	Nuclear ratios		Whole-tissue homogenate ratios		Uterus wet weight (mg)
		RNA/DNA	*PROTEIN/DNA*	*RNA/DNA*	*PROTEIN/DNA*	
			OVARIECTOMIZED ANIMALS			
0	0.98	0.23	2.20	0.43	2.10	68 ± 5
0.5	0.91	0.24	2.05	0.41	2.66	86 ± 7
1	0.85	–	–	–	–	79 ± 7
2	0.96	0.28	2.32	0.52	2.80	87 ± 6
4	0.92	0.27	2.30	–	–	102 ± 10
12	0.97	0.29	2.30	0.71	3.98	117 ± 9
24*	1.10	0.32	3.36	0.82	7.82	130 ± 8
36	1.22	–	–	–	–	135 ± 9
48*	1.20	0.32	3.64	–	–	140 ± 11
72*	1.24	0.33	3.78	–	–	210 ± 19
			NORMAL ANIMALS			
Diestrus	1.26	0.32	3.54	0.58	4.86	213 ± 16
Estrus	1.49	0.34	3.28	0.92	24.80	630 ± 44

*Hormone administered again at intervals of 24 hours each.
From Hamilton et al. 1968. *Proc. Nat. Acad. Sci. U.S.A.*, 59:1265-1272.

Ovariectomized adult rats were given (intraperitoneally) 10μg of 17-β-estradiol at zero time, and at later times in the experiments designated. Animals were killed, the uteri were weighed, and the nuclei were isolated. Each nuclear preparation was washed twice prior to determinations of ratios of RNA to DNA and of protein to DNA. Portions of the tissue homogenate were taken for DNA determination. Each control or experimental group consisted of six to eight animals, and their uteri were pooled for the subsequent determinations. With the exception of the data on uterine DNA, each value is the average of duplicate or triplicate experiments, with the range of variation being less than 5 percent.

mized rats is strongly indicative of an augmentation in ribosomal RNA synthesis. The process of formation of ribosomes may be rate-limiting in mammalian tissues, and any acceleration of growth processes, as would occur in the uterus of hormone-treated ovariectomized animals, should be accompanied by the formation of these cellular components. The biochemical data of Hamilton et al. (1968a) are supported by the electron micrographic observations of Laguens (1964). From 6 to 24 hours after administration of estrogen, an increase in both the size and number of nucleoli of the smooth muscle cells of the uterus may be observed.

Whether messenger RNA production is specifically enhanced in the uteri of estrogen-treated rats, although suggested in several experiments, cannot be answered with any degree of certainty. Wilson (1963) has shown that estradiol administration is attended by an increase in transfer RNA in the rat uterus.

Gorski and colleagues (Gorski et al., 1965) have shown that 17-β-estradiol administration has a very pronounced effect upon the enzyme that functions in the catalysis of RNA in rat uterine nuclei, RNA polymerase. The observation is only seen when the enzyme is assayed at low ionic strength; in the presence of high concentrations of ammonium sulfate, the effect is no longer apparent. The results were interpreted as indicating that the hormones did not produce any synthesis of new polymerase, but had some effect upon the template activity of the chromatin, i.e., deoxyribonucleoprotein, which is firmly attached to the RNA polymerase. Thus, we might consider this effect as a *genomic activation*. Similar results have been observed after treatment with a variety of other hormones as well as after administration of 3-methylcholanthrene (Bresnick et al., 1969; Bresnick, 1966).

EFFECTS OF ESTRADIOL UPON PROTEIN BIOSYNTHESIS

Estrogen administration results in a stimulation in the size of the uterine structure as well as an increase in the rate of turnover of cellular protein. The enzymes whose activities are augmented after estradiol administration have been the subject of a review by Segal and Scher (1967) and will not be discussed here further.

The uterine weight as well as the protein/DNA is subject to marked fluctuation, dependent upon the hormonal environment in that tissue. Thus, during diestrus, in the rat, the uterine weight is approximately one third the value seen in estrus (Table 1) (Hamilton et al., 1968b); the protein/DNA is only 20 percent of that seen in estrus. The protein/DNA is also sensitive to oblation of the ovary of the rat and falls precipitously (see Table 1). Administration of estradiol to the ovariectomized rat returns this value toward the normal range.

The effects of ovariectomy and hormone therapy upon the incorporation of labeled amino acids into uterine protein in vivo have been determined by Hamilton and his colleagues (Hamilton, 1968) and are presented in Figure 5. Initially, after hormone therapy, they observed a depression of the rate of incorporation of labeled methionine into nuclear mitochondrial and supernatant protein of the uterus of ovariectomized rats. By two hours after therapy, stimulation in the synthesis of nuclear protein was apparent. By eight hours, a 200 to 300 percent increase in incorporation into cytoplasmic protein was observed.

Teng and Hamilton (1967) have studied the cell-free incorporation activity of a polyribosomal fraction isolated from the uterus of overiectomized rats to which estradiol was administered. Within two hours after injection, a sharp increase in the incorporation of labeled leucine into polyribosomal protein was observed. Consequently, the in vitro system duplicated the effects seen in vivo.

SUMMARY OF EFFECTS.—Estradiol, administered to overiectomized rats, interacts with a receptor protein located in the target tissue, the uterus. The estradiol-receptor complex, in some manner, is able to react with a segment of the genetic information, at one or more loci. The latter interaction results in an activation of the genome, presumably by hastening the removal of blocking groups from the DNA. The activated chromatin is expressed by an enhanced nuclear RNA polymerase activity. The function of the latter enzyme is the elaboration of transfer RNA and ribosomal RNA required for the subsequent increase in protein

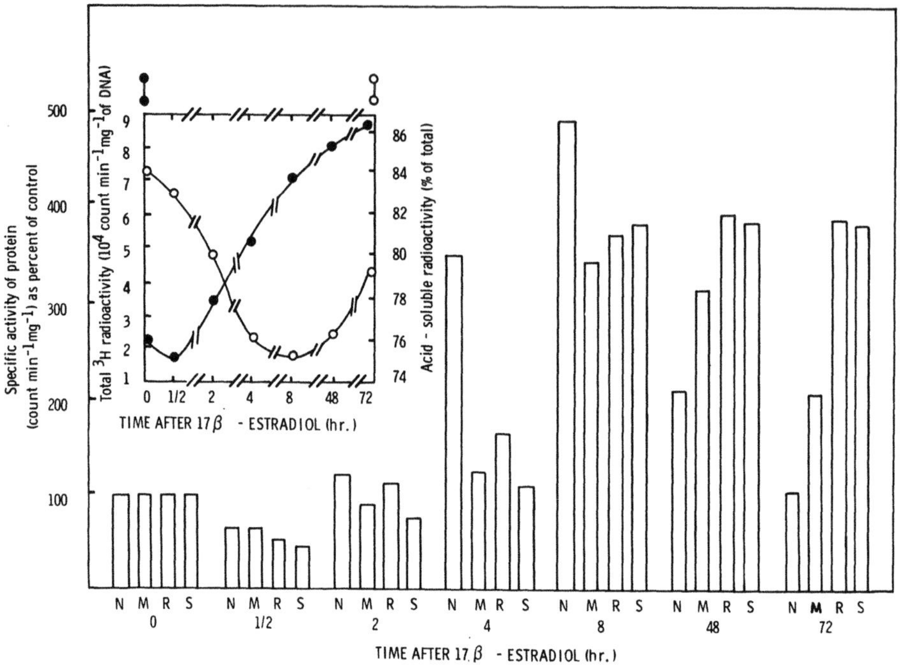

FIG. 5. Rates of synthesis of rapidly labeled protein of subcellular fractions of the uterus of the ovariectomized rat, as a function of time after treatment with estrogen in vivo. All animals were given 83 μc of tritiated L-methionine intraperitoneally 10 minutes before they were killed. Experimental animals were similarly given 10 μg of the hormone at zero time, and killed at the time indicated. Certain animals were given doses of the hormone at intervals of 24 hours thereafter. Uteri were pooled and homogenized, and the subcellular fractions were isolated for determination of protein and its radioactivity. Specific activity was expressed in counts per minute per milligram of protein. The data are expressed as percentages of the control values, which are nuclear protein (N), count/min 340; mitochondrial protein (M), 548 count/min; microsomal protein (R), 514 count/min; supernatant protein (S), 409 count/min. The insert shows the variation in tissue radioactivity and in the proportion of radioactivity that was in the acid-soluble fraction. (From Hamilton. 1968. *Science,* 161:649-661.)

synthesis, and perhaps an increase in specific messenger RNA formation. Finally, an increase in protein synthesis is observed within the uterus as an end result of hormone administration.

EXPERIMENTAL PROCEDURES

The experimental procedures from which the conclusions presented above may be drawn are extremely important. These procedures are rather ubiquitously employed in laboratories in which the effects of hormone administration upon biologic processes are under active investigation. Consequently, some additional experimental detail, particularly in procedure, might be beneficial to the reader. The remaining section of this chapter is devoted to this endeavor.

Procedure of Ovariectomy

Young adult female rats weighing 100 to 120 g are employed. In the rat, the whole estrous cycle lasts about five days, anestrus and estrus comprising three and two days, respectively. The uterus undergoes marked alterations in appearance during this time. During anestrus, the uterus is thin and pale in color, while in estrus it is full, perhaps distended with a fluid, pink in appearance.

Anesthetize the rat either under ether or by a subcutaneous injection of Nembutal (sodium pentobarbital), 50 mg/kg intraperitoneally. With the rat on its side, a localized incision is made about 2 cm lateral to the midline, from in front of the hip to a point just above the upper pole of the kidney. Laterally and interiorly to the upper pole of the kidney, a small aperture is made through the fascia of the abdominal rectus muscle. The aperture is widened by extension with forceps, and the ovary can be seen embedded in the fat layer just below the dorsal muscle mass or may be located by following the uterus upward.

Draw the ovary through the incision, clamp off the uterus with a bulldog clamp as a hemostat, and place a tie around the uterus just below the fallopian tube. Remove the ovary by cutting through the uterus on the ovarian side of the ligature. Suture the muscle and skin incisions and remove the other ovary similarly. Usually a week is allowed for the recovery of the rat from the surgery.

Interaction of Drug or Hormone with Receptor

One of the easiest ways to study the binding of labeled estradiol, or any drug, to a receptor present in the soluble fraction of a uterine homogenate is by means of gel filtration chromatography on Sephadex G-200. The method has been used with success in studying the binding of labeled polycyclic hydrocarbons to soluble proteins by this author (Bresnick et al., 1967a).

Sephadex is a modified dextran supplied in a form of minute beads. The dextrans are cross-linked into a three-dimensional network and are able to absorb a considerable quantity of water due to their high content of hydroxyl groups.

Sephadex chromatography or gel filtration became a routine laboratory tool in 1959 and has been extremely useful in the fractionation and separation of molecules according to size. Molecules that are larger than the largest pores of the Sephadex will not penetrate the gel particles and consequently will pass through the gel bed in the liquid phase outside of the particles. They are considered to be *above the exclusion limit* and are eluted first. On the other hand, smaller molecules penetrate the gel particles to varying degrees, which depend upon their size and shape. Consequently, these substances are eluted from the gel in the order of decreasing molecular size. The properties of the various Sephadex gels are given in Table 2. It is apparent from this table that each gram of Sephadex G-200 will absorb 20 grams of water and will form a column containing a bed volume of 30 to 40 ml.

TABLE 2

Type	Approximate Exclusion Limit (MW)	Water Regain ($g\ H_2O/g$ dry gel)	Wet Density (g/cm^3)	Particle Size (microns)	Bed Volume ml/g dry gel
Sephadex G-25	5,000	2.5 ± 0.2	1.13		5
Fine				20-80	
Coarse				100-300	
Sephadex G-50	10,000	5.0 ± 0.3	1.07		10
Fine				20-80	
Coarse				100-300	
Sephadex G-75	50,000	7.5 ± 0.5	1.05	40-120	12-15
Sephadex G-100	100,000	10.0 ± 1.0	1.04	40-120	15-20
Sephadex G-200	200,000	20.0 ± 2.0	1.02	40-120	30-40

From *Sephadex in Gel Filtration,* Uppsala, Sweden, Pharmacia Fine Chemicals Co., p. 3.

The useful range of separation of particles in terms of molecular weight is also given in Table 2. If one is interested in separating a molecule of molecular weight in excess of 5,000, either Sephadex G-100 or G-200 would be useful. In practice, we have found that Sephadex G-200 is extremely useful in the range from 5,000 to 400,000.

A quantity of Sephadex is weighed out and gradually added to a large volume of the aqueous eluting medium. The Sephadex is allowed to swell for a minimum of 48 hours in the latter. A column of Sephadex is prepared using a standard chromatography column. The dimensions of a column that has proven most useful in routine determinations for the gel filtration of 5 ml of supernate are 2.5 by 50 cm. With this column, it is possible to determine the approximate molecular weight of various proteins. An example of this aspect is given in Figure 6. After determining the elution volume, i.e., the amount of solvent required to pass through the Sephadex column and elute the solute, for a number of proteins of known molecular weight, it is possible to construct a graph relating the elution volume as a function of the log of the molecular weight. The resultant linear relationship (within the operable range of that Sephadex) remains a constant for that particular column of Sephadex. Hence, the approximate molecular weight of an unknown protein can be determined if the elution volume of the latter lies on the derived straight-line function.

It is also possible to take advantage of the difference in elution volumes of proteins whose mobilities on the Sephadex column are only partially retarded and of a low-molecular-weight material which essentially "dissolves" in the Sephadex and is completely retarded.* Consequently, the interaction between drugs or hormones and protein may be studied in this fashion.

The reaction mixture containing the hormone or drug which had been allowed to react with protein is slowly placed on the top of the Sephadex G-200 column, and the latter is rinsed twice with eluting buffer. Prior to each rinsing, the material is allowed to pass into the column.

*Another way of stating this is to utilize the concept of distribution coefficients (K_0). When $K_0 = 0$, the molecules are assumed to be large enough so as not to enter the stationary phase. When $K_0 = 1$, the molecules are small enough so that accessibility is complete. Intermediate retardation by the Sephadex yields K_0 values that are between 0 and 1.

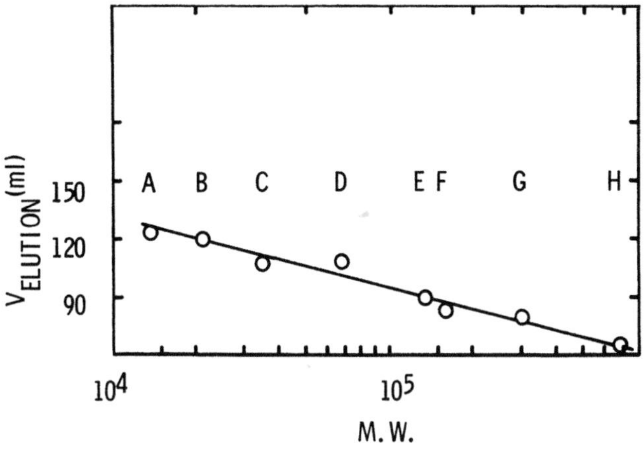

FIG. 6. Estimation of molecular weight of proteins with Sephadex G-200. The column of Sephadex G-200 is described in the text. The proteins employed in the calibration of the Sephadex G-200 included: *A*, ribonuclease; *B*, soybean trypsin inhibitor; *C*, pepsin; *D*, bovine serum albumin (monomer); *E*, bovine serum albumin (dimer); *F*, human γ-globulin; *G*, leucine aminopeptidase; and *H*, thyroglobulin. (From Bresnick and Thompson. 1965. *J. Biol. Chem.*, 240:3967-3974.)

The gel filtration is then begun with the proper eluent by collecting fractions of an appropriate volume. An example of the separation of labeled 3-methylcholanthrene (or its metabolites) from protein-bound material is presented in Figure 7. In this figure, the amount of protein, as the absorbancy at 280 mμ (A_{280}), is expressed as a function of the collection tubes; each fraction consisted of 2.5 ml. The radioactivity around fraction 20 is protein-bound material, whereas the radioactivity in fractions 65 to 85 represents methylcholanthrene or a derivative of methylcholanthrene. It is apparent from this figure that the protein-bound material separates quite nicely from the precursor. A similarly executed study could be performed using the supernatant fraction obtained from rat uterus after the in vivo administration of 17-β-estradiol of high specific activity. The uterus would be removed, homogenized in a suitable buffer, centrifuged at 100,000 × *g* for at least 60 minutes, and the radioactivity present in the supernatant fractions would be determined by standard techniques. An aliquot of the supernate would then be applied to the Sephadex G-200 and gel filtration conducted as previously described.

Isolation of Nuclei

Rats are lightly anesthetized under ether and then exsanguinated by transsection of the renal artery and vein. The livers are perfused via the portal system in situ with cold 0.25 M sucrose. The perfused livers are removed, blotted, and weighed. The remaining procedure is conducted in a cold room at 5°C. The perfused livers are minced in a Harvard tissue mincer, and the mince is then homogenized in 2.3 M sucrose containing 3 mM $CaCl_2$ (1:12, w/v) (Chauveau, et

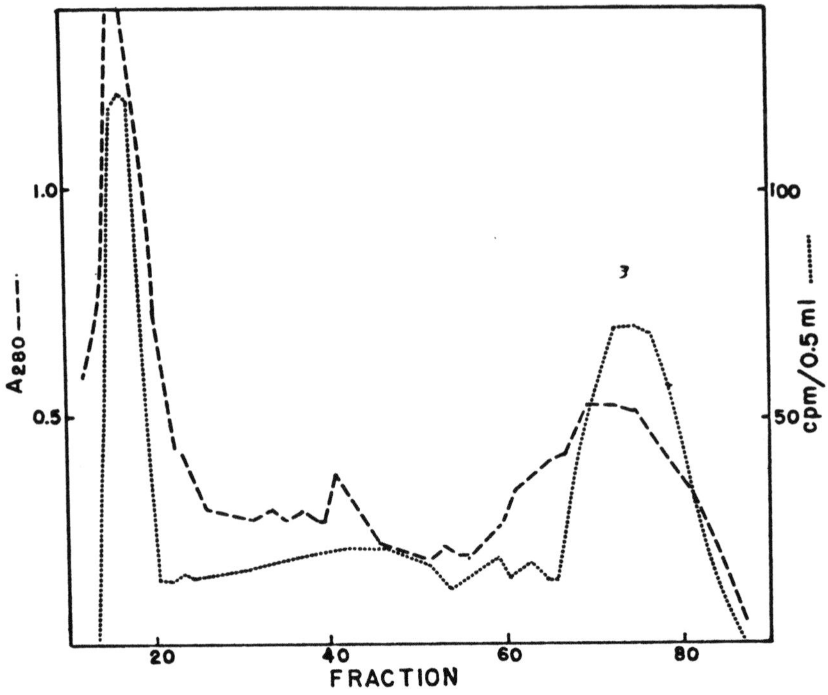

FIG. 7. Sephadex G-200 chromatography of the soluble cytoplasmic fraction. Rats were injected with methylcholanthrene-^{3}H (254 μc) and were sacrificed 10 hours later. Fractions of approximately 2.5 ml were collected. The livers were homogenized in 0.25 M sucrose to 20% and the homogenates were centrifuged at 100,000 $\times$ g for 60 minutes. The soluble fraction, 3.0 ml, was then applied to a column of Sephadex G-200, 2.5 $\times$ 40 cm, that had been equilibrated with 0.25 M sucrose. The column was eluted with 0.25 M sucrose at 4°C and fractions of 3.0 ml were collected. The void volume of this column was 47 ml. The radioactivity and absorbance at 280 mμ (A_{280}) of each fraction were determined. (From Bresnick et al. 1967. *Cancer Res.*, 27:462-468.)

al., 1957). The homogenate is centrifuged at 40,000 $\times$ g for 60 minutes to yield a crude nuclear pellet which is rehomogenized in 1 M sucrose plus 1 mM $CaCl_2$ (1 ml/g of uterus) and centrifuged at 900 $\times$ g for 10 minutes. The purified nuclear pellet is then utilized in the preparation of nuclear RNA. The purity of the nuclear preparation can be assessed by phase and light microscopy. For the latter, the nuclei are stained with a solution of 0.05 percent azure C in 0.25 M sucrose. A micrograph of purified liver nuclei isolated by this method is shown in Figure 8.

Preparation of Nuclear RNA

The method found most suitable for the isolation of nuclear RNA from mammalian tissues is the phenol-sodium dodecyl sulfate (SDS) method described in detail by Steele and Busch (1967). Nuclei isolated as previously described are suspended at 4°C in a medium containing 0.3 percent SDS, 0.1 M NaCl, and 0.05

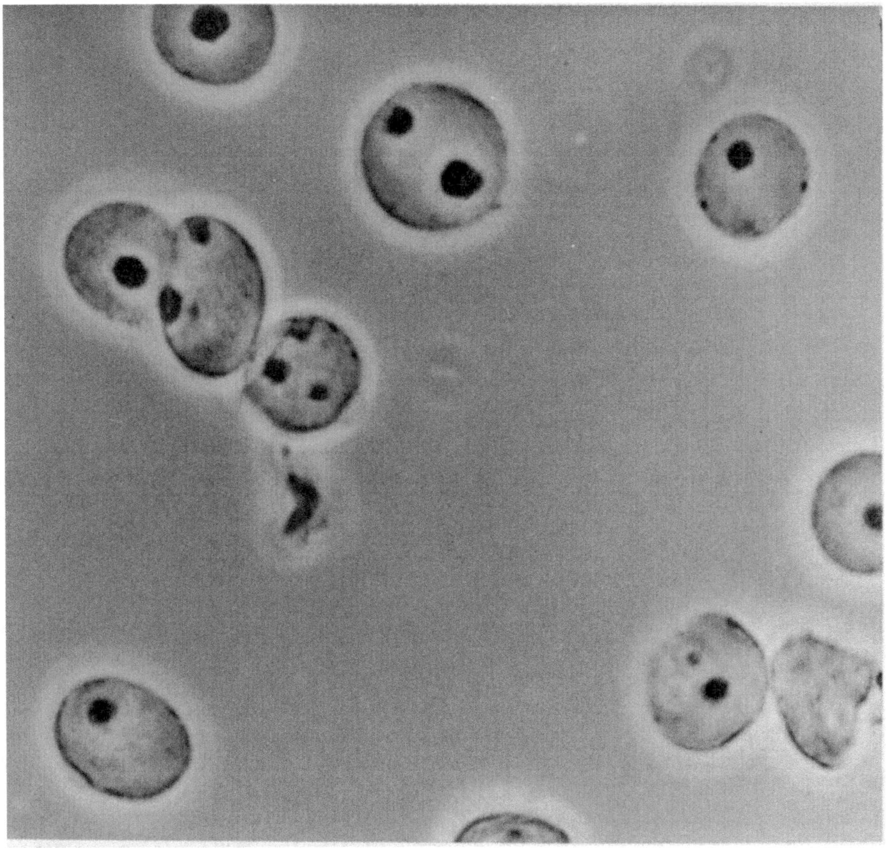

FIG. 8. Rat liver nuclei. (From Bresnick and Schwartz. 1968. *In* Functional Dynamics of the Cell, p. 168. Courtesy of Academic Press, Inc.)

M sodium acetate buffer, pH 5.0 (1 ml/g original tissue), by homogenization with a loose-fitting Teflon pestle, to yield a homogenous dispersion of gel (generally one minute of homogenization is required). An equal volume of phenol-*m*-cresol-8-hydroxyquinoline-water (3 liters-611 ml-3.87 g-400 ml) is added, and the mixture is homogenized to yield a uniform suspension. The mixture is tightly capped in a tube and shaken for five minutes at 4°C. The cap is loosened, the suspension is placed at 65°C for one to two minutes for equilibration, the cap is retightened, and the tube is incubated with vigorous shaking at the latter temperature for ten minutes. Following this treatment, the mixture is shaken for five to ten minutes at room temperature, and then centrifuged at 20,000 × *g* for ten minutes at 4°C. The upper aqueous layer containing the RNA is carefully removed by means of a Pasteur pipette and transferred to another centrifuge tube. A volume of the phenol mixture (see previous), one half of the original amount, is added, the mixture is shaken for five minutes at room temperature and recentrifuged at 20,000 × *g* for ten minutes at 4°C. The upper phase is again removed carefully, and two volumes

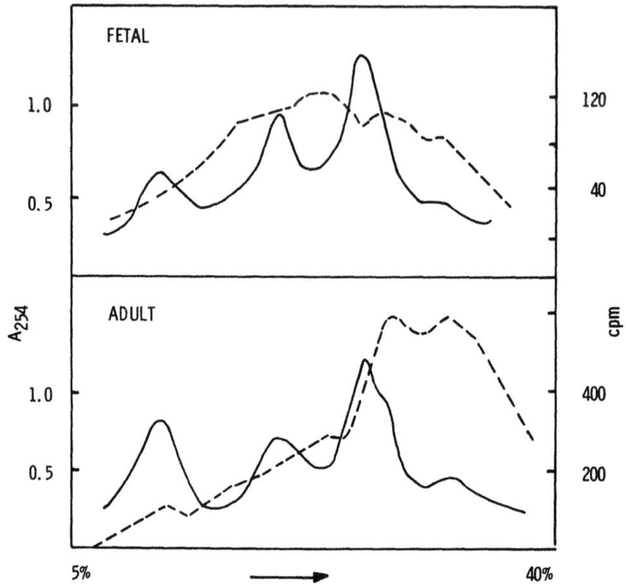

FIG. 9. Sedimentation analysis of liver nuclear RNA. See the text for some of the experimental details. Approximately 20 A_{254} units of nuclear RNA from fetal liver (top) or adult liver (bottom) were applied to 5-40% linear sucrose to gradients. The adult liver nuclear RNA had been labeled after the intraperitoneal administration of [6-^{14}C]orotic acid (5 μc/μmole, 2 μc) for 1 hour. The top of the gradient, i.e., 5%, is represented at the left of the figure. The direction of sedimentation is from left to right (arrow). The peaks of absorbance (solid line) correspond to 4-6, 18, 28, and 45 S with a shoulder at 35 S. The dashed lines indicate the radioactivity. (From Bresnick et al. 1967. *Biochemistry,* 6:2481-2488.)

of ethanol-2 percent potassium acetate are added. Precipitation of the RNA is allowed to proceed at −10°C overnight.

Following centrifugation to sediment the RNA, the latter is dissolved in a small volume of distilled water and once again precipitated with two volumes ethanol-potassium acetate. The final pellet is redissolved in dilute buffered solutions or in water and kept frozen at −20°C. The nuclear RNA may be examined by sedimentation analysis using a linear 5 or 10 to 40 percent sucrose density gradient containing 0.1 M NaCl, 0.01 M sodium acetate buffer pH 5.0, and 0.001 M EDTA. The gradients are centrifuged at 25,000 rpm in an SW 25.1 rotor for 16 hours at 5°C in a Spinco L-2 centrifuge. Optical density patterns at 254 mμ are facilitated by separation of the gradients into one-ml fractions with the aid of a model D Isco density gradient fractionator. The results of a sedimentation analysis of neonatal rat liver nuclear RNA are indicated in Figure 9. Four major peaks of ultraviolet absorption are apparent, with sedimentations at 4-6, 18, 28, and 45 S. A shoulder is always observed in the 35 S region.

The incorporation of a labeled precursor, i.e., orotic acid ^{14}C, into nuclear RNA may be followed using this technique. With a short pulse period, the regions of the gradient greater than 28 S possess the highest specific activity (bottom of

Fig. 9). With a longer interval between injection of the precursor and sacrifice, the pattern of radioactivity is seen to shift toward the lighter parts of the gradient, i.e., toward 18 and 28 S RNA.

Assay of "Aggregate" RNA Polymerase Activity

In some instances, it is necessary to ascertain the effects of a hormone upon the system responsible for the synthesis of RNA, the RNA polymerase. This aim may be achieved by employing a method that is used in our laboratory with considerable success (Bresnick, 1966). Nuclei obtained as previously described are lysed by the procedure of Busch et al. (1962) in 0.05 M tris-phosphate buffer, pH 7.4, and the resultant suspension is centrifuged at 10,000 × *g* for ten minutes.

The sediment that represents the "aggregate" enzyme consists of the enzyme RNA polymerase, to which deoxyribonucleoprotein, i.e., chromatin, is attached. Consequently, no exogenous DNA is required in the assay of activity. The RNA polymerase activity of the "aggregate" enzyme is determined in the following system: UTP-2-^{14}C (24μc/μmole),* 0.1 μc; $MnCl_2$, 1 μmole, or $MgCl_2$, 1.2 μmoles; ATP, GTP, CTP, 0.25 μmole each; tris buffer, pH 7.4, 40 μmoles; β-mercaptoethanol, 2 μmoles; "aggregate" enzyme (resuspended 0.05 M tris, pH 7.4, so that 0.2 ml contained approximately 20 mg of DNA); water to 0.25 ml. The incubation is conducted at 37°C for ten minutes. The reaction is terminated upon the addition of 0.1 ml of a solution containing 5 mg bovine serum albumin and 100 μg of unlabeled UTP and 5 ml of cold 5 percent trichloroacetic acid (TCA). The precipitate is sedimented by centrifugation at 1,000 × *g* for five minutes, washed three times with cold 5 percent trichloroacetic acid, and finally dissolved in 1 ml of 70 percent formic acid. An aliquot of the latter is dried on a stainless steel planchette at 80°C and its radioactivity determined in an end-window gas-flow counter.

Goldberg (1961) has shown that the "aggregate" RNA polymerase activity is markedly affected by ionic strength. Increasing the ionic strength by the addition of a saturated solution of ammonium sulfate produced a marked elevation in the amount of RNA produced. These results have been confirmed in this laboratory (Bresnick, 1966). We routinely assay the enzyme under two conditions of ionic strength–in the presence of magnesium ions (as previously described) and under high ionic strength conditions, i.e., in the presence of 0.7 M ammonium sulfate and manganese ions. A standard assay of "aggregate" RNA polymerase from liver and some of the requirements for its action are presented in Table 3. The incorporation of ammonium sulfate into the assay system does indeed result in an elevation in enzyme activity. Furthermore, it is also apparent that the divalent cation requirement differs under low and high ionic strength conditions. The omission of the nucleoside triphosphates produces a profound reduction in enzyme activity under both conditions.

*UTP is uridine-5-triphosphate; ATP, GTP, CTP are triphosphates of adenosine, guanosine, and cytidine, respectively.

TABLE 3
Requirements of the RNA Polymerase Reaction

Conditions	Nuclear RNA polymerase (mμmoles UTP incorporated/mg DNA) $-(NH_4)_2SO_4$	$+(NH_4)_2SO_4$
A. Complete system without Mg^{++} or Mn^{++}	< 0.5	< 0.5
$+MgCl_2$, 0.25 μmole	6.5	ND*
0.63 μmole	14.5	ND
1.25 μmoles	15.5	40.3
2.5 μmoles	18.0	ND
$+MnCl_2$, 0.5 μmole	5.0	ND
1.0 μmole	5.2	70.5
2.0 μmoles	2.3	ND
$+(MnCl_2$, 1.0 μmole; $+ MgCl_2$, 1.25 μmole)	3.3	56.4
B. Complete system without Mg^{++} or Mn^{++}	< 0.5	< 0.5
$+MnCl_2$, 1.0 μmole	6.4	79.0
$+MnCl_2$, 1.0 μmole; – (ATP, GTP, CTP)	3.0	3.0
$+MnCl_2$, 1.0 μmole; – mercaptoethanol	6.2	74.0
$+MnCl_2$, 1.0 μmole; ½ enzyme	3.1	41.0

*ND = not determined.
From Bresnick. 1966. *Molec. Pharmacol., 2:406-410*
The complete system included: UTP-2-^{14}C (24 μc/μmole), 0.1 μc; ATP, GTP, CTP, each 0.25 μmole; tris buffer, pH 7.4, 40 μmoles; β-mercaptoethanol, 2 μmoles; "aggregate" enzyme (see text), DNA content 16.9 μg (A), 19.0 μg (B); water, to 0.25 ml. The assays were conducted in the absence or presence $(NH_4)_2SO_4$, i.e., 0.7 M.

Assay for Template Efficacy

The assay of "aggregate" RNA polymerase activity does not distinguish between an enhanced efficiency of the attached chromatin template and the synthesis of additional RNA polymerase molecules. To establish definitively the former, it is necessary to isolate chromatin from tissue preparations and determine their ability to serve as a template for the production of RNA with a purified bacterial RNA polymerase enzyme, i.e., one that requires exogenous DNA or deoxyribonucleoprotein for activity. Such a procedure has been employed in determining the effect of administration of 3-methylcholanthrene on the ability of liver chromatin to catalyze the formation of RNA (Bresnick and Mosse, 1969).

In our hands, the method of choice for the preparation of chromatin is that of Dingman and Sporn (1964). The final chromatin preparation should be dialyzed overnight at 4°C against 0.01 M tris buffer, pH 8.0, to eliminate EDTA.

RNA polymerase can be either purchased from Miles Laboratories or purified from *Micrococcus lysodeikticus* by the method of Nakamoto et al. (1964). The RNA polymerase assay mixture contains tris buffer, pH 7.5, 10 μmoles; $MnCl_2$, 1 μmole; spermidine phosphate, 0.05 μmole; the four nucleoside triphosphates, i.e., ATP, GTP, CTP, UTP, 0.1 μmole each; the fourth nucleoside triphosphate, ^{32}P, 10 μc; RNA polymerase, 5 units (see above reference); DNA or chromatin, 0.1 to 10 μg, in a total volume of 0.25 ml. The amount of incorporation of nucleoside monophosphate-^{32}P into RNA after a 15-minute incubation at 37°C can be determined by a cellulose disc method (Madix and Bresnick, 1967).

The reaction is stopped by plunging the tubes in ice, and 1 mg of cold nucleoside triphosphate and 10 mg of bovine serum albumin are added to each reaction mixture. An aliquot of 0.025 ml is removed and placed on 2.5-cm discs of Whatman #1 paper. The discs are washed five times in cold 5 percent TCA-1 percent Na pyrophosphate, twice in 95 percent ethanol, and are then dried. The radioactivity present on the disc is determined in a Packard TriCarb liquid scintillation spectrometer.

Nearest Neighbor Frequency Analysis

If the chromatin isolated from hormone-treated rats exhibits enhanced template efficacy in the RNA polymerase systems, it is often necessary to ascertain whether different gene products are being made. Toward this end, one must ascertain the composition of the gene products. The composition of the RNA manufactured in the presence of the chromatin or uterine DNA may be determined by employing the principle of nearest neighbor frequency analysis. In this technique, the assay for RNA polymerase is conducted in the presence of a nucleoside triphosphate-a-^{32}P as precursor, 2.5 to 10 μc, and with an increased amount of RNA polymerase (9 units). The reaction mixture is terminated after the addition of 3 mg of yeast RNA, as carrier, by the addition of 2.5 ml of cold 5 percent trichloroacetic acid-1 percent sodium pyrophosphate. The precipitate is collected by centrifugation and is washed four times with cold 5 percent trichloroacetic acid to remove traces of the nucleotide precursor. The washed precipitate is then dissolved in 0.5 ml of 0.3 N KOH, and hydrolysis of the RNA is conducted at 37°C overnight. The hydrolysate is neutralized with 4 N $HClO_4$ with phenol red as an internal indicator. The neutralized material is maintained at 4°C for several hours to ensure the complete precipitation of $KClO_4$.

To 0.3 ml of neutralized extract, 0.2 ml of distilled water and 0.5 ml 0.1 HCl are added. The nucleotide composition is determined on Dowex-50-H^+ according to the method of Katz and Comb (1963); the ^{32}P content of the respective nucleotides can be determined in a liquid scintillation counter using Bray's phosphor mixture (Bray, 1960).

Assay of Template Activity in a Cell-Free Amino Acid Incorporation System

Often it is necessary to test for messenger RNA activity of mammalian RNA preparations. This aim may be achieved by employing the in vitro amino acid incorporation system of Nirenberg and Matthaei (1961), as modified for acceptance of exogenous messenger template. The assay system of 0.25 ml volume included tris buffer, pH 7.8, 25 μmoles, β-mercaptoethanol, 1 μmole; ATP, 0.25 μmole; GTP, 7.5 μmoles; magnesium acetate, 3 μmoles; ammonium chloride,

TABLE 4
L-Amino Acid Composition of the S-30 Assay

Alanine	Isoleucine
Arginine	Leucine
Asparagine	Lysine
Aspartic Acid	Methionine
Cysteine	Phenylalanine
Cystine	Serine
Glutamine	Threonine
Glutamic Acid	Tryptophan
Glycine	Tyrosine
Histidine	Valine

12.5 μmoles; KCl, 3 μmoles; phosphoenolpyruvate, 1.9 μmoles; pyruvate kinase, 4.0 μg; *E. coli* transfer RNA, 100 μg; 19 amino acids not including the labeled one, 0.5 μmole each; L-^{14}C-valine, 0.25 μc or L-^{14}C-phenylalamine, 0.25 μc; polyuridylic acid, nuclear RNA or cytoplasmic RNA; preincubated S-30 *E. coli* extract, 1 to 2 mg protein.

The S-30 extract is prepared from a strain of *E. coli* that is devoid of ribonuclease-I and polynucleotide phosphorylase, *E. coli* MRE 600. This organism also has the advantage of growing logarithmically to very high concentrations. The *E. coli* is grown in an inoculum consisting of 12 g of Difco yeast extract, 48.8 g of KH_2PO_4, 8.4 g of KOH diluted to 1.08 liters with distilled water. After autoclaving, 120 ml of 10 percent glucose is aseptically added, and the inoculum is grown overnight at 37°C with aeration. The inoculum is then transferred to a larger volume of the identical medium. The large volume is very briskly aerated until the optical density at 630 mμ reaches an absorbancy of 0.5. At this stage, the growth of the culture is arrested by pouring the suspension over cracked ice. The bacteria are sedimented by means of a Sharples centrifuge in the cold room and washed once by suspension in 0.01 M tris-0.02 M KCl-0.01 M magnesium acetate-4 mM β-mercaptoethanol, pH 7.8.

The S-30 extract is prepared immediately from the pelleted *E. coli* by grinding the bacteria with twice their wet weight by alumina (Alcoa 305) by means of a mortar and pestle at 5°C for five minutes until a smooth wet consistency is obtained. The buffer described above is added in a volume equal to twice the wet weight of the cells, and the mixture is centrifuged at 10,000 × *g* for 15 minutes. The supernatant fraction is removed, combined with 0.5 mg/ml of electrophoretically pure DNAase and allowed to stand at 5°C for five minutes. It is then centrifuged twice at 30,000 × *g* at 4°C for 15 minutes. After the first centrifugation, the supernatant preparation is aspirated to within 1 cm of the pellet and after a second centrifugation, four-fifths of the remaining supernate is aspirated. The combined supernates then constitute the S-30 extract.

Preincubation of the extract as suggested by Nirenberg (1963) was found necessary for the reduction of endogenous messenger activity. The preincubation of 10 ml of S-30 extract is conducted for 45 minutes at 37°C with gentle shaking

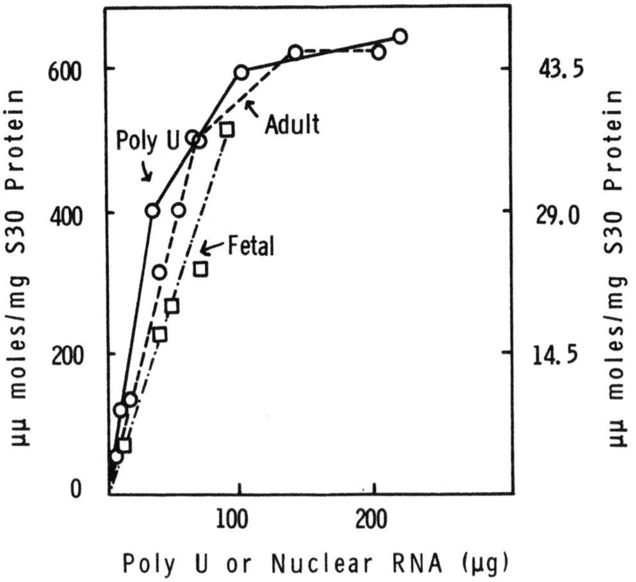

FIG. 10. Template ability of polyuridylic acid and nuclear RNA of fetal and adult rat liver in the *E. coli* S-30 system for protein synthesis. Stimulation of ^{14}C-phenylalanine incorporation by poly U (left ordinate) and of ^{14}C-valine incorporation by rat liver nuclear RNA (right ordinate) was determined for varying concentrations of the templates (abscissa). (From Bresnick et al. 1967. *Biochemistry*, 6:2481-2488.)

with the following components: 1.0 ml of buffer consisting of 0.6 M tris, 0.55 M KCl, 0.15 M magnesium acetate, and 0.06 M β-mercaptoethanol, pH 7.8; 0.38 ml of an amino acid solution containing 2 mM each of the 20 L-amino acids (as listed in Table 4); 0.29 ml of neutralized 0.07 M ATP, 0.13 ml of 0.75 M phosphoenolpyruvate; and 0.015 ml of pyruvate kinase (10 mg/ml). After the preincubation, the extract is dialyzed against the standard tris buffer in the cold room for five to six hours. The extract may be divided into 0.5- to 2-ml portions, quickly frozen by immersion of the tubes into acetone-dry ice, and stored in liquid notrogen. Under these conditions, the extract retains activity for at least four to five months.

The assay of template activity may be conducted in the mixture described above and incubated at 37°C with gentle shaking for 45 minutes. The reaction is stopped by plunging the tubes into ice water, and the amount of ^{14}C-amino acid incorporated into polypeptide material is determined by a disc method reported by Griffin et al. (1965). Aliquots of 0.05 ml are withdrawn and placed on Whatman 3 MM filter paper discs, 2 cm in diameter. The discs are allowed to dry momentarily, then are immersed in cold 5 percent TCA containing unlabeled amino acid and swirled for 10 minutes. This procedure is repeated with cold 5 percent TCA, with 5 percent TCA at 90°C (to extract any amino-acyl transfer RNA), and with two ethanol washes. The discs are dried at 80°C and counted in a Packard Tricarb liquid scintillation counter.

A typical titration curve of template activity with polyuridylic acid and with nuclear RNA of fetal and adult rat liver is shown in Figure 10. It is apparent that the bacterial assay system is extremely sensitive to synthetic messenger, i.e., poly-U, as well as to a more natural messenger, i.e., nuclear RNA.

CONCLUSION

The manner in which a low-molecular-weight chemical transmitter, a hormone, is able to trigger off a series of very specialized biologic events is still a mystery. The hormones appear to complex with specific proteins present in the target tissues, and it is this interaction that contributes heavily to the specificity of action. The hormone-protein complex presumably interacts with genetic "blockers" so that specific loci of the mammalian genome are activated. In this manner, specific messenger RNA molecules are elaborated in which the information for the construction of specific proteins is evident. These aspects have been discussed in the first part of this chapter, using the estrogen-induced events as the revolving point for discussion. In the second part, the methodology required for such studies has been presented. Although, in many cases, the tissue of choice was liver, the extrapolation to hormone-specific organs can be easily performed.

REFERENCES

Bray, G. A. 1960. A single efficient liquid scintillator for counting aqueous solutions in a liquid scintillation counter. Anal. Biochem., 1:279-281.

Bresnick, E. 1966. Ribonucleic acid polymerase activity in liver nuclei from rats pretreated with 3-methylcholanthrene. Molec. Pharmacol., 2:406.

—and Thompson, U. B. 1965. Properties of deoxythymidine kinase partially purified from animal tumors. J. Biol. Chem., 240:3967-3974.

—and Schwartz, A. 1968. Functional Dynamics of the Cell. New York, Academic Press, Inc.

—and Mosse, H. 1969. Activation of genetic transcription in rat liver chromatin after 3-methylcholanthrene. Molec. Pharmacol. (In press.)

—Liebelt, R. A., Stevenson, J. G., and Madix, J. C. 1967a. The distribution of radioactivity within the hepatic cell after administration of labeled 3-methylcholanthrene. Cancer Res., 27:462-468.

—Eckles, S. G., and Lanclos, K. D. 1967b. Nuclear ribonucleic acid in embryonic rat liver. Biochemistry, 6:2481-2488.

Busch, S., Chambon P., Mandel, P., and Weill, J. D. 1962. The effect of partial hepatectomy on the ribonucleic acid polymerase of rat liver. Biochem. Biophys. Res. Commun., 7:255-258.

Changeux, J. P., and Podleski, T. R. 1968. On the excitability and cooperativity of the electroplax membrane. Proc. Nat. Acad. Sci. U.S.A., 59:944-950.

—Thiery, J., Tung, Y., and Kittel, C. 1967. On the cooperativity of biological membranes. Proc. Nat. Acad. Sci. U.S.A., 57:335-341.

Chauveau, J., Moule, Y., and Rouiller, C. 1957. Isolation of pure and unaltered liver nuclei: Morphology and biochemical composition. Exp. Cell. Res. 11:317-321.

Dingman, C. W., and Sporn, M. B. 1964. Studies on chromatin. I. Isolation and characterization of nuclear complexes of deoxyribonucleic acid, and protein from embryonic and adult tissues of the chicken. J. Biol. Chem., 239:3482-3492.

Goldberg, I. H. 1961. Ribonucleic acid synthesis in nuclear extracts of mammalian cells grown in suspension culture; effect of ionic strength and surface - active agents. Biochem. Biophys. Acta, 51:201-204.

Gorski, J., and Mueller, G. C. 1963. Early effects of estrogen on acid-soluble nucleotides of the rat uterus. Arch. Biochem. Biophys., 102:21-25.

—and Nicolette, J. 1963. Early estrogen effects on newly synthesized RNA and phospholipid in subcellular fractions of rat uteri. Arch. Biochem. Biophys., 103:418-423.

—Noteboom, W. D., and Nicolette, J. A. 1965. Estrogen control of the synthesis of RNA and protein in the uterus. J. Cell Comp. Physiol., 66:91-110.

Griffin, A. C., Canning, L., Holland, B., and Malick, B. 1965. Further studies on tumors and liver amino acid incorporating systems. Cancer Res. 25:318-323.

Hamilton, T. H., 1968. Control by estrogen of genetic transcripton and translation. Science, 161:649.

—Widnell, C. C., and Tata, J. R. 1968a. Synthesis of ribonucleic acid during early estrogen action. J. Biol. Chem. 243: 408-417.

—Teng, C. S., and Means, A. R. 1968b. Early estrogen action: Nuclear synthesis and accumulation of protein correlated with enhancement of two DNA-dependent RNA polymerase activities. Proc. Nat. Acad. Sci. U.S.A., 59:1265-1272.

Jensen, E. V., Desombre, E. R., Hurst, D. J., Kawa-Shima, T., and Jungblut, P. W. 1967. Estrogen-receptor interactions in target tissues. Archives d'anatomie Microscopiqué et de Morphologie Experimentale (Suppl. 3-4), 56:547-569.

Jervell, K. F., Diniz, C. R., and Mueller, G. C. 1958. Early effects of estradiol in nucleic acid metabolism in the rat uterus. J. Biol. Chem., 231:945-949.

Karlson, P. 1961. Biochemical mode of action of hormones. Deutsch. Med. Wschr., 86:668-674.

Katz, S., and Comb, D. G. 1963. A new method for the determination of the base composition of ribonucleic acid. J. Biol. Chem., 238:3065-3067.

Laguens, R. 1964. Effect of estrogen upon the fine structure of the uterine smooth muscle cell of the rat. J. Ultrastruct. Res., 10:578-584.

Madix, J. C., and Bresnick, E. 1967. Increased efficacy of liver chromatin as a template for RNA synthesis after administration of 3-methylcholanthrene. Biochem. Biophys. Res. Commun. 28:445-452.

Markee, J. E. 1932. Rhythmic vascular uterine changes. Amer. J. Physiol., 100:32-39.

Mueller, G. C., Herranen A., and Jervell, K. 1958. Studies on the mechanism of action of estrogens. Recent Prog. Hormone Res. 8:95-139.

Nakamoto, T., Fox, C. F., and Weiss, S. B. 1964. Enzymatic synthesis of ribonucleic acid. I. Preparation of ribonucleic acid polymerase from extracts of *Micrococcus lysodeikticus.* J. Biol. Chem., 239:167-174.

Nirenberg, M. W. 1963. Cell-free protein synthesis directed by messenger RNA. *In* Methods in Enzymology. New York, Academic Press Inc., Vol. 6.

—and Matthaei, J. H. 1961. The dependence of cell-free protein synthesis in *E. coli* upon naturally occuring or synthetic polyribonucleotides. Proc. Nat. Acad. Sci. U.S.A., 47:1588-1602.

Noteboom, W. D., and Gorski, J. 1965. Stereospecific binding of estrogens in the rat uterus. Arch. Biochem. Biophys., 3:559-568.

Segal, S. J., and Scher, W. 1967. Estrogens, nucleic acids, and protein synthesis in uterine metabolism. *In* Cellular Biology of the Uterus. Wynn, R. M., ed. New York, Appleton-Century-Crofts, pp. 114-150.

Steele, W. J., and Busch, H. 1967. RNA: Isolation and fractionation. *In* Methods in Cancer Research. New York, Academic Press, Inc., Vol. 3, pp. 61-153.

Sutherland, E. W. and Rall, T. W. 1960. The relation of adenosine —3′, 5′-phosphate and phosphorylase to the actions of catecholamine and other hormones. Pharmacol. Rev., 12:265.

Talwar, G. P., Segal, S. G., Evans, A., and Davidson, O. W. 1964. The binding of estradiol in the uterus: A mechanism for depression of RMA synthesis. Proc. Nat. Acad. Sci. U.S.A., 52:1059-1066.

Teng, C. S., and Hamilton, T. H. 1967. Regulation of polyribosome formation and protein synthesis in the uterus. Effect of ovariectomy and administration of estradiol -17β in the amino acid-incorporation activity *in vitro* and the cytoplasmic concentration *in vivo* of polyribosomal preparation. Biochem. J., 105:1101-1109.

Toft, D., and Gorski, J. 1966. A receptor molecule for estrogens: Isolation from the rat uterus and preliminary characterization. Proc. Nat. Acad. Sci. U.S.A., 55:1574-1581.

—Shyamala, G. and Gorski, J. 1967. A receptor molecule for estrogens: Studies using a cell-free system. Proc. Nat. Acad. Sci. U.S.A., 57:1740-1743.

Ui, H., and Mueller, G. C. 1963. The role of RNA synthesis in early estrogen action. Proc. Nat. Acad. Sci. U.S.A., 50:256-260.

Volfin, P., Clauser, H., and Gautheron, D. 1957. Influence of estradiol and progesterone injections in the acid-soluble phosphate fractions of the rat uterus. Biochem. Biophys. Acta, 24:137-140.

—Clauser, H., Gautheron, D., and Eboue, D. 1961. Influence of estradiol and progesterone on the level of nucleotides and phosphocreatine in the rat uterus. Bull. Soc. Chim. Biol., 43:107-119.

Wilson, J. D. 1963. The nature of the RNA response to estradiol by the uterus of the rat. Proc. Nat. Acad. Sci., U.S.A. 50:93-100.

Yielding, K. L., and Tompkins, G. M. 1962. Studies on the interaction of steroid hormones with glutamic dehydrogenase. Recent Progr. Hormone Res. 18:467-489.

CHAPTER **16**

Chemical Transfer of Acquired Information

Georges Ungar

Departments of Anesthesiology and Pharmacology, Baylor College of Medicine, Texas Medical Center, Houston, Texas

INTRODUCTION

During the past two decades the concept of information has gained a dominant position in the biologic sciences. Processing of information is now recognized as one of the major biologic functions and the basic mechanism by which continuity of life on the globe is maintained.

The chemical nature of the code that handles genetic information is now universally admitted. There is still, however, a lively controversy over the possibility that a similar molecular mechanism operated in the acquisition, storage, and retrieval of the information that keeps biologic systems in touch with their environment. These processes, known usually under the designation of learning, allow living systems to adapt to their environment by modifying the inherited behavioral patterns and by creating new ones.

The original studies from the author's laboratory referred to in this chapter were supported by U.S. Public Health Service grant MH 13361.

The ability to learn is closely correlated with the degree of development of the nervous system, and it is usually assumed that the processing of acquired information takes place in nerve centers. One notable exception is immunologic "learning" which allows organisms to recognize foreign macromolecules. Although this type of acquired information has been chemically transferred for many years, it will not be considered in the present survey.

Hypotheses on possible chemical mechanisms of learning were formulated by Foerster (1948), Monné (1948), and particularly Katz and Halstead (1950); but the first experimental evidence was supplied by Hydén and his co-workers (1959). This is now supported by the results of Zemp et al.(1966, 1967), Bogoch (1968), and Shashoua (1968).

The chemical changes associated with learning and the effect of metabolic inhibitors on this process (Flexner, 1967; Agranoff, 1965; Barondes and Cohen, 1968) represent good circumstantial evidence, but the most decisive proof has been supplied by the experiments that succeeded in transferring acquired information from one animal to another by purely chemical means. These experiments are based on the same principle as the bioassay methods widely used in endocrinology and in the study of neurotransmitters. They have the same basic design as, for example, the experiments of Otto Loewi (1921) in which the effect produced by vagal stimulation of a donor heart was chemically transferred to a recipient heart. Loewi's experiments showed the existence of a chemical step in impulse transmission; transfer of learning aims at demonstrating a molecular mechanism in the processing of acquired information.

Chemical transmission of nerve impulses is now taken for granted, but for many years it was regarded as a dangerous heresy. Chemical transfer of learning seems to have provoked an even greater resentment, probably because of the greater complexity of the problem and also because it strikes closer to some cherished beliefs and well-entrenched dogmas.

The experiments to be discussed have been described under various names: (chemical) transfer of learning, of training, of acquired information, of learned behavior, of learned response; interorganism transfer of response tendencies; or memory transfer. If a neologism becomes necessary, I propose the term "diamnesis," from the Greek διαμνημονευω, to transmit memory. The first attempts at transferring learning were made in planarian worms (McConnell, 1962). These experiments have their own abundant literature (see Corning, 1970) and will not be reviewed here. The success of these widely publicized studies was the inspiration for the first experiments tried in mammals, published almost simultaneously from four laboratories (Reinis, 1965; Fjerdingstad et al., 1965; Ungar and Oceguera-Navarro, 1965; and Babich et al., 1965b). These observations were followed rapidly by others, and at present there are at least twenty-three laboratories that have obtained positive results. Several reviews of the problem are to appear shortly (Rosenblatt 1970b; Ungar, 1970a,c,d; Ungar and Chapouthier, 1970).

In this chapter we shall discuss only the published experiments and those about to be published in a volume edited by Byrne (1968). Some publications in the form of abstracts do not give sufficient technical information and will, therefore, be omitted. Since the main purpose of the chapter is to help workers who may wish to enter this challenging field, the main emphasis is on the experiments with positive results. The techniques used for obtaining negative results will be discussed in a separate section.

BEHAVIORAL METHODS

The basic design of the chemical transfer experiments includes the following steps: (1) training of donor animals, (2) preparation of the brain extracts and their administration to the recipients, (3) testing of recipients, and (4) evaluation of the results. In this section we shall examine the techniques used in steps 1 and 3.

Here are, first of all, a few rules for the choice of a paradigm suitable for transfer experiments:

1. The task given to the donors should be such that they can learn it completely in a reasonable period of time. When the recipients are of a different species, one must ascertain that they can also learn the task through training. It seems that donors that cannot learn the task completely do not yield active brain extracts (Reinis, 1966), and one would not expect a recipient to acquire a behavioral pattern through transfer if the pattern does not belong to its repertory.
2. The paradigm should be easily quantitated by objective criteria without requiring referees to adjudicate doubtful points. Preferably, but not necessarily, it should be possible to record automatically the critical parameter in the behavior of the recipients.
3. The behavioral trait to be transferred should either not occur spontaneously or if it does, it should have a constant and predictable occurrence in control animals. We shall see that this is one of the most difficult conditions to fulfill.

Before starting the detailed study of the methods used, a brief discussion on nomenclature will allow the definition of a few terms.

There have been, up to now, intraspecific transfers and interspecific transfers, such as rats to mice (in the author's laboratory) and hamsters to rats (Babich et al., 1965a).

In most experiments, recipients were tested for the same task for which the donors were trained. This shall be called homologous transfer. If the testing of recipients and training of donors include the same reinforcement, this is homologous transfer with reinforcement. The latter can be positive (reward of food or drink) or negative (punishment by electric shock or other painful stimulus). In homologous transfer without reinforcement, the recipients, although tested for the same task as the donors, do not receive any reinforcement that may supply a clue as to how they should behave.

In the case of transfer with reinforcement, the best one can hope for is to find that the recipients of trained brain learn the task faster than the controls injected with untrained brain. Only transfer without reinforcement gives direct evidence that information is actually transmitted from one animal to the other.

In some cases, the recipients were tested for a task different from the one for which the donors were trained. Such heterologous transfers were attempted to test the specificity of transfer. When two groups of donors were trained for tasks A and B, and the recipients of A are tested for B and the recipients of B are tested for A, this double heterologous transfer is referred to as cross-transfer (Ungar, 1967a, 1967b, 1970a). Sometimes, heterologous transfer takes place spontaneously—as, for example, the reversal observed in the transfer of spatial discrimination by several workers.

A final remark about the precautions to avoid self-deception or the risk of being deliberately misled by overzealous collaborators. It is essential that the experiments be conducted by a blind procedure. The persons testing the recipients should have no knowledge of the treatment received by the animals. This can easily be done by giving code numbers to the animals and testing control and experimental animals in a random order. This sort of secrecy can, of course, be overdone. Complicated coding systems may have been responsible for more errors than the bias of the observers. One should also keep in mind that self-deception can threaten not only those who believe in the possibility of a chemical transfer of learning but also its convinced and sometimes fanatical opponents.

Habituation

Defined as the loss of an innate response to repeated neutral stimuli, habituation is one of the simplest and most basic forms of learning. In the experiments of Ungar and Oceguera-Navarro (1965), which were among the first attempts at transferring learned behavior in mammals, the donors were trained to lose their startle responses to a sound stimulus repeated at 5-second intervals. After being submitted to this repetition of stimuli for 2 one-hour periods daily, the rats ceased to respond to 90 percent of the stimuli in 10 to 25 days, according to strain. When this criterion of habituation had persisted for three consecutive days, the donors were killed and their brain was extracted.

The recipients of the extract were tested with the same sound stimulus repeated 100 times daily. The startle responses were recorded by the observer who pressed a button every time the animal failed to respond. These signals, superimposed on the tracing of the stimuli, gave a permanent record of the tests. The observers who made these records had no knowledge of the treatment received by the animals. The controls, injected with extract of brain from nonhabituated donors, were intermingled with the recipients of trained extract. The recipients of habituated brain extract showed a loss of over 50 percent of their startle responses at the first test given 16 to 24 hours after injection, while the control animals were over 90 percent. The effect of the injections lasted usually about five to six days.

In further experiments (Ungar, 1967a,b), the specificity of this transfer of habituation was tested. Groups of donors were habituated either to sound, as just described, or to an air puff. This was delivered, under a pressure of 2 lb, by means of a valve connected to an oxygen tank and activated once every second by a solenoid. The same criteria of habituation were used as previously mentioned.

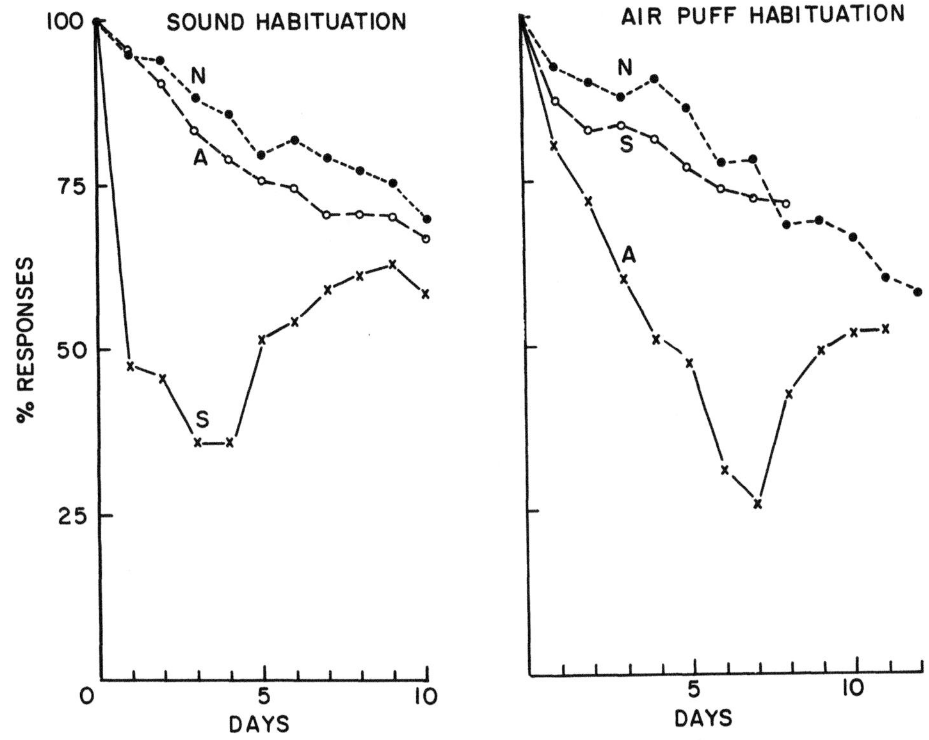

FIG. 1 Stimulus specificity of habituation transfer. Abscissa: Days after injection of extracts of brain from untrained rats (N), sound-habituated rats (S) and air puff-habituated rats (A). Ordinate: Number of startle responses to 100 stimuli by recipient mice. Each animal received the equivalent of 400 mg of donor brain dialyzate 20 hr before the first test. On the left, responses to sound; on the right, responses to air-puff. Each of the six groups consisted of at least eight animals. (From Ungar. 1967a. *Proc. Fifth Int. Cong. Colleg. Int. Neuropsychopharmacol.*, p. 169.)

When cross-transfer was attempted using brain extracts from these two groups of animals, it became evident that only homologous transfer was possible. Injection of brain extract from sound-habituated donors induced only sound-habituation and no habituation to air puff, and vice versa. (Fig. 1).

Dark-Light Discrimination

One of the first techniques to be used for transfer studies consisted of training donors in a two-alley runway and rewarding them when they selected the lighted alley (Fjerdingstad et al., 1965). The donors (male Wistar rats, weighing about 200 g) were deprived of water 24 hours before the first training session. In the course of each of these sessions, the animals were left in the box until they received, irrespective of the number of errors, 60 reinforcements of 0.1 ml of water each. One such session was given every day until the criterion of 10 percent or less errors was reached on two consecutive days.

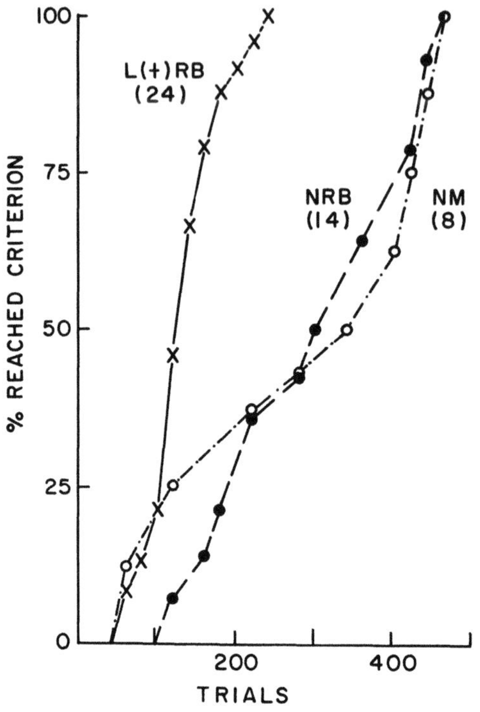

FIG. 2. Transfer of light-dark discrimination in escape training. Abscissa: Number of trials to criterion. Ordinate: Percent of recipients reaching criterion. L + RB, recipients injected with extract of brain (500 mg) from donors trained to escape into the lighted arm of the maze; NRB, recipients of untrained rat brain; NM, uninjected mice. Numbers of mice in each group are between parentheses. Recipients received the same reinforcement as the donors. (From Ungar, 1967b. *J. Biol. Psychol.,* 9:12.)

Recipients were tested by the same procedure, but on the first day (24 hours after injection) they were given two "short" sessions with 15 to 30 reinforcements. After the second day and for seven consecutive days, 60 reinforcements. After the second day and for seven consecutive days, 60 reinforcements were given, and the result was expressed in terms of percentage of errors. Transfer was assumed to have taken place when the number of errors made by the recipients of trained brain extracts was significantly smaller than that of the controls. Reverse effects were sometimes observed at the initial "short" trials, but, typically, transfer was most marked on the second day.

In some of the experiments, donors were trained both for light and for dark preference. The heterologous transfer experiments gave inconclusive results as far as specificity is concerned.

Dark-light discrimination with positive reinforcement was successfully used by Wolthuis (1969a, 1970). During training and testing, the subjects, previously fasted, were rewarded with food when they entered the lighted alley of a T-maze.

In the author's laboratory, donor rats were trained to escape electric shock by running into the lighted arm of a Y-maze (Ungar, 1967a, 1967b; Ungar and Irwin, 1967). The Y-maze was provided with a grid floor and electric lights at the end of

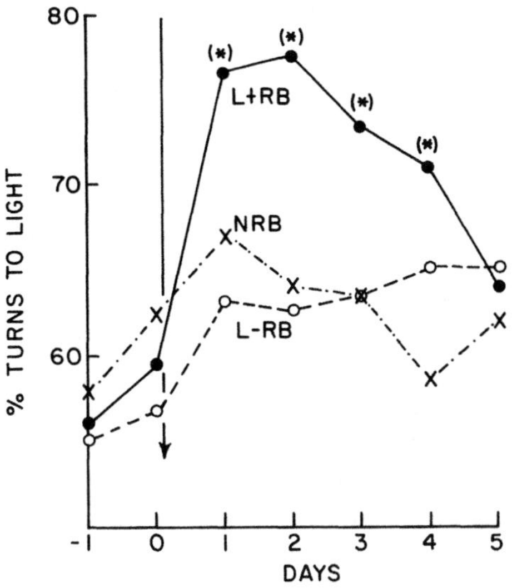

FIG. 3. Transfer of light-dark discrimination in escape training to unreinforced recipients. Abscissa: Days before and after injection of brain extracts (equivalent to 1.25 g of rat brain). Ordinate: Percent of turns to light of the unreinforced recipients. Arrow shows injections of extracts of brain from untrained donors (NRB), donors trained to escape into lighted arm of maze (L+RB), and into unlighted arm of maze (L—RB). Asterisks indicate significant differences of the mean from corresponding NRB value. It is obvious that, while L+ training was transferred, L— training of the donors failed to produce any effect on the recipients. (From Ungar. 1967b. *J. Biol. Psychol.*, 9:12.)

both arms. The animal was placed in the stem of the Y and the light was turned on in one of the arms. A few seconds later the shock was turned on in the stem and in the unlighted arm so that by running toward the light the animal was able to escape the shock. After having run into one or the other of the arms of the maze, the subject was replaced into the stem and the test started again. Twenty such tests were done daily with the light turned on in the arms in random sequence. The animals were shocked with a 60-cycle AC current with a 47 kohm resistance in series with the animals. Rats were given 100 V, mice 80 V. The donors were trained to a criterion of 90 percent correct responses maintained for at least three days, in some experiments longer.

In a first series of experiments, the recipient mice were treated identically with the donors; they were shocked when they had run into the unlighted arm of the maze. These experiments showed that the mice injected with trained rat brain learned to escape toward the light significantly faster than the controls which had received untrained brain or no treatment whatever (Fig. 2).

In the second series of experiments, the recipients were not reinforced. They received a shock in the stem of the Y, but both lighted and unlighted arms were shock-free. These animals were tested for their responses for two to four days before injection and for four days after. Transfer was considered to be successful when the recipients of trained brain made significantly more turns to the light after, than before, injection and when this did not take place in the controls. Figure 3 shows an example of these experiments.

Heterologous transfer was attempted in these light-dark discrimination experiments by training donors to escape into the dark arm of the maze and test the recipients with or without reinforcement. In neither case did dark preference appear to be transferable, so no valid conclusions could be drawn from these attempts at cross-transfer. Similar results were obtained by Chapouthier et al. (1969).

A complex two-choice discrimination problem was used by Jacobson et al. (1966). The subjects had the choice between alley A, which "had a fine mesh screen on the floor and a beaded chain hanging in the alley entrance," and alley B, having "white contact paper with black tape stripes on the floor and a vertical column of white jewel lights to one side of the alley entrance." Recipients of rats trained to be rewarded in A made 15 entries into A and 7 into B; those injected with brain from donors trained to B made 14 entries into B and 6 into A. The recipients were not reinforced. Left and right discrimination has probably played a role in this paradigm, since A and B were permanently on one or the other side. As we shall see in a moment, the innate left or right biases of the donors, as well as the recipients, represent a disturbing factor. The most appropriate discrimination situations would be those that avoid left or right choices.

Spatial Discrimination

The principle of these experiments is to train donors to discriminate between left and right sides by rewarding them if they turn to the desired side or press a bar on that side of a Skinner box or by punishing them if they choose the wrong side.

Rosenblatt (1966, 1970a,b) did a very large number of experiments with several designs, all based on rewarding the animals with food when they followed the correct direction or pressed a bar on the correct side of the box.

Similar experiments were carried out by Byrne and Hughes (1967) with some additional interesting features. Before being used, the animals (Holtzmann rats) were submitted to "environmental complexity," according to the method of Krech et al. (1962). They were placed, 20 or 30 at a time, in large enclosures provided with toys and other devices to develop the exploratory tendency of the animals. After a week of this preparation, the rats were deprived of food to reduce their weight by 15 percent. The first session of 20 minutes consisted of placing three rats at a time in a Skinner box but without reinforcement. This was followed by individual sessions in which pressing of both bars was rewarded with food. After several of these sessions, the training started in which only pressing of the left or right bar was reinforced. This was done on a progressive fixed ratio schedule, going from 1:1 to 9:1. Each training session either lasted 20 minutes or ended after 50 bar presses.

The recipients were similarly treated, and the injection of the extract took place after the unreinforced session. On the day following the injection, two other unreinforced periods of 10 minutes each were given. After this, the recipients were tested every day for 20 minutes with both bars being reinforced on a 1:1 schedule.

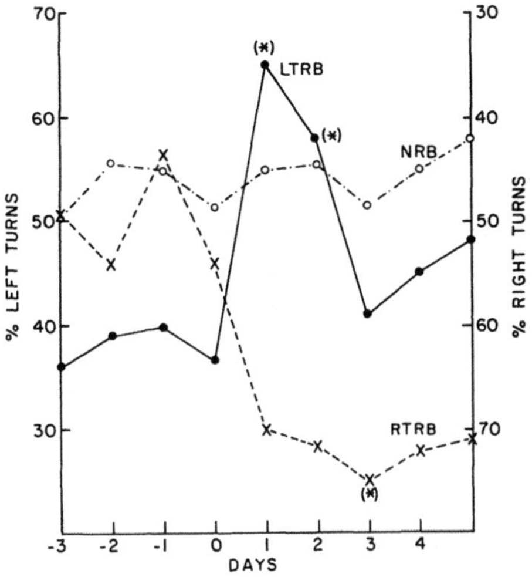

FIG. 4. Transfer of spatial discrimination in escape training to unreinforced recipients. Abscissa: Days before and after injection of brain extracts (equivalent to 750 mg of rat brain). Ordinate: On left, percent left turns; right, percent right turns. Arrow shows injection of extracts of brain from untrained donors (NRB), donors trained to escape to the left (LTBR), and to the right (RTRB). Asterisks indicate significant difference from preinjection mean. (From Ungar. 1967b. *J. Biol. Psychol.,* 9:12.)

In the author's laboratory, a spatial discrimination was used with negative reinforcement. The animals were trained and tested in a Y-maze provided with a grid floor. As previously described for the visual discrimination experiments, the donors were shocked when they entered the wrong arm of the maze. Groups of donors were trained to escape shock by running into the left arm; others were trained to run to the opposite side. For each animal, the side was selected so as to overcome its natural bias as shown in two preliminary sessions.

With 20 tests per day, the donors were trained to 90 percent criterion and maintained on it by continued training for an optimum number of days. This optimum duration of training, after criterion was reached, was found to be 6 days for the right side and about 12 days for the left.

The recipients were pretested for their side preference on four consecutive days. On the fourth day, they were divided into groups containing an approximately equal number of subjects with left bias, right bias, and no bias. After injection, the recipients were tested exactly the same way as before, without reinforcement, for four days. The results were evaluated by comparing the left and right turns of the animals before and after injections, and also the groups injected with brain extracts from left- and right-trained donors. In a few experiments, control recipients of untrained rat brain were also used (Fig. 4).

On the whole, these experiments, which promised to be among the simplest, gave variable and sometimes unexpected results. The most troublesome of these is the "reversal" phenomenon, observed by all the workers who used spatial discrimination (Rosenblatt, 1970a,b; Byrne and Hughes, 1967; Ungar, 1967b;

Ungar and Irwin, 1967). We found in this laboratory that, with prolonged training of the donors or after injection of supraoptimal amounts of brain extracts, recipients of right-trained donors had a tendency to increase their left turns, and vice versa. The dose-dependence of the phenomenon was also noticed by Rosenblatt, who described a complex dose-response curve with several inflections.

Another factor, studied by us systematically, was the bias of the recipients. This showed that transfer was most successful when, for example, left-biased animals were given brain extracts from donors trained to the right. Reversal occurred most readily when the bias of the recipients and the training of the donors were toward the same side. This suggested that the main message contained in the brain extract was to make the recipients act against their natural tendency. As mentioned earlier, the donors were always trained in the direction opposite to their bias.

This is probably only one of the many factors that make this paradigm so complex and difficult to reproduce. No doubt, at a later stage when transfer of learning is a widely accepted fact, studying the conditions of left-right transfer may become highly rewarding. At this point, however, when we still need clear and simple experiments to carry conviction, its usefulness is dubious.

Conditioned Reflexes

Two of the original paradigms that served to demonstrate transfer of learning represent conditioned reflexes with presentation of food as the unconditioned stimulus (US) and sound or light as the conditioned stimulus (CS).

Reinis (1965, 1966) trained fasted rats to open a gate leading to the food cup when the conditioned stimulus, light from a 15-watt bulb or a 2,000 c/s, 70 db sound, was presented. Each animal received 10 trials a day each, lasting 20 seconds, at two-minute intervals. The behavior of the animals, the number of correct and incorrect responses and their latencies, as well as the intertrial reactions, were automatically recorded. When the donors reached the criterion of 80 percent correct responses for three sessions, they were killed and their brain extracted.

The recipient rats were first tested 48 hours after injection of the extract and on the following days. Testing of the recipients was identical with the training of the donors. Control recipients received untrained rat brain or rat liver homogenates. Differences between the experimental and control groups, as expressed in the number of correct responses and their latencies, were significant throughout the 15 sessions when light was the CS. With sound, the difference was significant only on the first three sessions. No cross-transfer was attempted between the two stimuli.

Transfer could only be demonstrated if the recipients were deprived of food for 48 hours before the first test; 16 hours fasting was inadequate. In one of Reinis' experiments the donors were animals that were unable to learn the task; recipients of these brains behaved like the controls.

About the same time, Jacobson and his co-workers (Babich et al., 1965a, 1965b; Jacobson et al., 1965) attempted to transfer conditioned behavior under different conditions. They trained 48-hour fasted rats in a Skinner box to approach the food cup upon hearing the click produced by the operation of the pellet dispenser. Each of the rats was given 200 food-reinforced approaches per day for four days, followed by a last session of 100 tests on the fifth day.

The recipients, fasted for 28 hours were tested 4, 6, 8, 22, and 24 hours after injection. They were placed in the Skinner box and the click of the food magazine was sounded five times at one-minute intervals at each session. The response was considered positive if the animal put its nose inside an area surrounding the food cup within five seconds after the click. The food cup was empty, so that the recipients were not reinforced but food powder was sprinkled over the entire floor of the box. Control recipients, injected with untrained rat brain, gave significantly fewer responses than the experimental animals.

With the same technique, the authors have shown stimulus specificity of the transfer, using light as a second conditioned stimulus. They also did an interspecific transfer between hamsters and rats.

The experiments of the Jacobson group are still among the most controversial, and we shall return to them in the discussion of the negative experiments. They were repeated by Rosenblatt et al. (1966a) with minor modifications, among which was the introduction of some reinforced testing sessions given to the recipients after the unreinforced trials.

Dyal et al. (1967) have done experiments of the same type. They utilized the operant bar pressing response in a Skinner box. The number of bar presses and magazine approaches was automatically recorded.

The donors were given 8 or 10 days of training for 30 minutes each day. Bar presses were continuously reinforced; they were accompanied by a click of the magazine and a brief dimming of the light in the box. The controls were yoked to the experimental group in such a way that bar pressing by the experimental donors also activated the food delivery for the controls but the pellets fell outside the box. Food delivery was not activated when the control animal pressed the bar.

A special group of donors was trained, then extinguished for three days, followed by a period of reacquisition. These donors were to give the best results in transfer.

The recipients were on a food deprivation schedule for five days and were fasting for 48 to 56 hours at the time of the test, which took place 24 hours after injection. It consisted of two successive 30-minute sessions. During the first one, the bar was removed from the box and the magazine approaches to the click-light stimulus were recorded. The second session was for recording bar presses. These results were replicated by Golub and McConnell (1968) with even better results than in the original work.

Conditioned Avoidance

Rosenblatt et al. (1966a,b,c) described experiments performed in a shuttle box in which "rats were trained to stay on one side of the box to avoid a shock which was permanently connected to the 'wrong' side." One group was trained to stay on the lighted side of the box, another group on the dark side. In other experiments, the rats were "trained to avoid a shock by crossing the box within 2 seconds of a buzzer and light signal." The recipients "were given two preconditioning sessions and six unreinforced test sessions." Positive results were obtained with the extracts of donors trained to cross on the signal but not with the passive situation. No further details are available on these experiments.

In the author's laboratory (Ungar, 1967a,b) donor rats were trained to jump across a barrier to avoid electric shock within five seconds of a signal (buzzer). The recipients were naive mice without any pretraining, tested with the same reinforcement as the donors. When they were injected with trained brains they reached the criterion of 90 percent correct responses in 90 ± 34 (SD) trials, while those that received untrained brain required 151 ± 43 trials. Without reinforcement, no recipient jumped the barrier on the buzzer.

Adâm and Faiszt (1967) trained donors with the sound of a bell as conditioned stimulus. If within 5 seconds after the bell the rat did not jump to a shelf located at 12 cm above the floor, it received an electric shock. Four such trials were given at 1-minute intervals. There were three groups of donors with varying lengths of training: five sessions in 3 days, twelve sessions in 10 days, and twenty-four sessions in 20 days.

The recipients were all tested with reinforcement, as in the training of the donors. There were, however, differences in preliminary training; some animals were pretrained with both the conditioned and unconditioned stimuli, others only with the electric shock, and one group had no pretraining whatever.

Significant transfer was obtained with the extract taken from donors trained for 10 days. Shorter training gave less significant results and the 20-day training gave no transfer at all. The pretraining of the recipients also influenced the transfer; those that were pretrained with the conditioned stimulus gave the poorest results. With younger recipients, any pretraining had unfavorable effects.

Until recently, transfer of conditioned avoidance in unreinforced recipients was unsuccessful. Using goldfish, Fjerdingstad in my laboratory (unpublished experiments) was able to show that, without ever being shocked, recipient fish having received intracranial injections of brain extract from trained donors made significantly more avoidances in a shuttle box than the control fish treated with untrained fish brain. These results were confirmed by Braud (1970) who was able to transfer not only avoidance on a light stimulus but also the extinction of this learned behavior. Extracts taken from extinguished donors induced a significant decrease in the number of avoidances in pretrained recipients.

A very interesting paradigm was studied by Weiss (1970). Its main advantage lies in the fact that the animals, donors and recipients, were trained and tested in their normal environment, their home cages. They were placed individually in standard rat cages provided with a small signal light 7 cm above the glass water-delivery tube. When this light was on, and the animals attempted to drink, they received an electric shock through an electrode in contact with the drinking water and the wire cage floor. The same circuit allowed the recording of attempts made by the animals to drink during the lighted and unlighted periods.

During training of the donors each period lasted an average of 3 minutes. Following 48 hours of continuous exposure to these conditions, the rats showed 100 percent correct responses; they drank only when the light was off. However, training continued for an additional 50 days. No shorter training period was tried.

The recipients were placed in the same cages as the donors, and the lighted and dark periods were made to alternate exactly at 3-minute intervals. No shock was given to these animals at any time, but their approaches to the water-delivery tube were recorded under the two conditions of light or darkness. Control groups, untreated or injected with saline, were subjected to the same test for the same 48 hours duration. In the group treated with trained brain, the number of attempts at drinking was significantly higher during the unlighted than during the lighted period. In the control groups there was no significant difference.

Color Discrimination

The absence of color vision in laboratory rodents made it impossible to attempt the transfer of any behavior based on color discrimination. Zippel and Domagk (1969) trained goldfish to reverse their innate preference for red over green by feeding them at the side of the tank marked with a green light. When the donors were fully trained, their brains were extracted and the extract injected intraperitoneally into naive recipients. After 36 to 48 hours the fish injected with the trained brain extract showed a marked preference for green while the control fish, treated with untrained brain extract, continued to prefer the red.

These results have a considerable importance for demonstrating the specificity of transfer within the same sensory modality. We were able to confirm this specificity in my laboratory. We trained the fish by negative reinforcement; one group of donors was trained to prefer blue over red by receiving electric shocks at the red end of the tank with the possibility of escape to the blue end, while the other group was trained in the opposite direction. We injected the brain extracts by the intracranial route, particularly easy in the goldfish. The results were quite dramatic: the recipients of extracts of brain from fish that acquired a preference for the red avoided the blue and swam toward the red, and those injected with extracts from blue-preferring donors exhibited the opposite behavior. The differences between the two groups were highly significant; the effect had its maximum two to three days after injection and lasted for four to five days (Ungar, Galvan, and Johnson, unpublished experiments). We plan to repeat these experiments with colors lying closer and closer in the spectrum, to explore the limits of the specificity of color discrimination.

Passive Avoidance

A passive avoidance situation was successfully transferred by Gay and Raphelson (1967). The paradigm was based on the preference of rodents for dark over lighted enclosures. They used a set of three boxes (11 × 12 inches) linked

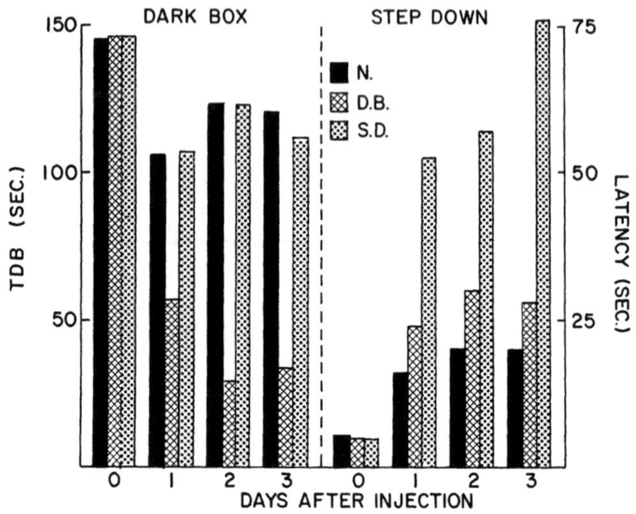

FIG. 5. Transfer of dark box avoidance, avoidance of step-down from platform, and failure of cross-transfer between the two. Abscissa: Days after injection of extracts of brain from untrained donors (N), donors trained to avoid the dark box (D.B.), and donors trained to avoid step-down (S.D.). Ordinate: Left, time spent in dark box by recipients; right, latency of step-down in recipients. (From Ungar. 1970.)

together with two runways (24 × 6 inches). The donors were placed in the middle or starting box, which had white walls and a transparent lid. This was connected on one side with a dark box and on the other with a white box. When the animals ran into the dark box, they received an electric shock through the grid floor for 5 seconds and were then allowed to run back into the starting box. This was repeated five times every day for 4 days. The donors seldom entered the white box.

The recipients were tested first 2 hours after injection and retested at 2-hour intervals, five times in all. The last test, therefore, took place 12 hours after injection. The recipients received no shock at any time, and the results were evaluated by recording the time spent in the dark box and the white box out of a total of 3 minutes.

In view of the good results reported by the authors, the experiments were repeated in this laboratory, and the results were confirmed and extended (Ungar et al., 1968). The apparatus was subsequently modified, particularly the connecting runways, which were reduced to short passages. (For a detailed description of the procedure see the Appendix.)

The conditions of training were specified. The best results were obtained with 6 to 8 days of training. Prolongation beyond 8 days decreased the probability of transfer. The testing procedure has remained essentially the same, but the time spent in each of the three boxes was recorded by a photoelectric system and the period of testing was extended to several days after injection. The effect was usually observable for at least four days (Fig. 5). These experiments have been replicated under slightly different conditions by Fjerdingstad (1969a), Wolthius (1969b), and Golub et al. (1969).

More recently a second passive avoidance paradigm was transferred successfully. Rats and mice, when placed on a narrow platform above a wider area, will rapidly step down. However, if they receive an electric shock on stepping down from the platform, they will stay on it after a small number of trials. Donor rats were placed on a platform (11.5 cm × 7.5 cm) 12.5 cm above the floor of a box (17 cm × 34 cm) provided with a grid floor, through which the animals were shocked when they stepped down. Five trials of 5-second duration, separated by a 10-second interval, were given for 6 days. After the first few trials, the rats had to be pushed down from the platform.

The recipient mice were tested twice or three times a day for 5 to 6 days, beginning 24 hours after injection. They were placed on a platform (3 cm × 9 cm) 3 cm above the floor and were given no shock when they stepped down. Latency of the stepdown and the total time spent on the platform out of 100 seconds were recorded. Transfer is usually detected 24 to 48 hours after injection and may last 2 to 3 weeks (Fig. 5). This figure also shows that the two passive avoidance paradigms are transferred specifically.

Miscellaneous Procedures

There have been a few experiments difficult to classify into any of the foregoing. Some of them deal with situations that do not represent learning in the accepted sense, although they are based on acquired information.

Transfer of *drug tolerance* was the first attempt in the writer's laboratory at transferring acquired information (Ungar and Cohen, 1966). Rats and dogs were made tolerant to morphine by administration of increasing doses of the drug over periods of several weeks. Brain extracts from these animals were injected into recipients without previous experiece of the drug. When these were tested for analgesic effect of morphine, they were significantly less sensitive than the controls injected with normal brain extracts. Recently, it was shown that these extracts shifted the LD_{50} of the drug to about four times that of the controls (Ungar and Galvan, 1969).

Revusky and DeVenuto (1967) proposed the *learned aversion to saccharine* as a paradigm to be transferred. Normally, rats when given the choice between a 0.1 percent solution of saccharine or water will prefer the former. However, if they receive, simultaneously with the access to saccharine, an x-irradiation sufficient to make them sick, the animals develop an aversion to saccharine. These results have recently been confirmed and extended by Moos et al. (1969).

Among the many learned behavioral patterns successfully transferred since 1965, I shall mention only maze-learning in chicks (Rosenthal and Sparber, 1968), the fixation time of postural asymmetry produced after unilaterial cerebellar lesion (Giurgea et al., 1969), alternation behavior in the Skinner box (Fjerdingstad, 1969), and the bar-pressing and door-opening discrimination (Rosenblatt, 1969).

There has been one attempt at transferring an *innate behavioral pattern* by Reinis (personal communication) who used the tendency to kill mice, a trait found in a number of rats. Extracts were prepared from the brains taken from such animals and injected into "nonkiller" rats. Tested at varying intervals up to four weeks, none of these animals exhibited the mouse-killing trait. The reverse attempt at changing the killing trait of rats by treatment with "nonkiller" brains was equally unsuccessful. Judging from these results and the generally unfavorable effects of prolonged training, it seems probable that only learned and recently acquired behavioral traits can be transferred. Once a memory trace is firmly consolidated, the transfer factors seem to have decreased in the brain.

PREPARATION OF THE EXTRACTS

Under this heading we shall consider not only the physical and chemical methods used for preparing the brain extracts but also the conditions under which the tissue is removed from the animals, handled, and stored.

The interval between the last training session and the removal of the brain is not specified in all the publications. When it is given, it varies from 15 minutes (Golub and McConnell, 1968) to 3 hours (Dyal et al., 1967). The interval most often mentioned is 2 hours. This is probably not a very critical factor. In the case of passive avoidance of the dark box, an analysis of this interval (Ungar et al., 1968) suggests that several hours are required for the synthesis of the transfer factor. This means that killing the donors too soon after the last session renders the effectiveness of that particular session questionable.

A few workers used anesthesia for the sacrifice of the donors (Babich et al; (1965b; Fjerdingstad et al., 1965; Dyal et al., 1967), but in the majority of published experiments the animals were decapitated and the brain removed. The brain is either frozen until the preparation is started or extracted immediately.

Most workers take the whole brain, usually without the olfactory bulbs. Babich et al. (1965), and after them other groups of workers, discarded "the frontal areas" and everything posterior to a line joining the superior colliculus to the rostral end of the pons. Others eliminated only the cerebellum (Dyal et al., 1967; Golub and McConnell, 1968). However, Rosenblatt et al. (1966) found practically equal activity in all parts of the brain. A few attempts made in the writer's laboratory to assay different parts of the brain reached the same conclusion.

There is also a difference in the way in which the brains of identically trained donors are pooled or kept individually, each being administered to a different recipient. It is unlikely that this is a critical difference but makes the basis for statistical treatment somewhat complex by increasing the number of variables.

Types of Extracts Used

Homogenates were used by Reinis (1965), Dyal et al. (1967), and in some of the experiments done in this laboratory (Ungar and Oceguera-Navarro, 1965). They were prepared in a glass homogenizer with distilled water, saline, or buffer solutions. This type of preparation has definite limitations as far as the amount of brain administered and the route of introduction are concerned.

Another type of crude extract is the supernatant obtained by centrifugation of the homogenate. This was used by several groups of workers (Ungar, 1967a, 1967b; Ungar and Irwin, 1967; Byrne and Hughes, 1967; Golub and McConnell, 1968). The activity of such preparations depends on a compromise between the thoroughness of extraction of all the soluble material and the necessity to prevent possible enzymic destruction of the active substance. At present, in the writer's laboratory the homogenate is stirred for 24 hours in an ice bath and then centrifuged at 60,000 × *g* for 1 to 2 hours.

"RNA" EXTRACTS.

Most of the transfer experiments were started with the avowed purpose of proving that the coded molecule, and consequently the transfer factor, was an RNA (Fjerdingstad et al., 1965; Babich et al., 1965b). The method used by the Danish group is based on the procedure described by Laskov et al. (1959), as modified by Haselkorn (1962). The frozen powder obtained from ten brains was mixed with 60 ml of 88 percent phenol and 60 ml of a 10^{-4} M solution of EDTA in 0.02 M phosphate buffer at pH 7.6. The mixture, maintained below 40°C, was stirred for 20 minutes and centrifuged at 2,500 × *g* for 10 minutes. The water phase was drawn off, and the bottom phase with the interphase was reextracted with the buffer. The combined water phases, assumed to contain all the RNA, were combined and centrifuged again. The supernatant was acidified with one drop of 1.0 M acetate buffer (pH 5.5) per ml and mixed with a slight excess of isopropanol. After thorough mixing, the precipitate formed was centrifuged down and dissolved in 20 ml of 10^{-4} M EDTA. This solution was dialyzed for 18 hours against three times 3 liters of 10^{-3} M NaCl. The retentate was again treated with isopropanol, and the precipitate was dried and kept frozen on dry ice until use.

In a later version (Røigaard-Petersen et al., 1968), the second water extraction was omitted and centrifugation was done for 20 minutes at 25,000 × *g*. It was claimed that this procedure reduced the protein content of the preparation from 50 percent with previous method to about 5 percent.

Prior to injection, the dry preparation was dissolved in a mixture of 0.145 M $NaHCO_3$ and 0.005 M $KHCO_3$ at the concentration of 1 mg RNA (estimated by UV absorption) per 50 μl.

The preparation of "RNA" used by Babich et al. (1965b) is described as follows:

> The tissue [part of one rat brain weighing about 1 g] was placed in a cold mortar with 5 ml of phenol (90 percent) and 5 ml of isotonic saline and was ground with purified sand for approximately 3 min. The mixture was then centrifuged at 18,000 rev./min. for 30 min. at 0°C. The aqueous phase was carefully drawn off to avoid contamination with phenol or with the interphase. The aqueous phase was then brought up to a concentration of 0.1 M $MgCl_2$, and 2 volumes of cold ethanol were added to precipitate the RNA. Precipitation time was 15 min. The suspension was centrifuged at 6,000 rev./min. for 15 min., after which the supernatant liquid was poured off. The remaining ethanol was evaporated off and the RNA was dissolved in 1.0 to 1.5 ml of isotonic saline.

The same procedure was used by Gay and Raphelson (1967) and, with some modifications, by Rosenblatt et al. (1966), Ádám and Faiszt (1967), and Weiss (1970).

Both methods claimed to obtain about 1 mg of RNA per gram of protein. Babich et al. (1965b) believed their preparation to be free of protein and DNA. They mention evidence from gel filtration data that RNA remains in a highly polymerized state, but no details are given. This claim is supported to a certain extent by the nondialyzability of the active material, mentioned previously.

One can probably admit that the final preparation in both cases contains most of the RNA present in the brain, but it is certainly far from being pure. Even if it were pure, it is only the mRNA or more precisely an infinitesimal fraction of this mRNA that contains the information relevant to the situation to be transferred. This point and the stability of the nucleotide sequence containing the information will be further discussed.

PEPTIDE EXTRACTS.—The nature of the active material was interpreted differently by the reviewer's group (Ungar and Oceguera-Navarro, 1965; Ungar and Irwin, 1967, 1968; Ungar, 1967a, 1967b, 1968) and by Rosenblatt et al. (1966a,b,c). Proceeding by successive stages of purification, both groups claim to have characterized the transfer factors as peptides or proteins.

In our laboratory, the first step was to dialyze the supernatant of the homogenate. In most cases, the activity was found in the dialyzate. After reducing the volume of the dialyzate by lyophilization, it was treated with an equal volume of 88 percent phenol. The active material was found in the phenol phase, and it was precipitated with 95 percent acetone. The transfer factor of sound habituation was destroyed by chymotrypsin and that of dark-box avoidance by trypsin, but the activity of neither of the extracts was affected by RNAase. The results of gel filtration on Sephadex G-25 suggest peptides with 8 to 12 amino acid residues. Passage through ion exchange resins so far has yielded positively charged active substances.

Rosenblatt et al. also found that the transfer factors were precipitated with acetone (90 percent) and destroyed by chymotrypsin and unattacked by RNAase. Gel filtration on Sephadex G-50 and G-25 indicated that the active material had a molecular weight between 1,000 and 5,000.

In two situations studied up to now, light-dark discrimination and conditioned avoidance, the transfer factor appeared in the nondialyzable fraction of the brain extract. A few attempts at purification by ammonium sulfate precipitation and gel filtration have yielded inconsistent results.

There is an apparent contradiction between the two series of studies just summarized: some of them obtained good results with RNA-type extracts while others characterized the transfer factors as peptides. I took advantage of the presence in my laboratory of Dr. Fjerdingstad, one of the early exponents of the RNA hypothesis, to solve this problem. We took a pool of brains from rats trained for dark avoidance and prepared an RNA extract and a peptide extract. Both preparations were about equally active and both were inactivated by trypsin but

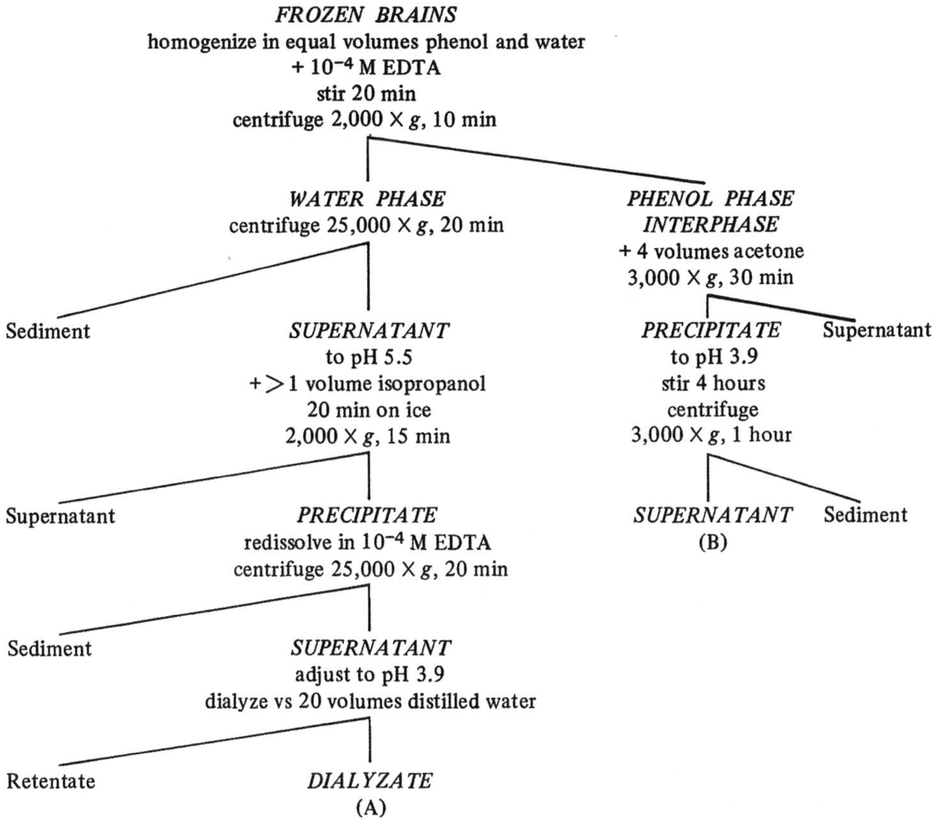

FIG. 6. Outline of purification procedure for the transfer factor of dark avoidance.

not by RNAase. It seemed probable that the active material was a peptide which formed a complex with RNA. We were able to dissociate this complex at low pH, dialyze out the peptide, and leave behind the inactive RNA (Ungar and Fjerdingstad, 1970). This procedure offered several advantages over the one outlined above and we adopted it for our large-scale extraction of dark-avoidance trained brain (Fig. 6).

Whatever extraction procedure is used, one should insist here on the precautions to be taken in the presence of substances with unknown stability. The brain should be brought to low temperature, preferably frozen, as soon as possible after the death of the donor animal, and all subsequent steps of the extraction procedure should be done as close as possible to 0°C. No preparation should be left at room temperature for more than a few minutes, and thawing and freezing should be kept to a minimum.

One should also bear in mind that both polynucleotides and peptides are easily hydrolyzed by enzymes present in the brain extracts. Enzymic destruction is probably reduced by low temperature treatment, but efforts should be made either to eliminate the enzymes from the preparation (e.g., by dialysis) or to find inhibitors or otherwise create unfavorable conditions for enzymic destruction. The latter can be achieved by selecting an appropriate pH for the extraction or by removal of some essential ion or other cofactor.

ADMINISTRATION OF THE EXTRACTS

Three important points have to be discussed in relation to the administration of the extracts: routes of administration, dose injected, and the interval between injection and testing of the recipients. Some other points will also be mentioned regarding the stability of the active material during and after administration.

Routes of Administration

Three main routes have been employed. In the majority of experiments intraperitoneal injections were given. In most of his experiments, Rosenblatt (1969, 1970) gave intravenous injections via the jugular vein. This required anesthesia and a small cutaneous incision.

The Danish group used the intracisternal route. In the early experiments this was done under ether anesthesia, but more recently they gave subcutaneous injections of chloral hydrate (0.7 ml of a 12 percent solution). Induction took about an hour, and the animal remained under deep anesthesia for a further period of one hour (Røigaard-Petersen et al., 1968).

The anesthetized animal was "placed with the neck over a roll of cotton to bend the neck maximally. The skin over the foramen magnum was opened by a cut of about 2 mm, thus preventing the tough skin from interfering with the fine movements of the needle." A tuberculin syringe containing 50 μl (equivalent to 1 mg of RNA), provided with a fine needle, is "held in the right hand and the tip of the needle thrust through the muscles and the connective tissue covering the foramen magnum and into the cisterna magna. The entrance into the cisterna could be felt distinctly as a decrease in resistance against the needle, and a too deep injection resulted in the animal's dying through damage to the respiratory center." During the injection, "a piece of sheet aluminum bent into an arch was placed over the back of the animal to give support for the hand during injection." Sterile precautions were taken after injection, and the skin was closed with a stitch. These workers have experienced some difficulty in keeping the extract active during the injection of the animals (Nissen et al., 1965) and they insist on speedy performance. It is probably essential even with the faster intraperitoneal injection to keep the extract cold until just a few minutes before administration.

Two other routes of introduction are worth mentioning. Rosenthal and Sparber (1968) administered brain extracts orally to newly hatched chicks which do not have digestive enzymes until the second day of their life. The intracranial route has been used in goldfish. This is a very convenient technique and allows the injection of at least 50 μl of fluid into the cranial cavity. The injection is done with a 30-gauge needle provided with a stop allowing only the tip of the needle to penetrate. The landmarks indicating the site of the injection are easily recognizable and with a minimum of practice a large number of fish can be injected in rapid succession.

There has been a great deal of discussion on the role of the blood-brain barrier in the transfer experiments. Doubts have been voiced on the possibility of macromolecules actually reaching the brain after intraperitoneal injections. This point has probably some validity as far as RNA is concerned. It is, however, well known that peptides and even proteins of the size of gamma globulins can cross the blood-brain barrier.

A second point concerning the fate of the injected material is the possibility of its enzymic destruction. The body fluids are rich in both ribonucleases and peptidases. The half-life of a nucleotide sequence injected intraperitoneally is unknown, but it is known that parenterally administered peptides (peptide hormones, bradykinin, substance P) remain intact long enough to produce their pharmacologic effects.

Dose of Brain Extract Injected

It is certain that only a small fraction of the active substances injected actually reach their site of action in the brain. This suggests that successful transfer probably requires the administration of a large excess of material, and the appropriate dose can be found only by injecting varying amounts. Nevertheless, in almost all of the early experiments a single arbitrarily chosen dose was given, usually the equivalent of one brain to each recipient (Reinis, 1965; Fjerdingstad et al., 1965; Babich et al., 1965a, 1965b). Rosenblatt et al. (1966a,b,c) used a variety of doses and found this factor to be critical. They obtained better results by giving higher amounts of brain extract. More recently (1970), however, with their spatial discrimination paradigm, these authors claim to have obtained effects with much lower doses following a complex dose-response pattern with several phases of reversal.

In the writer's experience, the optimum dose varies with the task to be transferred. In our work, recipients were mice whose brains weigh about 0.25 g. Administration of the equivalent of one recipient brain per mouse gave results only in the habituation experiments. In all other transfer situations, the minimum effective dose was about 0.5 g – that is, the equivalent of two recipient brains–and best results were obtained with approximately 0.75 to 1.0 g. In the case of spatial discrimination there was an optimum dose beyond which the results were unsatisfactory (Ungar, 1967b; Ungar and Irwin, 1967).

Dose-response curves were obtained in two situations: brightness discrimination in the Y-maze and passive avoidance of the dark box. In the former, the lowest effective dose was 0.75 g of donor brain per mouse, and the effect increased up to the highest dose used (1.25 g). In the latter situation the lowest effective dose was about 0.5 to 0.6 g (depending on the length of training of the donors). With increasing amounts the effect was dose-related (Ungar et al., 1968).

Schedule of Injection and Testing

There is no advance information that permits even a guess as to the onset and duration of the effect produced by the extract. It is, therefore, obvious that the interval between injection and testing, and the duration of the latter, must be varied until the best schedule is found.

Nevertheless, Babich et al. tested only between 4 and 24 hours after injection. This unfortunate precedent found many imitators, most of whom obtained negative results (see below). Several other workers limited their testing of recipients to a single session, usually 24 hours after injection (Dyal et al., 1967; Golub and McConnell, 1968). Most other publications, however, mention testing in several sessions from one to four or more days (Fjerdingstad et al., 1965; Rosenblatt et al., 1966a,b,c; Ádám and Faiszt, 1967).

In the writer's laboratory, the recipients were tested daily, beginning 24 hours after the injection, and for as many days as seemed necessary to show positive results or to demonstrate convincingly that no transfer has taken place. In the case of habituation, the maximum effect was obtained in 24 hours; in others (light-dark or spatial discrimination) the best effect took several days to appear. Only in dark-box avoidance was any effect detectable within a few hours after injection, and this became more marked at 48 hours.

It seems, therefore, that a single test session, at whichever interval, runs the risk of not showing any effect. Early effects are exceptional and, in most cases, the probability of transfer increases as time goes by up to about 2 to 3 days. Only when the chronology of a transfer is well established can testing be limited to the optimal period.

CONDITIONS OF SUCCESS AND THE NEGATIVE EXPERIMENTS

The problem of chemical transfer of learned information is basically the same as the one a pharmacologist faces when he studies the possible drug action of a material of animal or plant origin. He has to devise a procedure of extraction compatible with the physical and chemical properties of the active substance, particularly with its stability, and find a method for testing the activity of the hypothetical substance under optimal conditions of dose, onset, and duration of the effect. No pharmacologist would conclude that the material was inactive after having tested it at one arbitrarily chosen dose and interval.

This is, nevertheless, what happened in several of the attempts at reproducing the results of the first transfer experiments. Some of these (Gross and Carey, 1965; Gordon et al., 1966; Lambert and Saurat, 1967) were replications of the experiments of Babich et al. with only apparently minor changes. Others (Luttges et al.,

1966; Kimble and Kimble, 1966, and most of the group of workers who signed the collective paper of Byrne et al., 1966) also explored other paradigms.*

Critical Factors

After having reviewed the conditions under which positive results have been obtained, a number of factors appear to be quite critical. These factors may form a background against which the negative experiments can be examined.

ADEQUATE DONOR TRAINING.

It seems fairly well demonstrated that, to be good donors, the animals have to be trained beyond just having learned the task. In passive avoidance, training is completed on the first day, but several more days are required for the brain to accumulate the excess of material necessary for transfer (Ungar et al., 1968).

In repeating the experiments of the Jacobson group (who trained their donors for 8 to 10 days), Gordon et al. (1966) trained for 5 days and Lambert and Saurat (1967) for 4 days. In training for other tasks, Wagner et al. (1966) and Leaf et al. (1965) had schedules of 5 days and Corson and Enesco (1966) of 2 days.

A training period of fixed duration regardless of the performance of the trainees may not be satisfactory. Reinis (1966) showed that inadequately trained or untrainable animals are poor donors. It seems that training should be both prolonged and complete. In the negative experiments of Luttges et al. (1966) the training goal was deliberately set to the low level of 60 percent correct responses.

In some cases (Ungar and Irwin, 1967; Ungar et al., 1968; Ádám and Faiszt, 1967), unduly prolonged training also gave negative results. There may be, therefore, an optimum duration of donor training, somewhere between 8 and 12 days. This may vary with the task to be transferred and can only be found by trial and error.

PRESENCE OF ACTIVE MATERIAL IN THE EXTRACT.

Almost all the negative experiments used an RNA extraction procedure of the type described by Fjerdingstad et al. and Babich et al. Some of them (Kimble and Kimble, 1966; Wagner et al., 1966) used an improved technique with removal of the excess phenol with ether. In most of the negative experiments, the extraction procedure seems to have been handled more competently than in the original experiments of the Jacobson group, and they generally obtained a lower yield of "RNA-type" material with a presumably higher purity. If, as it now seems probable, the activity of the "RNA" extracts is due to the presence of traces of peptides, a purer RNA preparation would result in a decrease in activity.

In this same category, the care taken to avoid destruction of the active material was not always adequate. In some experiments of Corson and Enesco

*We had access to the detailed description of these experiments only for three groups: Corson and Enesco (1966), Leaf et al. (1966), and Wagner et al. (1966).

(1966) the volume of the extract was reduced by flash evaporation at 36°C. It is doubtful that any nucleotide or peptide sequence could resist such a treatment.

DOSE OF BRAIN EXTRACT.

In this respect, very few negative experiments attempted the administration of several amounts of donor brain in order to find an optimal dosage level. Almost all the experiments used one dose, the equivalent of one donor brain per recipient. Out of the 236 experimental recipients listed in the negative publications surveyed, only 40 received more than one donor brain equivalent. Luttges et al. (1966), in one of their experiments, gave up to three donor mouse brains to each recipient; Leaf et al. (1966) gave four brain equivalents to some of their recipients; and Corson and Enesco (1966) varied their dose from one to two brains per recipient.

SCHEDULE OF TESTING.

As mentioned earlier, there is no *a priori* reason to select one particular interval at which the injected recipients should be tested, since the onset and duration of the effect depends on many completely unknown factors.

Nevertheless, Gordon et al. tested only 4, 6, and 8 hours after injection; Gross and Carey 8 and 22 hours after; Luttges et al., in the one experiment in which adequate doses were given, tested the recipients only once, 4 hours after injection; in the others, testing was terminated 24 hours after administration of the extract. Only Lambert and Saurat (1967) tested for 4 days, and Kimble and Kimble (1966) every day until criterion was reached.

SELECTION AND PREPARATION OF THE RECIPIENTS.

This is often necessary in order to realize the best conditions. For example, if recipients are to be tested for avoidance of the dark box, one must ascertain that, before injection, they have a preference for the dark box. This sort of selection is perfectly permissible as long as the experimental and control recipients are selected in the same way.

Ideally, each recipient group should have the same mean learning ability. Since it is not possible to evaluate this directly, one should at least try to equalize all conditions. One of these conditions may be age. Ádám and Faiszt (1967) suggested that very young animals may not be as satisfactory recipients as the adults. This may also be true of very old subjects. Rosenblatt (1970) proposes older adults as donors and younger ones as recipients.

When the donors, in the course of training with positive reinforcement, were deprived of food or water, the recipients should be similarly deprived, even if they, themselves, are not reinforced. Reinis (1965, 1966) observed the transfer only in adequately fasted recipients.

It was seen previously that several groups of workers gave various types of pretraining to their recipients; some of them favored transfer, others had the opposite effect. If Ádám and Faiszt had done all their experiments with pretraining of their recipients (presentation of the conditioned stimulus), they would probably have drawn negative conclusions.

Optimal Conditions

Negative results are always easier to obtain than positive ones. This is particularly true in an area where many decisive variables are still unknown. It seems that the authors of the early experiments were just lucky to hit on the right conditions. At the present stage, however, the transfer experiments should be placed on a firmer foundation than fickle luck. Consistently successful transfers require extreme care and patience. They are not the sort of experiments set up by an unsupervised student with leftover animals and discarded pieces of equipment. They demand the organized and sustained effort of a team with a reasonable command of behavioral and biochemical methodology.

There have certainly been honest and conscientious efforts at replicating the successful experiments, but one cannot help feeling that in some of these studies the main purpose was to prove that somebody was wrong rather than to find out the truth. The verdict was decided before the trial, which became a perfunctory gesture. It is difficult to understand otherwise the "one-shot" experiments, done with a single dose and a single test. For example, in a replication of our experiments on transfer of morphine tolerance (Smits and Takemori, 1968), all the recipient mice were given uniformly 200 to 240 mg of tolerant rat brain and were all tested once 3 hours after injection of the extract. We did have success previously under the same conditions but only with highly potent extracts. Weaker preparations require higher doses and longer intervals, preferably both, to show their activity (Ungar and Galvan, 1969). In another attempt at repeating these same experiments (Tirri, 1967), in addition to using the one dose-one test procedure, one of the critical conditions was changed. Instead of using rats as donors, mouse brain was injected. This was tried also in our laboratory without success, probably because mice, able to tolerate much larger doses of morphine than rats, require a different injection schedule.

In the first three series of experiments published by Luttges et al. (1966), the experimental recipients, as far as one can judge from the mean values given in the publication, performed consistently better than the controls. Although the differences were small and failed to reach the criteria of statistical significance, they were consistent enough to encourage an unprejudiced worker to improve the conditions of the experiments. In most of the negative experiments, no special efforts seem to have been made to increase the chances of success. To avoid this taking place again in the future, it may be useful to summarize some of the conditions that seem to have contributed to the success of the experiments.

1. Donors should be trained for a period of between 6 and 12 days. They should be able to learn the task to a criterion of 90 percent or more correct responses; incompletely trained animals should not be used.
2. The initial experiments should be done with crude brain extracts, and purification should be guided by assays of activity. All preparative procedures should be done at low temperature.

3. The recipients should belong to a species, a strain, and an age group that can learn readily by training the task that is to be transferred to them. They should be screened individually so as to eliminate the subjects that do not exhibit normally the responses on which the transfer is based. If the response required deprivation in the donors, the recipients should be similarly deprived.
4. Usually, amounts equivalent to two or three recipient brains are necessary for significant transfer to take place, but the optimal dose should be determined by trial and error.
5. Recipients should be tested at widely spaced intervals after injection. Tests should be done from a few hours after administration of the extract and continued daily for four to six days.
6. Recipients should be tested under blind conditions, in random order, and preferably by automatic recording.
7. As a general and perhaps most important rule, all the conditions should be varied until the best procedure is found. Only after trying different modalities of training, a range of doses, and varying the testing schedules of the recipients can one conclude that, in that particular case, transfer has not taken place.

There have been, of course, several experiments with positive results in which all the conditions just enumerated were not fulfilled, and there may be others in the future. It is also possible that there are some critical conditions that were met more or less accidentally in the positive experiments and not fulfilled in the negative ones. This is one more reason why the experiments should be conducted under several widely different conditions.

STATISTICAL EVALUATION AND INTERPRETATION OF THE RESULTS

In the type of experiments considered in this chapter, the outcome depends essentially on the probability that the behavior of one group of animals is different from that of another group. In the vast majority of publications, this probability was computed by the nonparametric Mann-Whitney U-test (Siegel, 1956). When it is two-tailed, the results of this test are closely parallel with those of Student's t-test. The justifications for using the one-tailed test have been discussed at several meetings. It is considered permissible when the expected changes can take place in one direction only, and this clearly puts a severe limitation to its use.

In the writer's laboratory, whenever possible, the t-test or chi-square test has been used. Others used the Kruskal-Wallis analysis of variance (Siegel, 1956) and the Wilcoxon test (1964).

Rosenblatt et al. (1966) assumed that the population of recipients injected with trained brain was not homogeneous: "The injection had 'taken' on some of the rats, but not on others." Accordingly, they divided the animals into "high" and "low" categories and computed the U-test separately for the two groups. In a more recent publication (Rosenblatt, 1970a) this procedure seems to have been discontinued, and the results are computed using probit transformation, angular transformation, and shift scores (Finney, 1964).

The choice of the statistical method to be used depends largely on the type of parameter one wishes to compare. Correct versus incorrect responses can be handled by chi-square and probit transformation. Graded data (latency, time spent in a given space, etc.) can be treated with the t-test or the U-test.

The actual method used may be less critical than the relevance of the data to be compared. These are usually the parameters characterizing the simultaneous behavior of two or more groups of animals. In some experiments, Rosenblatt (1970a) compared the behavior of the same animals before and after injection of the extracts. This shift in behavior was also used in some of our experiments (Ungar, 1967b; Ungar and Irwin, 1967) but always coupled with the comparison of the postinjection behavior of the experimental and control groups. The shift, when it is marked, may be of great qualitative interest, but it is probably not reliable enough to serve as a basis for quantitative evaluation.

"Statistical significance" becomes easily a fetish and, provided that something is significantly different, one tends to lose sight of what is different from what. In a problem as complex as the one under review here, it may be useful to stop from time to time and examine the experimental data. They obviously represent an answer to some question, but one should keep in mind what the question was and what the meaning of the answer is.

Specificity of the Induced Behavior

To be able to assert that actual transfer of information has taken place, one has to answer the following two questions: Is the behavioral change produced in the recipients related to the training of the donors, and if so, is this a specific effect?

The first question is usually easy to answer, since the recipients are tested with the definite purpose of detecting a similarity with the donors. The results are more convincing when the testing is done without reinforcement. On the other hand, it is probably true, as suggested by Røigaard-Petersen et al. (1968), that reinforcement of the recipients makes the test more sensitive and less demanding. Specificity then can be ascertained by cross-transfer experiments.

Several of these experiments were attempted with varying degrees of success (Jacobson et al., 1965; Nissen et al., 1965; Ungar, 1967; Ungar and Irwin, 1967; Ungar, 1970a). (For our experiments, see Figures 1, 3, and 5.) The problem of specificity has been complicated by the reversal phenomenon, mentioned earlier (p. 487). It has been most consistently observed in the transfer of spatial discrimination (Ungar, 1967b; Ungar and Irwin, 1967; Rosenblatt, 1970a), but it was also seen in the light discrimination paradigm of Fjerdingstad et al. (1965), in which the "initial preference," observed on the first testing of the recipients, was in the direction opposite to the one shown by the trained donors.

In general, one can state that whenever specificity was tested with transferable situations and under conditions uncomplicated by reversal, it was possible to

1	2	3	4	5	6	7	8	9	10	11	12	13	14	15
SER	ASP	ASN												
		ASN	ASN											
			ASN	GLU										
				GLU	GLN									
					GLN	GLY								
						GLY	LYS							
						GLY	LYS	SER						
								SER	ALA					
									ALA	GLU				
										GLU	GLN			
											GLN	GLY		
											GLN	GLY	GLY	
												GLY	GLY	TYR-NH_2
SER	ASP	ASN	ASN	GLU	GLN	GLY	LYS	SER	ALA	GLU	GLN	GLY	GLY	TYR-NH_2
1	2	3	4	5	6	7	8	9	10	11	12	13	14	15

FIG. 7. Structure of scotophobin. Peptides found by mass spectrometry and final sequence (bottom line).

demonstrate it. The color discrimination experiments mentioned above (p. 491) represent probably the best evidence for specificity.

Chemical Identification

The single most significant point in the whole approach surveyed in this chapter is the possibility of using the behavioral transfer as a biologic assay method. Such an assay should enable us to guide the isolation, purification, and identification of the elements of the molecular code in which information is processed by the nervous system.

This has been attempted and perhaps successfully accomplished in the writer's laboratory for the coded molecule involved in dark avoidance. In an interval of slightly over two years (1967-1969) we collected about 5 kg of brain from almost 4,000 rats trained to avoid the dark. Most of the material was extracted by the method outlined in Figure 6. In the dialyzate of the RNA preparation we obtained about 1 mg of material (per kilogram of wet weight of brain) containing the active substance. After gel filtration on Sephadex G-25 the activity was concentrated twenty-fold. The active fraction was further purified by thin-layer chromatography which yielded a spot absent from identically prepared extracts of untrained brain. After elution, this material (about 0.2 μg per kg of brain) was found by the microdansylation method (Neuhoff et al., 1969) to contain the following amino acids: Ala, Asp or Asn (Asx), Gln or Glu (Glx), Gly, Lys, Ser, and Tyr with Ser as the N-terminal group. A quantitative amino acid analysis gave 4 Glx, 3 Asx, 3 Gly, 2 Ser, Ala, Lys, and Tyr. After trypsin hydrolysis, two fragments were obtained: T_1 contained Asx, Glx, Lys, and Ser; T_2 yielded Ala, Glx, Gly, Ser, and Tyr. The N-terminal group was Ser in both.

The amino acid sequence was established with the mass spectrometric method by Dr. D. M. Desiderio. Figure 7 shows the peptides identified by their masses and the sequence that was deduced from these data. Verification of this structure by synthesis is under way (Ungar et al., 1970).

I gave the name *scotophobin* to the pentadecapeptide extracted from the brain of dark-avoiding rats. Although it is impossible to say at present with certainty whether all the behavior-inducing substances formed in the brain are peptides, this is highly probable. It is hoped that an increasing number of these substances will be identified in the near future so that intelligent guesses can be made regarding the molecular code of acquired information.

CONCLUDING REMARKS

Although this chapter deals essentially with a discussion of methodology, it cannot evade some of the fundamental theoretical problems connected with the chemical transfer of acquired information. When, at the turn of the century, immunity was first passively conferred to animals never previously exposed to the specific antigen, the whole concept of the immune process had to be revised. The fact that passive immunization found subsequently some important medical applications is secondary to the theoretical significance of this transfer experiment.

The situation is strikingly similar regarding the transfer of learning. Whatever future uses may be found for these experiments, their basic importance is that, by "playing back" the code, they produce crucial evidence for its molecular nature. The real controversy is between those who believe that this is impossible–and therefore all attempts to prove it are "futile," "absurd," "ridiculous," "chimerical," "stupid" (all adjectives actually used by various critics, at least verbally)–and those who keep an open mind.

It is characteristic of the real issues of the debate that the collective paper signed by 23 authors from seven laboratories (Byrne et al., 1966) was published without any detailed evidence. Assuming that, before accepting the paper, the editors read carefully the "supplementary material" deposited in the Library of Congress, the ordinary reader still has to believe the authors without being given a chance to evaluate the evidence. Imagine now that the 75 authors from 23 institutions who have published positive results would have wanted to make a similar summary statement of their position, would they have been given this opportunity? Almost certainly not and quite rightly so.

The scientific method is poorly equipped for proving the negative because it is so deceptively easy to do. Any child can "disprove" the most firmly established facts of science by doing bad experiments. In the area of chemical transfer of information, the distinction between good and bad experiments was blurred by our ignorance of many of the variables. There have been some poorly designed and clumsily performed experiments, based on naive assumptions, on both the positive and negative sides. However, it seems that there have been enough positive data coming from many independent sources to justify further inquiry, in an unprejudiced frame of mind.

Since the real battleground of the debate is not in the experimental laboratory, but in the field of theory, one can wonder what the root of the prejudice is. Theories of learning and memory have been roughly classified into "connectionist" and "mass" or "field" hypotheses. According to the former, behavior is based on highly organized and more or less rigidly determined neural connections, whereas the latter, in the words of Hebb (1949), assume that the brain possesses as much structure as a "bowlful of porridge." When the molecular hypothesis was proposed, it came to be classified among the "field" theories because it gave the impression of a negation of structure; information appeared to be stored in the macromolecules of the porridge. This impression was reinforced by a curious semantic confusion. The "field" or "mass" theory is often called "molar" (from mass, *moles* in Latin) without implying any chemical connotation. For a nice example of the arbitrary use of these terms, see the review by Gaito and Zavala (1964).

At present, we often hear the connectionist view voiced as opposed to the molar or molecular conception, without clear distinction being made between the several meanings given to these terms. One must not forget that the problem we are discussing is at the borderline of psychology and biochemistry, disciplines that, until very recently, had no elements of a common vocabulary.

Semantics apart, is there a reason to believe that a molecular mechanism of learning is incompatible with the highly organized structure of the central nervous system? In an attempt at placing the chemical theory of memory and learning in a new conceptual framework, the author (Ungar, 1968) emphasized that the coded molecules designate specific pathways whose anatomy and physiology are genetically determined. Learning takes place when two or more of these pathways acquire new connections between them through a combination of their code substances, designated as "connectors." Closely similar conclusions were reached by Best (1968). For further discussion of the molecular code see recent surveys of the problem (Ungar, 1970b,c).

Since there is no further need to prove that chemical transfer of acquired information is possible, future research can concentrate on the most important issues such as specificity of the information stored in molecular structure, chemical identity of the code, and above all the study of the code itself. It may take the work of several generations to compile the vocabulary of code words and to discover the grammar and the syntax of the language in which the neurons transact their business.

APPENDIX: DETAILED PROCEDURE FOR TRANSFER OF DARK AVOIDANCE

The method is based on the observations of Gay and Raphelson (1967). It has been modified in some of the details, particularly in the preparation of the extract. The following is a description of the procedure used in our laboratory.

TRAINING AND TESTING APPARATUS.—This consists of a set of three boxes. The starting box (*S*), 30 cm long, 15 cm wide, 15 cm deep, has two openings

(7.5 cm on each side) leading on one side to the dark box ((*D*), 18 cm long, 8 cm wide, and 15 cm deep, and on the other side to the white box (*W*), which has the same dimensions as *S*. The boxes are linked by two passages, 7 cm on each side and 5 cm long; they can be closed by gates. *D* is made of dark plastic and has a dark lid. It is provided with a grid floor through which the donors receive electric shocks in the course of training. The recipients are never shocked. *S* and *D* are made of translucent plastic and have a transparent lid. When mice are used as recipients, the passage between *S* and *D* is closed by a gate provided with a mouse hole (semicircle with radius of 1.75 cm).

The time spent in each of the boxes by the animal under test can be measured by means of stopwatches or by automatic recording for which the gates are provided with photocells.

TRAINING OF DONORS.—Male Sprague-Dawley rats (200 to 250 g) are placed in *S* (see Fig. 1). As soon as they run into *D*, the gate is closed and the animal is given electric shocks (2 ma, 100 V on Variac dial) for 5 sec. Then the gate is opened and usually the animal runs out into *S*. If not, it is taken out from *D* through the top and placed again in *S*. If he runs back into *D*, the gate is closed and the animal is shocked as above. If he does not run back (this is the rule after the second session), he is pushed through the gate into *D* and shocked. Each daily session consists of 5 shock periods of 5 sec each, separated by intervals of 10 sec.

Good results have been obtained with six training sessions given on consecutive days or with a schedule of 3 days training and 2 days rest followed by 2 days of retraining.

PREPARATION OF THE EXTRACT.—The donors are killed 2 hours after the last training session by decapitation. The brain is removed and put on dry ice within 30 sec after death of the animal. Usually, all the brains of one series of donors are pooled. The frozen brains can be kept in the freezer (–20°C) for several weeks. The extracts are prepared as outlined in Figure 6.

TESTING OF RECIPIENTS.—In our experiments, the recipients have been male Swiss albino mice (20 to 25 g). We have tried other strains, but none of them offered serious advantages.

Before injection, the mice are tested for dark preference. Each mouse is allowed to explore the three compartments of the testing box for 3 to 5 min and then immediately tested for 3 min. Mice that do not spend at least 90 sec in *D* are eliminated.

Injections are done intraperitoneally. Volumes of 0.5 ml or less are injected into each mouse. No toxicity was observed up to 2 g of brain per mouse with the crude dialysate.

For testing, the animal is placed in *S*, right in the middle of the box, facing the side so that its head does not point to either of the gates. At this point a stopwatch is started or the recorder is activated. For manual testing a second stopwatch is used to record the time spent in *D* and a third for the time in *W*. It is preferable to use stopwatches that do not click, because the noise may disturb the animals.

We use the fluorescent lighting of the laboratory over *S* and *W*. Very bright light placed close to the boxes is not recommended.

We test each recipient twice a day for 2 or 3 days. Usually, we run all of them through once, then start over again. After the termination of each test, the animal is picked up in *S*, after the gates are closed.

With potent extracts, significant results can be obtained 6 hours after injection. The maximum effect is usually observed on the second day. Individual animals showed aversion to dark up to 8 days after injection, but the mean may not be significantly different from the controls after the fourth or fifth days.

Besides the significant decrease in the time spent in *D*, most recipients show typical behavior: putting their nose through the gate leading to *D* and hastily retreating, or running into *D* and rushing out to flee to the other end of *W*. This type of behavior is not observed in the controls.

Groups of 6 to 10 recipients are injected with the extract to be tested. A similar group is given a control extract made with the brain taken from untrained or pseudotrained donors (e.g., shocked in white box). Statistical analysis, comparing the experimental and control groups or their preinjection and postinjection behavior is done either by t-test or Mann-Whitney U-test.

REFERENCES

Adam, G., and Faiszt, J. 1967. Conditions for successful transfer effects. Nature (London), 216:198-200.

Agranoff, B. W. 1965. Molecules and memories. Perspect. Biol. Med., 9:13-22.

Babich, F. R., Jacobson, A. L., and Bubash, S. 1965a. Cross-species transfer of learning: Effect of ribonucleic acid from hamsters on rat behavior. Proc. Nat. Acad. Sci. U.S.A., 54:1299-1302.

—Jacobson, A. L., Bubash, S., and Jacobson, A. 1965b. Transfer of a response to naive rats by injection of ribonucleic acid extracted from trained rats. Science, 149:656-657.

Barondes, S. H., and Cohen, H. D. 1968. Memory impairment after subcutaneous injection of acetoxycycloheximide. Science, 160:556-557.

Best, R. M. 1968. Encoding of memory in the neuron. Psychol. Rep., 22:107-115.

Bogoch, S. 1968. The Biochemistry of Memory. Oxford University Press, Inc.

Braud, W. G. 1970. Facilitation of conditioning and extinction in goldfish by intracranial injection of "RNA" from brains of trained donors. Science. (In press.)

Byrne, W. L., ed. 1970. Molecular Approaches to Learning and Memory. AAAS Symposium. New York, Academic Press, Inc. (In press.)

—and Hughes, A. 1967. Behavioral modification by injection of brain extract from trained donors. Fed. Proc., 26:676.

—et al. Memory transfer. Science, 153:658-659.

Chapouthier, G., Pallaud, B., and Ungerer, A. 1969. Note préliminaire concernant l'effet sur l'apprentissage des broyats de cerveau conditionné. Rev. Comportement Animal, 3:55-63.

Corning, W. 1970. The planarian controversy: A question of replication. *In* Molecular Approaches to Learning and Memory. Byrne, W. L., ed. AAAS Symposium. New York, Academic Press, Inc. (In press.)

Corson, J. A., and Enesco, H. E. 1966. A failure to replicate inter-animal transfer of memory with intraperitoneal injections of brain extracts from trained rats. Supplementary material to W. L. Byrne et al. Science, 153:658-659.

Dyal, J. A., Golub, A. M., and Marrone, R. L. 1967. Transfer effects of intraperitoneal injection of brain homogenates. Nature (London), 214:720-721.

Finney, D. J. 1964. Statistical Method in Biological Assay. London, Griffin.

Fjerdingstad, E. J. 1969a. Chemical transfer of learned preference. Nature (London), 222:1079-1080.

—1969b. Chemical transfer of alternation training in the Skinner box. Scand. J. Psychol., 10:220-224.

—Nissen, T., and Røigaard-Petersen, H. H. 1965. Effect of ribonucleic acid (RNA) extracted from the brain of trained animals on learning in rats. Scand. J. Psychol., 6:1-5.

Flexner, L. B. 1967. Dissection of memory in mice with antibiotics. Proc. Amer. Phil. Soc., 6:343-346.

Foerster, H. v. 1948. Das Gedächtnis. Vienna, Deuticke.

Gaito, J., and Zavala, A. 1964. Neurochemistry and learning. Psychol. Bull., 61:45-62.

Gay, R., and Raphelson, A. 1967. "Transfer of learning" by injection of brain RNA: A replication. Psychon. Sci., 8:369-370.

Giurgea, C., Daliers, J., and Mouravieff, F. 1969. Pharmacological studies on an elementary model of learning: the fixation of an experience at spinal level. *In* Abstracts, Fourth International Congress on Pharmacology. Basel, Switzerland, Schwabe & Co., pp. 291-292.

Golub, A. M., and McConnell, J. V. 1968. Transfer of response bias by injection of brain homogenates: A replication. Psychon. Sci., 11:1-2.

Gordon, M. W., Deanin, G. G., Leonhardt, H. L., and Gwynn, R. H. 1966. RNA and memory: A negative experiment. Amer. J. Psychiat., 122:1174-1178.

Gross, C. G. and Carey, F. M. 1965. Transfer of learned response by RNA injection: Failure of attempts to replicate. Science, 150:1749.

Haselkorn, R. 1962. Studies on infectious RNA from turnip yellow mosaic virus. J. Molec. Biol., 4:357-367.

Hebb, D. O. 1949. The Organization of Behavior. New York, John Wiley and Sons, Inc., p. 17.

Hydén, H. 1967. Behavior, neural function, and RNA. Progr. Nucl. Acid Res., 6:187-218.

Jacobson, A. L., Babich, F. R., Bubash, S. and Goren, C. 1966. Maze preferences in naive rats produced by injection of ribonucleic acid from trained rats. Psychon. Sci., 4:3-4.

—Babich, F. P., Bubash, S., and Jacobson, A. 1965. Differential-approach tendencies produced by injection of RNA from trained rats. Science, 150:636-637.

Katz, J. J., and Halstead, W. C. 1950. Protein organization and mental function. Comp. Psychol. Monog., 20:1-38.

Kimble, R. J., and Kimble, D. P. 1966. Failure to find "transfer of training" effects via RNA from trained rats injected into naive rats. Worm Runner's Digest, 8:32-36.

Krech, D., Rosenzweig, M. R., and Bennett, E. L. 1962. Relations between brain chemistry and problem-solving among rats raised in enriched and impoverished environments. J. Comp. Physiol. Psychol., 55:801-807.

Lambert, R., and Saurat, M. 1967. RNA et transfert d'apprentissage: une réplique d'expérience. Bull. du C.E.R.P., 16:435-438.

Laskov, R., Margoliash, E., Littauer, V. Z., and Eisenberg, H. 1959. High molecular weight ribonucleic acid from rat liver. Biochem. Biophys. Acta, 33:247-248.

Leaf, R. C., Dutcher, J. D., Horovitz, Z. P., and Carlton, P. L. 1966. Failure to obtain memory transfer after intraperitoneal injections of RNA from trained rats. Supplementary material to W. L. Byrne et al. Science, 153:658-659.

Loewi, O. 1921. Über humorale Übertragbarkeit der Herznervenwirkung. Pflügers Arch. Ges. Physiol., 189:239-242.

Luttges, M., Johnson, T., Buck, C., Holland, J., and McGaugh, J., 1966. An examination of "transfer of learning" by nucleic acid. Science, 151:834-837.

McConnell, J. V. 1962. Memory transfer via cannibalism in planaria. J. Neuropsychiat., 3:1-42.

Monné, L. 1948. Functioning of the cytoplasm. Advances Enzym. 8:1-69.
Moos, W. S., LeVan, H., Mason, B. T., Mason, H. C., and Hebron, D. L. 1969. Radiation induced avoidance behavior transfer by brain extracts of mice. Experientia, 25:1215-1219.
Neuhoff, V., Von der Haar, F., Schlimme, E., and Weise, M. 1969. Zweidimensionale Chromatographie von Dansyl-Aminosäuren im pico-Mol-Bereich, angewandt zur direkten Charakterisierung von Transfer-Ribonucleinsäuren. Hoppe-Seyler's Z. Physiol. Chem., 350:121-128.
Nissen, T., Røigaard-Petersen, H. H., and Fjerdingstad, E. J. 1965. Effect of ribonucleic acid (RNA) extracted from the brain of trained animals on learning in rats. Scand. J. Psychol., 6:265-272.
Reinis, S. 1965. The formation of conditioned reflexes in rats after the parenteral administration of brain homogenate. Activ. Nerv. Sup. (Praha), 7:167.
—1966. Influence of brain homogenate injection on the speed of the formation of alimentary conditioned reflex in rats. Worm Runner's Digest, 8:7-24.
Revusky, S. H., and DeVenuto, F. 1967. Attempt to transfer aversion to saccharin solution by injection of RNA from trained to naive rats. J. Biol. Psychol., 9:18-22.
Røigaard-Petersen, H. H., Nissen, T., and Fjerdingstad, E. J. 1968. Effect of ribonucleic acid (RNA) extracted from the brain of trained animals on learning in rats. III. Results obtained with an improved procedure. Scand. J. Psychol., 9:1-16.
Rosenblatt, F. 1969. Behavior induction by brain extracts: a comparison of two procedures. Proc. Nat. Acad. Sci. U.S.A., 64:661-664.
—1970a. Experiments on behavioral induction by means of brain extracts. *In* Molecular Approaches to Learning and Memory. Byrne, W. L., ed. AAAS Symposium. 1967. New York, Academic Press, Inc. (In press.)
—1970b. Induction of behavior by mammalian brain extracts. *In* Molecular Mechanisms in Memory and Learning. Ungar, G., ed. New York, Plenum Press. (In press.)
—Farrow, J. T., and Herblin, W. F. 1966a. Transfer of conditioned responses from trained rats to untrained rats by means of a brain extract. Nature (London), 209:46-48.
—and Rhine, S. 1966b. The transfer of learned behavior from trained to untrained rats by means of brain extracts, I. Proc. Nat. Acad. Sci. U.S.A., 55:548-555.
—and Rhine, S. 1966c. The transfer of learned behavior from trained to untrained rats by means of brain extracts, II. Proc. Nat. Acad. Sci. U.S.A., 55:787-792.
Rosenthal, E., and Sparber, S. B. 1968. Transfer of a learned response by chick brain homogenate fed to naive donors. The Pharmacologist, 10:168.
Shashoua, V. E. 1968. RNA changes in goldfish brain during learning. Nature (London), 217:238-240.
Siegel, S. 1956. Non-parametric Statistics. New York, McGraw-Hill Book Company.
Smits, S. E. and A. E. Takemori. 1968. Lack of transfer of morphine tolerance by administration of rat cerebral homogenates. Proc. Soc. Exp. Biol. Med., 127:1167-1171.
Tirri, R. 1967. Transfer of induced tolerance to morphine and promazine by brain homogenates. Experientia, 4:278.
Ungar, G. 1967a. Chemical transfer of acquired information. Proc. of the Fifth Int. Cong. of the Collegium Internationale Neuropsychopharmacologicum. Amsterdam, Excerpta Medica, pp. 169-175.
—1967b. Transfer of learned behavior by brain extracts. J. Biol. Psychol., 9:12-27.
—1968. Molecular mechanisms in learning. Perspect. Biol. Med., 11:217-232.
—1970a. Chemical transfer of learned behavior. *In* Symposium on Protein Metabolism in the Nervous System. Lajtha, A., ed. New York, Academic Press, Inc. (In press.)
—1970b. Role of proteins and peptides in learning and memory. *In* Molecular Mechanisms in Memory and Learning. Ungar, G., ed. New York, Plenum Press. (In press.)
—1970c. Chemical transfer of learned behavior. Agents and Actions. (In press.)
—1970d. Chemical transfer of information. *In* Handbook of Neurochemistry. Lajtha, A., ed. New York, Plenum Press. (In press.)

—1970e. Molecular mechanisms in information processing. Intern. Rev. Neurobiol. (In press.)
—and Chapouthier, G. 1970. Mécanismes moléculaires de l'utilisation de l'information par le cerveau. L'Année Psychologique. (In press.)
—and Cohen, M. 1966. Induction of morphine tolerance by material extracted from brain of tolerant animals. Int. J. Neuropharmacol., 5:183-192.
—and Fjerdingstad, E. J. Chemical nature of the transfer factors; RNA or protein? Proceedings of the Symposium on Biology of Memory, Tihany, Hungary, September 1-4, 1969. Hungarian Academy of Science. (In press.)
—and Galvan, L. 1969. Conditions of transfer of morphine tolerance by brain extracts. Proc. Soc. Exp. Biol. Med., 130:287-291.
—and Irwin, L. N. 1967. Transfer of acquired information by brain extracts. Nature (London), 214:453-455.
—and Irwin, L. N. 1968. Chemical correlates of neural function. *In* Neurosciences. Ehrenpreis, S. and Solnitzky, O. C., eds. New York, Academic Press. Inc., Vol. 1, pp. 73-142.
—and Oceguera-Navarro, C. 1965. Transfer of habituation by material extracted from brain. Nature (London), 207:301-302.
—Galvan, L. and Clark, R. H. 1968. Chemical transfer of learned fear. Nature (London), 217:1259-1261.
—Ho, I. K., and Galvan, L. Isolation of a dark avoidance-inducing brain peptide. Fed. Proc. (In press.)
Wagner, A. R., Gardner, F., and Galambos, R. 1966. Preliminary report: An attempt to produce inter-animal transfer of brightness discrimination via brain extract. Supplementary material to W. L. Byrne et al. Science, 153:658-659.
Weiss, K. 1968. Measurement of the effects of brain extract on inter-organism information transfer. *In* Molecular Approaches to Learning and Memory. Byrne, W. L., ed. AAAS Symposium, 1967. New York, Academic Press, Inc. (In press.)
Wilcoxon, F. and Wilcox, R. A. 1964. Some Rapid Approximate Statistical Procedures. Pearl River, N.Y., Lederle.
Wolthuis, O. L. 1969. Inter-animal information transfer by brain extracts. Arch. Intern. Pharmacodyn., 182:439-442.
—Anthoni, J. F., and Stevens, W. F. 1969. Interanimal transfer of information by brain extracts. Acta Physiol. Pharmacol. Neerl., 15:93.
Zemp, J. W., Wilson, J. E., Schlesinger, K., Boggan, W. O., and Glassman, E. 1966. Brain function and macromolecules, I. Incorporation of uridine into RNA of mouse brain during short-term training experience. Proc. Nat. Acad. Sci. U.S.A., 55:1423-1431.
—Wilson, J. E., Schlesinger, K., and Glassman, E., Boggan, W. O. 1967. Brain function and macromolecules, II. Site of increased labeling of RNA in brains of mice during a short-term training experience. Proc. Nat. Acad. Sci. U.S.A., 58:1120-1125.
Zippel, H. P., and Domagk, G. F. 1969. Versuche zur chemischen Gedächtnisübertragung von farbdressierten Goldfischen auf undressierte Tiere. Experientia, 25:938-940.

CHAPTER 17

Phosphate Compound Analyses

G. Fawaz and E. N. Fawaz

Department of Pharmacology, School of Medicine, American University of Beirut, Beirut, Lebanon

INTRODUCTION

At the beginning of this century, phosphorus compounds were of interest mainly to the chemical anatomist. Phosphorus was known to be a constituent of phospholipids, nucleic acids, bone, and urine. The existence of free nucleotides in tissues was also known, for Liebig isolated inosinic acid more than a century ago. In 1905 Harden and Young were the first to discover the role of phosphorus in metabolism. They observed that inorganic phosphate stimulated carbohydrate breakdown in yeast juice. They subsequently isolated from these extracts fructose-1,6-diphosphate, the ester that still bears their name. The discovery of phosphocreatine (PC) and adenosine triphosphate (ATP) in 1927 and 1929 respectively emphasized the fundamental role of phosphorus in muscle biochemistry. Fiske and Subbarow, the Eggletons and Lohmann were the main pioneers in this field. In the early thirties the importance of phosphoric esters in intermediary metabolism became known due to the elucidation of the elaborate mechanism of glycolysis and fermentation in the laboratories of Embden, Meyerhof and Parnas. Fritz Lipmann, in the early forties, suggested that such phosphorylated intermediates represent a way by means of which cells store their chemical energy. He also introduced the concept of high- and low-energy phosphate bonds which was received enthusiastically and gave a tremendous impetus to research in all fields of biology.

We now know that practically all energy obtained from glycolysis or fermentation and from oxidation of metabolites as well as from photosynthesis is mainly stored in the form of adenosine triphosphate. The oxidation of one molecule of glucose, for instance, results in the synthesis of more than thirty molecules of ATP from adenosine diphosphate (ADP) and inorganic phosphate (oxidative phosphorylation). The energy in ATP is then utilized for all metabolic processes requiring energy, such as muscle contraction, glandular secretion, membrane transport, or synthesis of macromolecules. It is thus no wonder that pharmacologists are interested in phosphorus compounds in their attempt to elucidate the mechanism of action of drugs and toxins, and we often read of the effect of drugs on oxidative phosphorylation, membrane phenomena, muscle contraction, etc.

Inorganic phosphate can be estimated by chemical methods: gravimetric or colorimetric. These methods can also be applied to organic phosphorus compounds by splitting off their phosphate groups with acid. As the stabilities of organic phosphates vary greatly with the normality of the acid and with temperature, "differential hydrolysis" can serve as a basis for their estimation. The most generally known colorimetric method is that of Fiske and Subbarow (1925). It has been in use for over forty years and is quite reliable. In the past, one had to separate a compound in order to identify it. This was done by fractional precipitation. Such procedures often presented serious difficulties, and the separation was not clear-cut in all cases. The advent of chromatography, especially paper chromatography, was a great advance with regard to completeness of separation. The same can be said of enzymatic methods, introduced during the past decade, although the principles on which they are based (Warburg) are thirty years old. This is because crystalline enzymes and coenzymes with a great degree of purity became commercially available only recently. The enzymatic methods offer the advantage of sensitivity, speed, and specificity and do not require prior isolation of the P compounds. The combination of enzymology with fluorimetry has increased the sensitivity to such an extent that it is now possible to measure a 10^{-16} M solution of ATP, and thus determine the ATP content of a single cell!

In this chapter, chemical methods for estimation of phosphocreatine (PC), sum of inorganic phosphate and phosphocreatine (Pi + PC), hydrolyzable phosphorus (H), and total acid soluble phosphorus (T) are described. Enzymatic methods for the estimation of ATP and PC, ADP and AMP, inorganic phosphate (Pi), and the phosphorus-containing glycolytic intermediates are also described. For paper chromatographic methods, which require more time, the reader is referred to publications from Fleckenstein's laboratory (Gerlach et al., 1963).

PREPARATION OF TISSUES FOR ANALYSIS

The speed with which a tissue must be "fixed" depends on the tissue as well as the phosphorus compound to be analyzed. Enzymatically, phosphocreatine is the most labile phosphorus ester known so far. It is extremely sensitive to hypoxia, so much so that we use the level of phosphocreatine in the mammalian heart to tell us whether or not hypoxia of cardiac tissue had occurred.

To obtain specimens of heart tissue the chest should be opened under artificial respiration and a sample obtained by a method of freezing in situ. Eränkö (1954) first introduced this method for freeze-drying and he used two precooled aluminum blocks which formed the head of a forceps. Wollenberger's method (1958) employs pliers instead of forceps and is much better adapted for obtaining larger specimens, such as from a dog heart. The values for dog heart PC obtained by this method of "clamp-freezing" are about 25 percent higher than those obtained by the "cut-freezing" technique (Fawaz and Manoukian, 1962).

It is important to powder the frozen sample finely without allowing it to thaw *before* treating it with trichloracetic or perchloric acid. Failure to do so can result, depending on the size of the sample, in a loss of as much as 70 percent of the PC content. This was experimentally demonstrated by Fawaz and Hawa in 1953, yet low steady-state values of PC continue to be reported in the literature due to failure to observe this simple precaution.

To summarize, if 1 to 2 μ moles PC per g wet dog cardiac tissue is reported (normal 7 to 9) it could mean one of three things: (a) the heart suffered from ischemia or hypoxemia before obtaining the sample, (b) the method of fixation was not adequate, (c) the preparation of the extract was faulty.

Phosphocreatine in brain is most sensitive to hypoxia: scooping a sample with a spoon and dipping it immediately in liquid air results in hydrolysis of the major part of PC. The discovery of PC in brain was made possible by slowly pouring liquid air on the exposed skull or brain of an animal under artificial respiration (Kerr, 1935). For skeletal muscle it is permissible to cut a piece of tissue with a razor and immediately immerse it in liquid air provided the weight of the sample does not exceed 2 g.

PREPARATION OF PROTEIN-FREE EXTRACTS

REAGENTS:

1. Perchloric acid, about 0.65 N. Dilute 5.6 ml $HClO_4$ A.R. sp. gr. 1.67 (70 percent w/v) to 100 ml with glass-redistilled water.
2. Phenolphthalein, 0.5 percent in 50 percent alcohol. Dissolve 250 mg phenolphthalein in 25 ml of absolute ethanol and dilute to 50 ml with glass-redistilled water.
3. 15 percent KOH w/v.

NECESSARY EQUIPMENT FOR EXTRACTION OF ABOUT 1 g OF TISSUE:

Glass-stoppered Erlenmeyer flask of 25-ml capacity and a wide-necked funnel to fit loosely into its neck; porcelain mortar 10 to 12 cm inside diameter and a heavy pestle; forceps; spatulas.

PROCEDURE:

Pipette into an Erlenmeyer flask 6 ml of 0.65 N $HClO_4$ and weigh accurately. Dip spatulas and immerse a wide-necked funnel in liquid air. Pour successively portions of liquid air into the porcelain mortar to chill it well. Weigh quickly a piece of frozen tissue, about 1 g, on a torsion balance and pulverize it finely in the chilled mortar, adding liquid air at frequent intervals during the process to avoid thawing of the tissue. Transfer the powder into the preweighed flask containing acid using the chilled wide-necked funnel and spatulas without allowing the tissue powder to touch the warm neck of the flask. Stopper the flask, shake vigorously to disperse the powder, and reweigh. Place the flask in crushed ice and shake occasionally. In the meantime, readjust the volume of perchloric acid to obtain a 1:10 ratio of tissue to acid. (Weight of tissue powder in g × 9.2 gives the total volume of acid in ml to be used, considering the water content of the tissue to be 80 percent.) Allow 10 minutes for extraction, counting from the time of transfer of powder into acid. Filter quickly using dry fluted filter paper or centrifuge maintaining the temperature between 0° and 4°C all through. Neutralize in the cold, without delay adding 5 μl of phenolphthalein per 1 ml of acid extract and titrating carefully with 15 percent KOH until a faint pink color persists. It is important not to overneutralize. A total of about 0.25 ml KOH per 1 ml extract is required. Keep in ice for 15 minutes to allow the $KClO_4$ to settle. Centrifuge in the cold and store the filtrate in the refrigerator at around 4°C. If it is not possible to perform the necessary determinations within the next 12 hours, keep the neutralized extract frozen until use. It is clear that the frozen powder should not be allowed to thaw at any time before extraction.

If liquid air or liquid nitrogen is not available, a CO_2-snow-ether mixture (−90°C) may be used for freezing. The frozen sample is quickly blotted with filter paper, weighed quickly and accurately in a weighing bottle, powdered with sufficient CO_2-snow to prevent thawing and transferred quantitatively to the acid.

REMARKS:

Trichloracetic acid (10 percent w/v) instead of $HClO_4$ may be used for deproteinization. It is actually recommended when estimation of phosphorus is to be done only by the colorimetric method. Such extracts, however, are not suitable for any enzymatic determinations, as the trichloracetate ion inhibits and denatures many enzymes.

The 1:10 ratio of tissue to acid is arbitrary but convenient for calculation. However, any other ratio may be chosen, provided the acid is sufficient to denature the proteins and extract the soluble phosphorus fraction. With liver, for example, one may use a 1:5 dilution. Every gram of liver would then be extracted with 4.2 ml of acid. Liver tissue has a rather low phosphorus content, and it is advantageous to have a more concentrated extract. Some workers extract tissues with less concentrated acid, probably fearing the instability of PC in acid. In our experience, 10 minutes exposure of PC to 0.6 N $HClO_4$ in the cold results in no loss. In fact, Furchgott and De Gubareff (1958) observed no loss even after one hour. Although 0.3 N acid and a 1:10 dilution was used for some time in our laboratory, we found it unsatisfactory, since traces of some enzymes escaped denaturation and interfered with enzymatic assays.

Perchloric acid extracts are sometimes neutralized with K_2CO_3, instead of KOH, using methyl orange as indicator. This procedure has an advantage because some phosphorus compounds are unstable in alkaline solutions. Dihydroxyacetone phosphate (DHAP) is the best example. Its phosphate splits off within a few minutes in 1 N NaOH. Consequently, if an extract contains alkali-labile compounds they may not be stable at pH 9, which is the minimum pH obtainable in extracts neutralized to phenolphthalein, but sufficiently stable at pH 5 or 6.

Neutralization with K_2CO_3 has also a disadvantage. It sometimes results in faulty PC values when the Fiske and Subbarow method is used. This happens when freshly overneutralized extracts are used, in which case $CaCl_2$ fails to precipitate all the inorganic phosphate. As a result, we recommend careful neutralization with KOH. If any alkali-unstable compounds are to be determined, keep a portion of the acid extract aside and neutralize just a few minutes before it is needed. Alkali-labile compounds are generally stable in acid media.

The procedure described above is convenient for samples weighing as little as 300 mg of wet tissue. In order to powder smaller samples special devices have been used—e.g., the cartridge used for low-temperature powdering by Seraydarian et al. (1961).

DETERMINATION OF ACID-SOLUBLE PHOSPHORUS COMPOUNDS BASED ON THE COLORIMETRIC METHOD OF FISKE AND SUBBAROW

REAGENTS:

1. Phosphate standard of 1 μmole Pi per ml. Dissolve 136.1 mg KH_2PO_4 A.R., previously dried in a dessicator over concentrated H_2SO_4, in 1 liter of glass-redistilled water. This solution can also be used as a standard for the enzymatic assay of Pi.
2. 10 N H_2SO_4.
3. 5 N HCl.
4. Molybdate I: 2.5 percent ammonium molybdate in 5 N H_2SO_4. Dissolve 25 g of powdered $(NH_4)_6Mo_7O_{24} \cdot 4H_2O$ A.R. in 200 ml of water, transfer quantitatively into a liter volumetric flask containing 500 ml of 10 N H_2SO_4, dilute to the mark with distilled water and mix.
5. Molybdate II: 2.5 percent ammonium molybdate in 3 N H_2SO_4. Prepare as molybdate I but use only 300 ml of 10 N H_2SO_4.
6. Molybdate III: 8.3 percent ammonium molybdate in 3⅓ N H_2SO_4. Dissolve

50 g of powdered $(NH_4)_6Mo_7O_{24} \cdot 4H_2O$ A.R. in 400 ml of water and add 200 ml of 10 N H_2SO_4.

7. Reducer: 0.25 percent 1,2,4-amino-naphthol sulfonic acid with sodium sulfite and bisulfite.

   Powder mixture: Transfer into a mortar 2 g Na_2SO_3 A.R., 57 g $NaHSO_3$ A.R. and 1 g of 1,2,4-amino-naphthol sulfonic acid and mix thoroughly with a pestle but do not grind. Amino-naphthol sulfonic acid has to be of good grade. Eastman Grade of Eastman Kodak is satisfactory and no purification is necessary. Preserve powder mixture in a brown bottle.

   Solution: Dissolve 7.5 g of the powder mixture in 47 ml of water. Fresh solutions may not filter clear, so it is advisable to dissolve the powder a day before and filter before use. Store solution in a brown bottle at room temperature. It keeps for about a week.
8. 10 percent calcium chloride saturated with calcium hydroxide. Dissolve 10 g of anhydrous $CaCl_2$ A.R. in about 80 ml of distilled water in a glass-stoppered graduated cylinder, add 2 g $Ca(OH)_2$ A.R., shake vigorously, make up to 100 ml with distilled water. Transfer contents including the undissolved $Ca(OH)_2$ into a bottle and allow to settle. Use supernatant.

Principle of the Method of "Fractional" Hydrolysis

Only inorganic phosphate is estimated by the method of Fiske and Subbarow. The blue color that develops is due to reduction of phosphomolybdic acid, and its intensity is proportional to the amount of phosphate present. Organic phosphorus compounds have to be converted by acid hydrolysis to inorganic phosphate before they can be estimated. Since they differ in their stability to acid, this serves as a basis for their estimation. For convenience, one can group organic phosphorus compounds present in tissue extracts as follows:

1. Those that liberate inorganic phosphate at room temperature while in contact with the reagents
2. Those that are hydrolyzed by 1 N HCl at 100°C within 7 to 10 minutes
3. The remaining compounds which need more drastic methods to yield inorganic phosphate

Generally, four different types of determinations are carried out:

1. Sum of inorganic phosphate and phosphocreatine (Pi + PC)
2. Phosphocreatine alone (PC)
3. Hydrolyzable phosphorus (H)
4. Total acid-soluble phosphorus (T)

Phosphocreatine is hydrolyzed completely in 0.5 N H_2SO_4 at room temperature (20° to 25°C) in 30 minutes upon addition of molybdate, which acts as a catalyst. Under these conditions ATP is not hydrolyzed, and phosphocreatine values so obtained agree with those obtained by the more specific enzymatic method. Hydrolysis in 1 N HCl at 100°C for 7 minutes liberates, of course, all the phosphate from PC and in addition two thirds of the P of ATP and one half the P of ADP without affecting such stable esters as glucose-6-phosphate and glycerophosphate. This procedure gives fairly accurate values for resting muscle (as compared with enzymatic methods), since other labile compounds, like phosphopyruvic acid, dihydroxyacetone phosphate (DHAP) and fructose 1,6-diphosphate, occur in insignificant quantities. However, this method of estimation can yield entirely misleading results when some of the latter compounds accumulate—as, for instance, in an iodoacetate-poisoned frog muscle. Lundsgaard found in 1930 that such muscles when stimulated to contracture lose all their PC but retain the "pyrophosphate" (meaning ATP), since the value obtained by 10 minutes hydrolysis in 1 N HCl at 100°C was practically unchanged. We now know (unpublished work from this laboratory) that iodoacetate-poisoned muscles stimulated to contracture contain no ATP at all, and the compound hydrolyzed by hot acid is mainly fructose-1,6-diphosphate.

Several modifications of the original method of Fiske and Subbarow have appeared over the years. For instance, Lowry and Lopez (1946) published a method in which phosphomolybdate is reduced by ascorbic acid at pH 4. Gerlach and Deuticke (1963) adapted the method for use with paper chromatography.

Procedure

It is important to remember that the rate of color development depends on the acidity and on the temperature. The directions call for 0.5 N acid. If the normality is doubled, the rate of color development is slowed down significantly. The three molybdate solutions differ with regard to acidity, since during some determinations extra acid is used for hydrolysis or for digestion of the sample, and to compensate for this, a molybdate with correspondingly less acid is needed. Carefully note the kind and volume of each molybdate solution to be added for each determination:

Molybdate I is used for the determination of Pi in standard, for Pi + PC and for PC. Use 1 ml per final volume of 10 ml.

Molybdate II is used for the determination of "hydrolyzable phosphorus." Again use 1 ml per final volume of 10 ml.

Molybdate III is used for "total acid-soluble phosphorus." Use 0.75 ml for a final volume of 25 ml.

Before adding molybdate, always dilute the contents of the test tube to about two thirds the final volume with distilled water and mix. Watch for turbidity after addition of molybdate. In the determination of PC the turbidity is due to $CaSO_4$ and it is centrifuged off, not filtered (after the final volume has been adjusted). Any other turbidity demands centrifugation, and if the precipitate is blue the determination is of no value. One may obtain such a precipitate when the deproteinization is incomplete and the blue color is due to a protein-phosphomolybdate complex.

The same amount of reducer is used for all determinations: 0.4 ml per final volume of 10 ml. Start the stopwatch upon addition of reducer.

The color development is temperature-dependent, but 10 minutes is ample time at room temperature. After the 10-minute period the color continues to deepen but at a slow rate. If the measurements require a long time it is good practice to reread a standard in between measurements and at the end.

For colorimetric measurements any simple spectrophotometer may be used. The absorption is essentially the same in the range of 700 to 900 with the maximum at 860 $m\mu$ (Lowry). Lower ranges, however, give satisfactory results, and we use 660 $m\mu$ with the Coleman Junior spectrophotometer, which is very suitable for routine work. The newer model, Junior II, goes as high as 825 $m\mu$, and a higher wavelength may be chosen for measurement.

It is important to note that the color development follows Beer's law at all concentrations provided a high-quality instrument is used. When the simpler instruments are used, errors may occur when the color of the unknown solution is too deep. To remedy this, more than one standard solution is prepared so that the readings of standard and unknown do not fall too far apart.

Sum of Inorganic Phosphate and Phosphocreatine (Pi + PC)

Pipette an appropriate sample of neutralized tissue extract into a test tube graduated at 10 ml, dilute with distilled water, add 1 ml of molybdate I, mix and keep for one-half hour at room temperature (25° to 30°C) to allow the PC to be hydrolyzed. If room temperature drops below 25° keep the tube in a water bath at 30°, as the hydrolysis is strongly temperature-dependent. At the end of the half-hour period add 0.4 ml of reducer, adjust volume to 10 ml with distilled water, and mix thoroughly (this can be done by closing the tube with a clean thumb or palm of your hand and inverting three or four times) and allow 10 minutes for color development. Choose the sample according to the kind of extract analyzed. Since Pi does not vary much from tissue to tissue and is rather low, it is the PC level that determines the size of the sample. PC is high in skeletal muscle, lower in heart, and absent from liver (exception: cat liver). In case of rat tissue extracts, the volume of the sample should be around 0.3 ml for muscle, 0.7 ml for heart, and 1 ml or more for liver.

Phosphocreatine (PC)

In this estimation, all Pi is first precipitated at pH 9 with alkaline $CaCl_2$, and the PC that remains in solution is then hydrolyzed.

To 3 ml of neutralized extract (KOH and phenolphthalein) in a centrifuge tube, add 1 ml $CaCl_2$ saturated with $Ca(OH)_2$, mix, let stand for 10 minutes, centrifuge or filter through a dry filter paper. Pipette 3 ml of the above filtrate into a large test tube calibrated at 15 or 25 ml, dilute sample with distilled water, mix, and add molybdate I (1.5 ml if final volume is to be 15, and 2.5 ml if final volume is to be 25 ml). Follow then the procedure as described for Pi + PC. (Since 0.4 ml of reducer per 10 ml final volume is the prescribed quantity, use 0.6 ml for the final volume of 15, and 1 ml for the final volume of 25 ml.) Centrifuge off the precipitate of $CaSO_4$. This is done during the 10-minute period of color development.

The volume of extract suggested here is satisfactory for fresh skeletal muscles fixed and extracted properly. Where the PC is expected to be low, use a larger volume of extract if available and or reduce the final volume to as low as 5 ml so the optical density reading does not reach below 0.1.

PRECAUTIONS. Do not overneutralize the acid extract, as this would lead to precipitation of $Ca(OH)_2$ which usually carries with it a significant part of the PC. A similar situation may arise when there is too much Pi in the test solution. The voluminous phosphate adsorbs some of the PC. This does not happen normally in tissue extracts unless large amounts of Pi have been added to it.

Unreasonably high values of PC and "false positives" are obtained in tissues that may contain more than 2 percent glycogen, such as liver and diaphragm. In extracts of such tissues, $CaCl_2$ does not precipitate Pi completely. Under such conditions PC must be estimated enzymatically or by paper chromatography.

Hydrolyzable Phosphorus (H)

Unneutralized extracts are generally used in this determination. If a neutralized extract is used, add a measured amount of acid sufficient to decolorize phenolphthalein.

Pipette into a test tube, calibrated at 10 ml, a sample of extract. Suggested volumes for rat tissue extracts: skeletal muscle 0.3 ml, heart muscle 0.5 ml, liver 0.8 to 1 ml. For dog tissue extracts use larger samples, as the phosphorus content is normally lower than in rat. Now add distilled water to obtain a volume of 1.6 ml (if acid was used to decolorize sample, account for its volume), add 0.4 ml of 5 N HCl, mix, and immerse the tube in a large volume of briskly boiling water. Keep for exactly 7 minutes, immerse the tube immediately in cold water, dilute contents to around 7 ml with distilled water, add 1 ml of molybdate II, mix, then add 0.4 ml reducer, adjust volume to 10 ml, mix thoroughly, and allow 10 minutes for color development.

Total Acid-Soluble Phosphorus (T)

Total acid-soluble phosphorus is performed in large thick-walled Pyrex test tubes calibrated at 25 ml. For samples of low phosphorus content, small Kjeldahl flasks are recommended. Choose a size that contains 10 ml when the calibration mark can be drawn on the neck of the flask. The samples consist of neutralized or unneutralized trichloracetic or perchloric acid extracts.

Pipette into the test tube 0.5 ml of sample and 1 ml of 10 N H_2SO_4, add two small glass beads, and boil gently over a small flame (avoid bumping). Let the water evaporate, and when white fumes of SO_3 appear, cover the tube loosely with a glass stopper. Keep on digesting for 2 minutes. Remove tube from the flame, allow to cool, and add a drop of concentrated nitric acid. Boil again for 5 minutes. After cooling the tube, lift the glass-stopper cover and rinse the part exposed to fumes with distilled water, collecting rinsings into the tube. Rinse also the walls of the tube. Boil again for about 3 minutes to hydrolyze any pyrophosphate that might have been formed during the digestion process (avoid bumping).

Dilute with water, add 0.75 ml of molybdate III and mix, add 1 ml reducer, adjust volume to 25 ml, mix, and allow 10 minutes for color development. If Kjeldahl flasks calibrated at 10 ml are used, keep the above proportions: use 0.4 ml 10 N H_2SO_4 for digestion, 0.3 ml molybdate III and 0.4 ml reducer.

Blank and Standard

It is necessary to run in parallel a blank and a standard for each set of determinations. The blank is used to set the instrument at 100 percent transmittance and the standard is needed for the calculation.

To prepare the blank, add 2.5 ml of molybdate I into a test tube calibrated at 25 ml and dilute with distilled water. Do the same for the standard but include 1 ml of standard phosphate solution. An additional, more concentrated standard may also be prepared using 1 ml of standard in a final volume of 10 ml. The addition of reducer and final dilution are done simultaneously with the unknown samples and not before. Arrange all tubes in a certain order: blank, standard, unknown 1,2,3, etc. Add reducer to all, in succession, starting with the blank. Adjust volumes, mix, and read each one after 10 minutes (stopwatch) from the time the reducer was added. If color of any test solution is too deep, dilute 1:1 with the blank solution and read.

Calculations of Results

The following is an example of an analysis performed on a rat skeletal muscle extract.

Five ml of acid extract (dilution 1:10) were neutralized with 1.20 ml of 15 percent KOH after addition of 0.025 ml phenolphthalein. Thus 10 ml × 6.225/5 = 12.45 ml of neutralized extract correspond to 1 g tissue. Neutralized extract was used in all determinations. For the estimation of PC, 3 ml of neutralized extract were treated with 1 ml of $CaCl_2$ and 3 ml of filtrate were used, so that for PC estimation an extra dilution factor of 4/3 is used.

Type of determination	Volume of sample	Final volume	Optical density
Standard 1	2 ml standard	25 ml	0.285
Standard 2	1 ml standard	10 ml	0.360
Pi + PC	0.4 ml extract	10 ml	0.369
PC	3 ml of $CaCl_2$ filtrate	25 ml	0.277*
H	0.3 ml extract	10 ml	0.404
T	0.5 ml extract	25 ml	0.340

*Read after diluting 1:1 with the blank solution

To express phosphate in μ moles per 1 g of wet tissue, one calculates as follows:

$$\text{Pi + PC: } \frac{0.369}{0.360} \times 1 \times \frac{12.45}{0.4} = 31.8$$

$$\text{PC:} \quad \frac{0.277}{0.285} \times 2 \times \frac{12.45}{3} \times \frac{4}{3} \times 2 = 21.5$$

$$\text{H:} \quad \frac{0.404}{0.360} \times 1 \times \frac{12.45}{0.3} = 46.5$$

$$\text{T:} \quad \frac{0.340}{0.285} \times 2 \times \frac{12.45}{0.5} = 59.3$$

The amount of inorganic phosphate in the rat muscle is 10.3 μ moles per gram wet weight: (Pi + PC) - PC. The amount of phosphate that is liberated during a 7-minute period of hydrolysis in 1 N HCl at 100° is H - (Pi + PC), or 14.7 μ moles. Since hydrolysis releases 2 μ moles of phosphate per μ mole of ATP, and assuming that in this case the source of phosphate is only ATP, 14.7/2 = 7.35 gives the number of μ moles of ATP present in 1 g of tissue. In resting skeletal muscle the ADP content is low, and this value for ATP is not far from the true value as estimated by enzymatic methods. In the next part of this chapter, values of ATP, ADP, and AMP in this particular extract, obtained by enzymatic methods, are reported.

ENZYMATIC ASSAYS OF PHOSPHORUS COMPOUNDS IN TISSUE EXTRACTS

Principles of Enzymatic Analysis and Technical Details

Most phosphorus-containing metabolites can be determined by making them undergo a series of enzymatic reactions involving at one stage an oxidation or reduction of a pyridine nucleotide molecule. Di- and tri-phosphopyridine nucleotides (DPN and TPN) are the coenzymes of some dehydrogenases, and they exhibit, in their reduced but not in their oxidized form, a characteristic absorption maximum at 340 mμ, which is identical for both. Since proteins and common constituents of tissue extracts do not absorb at this wavelength, this property of pyridine nucleotides makes them useful tools for this type of analysis. A substance that in the course of one or several enzymatic reactions oxidizes or reduces a pyridine nucleotide will bring about a corresponding change in absorbancy at 340 mμ. For quantitative analysis, one uses a small, "limited" amount of a substrate (or cosubstrate) and a large excess of enzymes and reactants so as to "consume" all the substrate. Needless to say, this is only possible with reactions whose equilibria favor product formation. If the equilibrium is unfavorable, a quantitative utilization of the substrate may still be achieved by shifting the equilibrium, as by removing one of the products. For example, hydrazine or semicarbazide may be used to trap carbonyl-containing products. High alkalinity shifts equilibria of reactions involving proton formation, as is the case when DPN^+ and TPN^+ are reduced, during which process their quaternary nitrogen atoms change to the tertiary form, resulting in acid formation.

The activity of enzymes in tissue extracts can also be determined by applying the foregoing principles. Here, however, one uses a small, "limited" amount of nondeproteinized extract as the source of the enzyme, and a large excess of substrate. The initial rate of the reaction usually follows zero order kinetics, and the amount of substrate converted per unit time reflects the activity of the enzyme. Such determinations of enzyme activities are more complex than estimations of substrate levels.

It is rather simple to determine the activity of an isolated enzyme, and it is often necessary to do that—as, for example, when one uses enzymes as "reagents" for estimating phosphorus compounds. It may be necessary to check the purity of an enzyme or to find out how much activity has been lost owing to prolonged or improper storage. Commercial firms that sell enzymes usually provide directions for such assays. They also use the specific activity of each enzyme preparation as a criterion of purity. Specific activity is defined as the activity in units per mg enzyme protein. An "international unit" as defined by Racker (Cooper et al, 1958) is the amount of enzyme that converts 1 μmole of substrate per minute at 25°C and at optimum substrate concentration, optimum ionic buffer strength, and optimum pH. Racker units are used in this chapter. In 1959 the Enzyme Commission of the International Union of Biochemistry also proposed an international nomenclature for enzymes and coenzymes. For instance, the proposed names for DPN and TPN are NAD and NADP, respectively (nicotinamide adenine dinucleotide and nicotinamide adenine dinucleotide phosphate). The new names are chemically more meaningful, but we are retaining the old names in this chapter as they are probably more familiar to pharmacologists.

This section is devoted to the determination of phosphorus-containing metabolites and not enzyme activities. The latter will be described only as need arises. The methods described have been in use in this laboratory during the past ten years and are continuously revised. Some have been developed here (Fawaz and Fawaz, 1962; Fawaz et al., 1962, 1966) and others are modifications of methods developed in Professor Bücher's laboratory (Munich) or in the Boehringer laboratory (Tutzing). For a comprehensive treatise on enzymatic analysis consult Bergmeyer's *Methods of Enzymatic Analysis* (1963, New York, Academic Press).

EQUIPMENT:

Beckman spectrophotometer Model B or any equivalent instrument suitable for measurements at 340 mμ or proximity.

Cuvettes, semimicro, light path 10 mm, width 4 mm, height 45 mm, made of special optical glass (purchased from Hellma, Müllheim, Baden, Germany).

Marburg microliter pipettes for delivery of 5, 10, 20, 50 and 500 μl (obtainable from Eppendorf Gerätebau, Hamburg, Germany).

Plungers cut from thin polyethylene rods, bent and flattened at one end (preferably flattened with hot tweezers to give a groovy surface, convenient for holding small volumes of fluids).

REMARKS AND PRECAUTIONS: Semimicrocuvettes are used for reasons of economy. Since they are only 4 mm wide, one must make sure that the entire beam of radiation traverses them during the measurement. The Beckman spectrophotometer Model B was not designed for use with microcuvettes. Its simplicity of operation, however, makes it ideal for routine enzymatic work and a few precautionary measures will take care of its deficiencies. To check whether the semimicrocuvettes are in exact light-path, do the following: prepare two stock solutions of DPNH of measurable concentrations, one to give a high and one to give a low optical density. Read the two solutions using an ordinary-sized cuvette and a semimicrocuvette in all positions of the cuvette holder (carriage). If more than one carriage is in use, test them all out in a similar way, as their dimensions may differ. Subtract the low readings from the corresponding high readings and compare the values obtained. If they differ significantly, adjustment of the screws controlling the carriage holder and the entire sample compartment must be made. Switch to red light so as to make the beam visible.

It is important to use enough solution in a cuvette so that only light that passes through the solution will reach the photocell.

As frequent stirring of solution is required, glass rods should be avoided because these shorten the life of the cuvettes. Marburg microliter pipettes are very convenient for delivering small volumes of reagents into the cuvettes. If such pipettes are available, apply the enzyme solutions on to the foot of a polyethylene plunger, as this facilitates mixing in. Most of the procedures for assays of metabolites described by us are adapted for their use. To make the filling of cuvettes more efficient, the concentrations of reagents were designed in such a way that substrates for all assays demand a volume of 50 μl, salts as Mg-acetate and KCl a volume of 20 μl, pyridine nucleotides a volume of 10 μl, etc. If one is familiar with the principle of a method, he only needs to check which amounts of enzymes are to be added, and even this becomes unnecessary with a little experience.

For spectrophotometric measurements, control cuvettes are used to set the transmittance to 100 percent. They are filled with buffer and water in the same proportions used for the tests. Enzymes are introduced to the control cuvette, as they are added to the test cuvettes, but for general routine work this may be omitted in most cases. We also omit the enzyme from the control cuvette if a reagent blank is run with the test. A reagent blank contains everything except the test solution, and it measures the contamination of reagents with the substance that is tested for. Reagent blanks are needed, for instance, in the determination of inorganic phosphate (Pi).

A single reaction for a metabolite determination usually does not take more than 5 to 10 minutes, except the phosphorylase reaction used for Pi determination. Whenever a reaction begins to "drag" it probably means that the activity of the enzyme has deteriorated and more of it should be added. This is rarely necessary, however, since the prescribed amounts of enzymes are usually in great excess.

Only neutralized perchloric extracts should be used for metabolite determinations and to obtain good results a total change in absorption (E) should not exceed 0.400.

All glass equipment should be rinsed with glass-redistilled water after the regular washing procedure. Cuvettes must be frequently cleaned with acid, since traces of enzymes may be left over after insufficient washing, and this may result in serious trouble.

Methods

REAGENTS:

1. Tra-EDTA buffer pH 7.6 (Tra 0.12 M, EDTA 0.012 M). Dissolve 11.15 g of triethanolamine · HCl and 2.23 g of ethylenediaminetetraacetic acid, disodium salt · H_2O (EDTA-Na_2 · H_2O) in glass-redistilled water, transfer to a 500-ml volumetric flask and make up to volume adjusting pH to 7.6 with 2 N NaOH (about 12 ml required).
2. Tra buffer pH 7.6 (0.12 M). Prepare as No. 1 but use 2.23 g of triethanolamine · HCl, omit EDTA, and dilute to a volume of 100 ml with adjustment of pH to 7.6.
3. Glycine-EDTA-hydrazine buffer pH 9.5. Stock solution: weigh 2.9 g glycine, 2.0 g hydrazine · H_2SO_4 and 80 mg EDTA-Na_2 · $2H_2O$, dissolve in glass-redistilled water and dilute to 25 ml. Keep refrigerated.
   Buffer proper: to 7 ml of stock solution add 5 N NaOH (about 2.1 ml) and water to get a pH of 9.5 and a volume of 10 ml. Check pH with pH meter. Prepare buffer weekly as it gets turbid upon longer storage. It is used for α-glycerophosphate determination.
4. Glucose 0.024 M. Dissolve 47.7 mg of glucose monohydrate in glass-redistilled water and dilute to 10 ml.
5. 3-phosphoglycerate, about 0.12 M. Dissolve 65 mg of 3-phosphoglyceric acid, tricyclohexylammonium salt · $3H_2O$, in 1 ml glass-redistilled water.
6. Phosphoenolpyruvate, about 0.024 M. Dissolve 11 mg of phosphoenolpyruvic acid, tricyclohexylammonium salt, in 1 ml glass-redistilled water.
7. Glycogen, 2 percent. Dissolve 20 mg of glycogen in 1 ml glass-redistilled water.
8. Glutathione (GSH), about 0.1 M. Dissolve 31 mg of gluthione in 0.9 ml of glass-redistilled water, neutralize to about pH 7 with 2 N NaOH (about 0.050 ml required), and add water to a volume of 1 ml.
9. Magnesium acetate 0.3 M. Dissolve 645 mg of $Mg(C_2H_3O_2)_2$ · $4H_2O$ in glass-redistilled water and make up to a volume of 10 ml.
10. Potassium chloride 0.6 M. Dissolve 450 mg of KCl in glass-redistilled water and make up to a volume of 10 ml.
11. DPNH, about 0.015 M. Dissolve 11 mg of reduced diphosphopyridine nucleotide disodium salt in 1 ml of 0.12 M Tra buffer (pH 7.6, no EDTA). Prepare freshly each week.
12. DPN, about 0.075 M. Dissolve 50 mg of diphosphopyridine nucleotide in 1 ml of glass-redistilled water.
13. TPN, about 0.04 M. Dissolve 30 mg of triphosphopyridine nucleotide, monosodium salt, in 1 ml of glass-redistilled water.
14. ATP, about 0.024 M. Dissolve 15 mg of adenosine triphosphate, disodium salt · H_2O, in 1 ml glass-redistilled water.
15. ADP, about 0.024 M. Dissolve 12 mg of adenosine diphosphate, trisodium salt, in 1 ml glass-redistilled water.

16. AMP, about 0.05 M. Dissolve 20 mg of adenosine monophosphate, disodium salt, in 1 ml of glass-redistilled water.
17. Glucose-1,6-diphosphate, about 1.2 mM. Dissolve 1 mg of glucose-1,6-diphosphate, tetrahexylammonium salt · $4H_2O$, in 1 ml glass-redistilled water.
18. 2,3-diphosphoglycerate, about 1.2 mM. Dissolve 1 mg of 2,3-diphosphoglycerate, pentahexylammonium salt · $4H_2O$, in 1 ml glass-redistilled water.

ENZYMES:

Aldolase (ALD) sp. act. 9 units/mg (10 mg protein/ml)
Creatine phosphokinase (CPK) sp. act. 18 units/mg, suspend 20 mg lyophilized powder in 1 ml of 2 M $(NH_4)_2SO_4$ and keep not longer than a month
Enolase (ENOL) sp. act. 27 units/mg (10 mg protein/ml)
Glucose-6-phosphate dehydrogenase (G-6-PDH) sp. act. 140 units/mg (5 mg protein/ml), dilute 1:10 with water before use
Glyceraldehyde-3-phosphate dehydrogenase (GAPDH) sp. act. 36 units/mg (10 mg protein/ml)
α-Glycerophosphate dehydrogenase (GDH) sp. act. 36 units/mg (10 mg protein/ml)
Hexokinase (HK) sp. act. 140 units/mg (2 mg protein/ml)
Lactic dehydrogenase (LDH) sp. act. 360 units/mg (10 mg protein/ml), dilute 1:5 with 2 M $(NH_4)_2SO_4$ or water before use
Myokinase (MK) sp. act. 45 units/mg (5 mg protein/ml)
Phosphoglucomutase (PGluM) sp. act. 6.5 units/mg (10 mg protein/ml)
Phosphoglucoisomerase (PGI) sp. act. 390 units/mg (2 mg protein/ml)
3-Phosphoglycerate kinase (PGK) sp. act. 180 units/mg (10 mg protein/ml)
Phosphoglyceromutase (PGM) sp. act. 18 units/mg (2 mg protein/ml)
Phosphorylase-a (Pho-a): Boehringer Co. supplies 5 mg protein per bottle in form of lyophilized powder. Weigh an amount equivalent to 2 mg of protein (about 14 mg lyophilized powder) and suspend in 1 ml of 0.5 percent glycogen. Keep for 2 hours at room temperature with occasional stirring, then store at 4°C. Keeps for around a month. Always assay before use.
Pyruvic kinase (PK) sp. act. 125 units/mg (2 mg protein/ml)
Triosephosphate isomerase (TIM) sp. act. 2400 units/mg (2 mg protein/ml)
Enzyme mixtures:
GDH-TIM: mix 0.4 ml GDH with 0.1 ml TIM
PGK-GAPDH: mix 0.2 ml PGK with 0.3 ml GAPDH

All reagent solutions are stored in the deep-freeze when not in use except buffers, DPNH, and enzymes suspensions. These are stored at 2° to 4°C.

REAGENTS FOR ASSAY OF PHOSPHORYLASE ACTIVITY:

1. β-glycerophosphate-NaF-EDTA buffer pH 6.9 (β-glycerophosphate 0.035 M, NaF 0.02 M, EDTA 5 mM). Dissolve 1.07 g of β-glycerophosphate, disodium salt · $5H_2O$, 8.4 mg NaF and 186 mg EDTA-Na_2 · H_2O in glass-redistilled water and make up to 100 ml with adjustment of pH to 6.9 (2 N NaOH).

2. Substrate solution (glucose-1-P, about 0.128 M, AMP, about 4 mM). Weigh 47.7 mg of glucose-1-phosphate, dipotassium salt · $2H_2O$ and 1.56 mg AMP-Na_2. Add glass-redistilled water and some HCl (about 0.04 ml 1 N HCl) to get a pH of 6.9 and a volume of 1 ml.
3. 4 percent glycogen.
4. Molybdate 2.5 percent in 4.5 N H_2SO_4. Prepare as molybdate I (see p. 519) but decrease acid correspondingly. Prepare 100 ml only.

The following reagents were obtained from Merck Co. (Darmstadt, Germany): EDTA, glycogen, glucose, KCl, Mg-acetate, and β-glycerophosphate. All the others, including enzymes, were purchased from Boehringer Co. (Mannheim-Waldhof, Germany).

ADENOSINE TRIPHOSPHATE (ATP) AND PHOSPHOCREATINE (PC) DETERMINATION.

It is convenient to assay these two high-energy phosphorus compounds at the same time, in a sequential run. First ATP is made to transfer its terminal phosphate group to an acceptor. Adenosine diphosphate (ADP) so formed may be rephosphorylated by phosphocreatine (PC).

Two methods are in general use for the estimation of ATP. One utilizes hexokinase (HK) where ATP is made to react with glucose, and the other utilizes phosphoglycerate kinase (PGK) in which ATP reacts with 3-phosphoglycerate (3-PG). Both methods are satisfactory and both will be described so that, depending on the availability of enzymes and reagents, either can be used.

Hexokinase Method for ATP and PC

The following enzymes are needed for this method: glucose-6-phosphate dehydrogenase (G-6-PDH), hexokinase (HK), and creatine phosphokinase (CPK). It is best to describe an enzymatic method in terms of the reactions involved.

$$\text{glucose} + \text{ATP} \underset{\text{Mg}^{++}}{\overset{\text{HK}}{\rightleftharpoons}} \text{glucose-6-phosphate} + \text{ADP} \qquad (1)$$

$$\text{glucose-6-phosphate} + \text{TPN}^{+} \overset{\text{G-6-PDH}}{\rightleftharpoons} \text{6-phosphogluconate} + \text{TPNH} + \text{H}^{+} \qquad (2)$$

$$\text{phosphocreatine} + \text{ADP} \underset{\text{Mg}^{++}}{\overset{\text{CPK}}{\rightleftharpoons}} \text{creatine} + \text{ATP} \qquad (3)$$

In the presence of HK, Mg ions and an excess of glucose, ATP transfers a phosphate to glucose yielding glucose-6-phosphate (reaction 1). The latter generates TPNH from TPN^+ as it gets dehydrogenated (reaction 2). Equilibria of reactions 1 and 2 are in favor of the reaction products, and so ATP is quantitatively used up: 1 μmole of ATP forms 1 μmole of TPNH. Addition of CPK now starts reaction 3, in which phosphocreatine reacts quantitatively with the ADP generated by reaction 1, so that each μ mole of PC gives 1 μ mole of TPNH.

PROCEDURE:

Pipette into a semimicrocuvette the following reagents: 0.500 ml of Tra-EDTA buffer, 0.050 ml of 0.024 M glucose, 0.040 ml of 0.3 M Mg-acetate, 0.010 ml of 0.04 M TPN, test solution, and water to give a total volume of 1.200 ml including enzymes. Stir contents and measure absorbance at 340 mμ, adjusting first the instrument to 100 percent transmittance with a control cuvette containing 0.500 ml of buffer and 0.700 ml of water. Add enzymes, one at a time, to both control and test cuvettes and take measurements after each addition. First add 5 μl of G-6-PDH (0.5 mg enzyme protein/ml) containing about 0.35 unit. Any change in absorbance (ΔE) will be due to glucose-6-phosphate (G-6-P) present in the test sample. Follow by 5 μl of HK (2 mg enzyme protein/ml), about 1.4 units, and take readings until constant (5 to 10 minutes may be needed). ΔE will measure ATP. Finally add 10 μl of CPK (20 mg enzyme protein/ml), about 3.6 units, and take readings until constant. ΔE will measure PC.

When PC is to be determined in a pure solution, ADP must be included in the filling. Use 10 μl of 2.4 mM ADP freshly diluted from 24 mM ADP solution. Addition of ADP is also necessary for a PC run when ΔE for ATP is 0.05 or less. In that case ADP may be added before introducing CPK to the cuvette (10 μl of 2.4 mM solution).

Reaction 3 is strongly dependent on Mg^{++}. Note that this assay calls for 40 μl of 0.3 M Mg-acetate per cuvette or a final concentration of 10 mM. Only in assays that include PC determination is so much magnesium needed. Otherwise, half the amount is always used.

For calculations, let us consider an example of a neutralized perchloric acid extract obtained from rat skeletal muscle. Thirty microliters were used as a test sample and gave: $\Delta E = 0.093$ for ATP, $\Delta E = 0.270$ for PC. Since the original acid extract (dilution 1:10) was diluted through neutralization by a factor of

$$\frac{6.225}{5} = 1.245$$

1 g of tissue was equivalent to 12.45 ml of neutralized extract. Considering that the μ molar extinction coefficient for TPNH is 6.22 and that the reactions took place in a volume of 1.2 ml, 1 g of wet tissue contained:

$$\text{ATP: } \frac{0.093}{6.22} \times 1.2 \times \frac{12.45}{0.03} = 7.42\ (\mu\text{moles})$$

$$\text{PC: } \frac{0.270}{6.22} \times 1.2 \times \frac{12.45}{0.03} = 21.6\ (\mu\text{moles})$$

By the use of the colorimetric method similar values were obtained for this extract (see pp. 524-525).

PRECAUTIONS: G-6-PDH is practically always contaminated with glutathione reductase (GSSG-R). This enzyme catalyzes the following reaction:

$$\text{GSSG} + \text{TPNH} + \text{H}^+ \xrightarrow{\text{GSSG-R}} 2\,\text{GSH} + \text{TPN}^+$$

If extracts contain GSSG (example, liver), in the presence of the contaminating enzyme, some TPNH that is being generated by the assay system may be reoxidized. One may even observe the "back-run" if one takes readings at very short intervals. It is advisable, therefore, to use the minimum necessary amount of G-6-PDH. If liver extracts are used, take readings every 1 minute and consider the highest reading when calculating ΔE.

Phosphoglycerate Kinase Method

Enzymes needed: 3-phosphoglycerate kinase (PGK), glyceraldehyde-3-phosphate dehydrogenase (GAPDH), and creatine phosphokinase (CPK) if PC is also to be determined. Two more enzymes are optional: triosephosphate isomerase (TIM) and α-glycerophosphate dehydrogenase (GDH). The enzymes catalyze the following reactions:

$$\text{3-phosphoglycerate} + \text{ATP} \underset{\text{Mg}^{++}}{\overset{\text{PGK}}{\rightleftharpoons}} \text{1,3-diphosphoglycerate} + \text{ADP} \quad (1)$$

$$\text{1,3-diphosphoglycerate} + \text{DPNH} + \text{H}^+ \overset{\text{GAPDH}}{\rightleftharpoons} \text{glyceraldehyde-3-P} + \text{Pi} + \text{DPN}^+ \quad (2)$$

$$\text{glyceraldehyde-3-phosphate} \overset{\text{TIM}}{\rightleftharpoons} \text{dihydroxyacetonephosphate} \quad (3)$$

$$\text{dihydroxyacetonephosphate} + \text{DPNH} + \text{H} \overset{\text{GDH}}{\rightleftharpoons} \alpha\text{-glycerophosphate} + \text{DPN}^+ \quad (4)$$

$$\text{phosphocreatine} + \text{ADP} \underset{\text{Mg}^{++}}{\overset{\text{CPK}}{\rightleftharpoons}} \text{creatine} + \text{ATP} \quad (5)$$

The equilibrium of reaction 1 is not favorable for 1,3-diphosphoglycerate formation. The equilibrium of reaction 2 however, lies 65 percent to the right, and under the conditions of the assay to be described, utilization of ATP is complete in the presence of a good excess of 3-PG. For each μ mole of ATP, 1 μ mole of DPNH is oxidized. The sensitivity of the method is doubled when reactions 3 and 4 are included. Since equilibrium of reaction 4 lies far to the right, this represents an added advantage. Reaction 5 is used if PC is to be determined. Each molecule of PC will oxidize 2 molecules of DPNH when all the reactions are put to use.

PROCEDURE:

Pipette into a semimicrocuvette 0.500 ml Tra-EDTA, 0.050 ml of 0.12 M 3-PG, 0.040 ml of 0.3 M Mg-acetate, 0.020 ml of 0.1 M GSH, 0.010 ml of 0.015 M DPNH, test solution, and a calculated amount of water to give a final volume of 1.200 ml including enzymes. Stir contents and take an initial reading (E_1). Add 5 μl of GDH-TIM mixture, or about 1.5 units of GDH and 5 units of TIM. Take a few readings at intervals of 1 or 2 minutes until a steady reading (E_2) is obtained. Follow by 5 μl of PGK-GAPDH mixture, or about 3.5 units of PGK and 1.1 units of GAPDH and measure until a steady reading (E_3) is reached. Finally, add 10 μl of CPK, about 3.6 units, and measure until steady (E_4). Enzymes are added not only to the test cuvette but also to the control cuvette which contains buffer and water and serves for the adjustment to 100 percent transmittance before each test reading.

After addition of GDH-TIM, glyceraldehyde phosphate (GAP) and dihydroxyacetone phosphate (DHAP), if present, will "run." The first is not present in tissue extracts, and the second may be found at times if freshly neutralized extracts are used. After addition of PGK-GAPDH, ATP will "run" and $E_3 - E_2$ will give its ΔE value. With this enzymatic setup, 2 μmoles of DPNH will be oxidized for each μmole of ATP used up. After addition of CPK, PC will "run" and $E_4 - E_3$ will give its ΔE value. Here again the ratio of PC utilization to DPNH oxidation is 1:2.

The enzymes are added in pairs to shorten the time of assay. This is a safe procedure because neither 1,3-diphosphoglycerate (1,3-PG) nor glyceraldehyde phosphate (GAP) is found in tissue extracts. If an extract is expected to have a high ATP and PC level, addition of GDH-TIM may be omitted. Under these conditions GAP will be the final reaction product. We find it unnecessary to trap it with carbonyl compounds. It is also not necessary to use reduced glutathione in the filling when fresh enzymes are used.

The following procedure is advantageous with samples whose ATP and PC levels are difficult to predict: Add PGK-GAPDH first and, if the change in readings is satisfactory, follow up with CPK. Under these conditions the ratio of ATP or PC utilization to DPNH oxidation will be 1:1. If, on the other hand, ΔE for ATP is rather low, add GDH-TIM. The ΔE for ATP should double. Introduce, then, 10 μl of ADP into the cuvette (2.4 mM solution, freshly prepared) and follow up with CPK.

To compare the glycerophosphate method with the hexokinase method, we analyzed the same muscle extract that had been assayed with the hexokinase method and which was given as an example for calculation. Thirty μl of this extract with PGK-GAPDH only, gave: $\Delta E = 0.095$ for ATP and $\Delta E = 0.270$ for PC. These are in perfect agreement with the values obtained with the hexokinase method.

Just as one can double the sensitivity of the PGK method by the use of GDH-TIM, it is also possible to achieve the same thing with the hexokinase method by the use of an additional enzyme: 6-phosphogluconic dehydrogenase (6-PGDH), which catalyzes the following reaction:

$$\text{6-phosphogluconate} + TPN^+ \xrightarrow{\text{6-PGDH}} TPNH + H^+ + \text{ribulose-5-phosphate} + CO_2$$

In our laboratory we make use of this reaction but do not apply it to routine assays. We favor the phosphoglycerate method for ATP and PC determination as it gives no trouble with any extracts. The hexokinase method has to be used with caution if extracts contain glutathione.

Finally, it must be mentioned that although enzymes are the most specific reagents known today, some of them react with several chemically related substrates. Hexokinase (HK) and phosphoglycerokinase (PGK) are unfortunately among them. Consequently, both methods for ATP determination are not entirely specific and also measure some of the other triphosphonucleotides, if such are present in the test solution. Depending on the nature of the problem under study and the type of tissue used, this lack of specificity may or may not be neglected. With extracts of skeletal muscle and heart no serious errors arise, but with extracts of liver and kidney the errors may reach up to 20 percent, since the content of triphosphonucleotides, other than ATP, is much higher in the latter tissues. Enzymologists, however, have found a way out of this dilemma They couple a nonspecific reaction with a truly specific one, and thus the whole system becomes specific. In this case this is done by applying a reaction in which myokinase (MK) participates. MK is very specific for adenine nucleotides. For more information on this subject the reader is referred to the work of Gruber et al. (1966).

ADENOSINE DIPHOSPHATE (ADP) AND ADENOSINE MONOPHOSPHATE (AMP) DETERMINATION.

ADP and AMP are determined in the same assay system, in a sequential run. The following enzymes are needed: lactic dehydrogenase (LDH), pyruvic kinase (PK), and myokinase (MK). They catalyze the following reactions:

$$\text{phosphoenolpyruvate} + ADP \underset{Mg^{++}K^+}{\overset{PK}{\rightleftharpoons}} \text{pyruvate} + ATP \quad (1)$$

$$\text{pyruvate} + DPNH + H^+ \overset{LDH}{\rightleftharpoons} \text{lactate} + DPN^+ \quad (2)$$

$$ATP + AMP \underset{Mg^{++}}{\overset{MK}{\rightleftharpoons}} 2\,ADP \quad (3)$$

Phosphoenolpyruvate (excess) in the presence of PK, phosphorylates ADP to give ATP (reaction 1). Pyruvate thus formed oxidizes DPNH in the presence of LDH (reaction 2), and the change in absorption depends on the amount of ADP present in the sample.

To determine AMP, myokinase is used (reaction 3). Here, AMP is phosphorylated by the ATP generated in reaction 1. Note that for each molecule of AMP two molecules of ADP are formed, and consequently two molecules of DPNH are oxidized. The equilibrium of reaction 2 is very much in favor of lactate formation, that of reaction 1 is in favor of pyruvate formation, and so the two reactions combined tend to offset the slightly unfavorable equilibrium of reaction 3 (about 66 percent to the left) and AMP is quantitatively used up.

PROCEDURE:

Pipette into a semimicrocuvette the following reagents: 0.500 ml of Tra-EDTA buffer, 0.050 ml of 0.024 M phosphoenolpyruvate, 0.020 ml of 0.3 M Mg-acetate, 0.020 ml of 0.6 M KCl, 0.010 ml of 0.015 M DPNH, test solution, and a calculated amount of water to give a final volume of 1.200 ml including enzymes. Stir contents, take an initial reading and add enzymes, one at a time, in the following order: LDH, 5 μl (2 mg enzyme protein/ml) or about 3.6 units, PK, 5 μl (2 mg enzyme protein/ml) or about 1.3 units, and MK, 5 μl (5 mg enzyme protein/ml) or about 1.1 units. After addition of each enzyme stir and take readings until E becomes steady. ΔE obtained with LDH measures the sum of pyruvate present in sample and reagents, ΔE obtained with PK measures ADP, and ΔE with MK measures AMP of test solution and reagents. To correct for the presence of contaminants in the reagents, run a reagent blank in parallel with the test. The reagent blank contains everything except the test solution. Small amounts of AMP and ATP are generally present in DPNH and PEP solutions and produce a change in absorbance after addition of MK. To correct for this, subtract ΔE obtained for reagent blank from the corresponding ΔE obtained for the test.

When a reagent blank is used, addition of enzymes to the control cuvette, which serves for the adjustment of 100 percent transmittance, is omitted.

For the estimation of AMP in pure solutions or in test samples that do not contain any ADP or ATP, one must provide theoretically some ATP to the assay system. In practice, however, this is rarely necessary, as the reagents are usually contaminated with a sufficient amount of ATP. To make sure of this point, check your reagents by assaying an AMP solution of known concentration with and without addition of ATP. Run a reagent blank for each assay. You may use 10 μl of 2.4 mM ATP solution (prepared by freshly diluting a 24 mM solution). Such an experiment will show whether you need to add ATP along with other reagents for estimation of AMP.

As an example for calculation, consider the same rat skeletal muscle extract in which ATP was determined; 0.200 ml of this extract was used as test. After addition of PK, no change in absorbance was noted in the reagent blank and in the test cuvette a ΔE of 0.060 was obtained. After addition of MK, the reagent blank gave a ΔE of 0.040 and the test a ΔE of 0.055. Therefore, 0.055 − 0.040 will represent a ΔE value which measures the AMP present in the test solution. Since 1 μ mole of DPNH in a volume of 1 ml has an absorbancy of 6.22 at 340 mμ and 12.45 ml of the neutralized extract are equivalent to 1 g of tissue, the ADP and AMP contents of this muscle are:

$$\text{ADP: } \frac{0.060}{6.22} \times 1 \times 1.2 \times \frac{12.45}{0.2} = 0.72\ (\mu\text{moles/g wet tissue})$$

$$\text{AMP: } \frac{0.015}{6.22} \times \frac{1}{2} \times 1.2 \times \frac{12.45}{0.2} = 0.09\ (\mu\text{moles/g wet tissue})$$

The foregoing method is very specific for AMP but not specific for ADP, since pyruvic kinase may utilize not only ADP but other diphosphonucleotides such as inosine diphosphate (IDP), uridine diphosphate (UDP), etc. To ensure complete specificity apply the method of Gruber et al. (1966).

INORGANIC PHOSPHATE (Pi) DETERMINATION.

This method utilizes the phosphorylase reaction. In addition to phosphorylase (Pho), either form a or b, phosphoglucomutase (PGluM) and glucose-6-phosphate dehydrogenase (G-6-PDH) are needed. The reactions involved are as follows:

$$\text{glycogen} + \text{Pi} \xrightleftharpoons{\text{Pho}} \text{glucose-1-phosphate} \quad (1)$$

$$\text{glucose-1-phosphate} \xrightleftharpoons[\text{Mg}^{++}]{\text{PGluM}} \text{glucose-6-phosphate} \quad (2)$$

$$\text{glucose-6-phosphate} + \text{TPN}^{+} \xrightleftharpoons{\text{G-6-PDH}} \text{6-phosphogluconate} + \text{TPNH} + \text{H}^{+} \quad (3)$$

Reaction 1 is freely reversible, reaction 2 favors glucose-6-P formation, and reaction 3 proceeds virtually completely to the right under the conditions of the assay. Thus a small, "limited" amount of Pi in the presence of excess of glycogen, which serves as donor of glucose units, is quantitatively converted to 6-phosphogluconate. The formation of the latter is measured by TPN reduction.

The success of this determination depends on the reagents. They must be carefully selected so as to contain as little Pi as possible. Test products of different companies (determine Pi content by the colorimetric method) and choose the best. The reagents most likely to contain more Pi than the method can tolerate are: TPN, G-6-PDH, and Pho. It is not difficult to find a grade of TPN that has a low Pi content. G-6-PDH is often dialyzed against phosphate buffer during its purification stage. Such preparations must be dialyzed prior to use against glass-redistilled water containing 1 mM EDTA. The method for Pi in this laboratory has been worked out with Pho-a preparation generously provided by Dr. Edwin G. Krebs (Seattle). Recently Pho-a and Pho-b became available at Boehringer Co., and we recommend the a form for this determination. Pho-a of Sigma Chemical Co. is also suitable provided it is dialyzed and activated prior to use (Fawaz et al., 1966). The phosphorylases keep best when stored in the form of lyophilized powders. To prepare a solution of Pho-a, weigh an amount equivalent to 2 mg of protein and suspend in 1 ml of 0.5 percent glycogen (see reagents). We use for this purpose glycogen of Merck (Darmstadt) without any purification. Determine activity of phosphorylase next day. If it is low, the preparation must have aged and the enzyme can be reactivated by addition of 0.100 ml of 0.3 M cystein (neutralized to pH 7) followed by warming at 30°C for 2 hours. If Pho-b is to be used for Pi determinations, suspend the Boehringer lyophilized powder equivalent to 5 mg protein in 1 ml of water, keep at room temperature with occasional stirring for around 2 hours and later store at 2° to 4°C. Assay next day and, if the preparation shows poor activity, add mercaptoethanol (Eastman Organic Chemicals) to a final concentration of 0.01 M. Solutions of both phosphorylases prepared as described keep well for at least a month, but better results are obtained with preparations not more than 2 weeks old.

Each phosphorylase solution should be tested for activity before it is used for a Pi determination. According to the directions to be given, only the so-called total activity of Pho-a is measured. This is permissible as Pi determinations are carried out in the presence of AMP. Such a procedure does not require AMP-free glycogen which is difficult to obtain and can also be used for assay of Pho-b, which needs AMP for activity.

ASSAY OF PHOSPHORYLASE ACTIVITIES:

Pipette into a centrifuge tube the following solutions: 0.1 ml of 4 percent glycogen, 0.2 ml of β-glycerophosphate-NaF-EDTA buffer pH 6.9, and 0.1 ml of substrate solution (see Reagents for assay of phosphorylase activity). Preincubate at 30°C for 10 minutes and add 5 μl of Pho-a which has been diluted, just before use, to a concentration of 0.5 mg protein/ml. (For dilution preincubate a small amount of the enzyme containing 2 mg protein/ml for 5 minutes at 30°C and then dilute with glass-redistilled water of the same temperature.) Exactly 5 minutes later withdraw a sample of 0.2 ml and pipette it into a test tube, graduated at 10 ml, containing 7 ml of 0.07 N H_2SO_4. As liberation of Pi from glucose-l-P serves to measure the activity of the enzyme, it is important to determine the initial level of Pi in the system. This is done as follows: glycogen, buffer, and substrate solutions are pipetted into 7 ml 0.07 N HSO_4 in the same amounts as used for the activity test. After mixing, 5 μl of Pho-a solution are added. This is called the reagent control. Note the "reagent control" contains 0.4 ml of assay mixture and 5 μl of enzyme, while the test contains half the amounts because after incubation for 5 minutes a sample of 0.2 ml was withdrawn and added to the acid.

The assay of Pho-b is done the same way, but since a solution of higher protein concentration was prepared, the enzyme is added to a larger volume of assay mixture. Preincubate a small sample of Pho-b (5 mg protein/ml) for 5 minutes at 30°C, dilute with an equal volume of water of the same temperature, mix, and immediately add 5 μl to 1 ml of assay mixture (0.25 ml glycogen, 0.50 ml buffer, and 0.25 ml substrate). The usual amount of 0.2 ml is withdrawn after exactly 5 minutes of incubation at 30°C and pipetted into 7 ml of 0.07 N H_2SO_4. For reagent control use same amounts of glycogen, buffer, and substrate as used for incubation and 5 μl of enzyme. Note that in this case the reagent control contains five times the amounts of reagents and enzyme present in the test.

Pi is determined in reagent controls and tests by the colorimetric method. As acid was used to inactivate the enzyme (7 ml 0.07 N), a less acidic molybdate is needed for this purpose (2.5 percent in 4.5 N H_2SO_4). Use 1 ml of this molybdate, 0.4 ml reducer, dilute to 10 ml, and allow 10 minutes for color development. Run a blank and standard along with the unknowns. Do not allow your reagent controls and tests to stand too long in 0.07 N H_2SO_4. Some glucose-l-P, which is present in large concentration, may split if kept in 4.5 N H_2SO_4 for over one-half hour. Any small amounts of Pi thus liberated will affect the value of the reagent control considerably, as the latter is generally low.

CALCULATION OF ENZYME ACTIVITIES:

Pho-a (2 mg protein/ml) and Pho-b (5 mg protein/ml) both prepared from lyophilized powders of Boehringer Co. were assayed according to the directions given. A phosphate standard contained 0.5 μ mole of Pi in a final volume of 10 ml.

Optical density measurements taken at 660 mμ were as follows:

Standard	0.170
Pho-a (T)	0.195
Pho-a (T) reagent control	0.070
Pho-b	0.245
Pho-b reagent control	0.180

Correcting the optical densities for Pi present before the incubation started, we get:

$$\text{for Pho-a: } 0.195 - \frac{0.070}{2} = 0.160$$

$$\text{for Pho-b: } 0.245 - \frac{0.180}{5} = 0.209$$

The value of 0.160 represents optical density for phosphate which has been liberated from G-1-P by 2.5 μl of Pho-a solution diluted 4 times, and the value of 0.209 refers to 1 μl of our Pho-b solution diluted 2 times.

Since by definition one unit of enzyme converts 1 μmole of substrate per minute, the phosphorylase solutions contain:

$$\text{Pho-a: } \frac{0.160}{0.170} \times 0.5 \times \frac{1000}{2.5} \times 4 \times \frac{1}{5} = 150 \text{ (units/ml or 2 mg protein)}$$

$$\text{Pho-b: } \frac{0.209}{0.170} \times 0.5 \times \frac{1000}{1} \times 2 \times \frac{1}{5} = 246 \text{ (units/ml or 5 mg protein)}$$

One cannot expect a higher specific activity for Pho-a than the one obtained with this preparation. The contamination with Pi is also not too high. The highest specific activity for Pho-b obtained in this laboratory with some samples kindly provided by Boehringer was also in this range (around 80 units/mg protein). The commercial preparation used to illustrate the preceding calculation is less active (around 50 units/mg protein). More testing has to be done on newer batches of Pho-b before deciding whether it is as suitable as the Pho-a preparation.

It must be pointed out that phosphorylase is sometimes assayed by a spectrophotometric method which involves reactions identical with those used for Pi determination, except that an excess of Pi and a limited amount of phosphorylase are added. The rate of TPN reduction measures the activity. This method is used at Boehringer and gives around 50 percent lower specific activity than the colorimetric one starting with G-1-P.

For a Pi determination done in a final volume of 1.200 ml, 1.5 to 3 units of Pho-a and 4.5 to 6 units of Pho-b, as assayed by the colorimetric procedure, are recommended. With the aforementioned preparations one must therefore use 10 to 20 μl of Pho-a and 20 to 25 μl of Pho-b.

There are several reasons why a definite amount of phosphorylase must be used for Pi determination and not what is just thought to be an excess, as is done in other determinations. One must avoid using more enzyme than necessary in order not to increase the value of reagent blank and also to minimize the error due to impurities of phosphatases if such are present in the preparation. As phosphorylase solutions do not keep very well, there is always a possibility that too little of the enzyme is added. This is very dangerous, as phosphorylase upon high dilution in the cuvette may get inactivated to such an extent that the Pi present in the reagents and sample will not be completely esterified. The reaction may consequently come to a stop or it may drag. The dragging might be incorrectly attributed to the presence of an impurity of a phosphatase, when in reality a low activity of the enzyme may be responsible.

For these reasons, it is advisable not only to test the activity of a phosphorylase solution every 10 days or so, but also to test the method itself by using a standard solution of Pi with every new batch of an enzyme. Fifty μl of Pi standard (see Reagents, p. 519) should give a ΔE of 0.260. The reaction must come to a complete stop within 30 minutes after adding phosphorylase. If this is not the case and the readings of reagent blank and Pi standard continue to increase at a steady rate, thus giving the same ΔE for the standard, it means that the enzyme preparation is contaminated with a phosphatase. It would still be suitable for use provided a correct ΔE for the standard is obtained and the reagent blank is not too high. The latter should give a ΔE of around 0.100 but not more than 0.200. If all the conditions mentioned are satisfied, the preparation of phosphorylase is suitable for use with extracts.

PROCEDURE:

Pipette into the test cuvette the following solutions: 0.500 ml Tra-EDTA buffer pH 7.6 (in the original publication, Fawaz et al., 1966, due to a printing error, the pH of the buffer was given as 6.7; at this pH the method does not work), 0.050 ml of 2 percent glycogen, 0.020 ml of 0.3 M Mg-acetate, 0.010 ml of 0.04 M TPN, 0.005 ml of 0.05 M AMP, 0.005 ml of 1.2 mM glucose-1,6-diphosphate, a sample to be analyzed, and water to a final volume of 1.200 ml including enzymes. Prepare a reagent blank in the same way, but omit the sample. Take an initial reading and add to both, reagent blank and test cuvette, 5 μl of G-6-PDH (0.5 mg enzyme protein/ml), or about 0.35 unit. Stir and follow with 5 μl of PGluM (2 mg enzyme protein/ml obtained by freshly diluting a 10-mg suspension with cold water), or about 0.07 unit. Take readings until steady. Finally add either Pho-a, 1.5 to 3 units, or Pho-b, 4.5 to 6 units, stir and take readings every 5 minutes until steady. With good grade phosphorylase preparations, the reactions come to a complete stop within 20 minutes. If the readings of reagent blank and test continue to increase, but a steady ΔE for test cuvette is obtained, use this value for calculation. Always substract the ΔE of reagent blank from ΔE of the unknown, as in case of ADP and AMP determination. For every μmole of Pi esterified, 1 μmole of TPN is reduced.

DETERMINATION OF GLYCOLYTIC INTERMEDIATES

Hexose Monophosphates

Glucose-1-, glucose-6-, and fructose-6-phosphate (G-1-P, G-6-P, and F-6-P), the primary intermediates of the anaerobic breakdown of carbohydrates, can be determined along with Pi. Since, however, their levels are generally much lower than that of Pi, a separate assay using a larger volume of extract is preferred. In this assay G-6-P is first converted to 6-phosphogluconate (6-PG), and then G-1-P and F-6-P are converted in separate reactions to G-6-P and subsequently to 6-PG. The stepwise reduction of TPN is followed. The reaction scheme can be represented as follows:

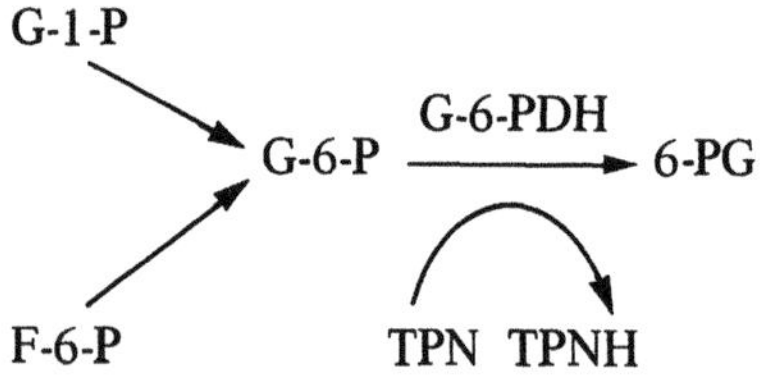

PROCEDURE:

Pipette into a semimicrocuvette the following reagents: 0.500 ml Tra-EDTA buffer, 0.020 ml of 0.3 M Mg-acetate, 0.010 ml of 0.04 M TPN, test solution, and water to give a total volume of 1.200 ml including enzymes. After taking an initial reading, add enzymes, one at a time, in the following order: G-6-PDH, 5 μl (0.5 mg enzyme protein/ml), or about 0.35 unit, PGluM, 10 μl (2 mg enzyme protein/ml), or about 0.13 unit, and 5 μl of phosphoglucoisomerase (PGI, 2 mg enzyme protein/ml), or about 4 units. The ΔE obtained after addition of G-6-PDH measures G-6-P, ΔE after PGluM measures G-1-P, and ΔE after PGI measures F-6-P.

The equilibria of the reactions that convert G-1-P and F-6-P to G-6-P favor the formation of the latter; hence one expects to find in normal extracts mainly G-6-P and in small amounts. As larger test volumes are required, the presence of GSSG (example, liver extracts) is especially troublesome. To avoid a "back-run" under such conditions, it is recommended (Fawaz and Fawaz, 1962) to inhibit GSSG-R, the contaminating enzyme present in G-6-PDH, with $ZnSO_4$ (add 0.01 ml of 1 mM $ZnSO_4$ solution along with the reagents and use Tra buffer without

EDTA to make the Zn^{++} effective). If the back-run is not too strong, $ZnSO_4$ need not be used: after introducing enzymes into the cuvette, readings may be taken at short intervals and the highest ΔE obtainable may be used for calculation as described for ATP and PC determination with HK.

G-6-P is resistant to acid hydrolysis (t ½ in 1 N HCl at 100°C is 1,300 min). In case hexose monophosphates are of no particular interest, one performs this assay only when the difficultly hydrolyzable fraction (T-H: see Fractional Hydrolysis) appears abnormally high.

Fructose Diphosphate (FDP), Glyceraldehyde Phosphate (GAP), and Dihydroxyacetone Phosphate (DHAP)

FDP is cleaved by aldolase (ALD) to two triosephosphates: GAP and DHAP. These are interconvertible in the presence of triosephosphate isomerase (TIM). It is possible to determine the parent compound and the breakdown products without difficulty, as another enzyme, glycerophosphate dehydrogenase (GDH), converts DHAP to α-glycerophosphate (α-GP) with the resulting oxidation of DPNH. The equilibrium of the latter reaction at pH 7.6 lies far to the right, so that all participating substrates are quantitatively transformed to α-GP according to the following scheme:

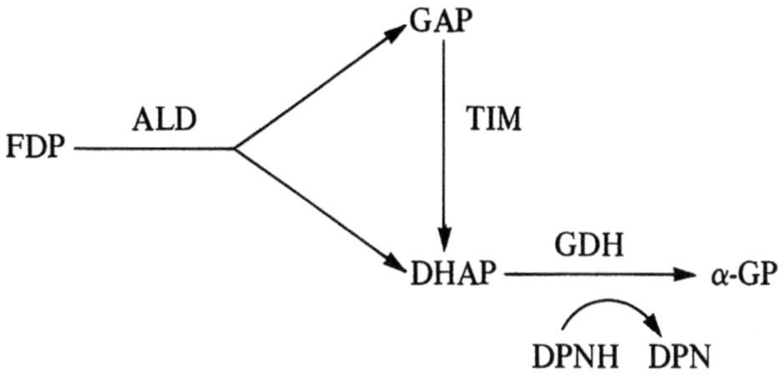

It is clear that for each μ mole of FDP used up, 2 μ moles of α-GP are formed, and thus 2 μ moles of DPNH are oxidized, while for the trioses the ratio is 1:1.

PROCEDURE:

Pipette into a semimicrocuvette 0.500 ml Tra-EDTA buffer, 0.010 ml of 0.015 M DPNH, test solution, and a calculated amount of water to give a final volume of 1.200 ml including enzymes. Start assay by adding 5 μl of GDH (10 mg enzyme protein/ml), or about 1.8 units: ΔE measures DHAP. Next add 5 μl of TIM (0.4 mg enzyme protein/ml, obtained by appropriate dilution with cold water from a more concentrated solution), or about 5 units: ΔE measures GAP. Finally add 5 μl of ALD (10 mg enzyme protein/ml), or about 0.45 unit: ΔE measures FDP.

These directions, as given, are meant for assays of test solutions containing all three substrates. If not all are present, as is mostly the case with tissue extracts, one may shorten the period of assay by adding a GDH-TIM mixture, 5 μl (see

Reagents). This is permissible because GAP is not present in detectable amounts in tissues. DHAP ordinarily is not found either, but may accumulate under certain conditions. To determine it, one must neutralize the $HClO_4$ extract to methyl orange with K_2CO_3, or neutralize to phenolphthalein with KOH but proceed with the assay without delay as the ester is unstable at pH 9.

The assay for these intermediates is important, as all three are partially hydrolyzed by 1 N HCl at 100° during the 7-minute period and would, if present, render the estimation of ATP by fractional hydrolysis erroneous.

α-Glycerophosphate (α-GP)

In the determination of α-GP the GDH reaction is again utilized, but in this case it is driven against an unfavorable equilibrium. This is achieved by using a hydrazine-containing buffer of pH 9.5 and by applying high enzyme and coenzyme "pressure." Hydrazine serves to trap the ketone as hydrazone, and the high pH buffer takes care of the H^+ formed during the reaction:

$$\alpha\text{-GP} + \text{DPN}^+ + \text{hydrazine} \xrightarrow{\text{GDH}} \text{DHAP-hydrazone} + \text{DPNH} + \text{H}^+$$

PROCEDURE:

Pipette into a semimicrocuvette 0.500 ml of glycine-hydrazine-EDTA buffer pH 9.5, 0.050 ml 0.075 M DPN, test solution, and a calculated amount of water to give a final volume of 1.200 ml including the enzyme. Take an initial reading against blank cuvette containing 0.500 ml of the above buffer and 0.700 ml water. Now add 0.020 ml of GDH (10 mg enzyme protein/ml), or about 7.2 units to the test cuvette, and take readings every 5 minutes until reaction comes to a stop.

PRECAUTIONS:

As this determination is carried out at pH 9.5, presence of phenolphthalein in a test sample interferes. Alkalinize for this purpose a small portion of an extract using no indicator. Check pH (with pH paper) in individual cuvettes before experiment is terminated. Absence of a "run" with final pH lower than 9.3 may not necessarily mean absence of α-PG, but it may mean that conditions for reversal of GDH reaction are not favorable. This may also be the case when the reaction does not come to a stop within 15 minutes. Check pH first, and if it is 9.3 or above, add an additional 5 to 10 μl of GDH. The "dragging" may be due to either too low a pH or an insufficiently active enzyme preparation.

α-GP is resistant to acid hydrolysis and is assayed for when the fraction T-H (see Fractional Hydrolysis) is abnormally high.

2- and 3-Phosphoglycerates (2-PG and 3-PG)

In one of the methods described for ATP determination, 3-PG served as phosphate acceptor. Here, this method is adapted for the estimation of a small, limited amount of the substrate, by using an excess of ATP. Phosphoglyceromutase (PGM), in the presence of a cofactor, 2,3-diphosphoglycerate (2,3-PG), converts 2-PG to 3-PG, the overall reaction scheme being as follows:

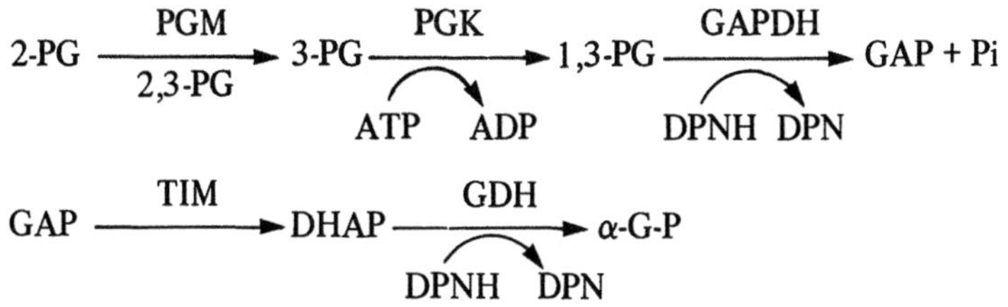

The commercially available GAPDH has some PGM activity; hence this test measures the sum of 2-PG and 3-PG.

PROCEDURE:

Pipette into a semimicrocuvette 0.500 Tra-EDTA, 0.050 ml of 0.024 M ATP (freshly prepared), 0.020 ml of 0.3 M Mg-acetate, 0.010 ml of 0.015 M DPNH, 0.005 ml of 1.2 mM 2,3-PG, test solution, and water to give a final volume of 1.200 ml including enzymes. Stir contents and take an initial reading against blank cuvette containing Tra-EDTA and water in the usual proportions. Then introduce the enzymes to the test cuvette: 5 μl of PGK-GAPDH mixture (see Reagents and ATP Determination) and 10 μl of PGM (2 mg enzyme protein/ml), about 0.36 unit. Take readings until there is no further decrease in optical density: ΔE measures the sum of 2-PG and 3-PG. The sensitivity of the method is doubled by the use of two additional enzymes: GDH and TIM (add 5 μl of GDH-TIM mixture). This enzyme mixture may be added last, but it is safer to add it at the beginning, as the test solution may contain some DHAP.

Like α-GP, 2-PG and 3-PG are both "acid-resistant" and appear in the T-H fraction.

Phosphoenolpyruvate (PEP) and an Alternative Method for 2- and 3-Phosphoglycerates (2-PG and 3-PG)

PEP in the presence of an excess of ADP, pyruvic kinase (PK), and lactic dehydrogenase (LDH) is quantitatively transformed to lactate with a resulting oxidation of DPNH in a mole-to-mole ratio. This method is a variation of the one described for estimating ADP except that in this test PEP is used in a limited amount and ADP in excess. As 3-PG is converted to 2-PG by phosphoglyceromutase (PGM) and 2-PG to PEP by enolase (ENOL), these two esters may also be determined along with PEP. This is done when the amount of PEP relative to the glycerate esters is not too high in the test sample and also when the pyruvate content is low. The reactions involved are as follows:

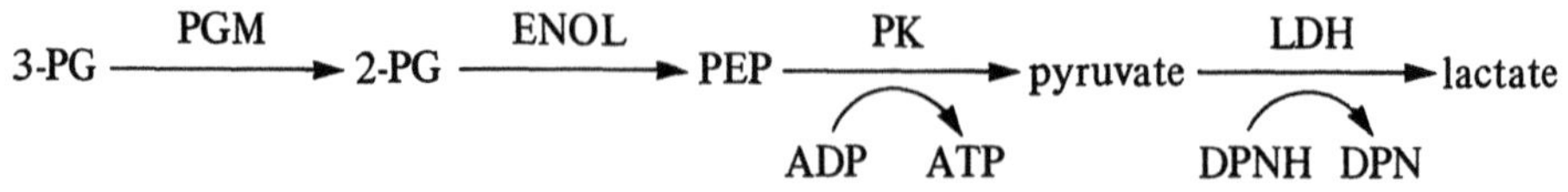

If a known solution of 3-PG is analyzed according to the foregoing scheme, and all the enzymes except PGM are added in succession, starting with LDH, a slow run in most cases is observed, indicating that the enzymes used are contaminated with PGM. For this reason 2-PG and 3-PG cannot be determined separately, unless all three enzymes (LDH, PK, and ENOL) are free of PGM.

PROCEDURE:

Pipette into a semimicrocuvette 0.500 ml Tra-EDTA, 0.050 ml 0.024 M ADP, 0.020 ml of 0.3 M Mg-acetate, 0.020 ml of 0.6 M KCl, 0.010 ml of 0.015 M DPNH, test solution, and a calculated amount of water to give a final volume of 1.200 ml including enzymes. If, in addition to PEP, 2-PG and 3-PG are to be determined, include in the filling 0.005 ml of 1.2 mM 2,3-diphosphoglycerate. Take an initial reading and add 5 μl of LDH (2 mg enzyme protein/ml), or about 3.6 units. Take readings until steady: ΔE measures pyruvate in the sample. Follow with addition of 5 μl PK (2 mg enzyme protein/ml), or about 1.3 units: ΔE measures PEP. Finally add 5 μl of ENOL (10 mg enzyme protein/ml), or about 1.3 units, and 10 μl of PGM (2 mg enzyme protein/ml), or about 0.36 unit: ΔE measures the sum of 2-PG and 3-PG.

PEP may be found in tissue extracts when PK is blocked, as by malonate (Fawaz and Fawaz, 1962). It accumulates only in those tissues where the GDH enzyme operates for the following reason: during the formation of PEP by way of the glycolytic pathway, DPN is reduced. As the level of this coenzyme is very low, it must be continuously reoxidized in order to produce relatively large amounts of PEP. Normally this is done by pyruvate, but as the latter does not form when PK is inhibited, another glycolytic intermediate, namely DHAP, must oxidize DPNH. Thus, whenever PEP accumulates, a test for α-GP is indicated.

In 1 N HCl at 100°C around 50 percent of PEP is dephosphorylated during a period of 7 minutes. Hence, when ATP is estimated by the method of fractional hydrolysis and PEP is present, it will increase the actual value of ATP.

COMMENT ON THE RELATIVE MERITS OF THE COLORIMETRIC AND ENZYMATIC METHODS

The two methods are not mutually exclusive but rather supplementary. Total phosphorus of tissues and total acid-soluble phosphorus of tissue extracts are performed by wet ashing followed by colorimetry. The importance of these determinations cannot be overemphasized, as they may also serve to demonstrate or exclude tissue edema, leakage of phosphorus compounds into the perfusion medium, or indicate if an exchange between acid-insoluble and acid-soluble fraction occurs. Inorganic phosphate and phosphocreatine can be determined accurately according to the colorimetric procedure of Fiske and Subbarow or a modification thereof, the advantage of the enzymatic methods being mainly greater sensitivity. PC is stable in 0.6 N $HClO_4$ in the cold for at least one hour. Besides PC, the more labile 1,3-diphosphoglyceric acid may be hydrolyzed during acid extraction or by acid molybdate at room temperature, but it is not found in measurable amounts in tissues. Also, unpublished extensive work in this laboratory in search for other "ultralabile" compounds, like phosphorylated amino acids, which are stable only in neutral or alkaline media, have yielded only negative results. In the light of this knowledge, we do not see the need for introducing new and "mild" procedures to extract inorganic phosphate, such as the avoidance of acid treatment and the use of organic solvents at low temperature at the risk of failing to extract all the inorganic phosphate.

The so-called acid-labile fraction (H–[Pi + PC], according to our nomenclature) or organic phosphorus hydrolyzed in 1 N HCl, during 7 minutes at 100°C from other sources than PC, yields useful information, since in "resting" skeletal and cardiac muscle it measures two thirds of ATP and one half of ADP phosphorus. However, under the influence of certain metabolic inhibitors, some compounds may accumulate which contribute to this fraction significantly and thus render such calculations invalid. The "acid-resistant fraction" (T-H), in resting tissue, in addition to the remainder (or unhydrolyzed phosphorus) of ATP and ADP, includes: AMP, G-6-P, and some other difficultly hydrolyzable compounds, some of which have not been identified so far. A substantial increase in this fraction may be obtained after treating tissues with certain chemicals. An experiment taken from unpublished work done in this laboratory is chosen to show that values calculated from the acid-labile fraction have to be checked by enzymatic tests. This experiment also illustrates how both the acid-labile and acid-resistant fractions yield useful information that tells what additional specific enzymatic determinations should be carried out in order to obtain a complete picture.

A pithed frog was treated with iodoacetate (IAc) according to the classical experiments of Lundsgaard (1930). The gastrocnemius muscles were removed and hung on levers to provide for direct electrical stimulation. One muscle was stimulated by single shocks at the rate of one per second until exhaustion and contracture. The other muscle was not stimulated and served as a control. The experiment was terminated by dipping both gastrocnemii into liquid air. Protein-free extracts were prepared, and the acid-soluble P compounds analyzed by fractional hydrolysis followed by colorimetry as well as by the individual enzymatic tests as described in preceding sections. The results obtained by the colorimetric method are summarized in Table 1 and those of the enzymatic methods in Table 2.

The resting values for frog gastrocnemii (not treated with IAc) in that particular shipment of frogs were, on the average, 16 μmoles of PC/g and 6 μmoles of ATP/g. It can be seen from Tables 1 and 2 that in the nonstimulated muscle IAc treatment reduced the level of these two high-energy compounds. In the stimulated muscle PC was almost completely hydrolyzed and so was ATP, as shown by the enzymatic determination.

TABLE 1

Analysis of Gastrocnemius Muscles from Iodoacetate-Treated Frog: Colorimetric Method.

Type of determination	Control muscle*	Stimulated muscle*
Pi + PC	17.3	6.7
PC	11.8	0.8
H	26.7	13.7
T	46.7	46.2
Pi ([Pi + PC] – PC)	5.5	5.9
Acid-labile (H – [Pi + PC])	9.4	7.0
Acid-resistant (T – H)	20.0	32.5

*Values are expressed in micromoles P per g wet tissue.

TABLE 2

Analysis of Gastrocnemius Muscles from Iodoacetate-Treated Frog: Enzymatic Methods.

Type of determination	Control muscle*	Stimulated muscle*
ATP (μmoles of ATP × 3)	9	traces
ADP (μmoles of ADP × 2)	1.6	1.4
AMP	0.1	0.3
FDP (μmoles of FDP × 2)	10.8	20.2
G-6-P	1.9	7.5
F-6-P	0.3	1.6
GAP	traces	traces
DHAP	traces	1.5
α-GP	traces	traces
G-1-P	traces	0.5

*Values are expressed in micromoles P per g wet tissue.

Closer consideration of the data in both tables reveals that not only in the stimulated but also in the control muscle, the acid-labile fraction as determined by the colorimetric procedure must represent some phosphate from sources other than ATP and ADP. The latter compounds, by calculation from enzymatic findings, should give upon hydrolysis 6.8 μ moles P/g for the control muscle (2 and 1 μ moles of P are released per 1 μ mole of ATP and ADP respectively), but 9.4 μ moles P/g were actually obtained. It is now known that IAc blocks the enzyme GAPDH. One must therefore expect an accumulation of GAP, DHAP, or their predecessor, FDP. All three compounds are partially hydrolyzed by 1 N HCl at 100°C during 7 minutes (around one half of the phosphate of GAP and DHAP and one fourth of the phosphate of FDP are released under such conditions). Enzymatic tests did indeed show accumulation of FDP in both muscles. Adding the contributions of ATP and ADP along with those of FDP and DHAP to the acid-labile fraction, one obtains for the control muscle extract 9.5 and for the stimulated 6.5 μ moles of P/g, values that agree with those obtained by the hydrolysis procedure. One can thus conclude that no other "semilabile" compounds have accumulated in the two extracts.

In the early thirties when Lundsgaard performed his experiments, the site of IAc inhibition was not known, nor were any specific methods for determining ATP available. On the basis of experiments similar to the one quoted, in which the IAc-poisoned muscle stimulated to exhaustion lost all its PC but retained the major part of the ATP (actually "retained" the hydrolyzable fraction or what was then called the pyrophosphate fraction), Lundsgaard concluded that the energy for contraction was provided by PC and not ATP.

Further examination of the results shows that, although all the PC was hydrolyzed in the stimulated muscle, there was no corresponding increase in Pi, but an increase in the acid-resistant fraction instead (see Table 1). As the increase in the level of FDP in the stimulated muscle over that of the control cannot account for the difference of 12.5 μmoles P/g between the two acid-resistant fractions, one must assume that some difficultly hydrolyzable compounds must have also been formed. Among the acid-resistant glycolytic intermediates are G-6-P, F-6-P, and α-GP. Enzymatic tests for these revealed that some G-6-P, and to a smaller extent F-6-P, accumulated. Adding up all the contributions to the acid-resistant fraction from our enzymatic data (1/3 of ATP, 1/2 of ADP, 3/4 of FDP, 1/2 of DHAP, and all phosphate of G-6-P, F-6-P and AMP), we obtain 14.2 μmoles P for the control and 25.0 μmoles P for the stimulated muscle. The difference between these two values is less than 12.5 μmoles, as required from Table 1, but the agreement may be considered satisfactory as the stimulated muscle is expected to contain more inosinic acid which was not estimated. Glucose-1-phosphate belongs to the acid-labile group of phosphorus compounds, and its contribution brings the level of the acid-labile fraction to 7 μmoles P/g, a value that agrees perfectly with that obtained by fractional hydrolysis (Table 1).

The conclusion to be drawn from this experiment is that IAc inhibited glycolysis in the control as well as in the stimulated muscle, as evidenced by the accumulation of intermediates preceding the site of blockade. The energy provided by glycolysis was eliminated, and stimulation brought about complete hydrolysis of ATP and PC with resulting exhaustion. The question arises as to why the control muscle accumulated less FDP than the stimulated muscle and why the level of G-6-P rose only in the stimulated muscle. The answer may be as follows: In iodoacetate poisoning the inorganic phosphate derived from the hydrolysis of PC and ATP is trapped in the form of FDP. Stimulation increases the rate of hydrolysis of ATP and PC, and more FDP accumulates. The accumulation of G-6-P and F-6-P may be due to "overflooding" or to the fact that during the later stages no ATP was available to phosphorylate F-6-P. More G-6-P accumulates than F-6-P because the isomerization reaction between these two compounds favors G-6-P formation.

PHYSIOLOGIC AND PHARMACOLOGIC APPLICATIONS

The central role occupied by phosphorus compounds in cell biology has led many investigators to anticipate and search for changes in the levels of these compounds, particularly the high-energy ones, under various physiologic and pathologic conditions and under the influence of drugs and toxins. The pertinent literature is enormous but the yield has been meager.

Heart failure may be produced acutely, as by the action of barbiturate on a heart-lung preparation, or chronically, as by pulmonary artery or aortic constriction. In some cases, such failing hearts show insignificant changes in the levels of PC and ATP. However, severely failing hearts do exhibit significant depressions of PC and ATP (Feinstein, 1962). The conclusion has been drawn that, since failure may not be associated with a decrease in the levels of high-energy phosphate compounds, it must be due to lack of *utilization* of these compounds. Recent work indicates that the utilization of high-energy phosphorus in failure proceeds with normal efficiency but that the rate of conversion of energy to work proceeds slowly. This may be due to a reduction in the activity of myofibrillar ATPase. For literature see Pool and Braunwald (1968). Recently, however, the concept that there is no defect in energy production in heart failure has again been challenged (Lindenmayer et al., 1968).

In 1957 we produced anoxic heart failure in the dog heart-lung preparation by gradual asphyxia and in intact open-chest dogs by ligating the anterior descending and circumflex branches of the left coronary artery (Fawaz et al., 1957; Fawaz and Tutunji, 1957). In both cases the onset of heart failure was associated with a decrease in PC without a significant change in ATP. Prolonged total anoxia resulted in hydrolysis of ATP also. In the light of these experiments we posed the following question: "Phosphocreatine breakdown may or may not have the function of replenishing the ATP reserves, but it is difficult to visualize why the heart should not continue its action if, as in all those cited cases of failure, its ATP stores are intact." These experiments have been amply confirmed in recent years, and a plausible answer to our question was proposed by assuming that only an insignificant and unmeasurable portion of the ATP is in equilibrium with PC, the major bulk of the measurable ATP being in different cell compartments. The rate of loss of high-energy phosphorus compounds after anoxia may be decreased, as by hypothermia. A more effective way of decreasing this rate has been described by Bretschneider (1964). It involves a combination of hypothermia and perfusion of the heart with a solution containing procaine and free of Na^+ and Ca^{++}. This treatment also markedly prolongs the so-called resuscitation period–i.e., the maximum period of complete anoxia that the heart can endure and still be capable of resuscitation. The importance of these findings for heart surgery cannot be overestimated.

It is clear from the foregoing that anoxic heart failure is associated with a decrease in the high-energy phosphorus content and that a prolongation of the "resuscitation period" is accompanied by a decrease in the rate of hydrolysis of PC and ATP. Yet it is difficult to assume a cause-and-effect relationship between heart failure and decrease in high-energy phosphate content. The following unpublished experiments from this laboratory may serve to illustrate this difficulty. Failure in a dog heart-lung preparation was produced by asphyxia. After a period of standstill amounting to about 30 minutes in which the PC level was reduced to zero and a major part of ATP had decomposed, resuscitation was achieved by reperfusion with blood and defibrillation. The heart resumed its activity, and although it could maintain a normal blood pressure, it was evidently in failure, judging by its markedly reduced output. Such resuscitated but failing hearts show a perfectly normal phosphocreatine content, although here the ATP values remain markedly reduced.

Fluoroacetate, an inhibitor of the Krebs cycle, can also cause failure in a dog heart-lung preparation (Fawaz, 1956) which is not due to tissue hypoxia. The degree of failure is proportional to the dose of fluoroacetate and also to the degree of citrate accumulation in the heart. The phosphocreatine content progressively decreases with the degree of failure, yet one cannot correlate the degree of failure with the decrease in PC in each case. Here again, ATP decreases only when failure is severe.

Dinitrophenol, an uncoupler of oxidative phosphorylation, can also produce failure in a heart-lung preparation, yet the first experiments reporting such failure were faulty in that the failure was evidently due to hypoxia. The lungs in a heart-lung preparation do not function properly and cannot even support one tenth of the oxygen exchange they do in an intact animal. Even an "unloaded" heart-lung may have to be ventilated with pure oxygen, or oxygen has to be vigorously bubbled through the venous reservoir to ensure proper oxygenation of the blood. If dinitrophenol is added to a heart-lung preparation, the blood gets dark within a few minutes and the heart fails. This is due to an increase in heart oxygen consumption (two- to four-fold, depending on the dose), so a relative hypoxia developed. Whenever proper oxygenation is ensured (Fawaz and Tutunji, 1957), the survival period is prolonged. Hearts examined at the onset of failure or even *before* failure show a 50 percent decrease in PC content without a change in ATP. Yet it is difficult to exclude relative hypoxia as being the cause of the PC decrease. The blood was oxygenated to give normal arterial oxygen levels–more cannot be achieved. Yet the coronary venous oxygen content was in the range of 5 percent, which is normal for an unloaded heart but may be insufficient for a heart whose oxygen consumption increased severalfold.

What has been said regarding the danger of producing hypoxia in a heart-lung preparation applies with greater force to those hearts perfused with salt solutions or to the experiments in which heart strips are suspended in such solutions. Such hearts may show no hypoxia as long as they are unloaded, and indeed their PC content may be normal. Yet if the oxygen consumption is increased, as by toxic doses of digitalis or high doses of catecholamines or by increased mechanical work–especially pressure work–the observed decrease in high-energy phosphorus levels is most likely due to relative hypoxia. Clearly, a salt solution cannot store as much oxygen as hemoglobin. In well-oxygenated dog heart-lung preparations, digitalis and catecholamine doses that raise oxygen consumption as much as 70 percent and 200 percent, respectively, do *not* decrease the high-energy phosphate level (Fawaz and Tutunji, 1959; Fawaz and Tutunji, 1960). In conclusion, we cannot overemphasize the necessity of excluding tissue hypoxia when changes in the level of high-energy phosphorus compounds are reported.

REFERENCES

Bretschneider, H. J. 1964. Überlebenszeit und Wiederbelebungszeit des Herzens bei Normo- und Hypothermie. Verh. Deutsch. Ges. Kreislaufforsch. 30:11-34.

Cooper, J., Srere, P. A., Tabachnick, M., and Racker, E. 1958. The oxidative pentose phosphate cycle. II. Quantitative determination of intermediates and enzymes. Arch. Biochem., 74:306-314.

Eränkö, O. 1954. Quenching of tissues for freeze-drying. Acta Anat., 22:331-336.

Fawaz, E. N., and Fawaz, G., 1962. Inhibition of glycolysis in rat skeletal muscle by malonate. Biochem. J. 83:438-445.

—Fawaz, G., and von Dahl, K. 1962. Enzymatic estimation of phosphocreatine. Proc. Soc. Exp. Biol. Med., 109:38-41.

—Roth, L., and Fawaz, G. 1966. The enzymatic estimation of inorganic phosphate. Biochem. Z. 344:212-214.

Fawaz, G. 1956. Die Wirkung von Fluoressigsäure auf Leistung und Stoffwechsel des Herzlungenpräparates des Hundes. 1956. Naunyn Schmiedeberg Arch. Pharm. Exp. Path., 228:377-386.

—and Hawa, E. S., 1953. Phosphocreatine content of mammalian cardiac muscle. Proc. Soc. Exp. Biol. Med., 84:277-280.

—and Manoukian E., 1962. Steady-state level of phosphocreatine in the heart. Cir. Res., 11:115-118.

—and Tutunji, B. 1957. The mechanism of dinitrophenol heart failure. Brit. J. Pharmacol., 12:273-278.

—and Tutunji, B. 1959. Ouabain-induced ventricular tachycardia and its effect on the performance and metabolism of the dog heart. Brit. J. Pharmacol. 14:355-357.

—and Tutunji, B. 1960. The effects of adrenaline and noradrenaline on the metabolism and performance of the isolated dog heart. Brit. J. Pharmacol., 15:389-395.

—Hawa, E. S., and Tutunji, B. 1957. The effect of dinitrophenol, hypoxaemia and ischaemia on the phosphorus compounds of the dog heart. Brit. J. Pharmacol., 12:270-272.

Feinstein, N. B. 1962. Effects of experimental congestive heart failure, ouabain, and asphyxia on the high-energy phosphate and creatine content of guinea pig heart. Circ. Res., 10:333-345.

Fiske, C. H., and Subbarow, Y. 1925. The colorimetric determination of phosphorus. J. Biol. Chem., 66:375-400.

Furchgott, R. F., and De Gubareff, T. 1958. High energy phosphate content of cardiac muscle under various experimental conditions which alter contractile strength. J. Pharmacol. Exp. Ther. 124:203-218.

Gerlach, E., and Deuticke, B. 1963. Eine einfache Methode zur Mikrobestimmung von Phosphat in der Papierchromatographie. Biochem. Z., 337:477-479.

—Deuticke, B., and Dreisbach, R. H. 1963. Zum Verhalten von Nucleotiden und ihren dephosphorylierten Abbauprodukten in der Niere be: Ischämie und kurzzeitiger postischämischer Wiederdurchblutung. Pflüger Arch. Ges. Physiol., 278:296-315.

Gruber, W., Moellering, H., and Bergmeyer, H. U. 1966. Analytische Differenzierung von Purin- und Pyrimidin-Nucleotiden. I. Bestimmung von AMP, ADP und ATP sowie GTP + ITP. Enzym. Biol. Clin. (Basel), 7:115-129.

Kerr, S. E. 1935. Studies on the phosphorus compounds of brain, I. Phosphocreatine. J. Biol. Chem., 110:625-635.

Lindenmayer, G. E., Sordahl, L. A., and Schwartz A. 1968. Reevaluation of oxidative phosphorylation in cardiac mitochondria from normal animals and animals in heart failure. Circ. Res., 23:439-450.

Lowry, O. H., and Lopez, J. A. 1946. Determination of inorganic phosphate in the presence of labile phosphate esters. J. Biol. Chem., 162:421-428.

Lundsgaard, E. 1930. Untersuchungen über Muskelkontraktionen ohne Milchsäurebildung. Biochem. Z., 217:162-177.

Pool, P. E., and Braunwald, E. 1968. Fundamental mechanisms in congestive heart failure. Amer. J. Cardiol., 22:7-15.

Seraydarian, K., Mommaerts, W. F. H. M., Wallner, A., and Guillory R. J., 1961. An estimation of the true inorganic phosphate content of frog sartorius muscle. J. Biol. Chem., 236:2071-2075.

Wollenberger, A., Krause, E. G., and Wahler, B. E. 1958. Orthophosphat- und Phosphokreatingehalt des Herzmuskels. Naturwissenschaften, 45:294.

CHAPTER 18

The Use of Microelectrode Techniques in Muscle

Kalman Greenspan and Robert E. Edmands

Krannert Institute of Cardiology, Marion County General Hospital
Indiana Univeristy School of Medicine, Indianapolis, Indiana

THE INTRACELLULAR MICROELECTRODE

Introduction

The clinical electrocardiogram has for decades been of immense utility in the diagnosis and treatment of cardiac disease. However, much of the art of electrocardiographic interpretation remained largely empirical prior to 1949. The electrocardiogram is in essence a composite or aggregate record of the electrical activity of all cardiac cells, recorded both in parallel and in series, while the activity of the specialized conduction system, by virtue of its relatively small mass, is only indirectly apparent on the conventional electrocardiogram. The advent of the Ling-Gerard microelectrode (Ling and Gerard) in 1949 has provided a means for recording the electrical activity of the single cell, however. Thus, a more objective basis has become available for evaluating drug therapy and the effect of noxious agents, as well as for the interpretation of cardiac arrhythmias. Moreover, this method of study has indeed proven to be fruitful in this regard, evidence of which will be cited in the following description of the experimental procedure commonly followed.

The technical aspects of microelectrophysiology vary in some detail from laboratory to laboratory, but are essentially comparable in all. As a consequence, the subsequent description of microelectrode techniques will refer specifically to those employed in our laboratory, while noting salient departure from generally used methods only where such is appropriate.

Tissue Preparation

The appropriately anesthetized experimental animal is first subjected to thoracotomy and cardiac excision, following which the intact heart is immediately placed in warm, oxygenated Tyrode solution in order that excess blood may be removed. The heart is then placed in a second container of warm, fresh, oxygenated Tyrode solution, and an appropriate segment (ventricular or atrial muscle, His Purkinje network [false tendons], SA nodal tissue, or AV junctional tissue), 1 and 2 cm in size, is excised and placed in 30-ml bath chamber continuously perfused with fresh Tyrode solution aerated with 95 percent oxygen and 5 percent carbon dioxide. The Tyrode solution, in millimoles per liter, is of the following composition:

NaCl	37.0
KCl	2.7
$NaHCO_3$	12.0
$MgCl_2$	0.5
$CaCl_2$	2.7
NaH_2PO_4	1.8
Glucose	5.5

A variety of solutions, Krebs' or Ringer's e.g., are used by other investigators, without apparent difference in the results obtained.

The temperature of the solution entering the tissue chamber is maintained constant at 37°C ± 1° (32°C ± 1° is more appropriate for studies of contractile behavior). The tissue chamber itself is maintained partially filled with paraffin, to which the tissue specimen is affixed by four or five stainless steel pins. Such immobilization of the tissue specimen is of considerable importance to adequate recording of the transmembrane action potential, as a freely contracting specimen may preclude maintenance of intracellular position of the recording microelectrode. Some laboratories have employed a "floating" electrode technique, however, with which action potentials may be recorded from an actively contracting ventricle.

Preparation of Tyrode Solution

Each of the Tyrode ingredients is made as a stock solution from which two main solutions are made that are eight times the strength of the "working" solution. The stock solution is made as follows:

Solution	Stock	Withdraw (in ml)	Preparation	
Solution A	NaCl	274.0	Pipette these in to 1-liter volumetric flask. Add 640 mg penicillin and 1,280 mg dihydrostrep-tomycin	Label flask "8X" and refrigerate
	$NaHCO_3$	192.0		
	Dextrose	176.0		
	KCl	21.6		
	$MgCl_2$	8.0		
	NaH_2PO_4	14.4	Dilute up to mark	
Solution B	$CaCl_2$	43.2	Pipette in to 1-liter volumetric flask and dilute to mark	Label flask "8X" and refrigerate

Compound	Molecular Weight	Weight out (in g)	Dilute to (ml)	Molarity
NaCl	58.448	116.9	500	4.00
$NaHCO_3$	84.01	21.0	500	0.50
Dextrose	180.16	22.52	500	0.25
KCl	74.55	37.275	500	1.00
$MgCl_2 \times 6H_2O$	203.33	50.83	500	0.50
NaH_2PO_4	138.00	34.50	500	0.50
$CaCl_2 \times 2H_2O$	147.00	36.75	500	0.50

All dilutions should be made with triple-distilled water.

When the Tyrode solution is required for a given experiment, the following procedure is followed:

1. Remove Solutions A and B from the refrigerator and allow to come to room temperature.
2. Withdraw 125 ml of Solution A and place in a 500-ml volumetric flask. Dilute up to mark.
3. Pour into 2-liter bottle and aerate with 95 percent O_2–5 percent CO_2 gas mixture. Label the solution A_1.
4. Withdraw 125 ml of Solution B and place in 500-ml volumetric flask. Dilute up to mark. Label the solution $B_1$1.
5. Pour Solution B_1 slowly into bottle containing the gas-aerated Solution A_1. Stir.

The mixed Solution A_1 and B_1 is the working or "ready to use", Tyrode solution with which the isolated tissue is to be perfused.

Recording Apparatus

A glass microelectrode (Fig. 1; for preparation, see p. 558), with an open tip diameter of about 0.5 μ, is filled with 3 M KCl and placed on an electrode holder, over a silver-silver chloride wire. The electrode is then lowered into the bath

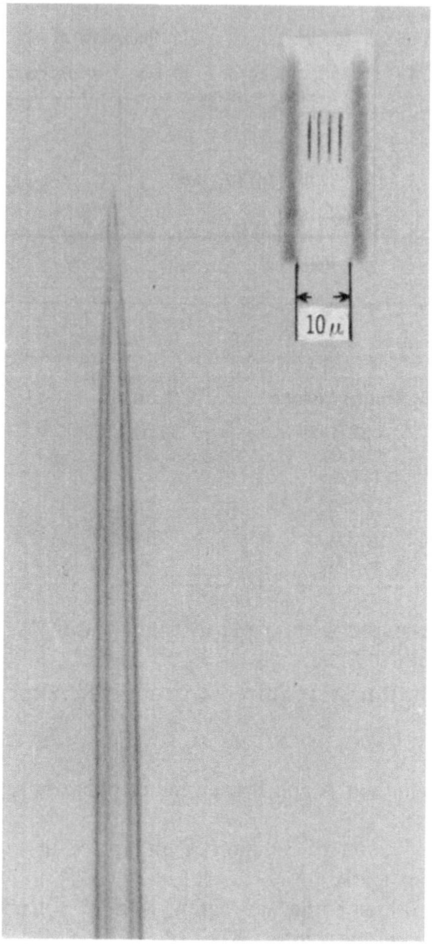

FIG. 1. Photograph of a glass microelectrode (×450) with a reference scale of 10 μ.

solution by a Brinkman micromanipulator. The microelectrode is coupled to the input of a Bioelectric Instruments electrometer (or Philbrick preamplifier), by a silver-silver chloride lead of minimal length. This preamplifier has sufficient input capacitance neutralization at the operating point (gain = 3.0) to neutralize the capacitance associated with any reasonable lead length. Ground return on the input circuit is accomplished by a silver-silver chloride reference cell immersed in the perfusing solution, and a low impedance calibrator (it is important, to preclude junction potentials, that the composition of the microelectrode lead and the reference cell be identical; chloriding of the wires is equally important in order that an equilibrium be achieved between the metal leads and the bath solution to avoid "DC shifts" during the experiment). The low impedance calibrator, so situated, permits calibration of microelectrode resistance and voltage sensitivity of

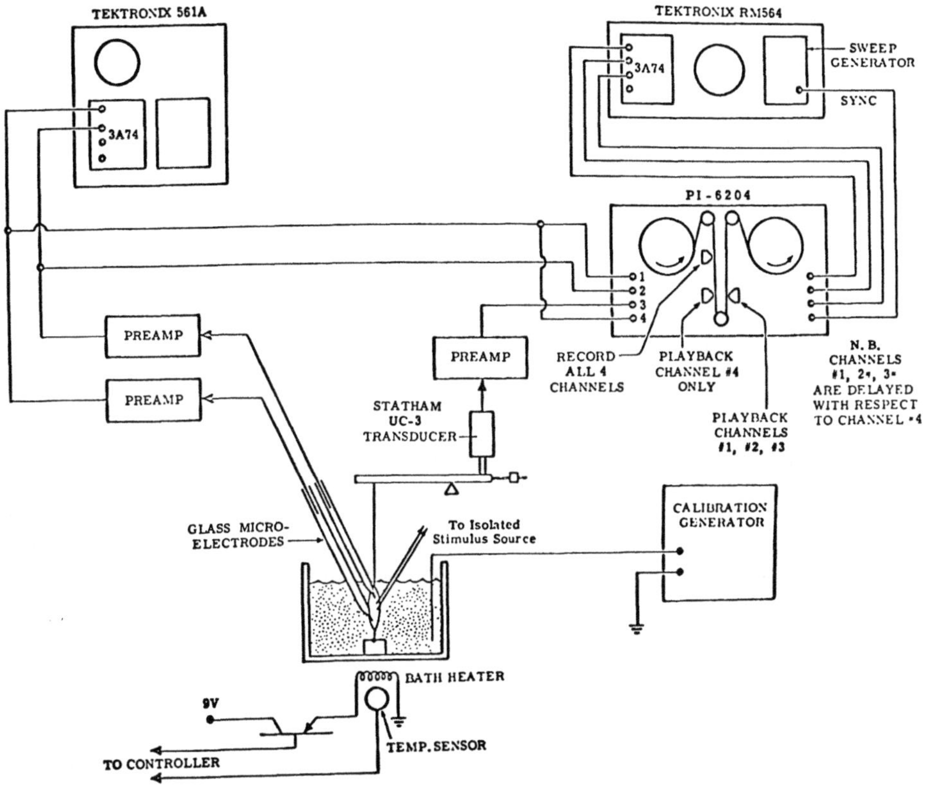

FIG. 2. Schematic diagram of stimulating and recording apparatus.

the recording system with all components in normal operating position. The output of the preamplifier is used to drive simultaneously two Tektronix 561A oscilloscopes. One is used for monitoring and the second for photographic recording with a grass kymograph camera. Alternatively, the preamplifier output may be used to drive the monitoring oscilloscope and either one channel of an eight-channel Electronics for Medicine oscilloscope or one channel of a Precision Instruments magnetic tape recorder (Fig. 2).

A system of Tektronix 161 pulse generators and Tektronix 162 wave-form generators is used to provide synchronized stimulus pulses, scope triggering pulses, and a 100 msec standard time display for the photographic records. The time pulse display may be set to appear under each action potential and its amplitude adjusted to a predetermined voltage scale for continuous record calibration (15 to 20 mv amplitude, e.g.). Stimulus pulses, at rates varying from 20 to 300 per minute, are administered through isolated bipolar electrodes made of 0.005-inch stainless steel wire. Isolation is achieved by a Bioelectric Instrument, Inc., Model 15A-100 stimulus isolator. If desired, two synchronized stimulus generators may be used to introduce stimuli of variable prematurity; in this manner extrasystoles may be introduced by switching from one generator to the other.

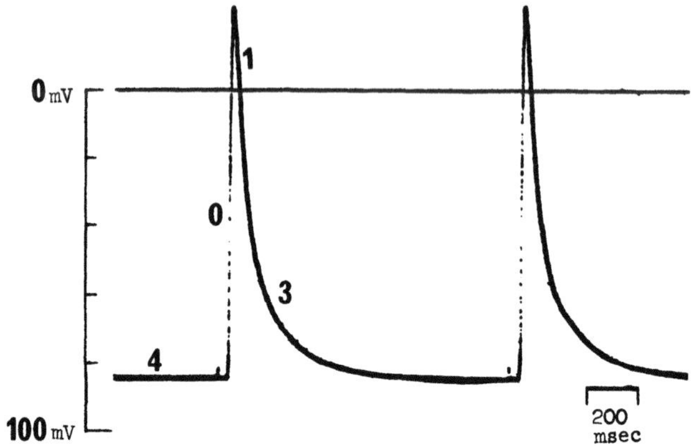

FIG. 3. A characteristic action potential recorded from a canine atrial cell. The various phases of the complex are labeled accordingly. The initial upstroke of depolarization is referred to as phase 0 including the "overshoot." The rapid but short initial repolarization is referred to as phase 1, slowing then to form a variably distinct plateau (phase 2). Many atrial cells do not show a distinct phase 2. Following phase 2, repolarization occurs more rapidly (phase 3), with which the transmembrane potential returns to its resting state.

Microelectrode Preparation

The preparation of glass microelectrodes is a most critical aspect of this experimental technique, for the integrity of the intracellular electrode is most susceptible to damage or dysfunction. The glass pipettes are initially drawn by an Industrial Science Association, Inc. (or other commercially available) Micropipette Puller, from 2½-inch lengths of 1 to 1.5 mm internal diameter soft Pyrex glass capillary tubing. The pipette puller may be adjusted to yield, reproducibly, microelectrodes with an open-tip diameter of about 0.5 μ and with tip-to-shank length of 3 to 3.5 mm. About 15 to 20 such microelectrodes are tied, with string, on a conventional microscope slide. Two or three slides are then placed horizontally on a wire rack which is immersed in a beaker containing 3 M KCl. Filling of the microelectrode with 3 M KCl is produced by gently heating the solution to boiling point (about 5 minutes), which is usually sufficient to produce uniform filling without air bubbles occluding the lumen. Subsequently, microelectrodes with a resistance of 20 to 60 megohms are accepted for experimental purposes (tested by a 100-mv calibration across a 10^6-megohm resistor). The electrodes are routinely kept in a 3 M KCl solution under refrigeration, prior to use. For more detailed steps of the foregoing techniques, see Bures et al. (1967).

Experimental Technique

In an experiment designed merely to record action potentials from a single intracellular microelectrode, the microelectrode is first positioned on the electrode

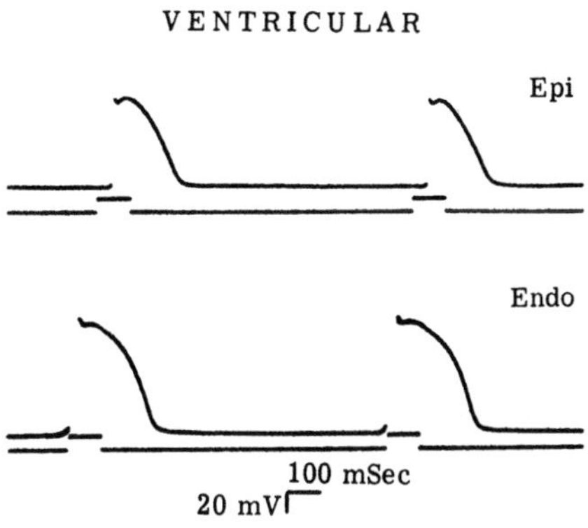

FIG. 4. Characteristic action potential recorded from canine ventricular cells. The upper tracing is recorded from the epicardial surface; the lower tracing is recorded from the endocardial surface.

holder and lowered into the bath solution. Electrode resistance is first tested for acceptability, as previously described; then the microelectrode is "balanced" (i.e., the oscilloscope beam is adjusted until no potential difference is recorded between the microelectrode, in the "intracellular space," and the reference electrode). Cell impalement is then produced by further gradual lowering of the microelectrode, while observing the monitor oscilloscope. An intracellular position of the electrode is recognized when a transmembrane potential of 80 to 100 mv is observed on the oscilloscope (the oscilloscope is customarily calibrated for a 100-mv signal to yield a 5-cm deflection). A threshold stimulus (achieved by adjustment of voltage with the pulse generator and stimulus isolator) is then used to elicit transmembrane action potentials (Figures 3 and 4 illustrate characteristic action potentials recorded from canine atrial and ventricular fibers).

The effect of drug and electrolyte alteration upon the cardiac action potential may then be assessed either pharmacologically (by direct injection of an appropriate solution into the bath) or physiologically (by constant perfusion of the tissue with Tyrode solution containing the appropriate drug or altered electrolyte composition).

Application of Technique

ATRIAL AND VENTRICULAR CELLS.—Studies of this nature have demonstrated characteristic changes in the cardiac monophasic action potential upon exposure to such environmental changes. The monophasic action potential changes may be quite variable from species to species, however, as well as from one tissue type to another. Acetylcholine administration, e.g., produces a striking abbreviation of action potential duration in mammalian atrial tissue without loss of resting transmembrane potential, while the ventricular myocardial cells of the same species are affected little if at all by acetylcholine. Cardiac glycosides, similarly, exert a more rapid and striking effect on atrial than on ventricular tissue,

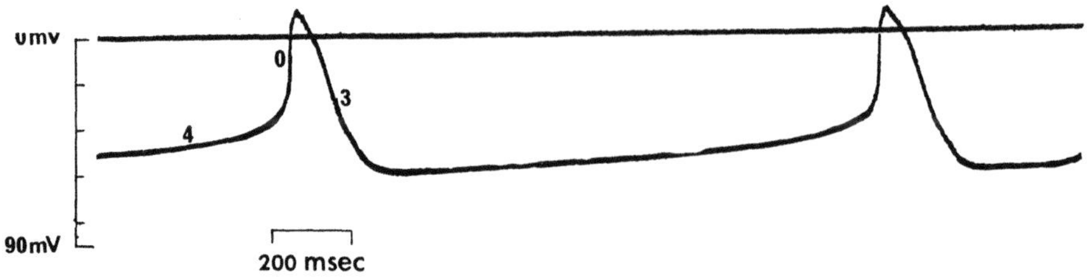

FIG. 5. Sino-atrial cell action potentials from a canine heart. It is to be noted that there is no true resting potential but that following repolarization there is a continuous slow diastolic depolarization (phase 4) which, on reaching the threshold potential, depolarizes rapidly in a regenerative fashion (phase 0).

ATRIUM

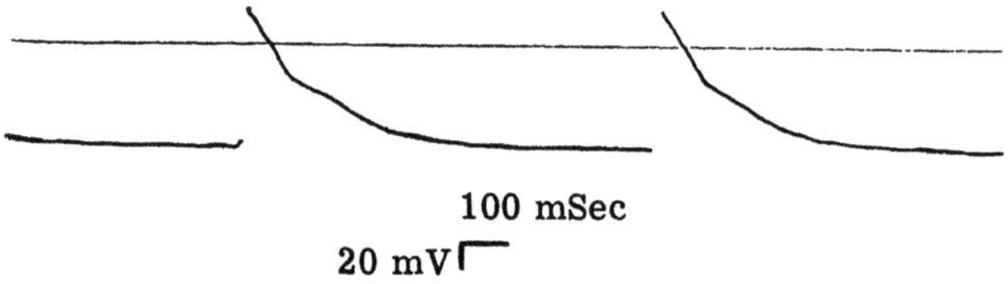

FIG. 6. This action potential recorded from canine atrium, is identical to that described by Wagner et al. (1966) as a specialized conduction fiber. No spontaneous diastolic depolarization is exhibited by this cell at the time of this recording.

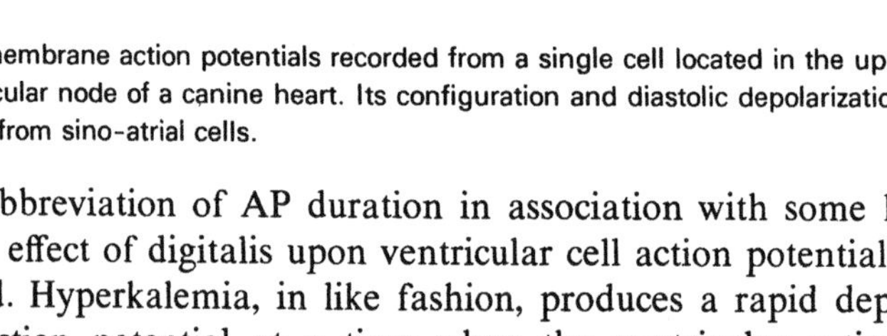

FIG. 7. Transmembrane action potentials recorded from a single cell located in the upper to mid portion of the atrioventricular node of a canine heart. Its configuration and diastolic depolarization are very similar to that recorded from sino-atrial cells.

yielding an abbreviation of AP duration in association with some loss of resting potential; the effect of digitalis upon ventricular cell action potential is similar but much delayed. Hyperkalemia, in like fashion, produces a rapid depolarization of atrial fiber action potential at a time when the ventricular action potential is relatively unchanged. The demonstration of such characteristic change in action potential configuration, by the microelectrode technique, has helped to explain the clinical behavior of numerous drugs and electrolyte alterations and to provide a rationale for even more effective therapy.

SPECIALIZED CONDUCTION SYSTEM.—Certain cardiac cells, in all mammalian species, possess the capacity, overt or latent, to initiate impulses

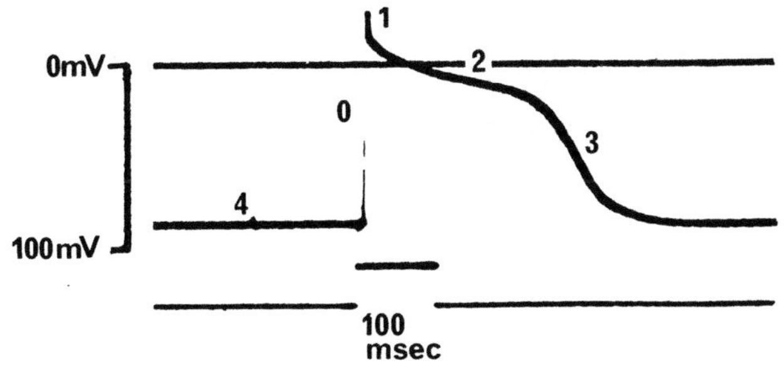

FIG. 8. Transmembrane action potential of a canine Purkinje cell. The plateau or phase 2 is most prominent in these specialized conduction fibers.

spontaneously. Among such tissues are included the sinoatrial node (Fig. 5), the specialized conduction fiber of the atrium (Fig. 6), the atrioventricular junctional tissue (Fig. 7), and the His Purkinje system (Fig. 8). These cells may exhibit spontaneous depolarization ("phase 4" depolarization) constantly (sinoatrial cells, e.g., and certain AV junctional cells), or they may do so under appropriate stimulation (specialized atrial conduction fibers and the cells of the His Purkinje system under the influence of digitalis [Fig. 9], or hypokalemia, e.g.). Microelectrophysiologic studies have clearly demonstrated this characteristic property of specialized conduction cells (i.e., the property of automaticity or spontaneous depolarization), and have helped to define the role that various factors play in affecting the rate at which these specialized fibers may initiate impulses. In addition to the slope of phase 4 depolarization, affected by acetylcholine, catecholamines, digitalis, quinidine, and variations in extracellular K^+ concentration, such factors as the level of transmembrane potential and the threshold potential (i.e., that level of transmembrane potential at which spontaneous *regenerative* depolarization occurs, producing the rapid upstroke or phase 0) play a significant role in the frequency of ectopic impulse formation. And this latter knowledge, again gleaned from microelectrophysiologic studies, has been and continues to be of major importance in understanding the genesis of cardiac arrhythmias as well as in devising a rational approach to therapy.

A further application of microelectrode technique to the study of cardiac muscle stems from the observations of Edmands et al. (1966) and

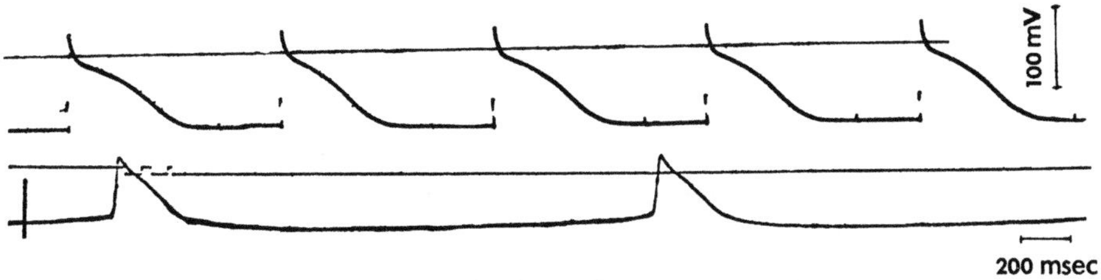

FIG. 9. The upper tracing is recorded from a canine Purkinje cell. The lower tracing, recorded from the same cell, reveals the development of spontaneous diastolic depolarization under the influence of digitalis.

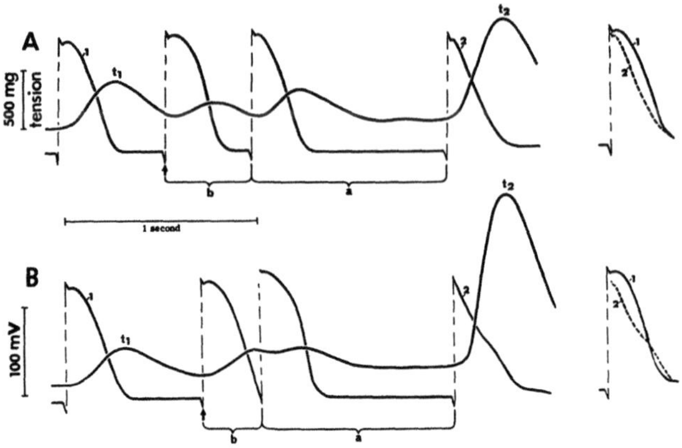

FIG. 10. Simultaneous recordings of isometric contractile tension and ventricular action potentials from canine myocardium. The basic stimulus rate is 60/minute in each strip. Premature stimuli are interpolated in both A and B (marked by arrows). In each case, the *second* contraction after the interpolation is enhanced and is associated with an AP that exhibits acceleration of early repolarization (i.e., phase 2). In strip 3, the contractile enhancement is more marked and is associated with a more marked abbreviation of phase 2 (the changes are illustrated by superimposition at the end of each trace). Both the AP and contractile changes appear related to the degree of relative cycle-length prolongation (i.e., the ratio a/b). See Greenspan et al. (1967) for a more detailed discussion. (From Greenspan et al. 1967. *Circ. Res.,* 20:311. Reprinted with permission of the American Heart Assn., Inc., New York.)

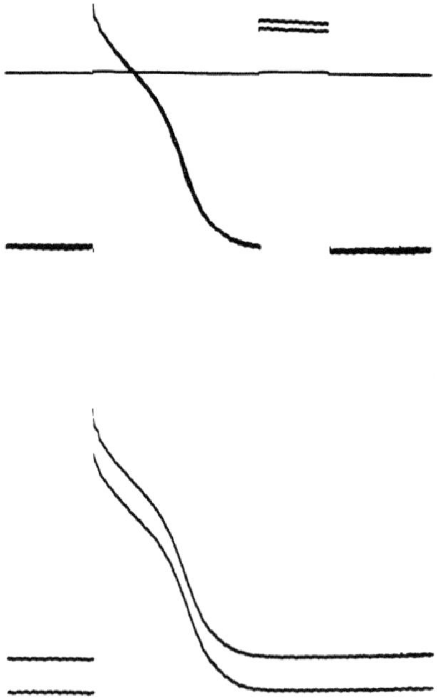

FIG. 11. This figure illustrates two Purkinje cell action potentials elicited from a single stimulus and recorded simultaneously. In trace A (top), the two AP's are superimposed. A 100 mv calibration deflection is shown. In trace B (bottom), the lower beam has been further lowered to illustrate more clearly the two complexes.

Greenspan et al. (1967) concerning an apparent temporal relation between action potential configuration and the inotropic state of canine and human ventricular muscle, under a variety of circumstances. These studies have noted at least a semiquantitative relation between the duration of phase 2 of the action potential and the contractile state of the myocardium (Fig. 10). The method of study here involved the recording of isometric contractile tension simultaneously with the transmembrane action potentials. In this case, a thin trabecular muscle (0.5 to 1 mm in diameter) was isolated from the right ventricle and placed in a 30-ml bath filled with Tyrode solution as previously described. One end of the muscle was clamped to a plastic block by coated steel springs, while the other end was impaled by a steel hook and attached to a UC3 (Statham) transducer via a gold chain. Stimuli were provided by bipolar steel electrodes as before, while both the action potential and the concomitant contractile tensions were recorded on Electronics for Medicine paper at a speed of 100 mm/sec. The effect of various inotropic agents, including abrupt rate change, was then directly assessed. It has been suggested, on the basis of prevalent electrophysiologic concepts, that the action potential change associated with contractile enhancement may reflect an increased efflux of K^+ ions. This remains to be determined beyond equivocation, however. In any case, delineation of the fluxes apparently associated with contractile variation may aid in a more precise characterization of the contractile phenomenon itself.

Multiple Electrode Recording

It has been demonstrated in a number of electrophysiologic studies that cardiac impulse conduction between two or more discrete points may be assessed by the use of two or more electrodes recording action potentials consequent to a single impulse (Fig. 11). Numerous factors are involved in the production of cardiac conduction disturbances (sinoatrial, interatrial and intraatrial, atrioventricular and intraventricular). Fundamentally, slowed conduction stems from a decrease in the rate and amplitude of phase 0 depolarization. The latter may be produced by several factors, however—a reduction in transmembrane potential, a lesser magnitude of the threshold potential, and even an increase in the rate of spontaneous phase 4 depolarization in specialized conduction tissue such as the AV junction. The concept of decremental conduction, fundamental to an understanding of conduction disturbances, stems from the observation of Hoffman and Cranefield (1960) that a reduction in the upstroke velocity of the transmembrane action potential may yield a progressively greater reduction in the amplitude and rate of rise of subsequent action potentials, until conduction ceases. Such an end result may stem from a variety of factors: acetylcholine administration, digitalis "toxicity," hyperkalemia, hypercalcemia, hypoxia, etc.

Further clarification of the mechanism of some arrhythmias awaits still more microelectrophysiologic study, to identify the physiologic basis of such apparent clinical electrocardiographic entities as reciprocal rhythm and "supernormal" conduction. This type of study would undoubtedly entail the employment of multiple microelectrode impalements.

Still more sophisticated evaluation of action potential change associated with environmental alteration may lie in the application of techniques employed in high-frequency electrocardiography to the recording of intracellular action potentials. Such a technique has been described by Anderson et al. (1967). In this method, the intracellular potentials are recorded on magnetic tape with displaced reproduce heads for accurate synchronization and displayed on a Tektronix memory oscilloscope (Fig. 2). Direct photography of phase 0 may thus be performed with reliable sweep speeds ranging from 2×10^6 to 5×10^7 mm/sec. Using this technique, the administration of hyperkalemic solutions (Anderson et al., 1967) has been shown to be associated with a significant initial increase in the maximum rising velocity of phase 0, without a discernible change in the transmembrane resting potential. While they are significant and reproducible, these changes are not sufficiently gross to be detected by conventional methods that employ differentiation to assess the velocity of the action potential upstroke. Such an observation may nevertheless explain the initial acceleration of AV conduction as well as the decrease in threshold requirements for external stimulation, observed in humans during K^+ infusion. In any case, the application of this technique to the recording of cardiac transmembrane action potentials may yield information of substantial value, not hitherto available, concerning the mechanism of action of a variety of cardiotonic agents.

TECHNIQUE OF POLAROGRAPHY: THE OXYGEN CATHODE

Introduction

The mammalian heart and its cellular components have been subjected to a variety of studies. Its embryology, histology, and anatomy are well defined. Furthermore, the electrophysiologic properties of the single cardiac cell have been extensively investigated and the technique of recording these potentials has been previously described. In addition, attempts have been made to elucidate the metabolic requirements of the normal myocardium in order to serve as a basis for differentiating the deficiencies that may or may not exist in a decreased or failing heart. Inherent in these latter studies is the prerequisite of determining the oxygen metabolism of the heart as a whole and its parts in particular. The significance of such studies on the cardiac oxygen requirement is evident, for it can define, indirectly, the energy cost of the work done by the heart and the efficiency of the myocardium under normal and stress conditions and during failure. Despite the importance of this parameter there exists a paucity of information on the resting oxygen uptake of myocardial tissue. This is particularly true for the specialized conducting tissue of the mammalian heart.

Many methods are available for the study of metabolic processes of excised tissues. Techniques in microrespirometry have been developed which aim at simplicity, high sensitivity, and rapidity of response without affecting stability and reliability. However, strict adherence to all of the foregoing criteria is not always essential. In studies on the oxygen uptake of excised tissue involving measurements over a long period of time, the stability of the measuring device becomes more important than the rapidity of response, whereas the latter assumes dominance during short time studies. In both cases, however, sensitivity and reliability are at a premium. Specifically, it is felt by us that in studies involving the determination of oxygen uptake of small intact viable tissue over a relatively long time the method of oxygen polarography coupled with a flow-type microrespirometer is best for its stability, sensitivity, and reliability.

The technique of polarography was first developed by Heyrovsky (1923) and by Heyrovsky and Shikata (1925). In 1940, Kolthoff and Laitinen replaced the dropping mercury electrode with a platinum wire microelectrode and demonstrated its use for polarographic determination of oxygen dissolved in solution. The applicability of this method for the study of oxygen metabolism was further advanced with the development of a microrespirometer that incorporated the platinum microelectrode (Davies and Brink, 1941).

The Oxygen Cathode

The microelectrode itself consists of a platinum wire encased in soft glass tubing with one end ground so that the platinum surface is flush with the soft glass tubing. The other end of the platinum wire is connected to the negative terminal of an adjustable source of voltage. The electrical circuit is completed through a chopper amplifier to a nonpolarizable reference electrode such as a calomel half-cell. When the platinum microelectrode is made electronegative to the calomel half-cell, the oxygen that is dissolved in the medium at the surface of the platinum wire is reduced, resulting in a flow of current. This current is amplified by a chopper amplifier, which in turn drives an ink-writing recorder.

The oxygen polarographic method of analysis is based upon a current-voltage curve in which the current is eventually limited by the diffusion of fresh oxygen from the source to the platinum tip. A typical current-voltage curve is shown in Figure 12. On the ascending limb of the curve there is a partial but progressive disappearance of the dissolved oxygen with increasing voltage which permits the oxygen from the bulk solution to diffuse toward the electrode tip. However, at potentials of about 0.6 to 0.9, the curve plateaus out because the electrolysis is sufficiently rapid to permit all of the oxygen diffusing toward the tip to be reduced. Hence the rate of the reaction becomes limited by diffusion. It is this diffusion limitation that results in the plateau. Thus during this plateau the oxygen concentration at the microelectrode surface is practically equal to zero; otherwise oxygen diffusion would not be at its maximum and a plateau would not occur. Hence the current recorded is proportional to the oxygen concentration in the bulk of the fluid. For this reason, plus the fact that in the region of the plateau the slope is at a minimum, the potential is always adjusted to some value on the plateau. The current increase that occurs again at the higher voltages is due to a second reaction in which ionic hydrogen is reduced to molecular hydrogen.

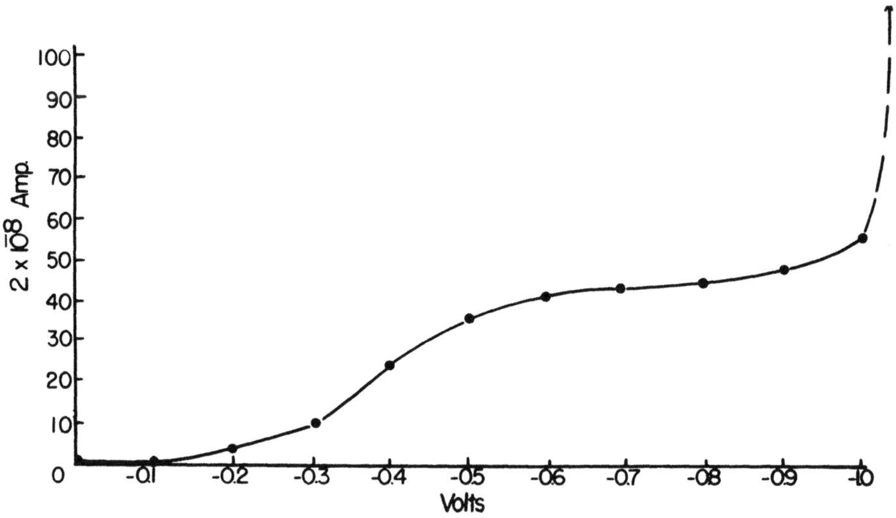

FIG. 12. Current-voltage curve for a collodion-coated oxygen cathode in 0.15 M NaCl. Solution equilibrated with a gas mixture containing 5% CO_2 and 95% O_2. Respirometer flow rate was 0.3 cc/hour and at a temperature of 30°C.

In the use of a platinum microelectrode for oxygen determination there are two important points to bear in mind. First, the platinum microelectrode acts as an amperometric device that irreversibly consumes the material whose concentration it is measuring. For this reason it is best to call this device an oxygen cathode rather than an oxygen electrode. Second, measurements with an oxygen cathode are strictly empirical, and hence the cathode must be calibrated under conditions essentially similar to those under the experimental conditions. This calibration is done in two steps. The first is the establishment of a current-voltage curve as previously described and shown in Figure 12. The second step in calibration involves the adjustment of the polarizing potential to a value in the plateau region and measuring the current to the cathode when the surrounding solution is equilibrated with different gas mixtures of known oxygen content. A typical current-oxygen concentration curve is shown in Figure 13. The establishment of these curves is essential to demonstrate the hypothesis that the current is directly proportional to the concentration of the dissolved oxygen or to the oxygen tension of the equilibrating gas. Thus, with a constant polarizing voltage, a constant flow velocity past the cathode tip, and at a constant temperature, the current will remain constant for a given oxygen tension. When viable tissue is added to the system under the foregoing conditions there will be a decrease in current resulting from the decrease in oxygen concentration due to respiration by the tissue. This change in oxygen tension can then be accurately determined.

There is, however, an exception to the preceding in which a reduced current reading can not be totally attributed to active oxygen uptake by the tissue. There is a tendency for the cathode current to decrease with time even though the oxygen

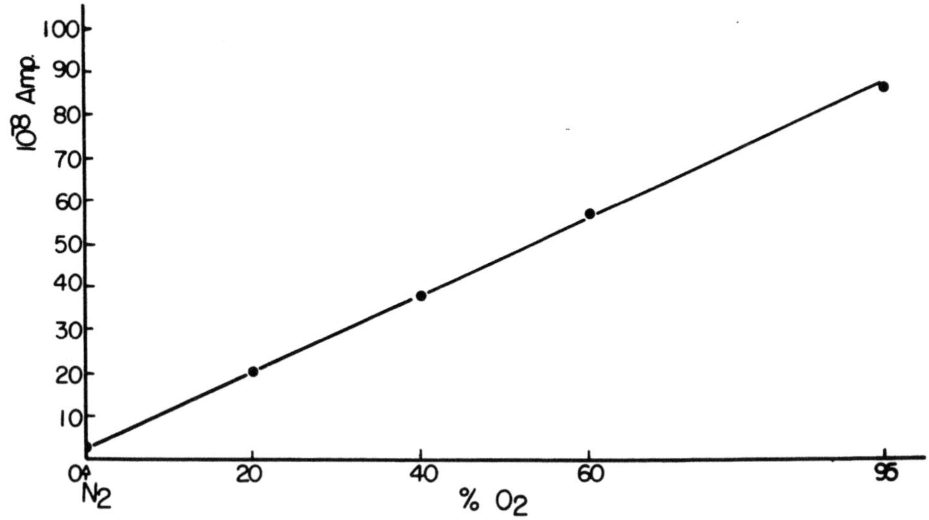

FIG. 13. Calibration curve for a collodion-coated oxygen cathode in 0.15 M NaCl. Polarizing potential set at 0.7 volts, temperature 30°C, and respirometer flow rate at 0.3 cc/hour.

tension in the solution is maintained at a constant level. This decline in sensitivity is called "aging." The mechanism(s) that produce(s) the aging is not fully understood. There are, however, two possibilities that can initiate this condition:

1. A change in the number of electrons reacting during oxygen reduction.
2. Oxygen cathode surface occlusion by precipitation of insoluable salts.

When dissolved oxygen is reduced by the polarizing voltage the reactions that can occur are:

$$O_2 + 2H^+ + 2e^- \longrightarrow H_2O_2$$
$$H_2O_2 + 2H^+ + 2e^- \longrightarrow 2H_2O$$

There is still some controversy as to whether there is a 2- or 4-electron reaction; if only the first reaction occurs, then 2 electrons flow in the circuit for each oxygen molecule that reacts. Hill (1948) observed that as soon as peroxide was formed it was immediately reduced to water by the second reaction. On the other hand, Davies and Brink (1942) noted a 2-electron reaction for some of their cathodes but a 4-electron reaction for other cathodes. Assuming that a 4-electron reaction is normal, then during a determination a cathode shift to a 2-electron reaction will result in a temporal decrease in cathode sensitivity. Furthermore, the reaction(s) require that the medium near the cathode supply hydrogen ions. Actually, from a physiologic point of view, it is more meaningful to write the reactions as producing hydroxyl ions. This base production will result in a change in pH that in turn could result in a precipitation of insoluble salts. The net result would be an occlusion of the cathode surface and a decrease in sensitivity. In order to reduce the aging process to a minimum, the oxygen cathodes used in most investigations are coated with a layer of collodion or encased with some polyethylene cover. This serves to reduce the current density at the cathode surface. In addition, the polarizing voltage is applied intermittently, so that the cathode operates about 8 seconds out of every minute. Since the rate of hydroxyl production, and therefore the intensity of alkalinity, varies with the cathode current density it is conceivable that reducing the time the polarization is on will delay the onset of decay in sensitivity. The coating and intermittent polarization thus virtually eliminates the problem of drift in the cathodes.

In general, the oxygen cathode represents an excellent tool for oxygen tension determinations. By intermittent polarization and enclosing the cathode with a membrane, the problem of drift is virtually eliminated. The net result is a method that is reliable, stable, and highly sensitive for the measurement of oxygen uptake of excised tissues.

The Flow-Type Microrespirometer

The foregoing description of the calibration of an oxygen cathode is based upon the establishment of a diffusion equilibrium of oxygen from an external source to the cathode surface. Although this equilibrium can be attained in the static type of respirometer (the volume is fixed), there are certain undesirable features in the use of such microrespirometers. In static respirometers no provision is made for the removal of waste materials produced by the metabolic processes of the tissue. Nor is the tissue presented with a constant fresh supply of its essential nutrients. Hence with time the normal substrates are utilized by the metabolizing tissue, and ultimately the energy provided by the oxidation of these substances is reduced. In addition, the accumulation of metabolic waste products may have a deleterious effect on the enzymatic reactions in the tissue. Under such conditions the tissue may never reach a steady state of metabolism, which is essential if one desires to measure the resting rate of oxygen consumption.

Moreover, the use of tissue slices with the possible destruction of some of the enzyme systems might cause a lower oxygen uptake. It is possible that the tissue samples used in many previous studies were anoxic at the start of the experiments. It may be that the use of tissue slices and the employment of a static type of respirometer are inappropriate for determining the "resting" oxygen consumption of metabolizing heart tissue, and in particular the QO_2 of actively conducting muscle. All of the foregoing undesirable properties may be avoided by the use of intact preparation, such as Purkinje fibers and papillary muscles, and the employment of a flow respirometer coupled with an oxygen electrode as the sensing device.

The basic aim in physiologic research is ultimately to comprehend the various activities on a cellular level. Ideally the unknown variables should be studied in

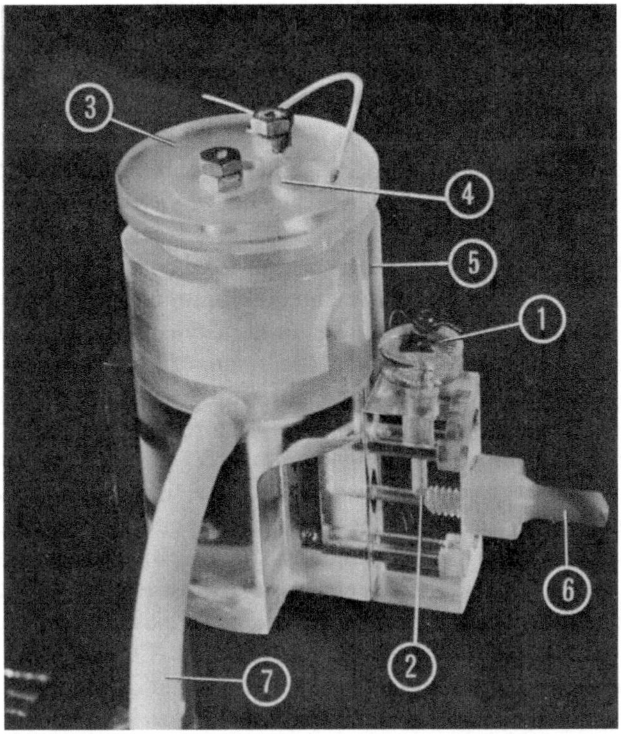

FIG. 14. Photo of the tissue flow type microrespirometer. The component parts are: (1) Holder containing oxygen cathode. (2) Capillary in which oxygen cathode is placed. (3) Cap of respirometer rod to which one end of the tissue is attached. (4) Area through which muscle tie is led to be attached to the transducer pin (see Fig. 15, 1). (5) Respirometer reservoir. (6) Tubing leading to precision syringe for constant flow. (7) Tubing for rapid emptying of solution in respirometer reservoir.

vivo. However, this is not always feasible, and hence, in vitro studies must be employed. In the latter case, therefore, it is desirable to produce an environment that is almost identical to the tissue's in vivo surroundings. Hence, a respirometer becomes the integument of the excised tissue, and from there the following conditions must be provided:

1. A normal thermal environment
2. A constant supply of oxygen
3. A constant supply of essential nutrients and substrates
4. A means for the removal of CO_2, heat, and other diffusable material produced by the metabolic processes of the tissue

In effect the respirometer should provide a constant thermal and chemical environment which will maintain a steady state of metabolism. All of these conditions cannot be met by the static type of respirometers but, in essence, are met with a flow type of respirometer. Such a microrespirometer was developed by

Carlson et al. (1950). The respirometers used in the studies of Cranefield and Greenspan (1960) and Greenspan and Cranefield (1963) were essentially similar in design and performance to that described by Carlson et al. (1950), except for the following modifications. The respirometer, utilized for papillary muscles (Figure 14), made of Lucite, consists of a well containing Tyrode solution and a capillary of diameter 2.4 mm in which the tissue is eventually placed for the measurement of oxygen uptake. The respirometer used for Purkinje fiber studies (Greenspan and Cranefield, 1963) should have a capillary diameter no greater than 1.6 mm. Thus, depending on the tissue to be studied, the capillary diameter is specifically adjusted so that the volume of the capillary can be restricted in order to reduce the time required for the establishment of diffusion equilibrium between the gas phase and the tissue. The Tyrode solution is drawn through the respirometer at a constant flow rate of either 9.3 ml/hour, 0.6 ml/hour, or 1.23 ml/hour by means of a precision syringe drive mechanism. This motor-driven syringe is custom-made so that constancy of flow is maintained. Furthermore, the syringes are made of precision-ground glass with close-fitting stainless steel plungers to prevent leakage, and again maintain the constancy of flow past the tissue. The constancy of the oxygen tension is maintained by the continuous bubbling of a gas of known oxygen concentration through the solution in the reservoir. The oxygen cathode is placed in the capillary at a point far enough downstream from the end of the respiring tissue so that all the concentration gradients existing across the stream as they leave the end of the tissue become equilibrated. Carlson et al. (1950) have shown that the distance, L, in cm should be greater than that given by the equation:

$$L = \frac{12r^2 D}{V - (V^2 + 145\, r^2 D^2)^{1/2}}$$

where

V = volume flow rate in cm^3/sec
r = radius of the capillary in cm
D = diffusion coefficient of oxygen in cm^2/sec

According to these investigators, at this distance from the tissue the oxygen concentration across the area of the capillary will be constant to within 2 percent of its average value.

The entire respirometer may be contained in a large insulated box (or any device) that maintains a constant temperature that is thermostatically controlled to within ± 0.3°C. The housing temperature is continuously monitored by a thermistor, which when necessary activates a controller to increase or decrease the temperature to maintain a constant bath temperature. The latter in turn is continuously monitored by a thermistor embedded in the respirometer reservoir.

The Tissue Preparation

The appropriately anesthetized experimental animal is subjected to thoracotomy and cardiac excision, following which the intact heart is placed in warm Tyrode solution oxygenated with gas composed of 5 percent CO_2 and 95 percent O_2. All subsequent dissection is carried out under the stream of gas. This procedure assists in maintaining oxygenation of the tissues and also prevents tissue CO_2 from falling rapidly (Cranefield et al., 1957; Monnier, 1952). The left or right ventricle chamber is opened and a papillary muscle, trabecula, or a free running Purkinje fiber (false tendon) is selected. The small papillary muscles are always obtained from the right chamber, while the left chamber contains the "better" Purkinje fiber. A fine thread is tied around each end of the tissue, which is then cut free from its attachment to the heart and placed in a thermostatically controlled bath containing Tyrode solution. The Tyrode solution has a composition similar to that previously given and a pH of 7.2 at 35°C when in equilibration with the gas mixture containing 5 percent CO_2. The thread attached to one of the tissues is tied to a thin rod which is an extension of the reservoir cap and which fits in the center of the respirometer capillary that is vertical to the reservoir. After washing and thermal equilibration, the muscle is placed in the respirometer reservoir. The oxygen tension of the fluid flowing from the reservoir is determined, and then the tissue is placed into the capillary by inserting the rod to which the tissue is tied. This maneuver can be accomplished without marked disturbance of the flow through the capillary. With the muscle in the capillary, one end of the muscle is thus held in place because it is fixed to the rod which in turn is attached to the cap of the reservoir. The thread tied to the other end of the muscle is brought through the top end of the capillary into the reservoir and straight up to a fine glass hook attached to the pin of an RCA-5734 mechanoelectric transducer tube (Figure 15). Recording from the transducer (Ross, 1958) is accomplished, with appropriate amplification, on the usual recorders. The entire transducer assembly, as shown in Figures 14 and 15, is mounted on a pair of micromanipulators, which in turn is clamped to a stand. This clamp and one of the micromanipulators enables rotational and horizontal movement of the transducer assembly and thus makes it possible to position the thread and muscle in the center of the capillary. The other micromanipulator moves the transducer assembly vertically so that stretch could be applied to the muscle. Initially for the determination of resting QO_2 the position of the tissue is such that it rests under no tension in the center of the capillary. After the stabilization and determination of the "rest" QO_2, the tissue could be stretched, electrically stimulated, or drug added to the perfusion fluid, etc. Then the QO_2 of the various cardiac tissue types can be measured under a variety of experimental conditions.

The calculation of the rate of oxygen uptake is performed in the usual manner, as described by Carlson et al. (1950) and Cranefield et al. (1957) (for the mathematical consideration of this calculation, see pp. 573-574).

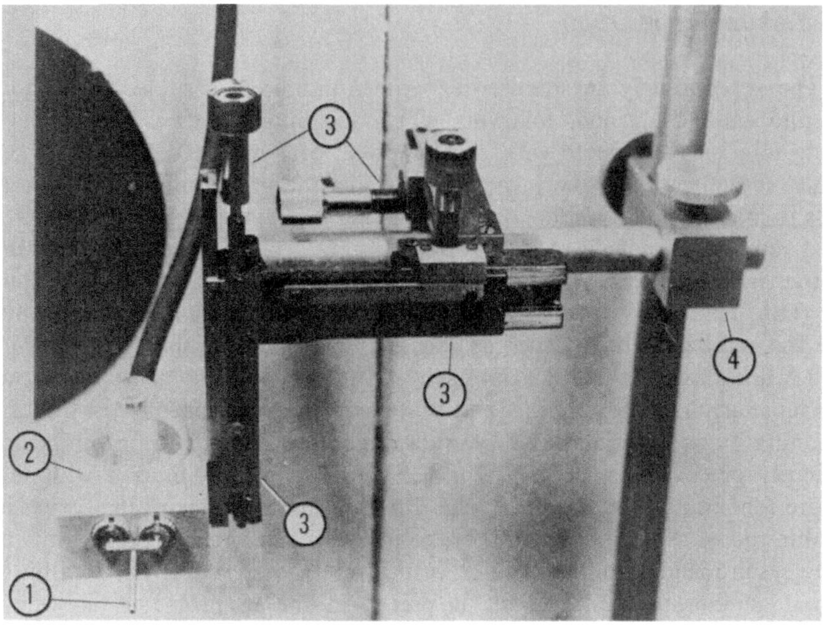

FIG. 15. Photo of the unit for recording of isolated myocardial tension development. The component parts are: (1) Pin of transducer (RCA 5734) to which muscle is attached via its string or gold chain (see Fig. 14, 4). (2) Transducer assembly. (3) Micromanipulator for movement of transducer in various planes. (4) Clamp for attachment of micromanipulator to stand and for rotational movement of entire unit.

Determination of Tissue Diameter by Calculation

The diameters of Purkinje fibers and papillary muscles may be calculated on the basis of their length and wet weight. One assumption, however, must be made, and that is that these tissues are cylindrical in shape. Although this is not always the case for many papillary muscles, they do, nonetheless, more closely approximately cylinders than any other types of geometrical shape.

It is possible to determine the radius of a cylinder from the equation:

$$\text{volume} = \text{surface area} \times \text{length}$$

Since the surface area of a cylinder is equal to πr^2, then substituting in the above equation it becomes: volume = $\pi r^2 L$. As the volume of a cylinder is also equal to weight/specific gravity, then the equation after substitution and rearrangement becomes:

$$r^2 = \frac{\text{weight/specific gravity}}{\text{length} \times \pi}$$

The weight and length of the tissue can be measured directly. To determine the volume, a number of muscles are first weighed in air and then in distilled water with the difference in weight representing the weight of water that is displaced, and this is volume (the density of water being 1). The ratio of weight to volume, and hence specific gravity, was observed by one of us (Greenspan) to be rather constant, and the value determined was very close to 1.1. This figure may be used in all of the diameters to be calculated. These calculated diameters, by and large, are in almost perfect agreement with the direct measurements. In fact, such calculated diameters never vary from the measured diameters by more than the experimental error of the measurement involved in measuring diameter directly.

Calculation of the Rate of Oxygen Uptake

The oxygen uptake of viable tissue is often expressed by the term QO_2. In this discussion the units of QO_2 are in mm^3 or microliters of oxygen consumed per mg of wet weight in one hour. The QO_2 is determined in the following manner. Since the calibration curve of cathode current as a function of oxygen concentration is linear (Fig. 13), it establishes the strict proportionality between oxygen tension and the cathode current. Hence, a proportion can be set up in which:

$$\frac{\text{cathode current without tissue}}{\text{cathode current with tissue}} = \frac{\text{oxygen concentration in reservoir}}{\text{oxygen concentration in capillary beyond tissue and near cathode surface}}$$

The difference between the two oxygen concentrations represents the oxygen concentration consumed by the tissue. This oxygen concentration is multiplied by the solubility of 100 percent oxygen in water at the experimental temperature (Lange, 1941). The product, in units of microliters of oxygen/ml of water, is multiplied by the volume flow rate in units of ml/hour, to yield the total amount of oxygen utilized by the tissue sample. This product, in units of microliters of oxygen/hour, is divided by the wet weight of the tissue in mg to yield microliters of oxygen consumed per mg of wet weight in one hour.

Since the volume flow rate is critical in the determination of uptake it must, therefore, be absolutely constant throughout the experiment, and from experiment to experiment. This constancy is established by means of a precision syringe-drive mechanism (see Methods). The volume flow rate is obtained by determining the distance the fluid traversed in unit time across the capillary area. Thus:

$$\text{volume flow rate} = L\pi r^2/t$$

In the studies by Cranefield and Greenspan (1960) and Greenspan and Cranefield (1963), r, the radius of the capillary, was 0.079375 cm and the distance the fluid traveled in unit time, L/5, was 15.24 cm/hour. Substituting in the preceding equation:

$$\text{volume flow rate} = (15.24\ \text{cm/hour}) \times (3.14) \times (0.079375\ \text{cm})^2 = 0.301\ \text{cm}^3/\text{hour}$$

This can be verified by determining the distance the plunger in the syringe drive moves per unit time, which was found, in the foregoing studies, to be 1.55 cm/hour. The radius of the plunger was 0.24892 cm. Hence, volume flow rate equals (1.55 cm/hour) times (3.14) times $(0.24892\ \text{cm})^2$, which yields 0.304 cm^3/hour.

Application

The in vitro studies, which had been performed by a number of investigators, showed a wide range of mean values for cardiac oxygen consumption. Muus et al. (1939) reported that the oxygen uptake of rat atrial slices was 15.7 microliters/mg dry weight/hour, while ventricular strips gave QO_2 of 7.8. On the other hand, Olson and his co-workers (1948) observed much higher values for their rat ventricular slices. These investigators reported a ventricular QO_2 of 10.27 as compared to 14.77 for their atrial slices. Ranson and Loomis (1952) noted that rat atrial slices under no tension had an uptake of 4.2 microliters/mg dry weight/hour. Much lower oxygen uptakes were reported by Webb et al. (1951), especially considering the fact that their rat atrial and ventricular strips were being electrically driven and thus were contracting. Values of 5.0 and 4.3 for atrium and ventricle, respectively, were observed. Burdette and Wilhelmi (1946), using thin slices of rat heart, noted a value of 7.9 microliters/mg dry weight/hour. Furhman et al. (1945) determined the oxygen consumption of rat ventricle and observed a QO_2 of 10.0. Much lower values of 3.4 and 2.6 were reported for cat papillary muscle by Whalen (1957) in utilizing the solutions of Cattell and Gold (1938) and Gardner et al. (1954). Hence, the reported values of cardiac oxygen consumption range from 2.6 to about 16.0 microliters/mg dry weight/hour.

The disagreement in values, as stated, can be explained on the basis of one or more of the following counts. All of the foregoing investigators, in their determinations of the oxygen metabolism of cardiac tissue, utilized the Warburg apparatus or a modification of this method. However, the use of static-type respirometers lend themselves to criticism. How such respirometers can abet a low oxygen uptake was discussed in the description of a flow type of respirometer.

A second factor that can affect the oxygen uptake of viable tissue is the time elapsed between the obtaining of tissue and the start of oxygenation. Thus, in vitro observations by Bernheim and Bernheim (1944) showed that a 5-minute incubation of rat heart at body temperature in semianaerobic conditions resulted in a rapid diminution of oxygen uptake. However, if the slices were made as rapidly as possible upon immediate removal of the heart from the animal, the uptakes were higher and, moreover, remained constant over a period of six hours. Similar observations were made by Pearson et al. (1949) on rat myocardium.

Another factor that may affect the oxygen uptake is the ionic concentration of the bathing fluid. The effect of K^+, Na^+, and Ca^{++} on the electrical and mechanical properties of the heart are well known (Burgen and Terroux, 1953; Green et al., 1953; Hoffman and Suckling, 1956; Ringer, 1880-1882). Whether the changes in the excitability and mechanical response brought about by these ions also affect the oxygen consumption is not completely known, since few studies have been done to correlate their effects. It has been shown by Murray (1954) and Pearson et al. (1949) that a decrease in the Ca^{++} concentration had no effect on the respiration of beef Purkinje fibers and rat ventricle. Pearson et al. (1949) stated, on the other hand, that when the K^+ concentration was greater than 77 MEq/L, the QO_2 of rat ventricle was reduced by as much as 78 percent. However, close scrutiny of their values indicates that the QO_2 of their ventricle slices in normal Na^+ and K^+ concentrations was lower to begin with when compared to values given by these workers when the phosphate concentration was high and care was taken to determine the thickness of the slices. Thus, they reported that when the phosphate concentration was reduced from 20 mm/liter to 2.5 mm/liter the QO_2 (high to begin with at 12.8 microliters/mg/dry weight/hour) fell by about 50 percent. Since the media used by all of the preceding investigators differed as to their compositions, such might possibly be a factor contributing to the variability in cardiac respiration of the in vitro studies reported in the literature. The studies of Sonnenblick et al. (1965), suggesting a dependency of myocardial oxygen requirements upon the inotropic state of the myocardium, suggest that electrolyte alterations may indeed be relevant to the disparate results in the foregoing studies.

Additional factors that must be taken into account are the state of activity of the tissue during the experiment and the age of the animal from which the myocardial sample was obtained. The higher uptakes may be due to the fact that the tissue may have been contracting spontaneously. Furthermore, age appears to be a determinant in the amount of oxygen a tissue will consume. It is well known that young animals have a higher metabolic rate than do adults. Villee (1953, 1960) has demonstrated that the QO_2 of human placenta decreases with age. Additional evidence that age does affect oxygen uptake was demonstrated by Cranefield and Greenspan (1960) in their studies on kitten and adult cat papillary muscles.

Probably the most important aspect in determining the factors that could explain the wide range of reported oxygen uptakes is the thickness of the tissue sample employed in the experiments. In order to measure the true resting oxygen uptake of any tissue, there must exist the certainty that the core of the tissue is being supplied with oxygen by diffusion. Clark and White (1930) noted that the frog auricle suspended in an atmosphere of oxygen was just thick enough to be supplied by diffusion. However, they found that tissues of greater than 0.2 mm in thickness would not allow an adequate supply of oxygen. For liver slices, however, optimal respiration occurs when the maximal thickness is between 0.5 mm and 0.6 mm, while slices that are thinner or thicker showed a reduced rate of oxygen uptake (Fuhrman and Field, 1945). Similar observations were made for rat ventricular slices (Pearson et al., 1949). The reduced uptake noted for the thinner slices was probably due to the slicing and its inherent destruction of cells and their

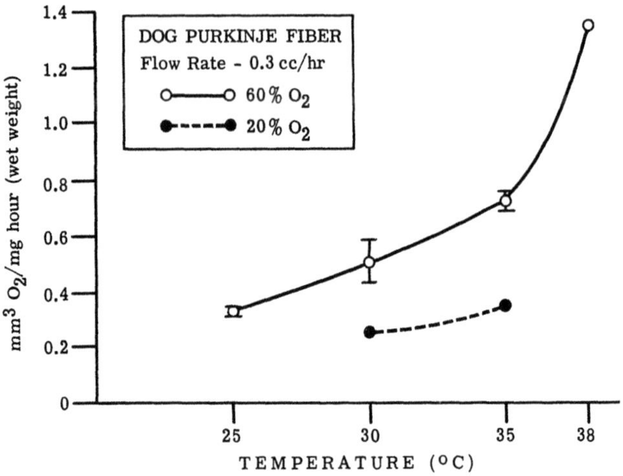

FIG. 16. The apparent rate of oxygen uptake of quiescent Purkinje fibers of the adult dog heart as a function of temperature in 60% oxygen and 20% oxygen. Each point in the 60% oxygen curve represents the average uptake of a group of fibers at each temperature. The bars indicate the range of observed values. (Adapted from Greenspan and Cranefield. 1963. *Amer. J. Physiol.*, 204:5. Reprinted with permission of Waverly Press, Inc., Baltimore, Md.)

enzyme systems. Furthermore, the lower respiration of the thicker slices was presumably due to an inadequate diffusion of oxygen. This diffusion limitation probably explains many of the low uptakes reported in the literature, particularly the uptakes of the cat papillary muscles (Lee, 1953; Whalen, 1957), since the muscles utilized had diameters of 1.2 mm or greater. Indeed, the results obtained by Cranefield and Greenspan (1960) demonstrated that the maximal thickness for cat papillary muscle that will allow adequate diffusion of oxygen is similar to that found for liver slices (Fuhrman and Field, 1945) and ventricular strips (Pearson et al, 1949). This thickness is considerably greater than that recommended by Clark and White (1930) for frog auricle (i.e., 0.2 mm). However, for contracting hearts in situ, the maximal thickness does indeed become reduced to about 0.2 mm. This is so because of the high oxygen requirement of contracting tissue. This figure becomes highly important in relation to the in vitro perfused whole heart preparation. Such a preparation may be anoxic unless there is complete capillary bed patency coupled with a coronary flow rate equal to that of the in situ heart.

In any case the technique of polarography has been and is being utilized for studies on the metabolic requirements of the myocardium. Thus, a number of the factors previously discussed were investigated by Greenspan and Cranefield (1960; 1963) on canine Purkinje fibers and on feline papillary muscles utilizing the technique of polarography. Their determinations of resting QO_2 of these isolated tissues were accomplished in a flow microrespirometer with the use of the oxygen cathode. The results obtained by the utilization of the technique indicated that the apparent resting oxygen consumption of the specialized conducting tissue was extremely sensitive to temperature (Fig. 16) and to the ambient oxygen concentra-

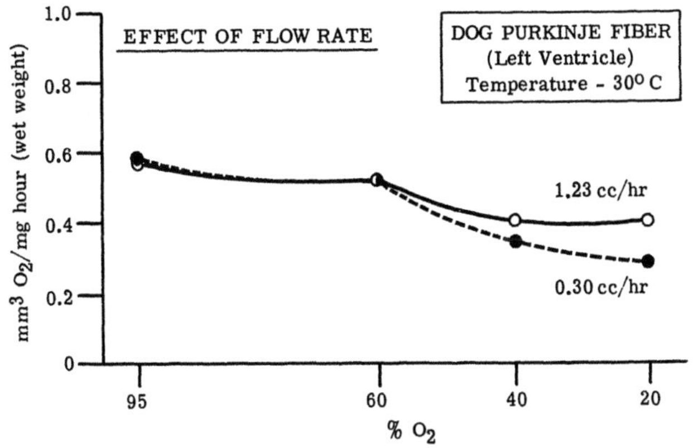

FIG. 17. The apparent oxygen uptake of quiescent Purkinje fibers of the adult dog heart as a function of flow rate; 1.23 cc/hour and 0.3 cc/hour. At each oxygen concentration the same Purkinje fiber was exposed to both flow rates. The uptakes were determined at 30°C. (From Greenspan and Cranefield. 1963. *Amer. J. Physiol.*, 204:5. Reprinted with permission of Waverly Press, Inc., Baltimore, Md.)

tion (Fig. 17). Furthermore, at equal temperature and aerated at any given oxygen concentration, the mammalian papillary muscle has a greater resting QO_2 than do Purkinje fibers. In addition, the diameter of the tissue is extremely important in the determination of QO_2. An inverse relationship appears to exist between rest QO_2 and diameter (Fig. 18). Thus there exists a limit to tissue diameter beyond which the QO_2 decreases, indicating a diffusion limitation. This was further

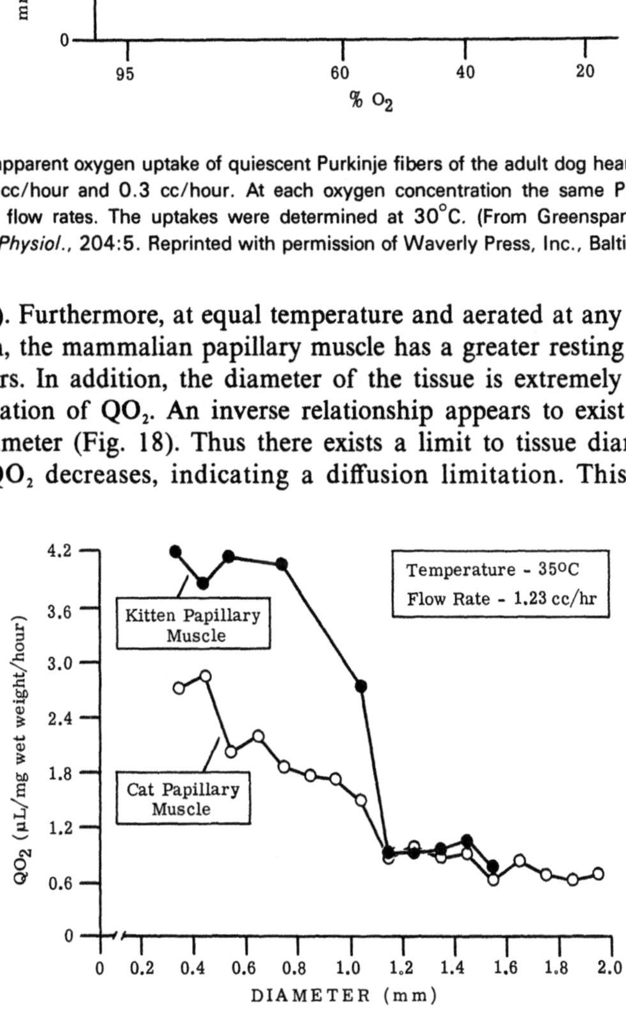

FIG. 18. The apparent oxygen uptake (in microliters/mg wet weight/hour) of quiescent papillary muscles from kitten hearts and from cat hearts. Diameters are combined into groups with a range of 0.1 mm, and the average oxygen uptake for each diameter range is plotted above the diameter which represents the midpoint of the diameter range of the group. The uptakes were measured at 35°C. (From Cranefield and Greenspan. 1960. *J. Gen. Physiol.*, 44:235. Reprinted with permission of The Rockefeller University Press, New York.)

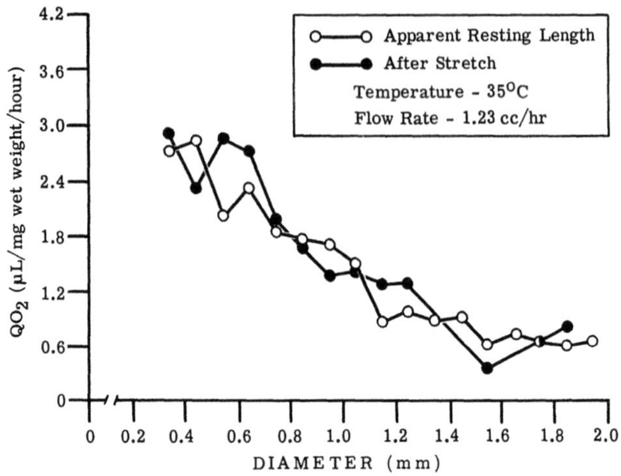

FIG. 19. Apparent oxygen uptake (in microliters/mg wet weight/hour) of quiescent unstretched papillary muscles and of quiescent papillary muscles stretched to a length 50% greater than their rest length. Diameters are combined into groups with a range of 0.1 mm, and the average oxygen uptake for each diameter range is plotted above the diameter which represents the midpoint of the diameter range of the group. The oxygen uptake of the unstretched muscles is plotted above the diameter of the unstretched muscle; the oxygen uptake after stretch is plotted above the diameter after stretch. Not all muscles were stretched and there are thus more muscles represented in the averages of the unstretched groups than in the averages of the stretched groups. The papillary muscles were taken from the hearts of adult cats. The uptakes were determined at 35°C. (From Cranefield and Greenspan. 1960. *J. Gen. Physiol.*, 44:235. Reprinted with permission of The Rockefeller University Press, New York.)

indicated by stretching the muscle, thereby reducing diameter, and resulting in an increased oxygen uptake (Fig. 19).

These findings revealed that the muscles with initial diameter of 0.6 to 0.7 mm were the only ones to show increased oxygen uptake following stretch because the stretching permitted their attaining a diameter less than the critical diameter apropos to the new and reduced oxygen tension in the effluent. However, the larger muscles (initial diameter of 0.8 mm and greater) were much too thick to allow for normal oxygen diffusion and hence did not show an increased QO_2 following a stretch equal to that of those muscles that were small enough to be supplied by diffusion. It can thus be concluded that stretch itself plays little or no role in the rate of oxygen consumption except that it permits a reduction in normal thickness approaching a diameter at which the tissue may be adequately supplied with oxygen by diffusion.

The findings described have, of course, important research implications in the physiology and pharmacology of cardiac metabolism. It is quite difficult to find muscles in the heart that are small enough (0.65 mm or less in diameter) to permit oxygen diffusion in an in vitro environ. It is likely that most prior studies on the electrical and mechanical properties of the isolated papillary muscle were performed on tissues that contained an anoxic core. The situation is, of course, appreciated in an actively contracting muscle where the critical diameter approaches 0.45 mm or less. This situation may explain the variability in response and the viability of an in vitro contracting muscle. The investigator should be especially careful for the whole heart perfused in vitro where the probability of anoxia is great unless adequate measures are taken to permit a complete capillary bed patency and a coronary fluid flow rate equal to that of the intact contracting myocardium.

REFERENCES

Abbott, B. C., and Mommaerts, W. F. H. M. 1959. A study of inotropic mechanism in the papillary muscle preparation. J. Gen. Physiol., 42:533-551.

Adrian, E. D. 1921. The recovery process of excitable tissues. Part II. J. Physiol. (London), 55:193-225.

Anderson, G. J., Greenspan, K., Edmands, R. E., and Fisch, C. 1967. The effect of K^+ on human monophasic action potential. Circulation, 36:II 53.

Baudze, S., and Wertheimer, E. 1928. Der glykogengehalt des reizleitungs-systems im herzen. Pflügers Arch. Ges. Physiol., 219:233-237.

Bernheim, F., and Bernheim, M. L. C. 1944. The effects of various conditions on the respiration of rat heart muscle in vitro. Amer. J. Physiol., 142:195-199.

Bing, R. J., Maraist, F. M., Dammann, J. F., Jr., Heimbecker, R., Daly, R., Gerard, R., and Calazel, P. 1950. Effect of strophantus on coronary blood flow and cardiac oxygen consumption of normal and failing human hearts. Circulation, 2:513-516.

—Hammond, M. M., Handelsman, J. C., Power, S. R., Spencer, F. C., Eckenhoff, J. E., Goodale, W. T., Hafkenschiel, J. H., and Kety, S. S. 1949. The measurement of coronary blood flow, oxygen consumption, and efficiency of the left ventricle in man. Amer. Heart J., 38:1-24.

Brink, F., Bronk, D. W., Carlson, F. D., and Connelly, C. M. 1952. The oxygen uptake of active axons. Cold Spring Harbor Symposium on Quantitative Biology, 17:53-67.

Burdette, W. J., and Wilhelmi, A. E. 1946. Respiration of heart muscle slices from rats in the terminal stage of hemorrhagic shock. Proc. Soc. Exp. Biol. Med., 61:411-413.

Bures, J., Petran, M., and Zachar, J. 1967. Electrophysiological methods in biological research. 3rd ed. New York, Academic Press, Inc.

Burgen, A. S. V., and Terroux, K. G. 1953. The membrane resting and action potentials. J. Physiol. (London), 119:139-152.

Bryant, R. E., Thomas, W. A., and O'Neal, R. M. 1958. An electron microscopic study of myocardial ischemia in the rat. Circulation, 6:699-709.

Carlson, F. D., Brink, F., and Bronk, D. W. 1950. A continuous flow respirometer utilizing the oxygen cathode. Rev. Sci. Instrum., 21:923-932.

Cattel, McK., and Gold, H. 1938. The influence of digitalis glycosides on the force of contraction of mammalian cardiac muscle. J. Pharmacol. Exp. Ther., 62:116-125.

Clark, A. J., and White, A. C. 1930. The oxygen consumption of the auricles of the frog and of the tortoise. J. Physiol. (London), 68:406-440.

Cranefield, P. F., and Hoffman, B. F. 1958. Electrophysiology of single cardiac cells. Physiol. Rev., 38:41-76.

—and Greenspan, K. 1960. The rate of oxygen uptake of quiescent cardiac muscle. J. Gen. Physiol., 44:235-249.

—Brink, F., and Bronk, D. W. 1957. The oxygen uptake of the peripheral nerve of the rat. J. Neurochem., 1:245-249.

Davies, P. W., and Brink, F. 1941. A new microrespirometer for nerve. Amer. J. Physiol., 133:257-258.

—and Brink, F. 1942. Microelectrodes for measuring local oxygen tension in animal tissues. Rev. Sci. Instrum. 13:524-533.
Draper, M. H., and Weidmann, S. 1951. Cardiac resting and action potentials with an intracellular electrode, J. Physiol. (London), 115:74-94.
Edmands, R. E., Greenspan, K., and Fisch, C. 1966. The effect of cycle-length alterations upon the configuration of the canine ventricular action potential. Circ. Res., 19:602-610.
Fenn, W. O. 1927. The oxygen consumption of frog nerve during stimulation. J. Gen. Physiol., 10:767-779.
Fuhrman, F. A., and Field, J. 1945. Factors determining the metabolic rate of excised liver tissue. I. Effect of slice thickness and tissue injury on oxygen consumption. II. Effect of glycogen content on oxygen consumption. III. Effect of temperature on oxygen consumption. Arch. Biochem., 6:337-349.
—Fuhrman, G. J., and Field, J. 1945. Oxygen consumption of excised rat tissue following acute anoxic anoxia. Amer. J. Physiol., 144:87-90.
Furchgott, R. F., and Shorr, E. 1958. The effect of succinate on respiration and certain metabolic processes of mammalian tissues at low oxygen tensions in vitro. J. Biol. Chem., 175:201-215.
Gardner, E. A., Wilson, M., and Farah, A. 1954. The action of iodoacetate on the isolated rabbit auricle. J. Pharmacol. Exp. Ther. 110:166-179.
Green, J. P., Giarman, N. J., and Salter, W. T. 1953. Combined effects of potassium and calcium on contractibility and excitability of the mammalian myocardium. Amer. J. Physiol., 171:174-177.
Greenspan, K., and Cranefield, P. F. 1963. Influence of some factors on oxygen uptake of canine cardiac Purkinje fibers. Amer. J. Physiol., 204:5-8.
—Edmands, R. E., and Fisch, C. 1967. The relation of contractile enhancement to action potential change in canine myocardium. Circ. Res., 20:311-320.
Heyrovsky, J. 1923. *As cited in* Polarography. 2nd ed. Kolthoff, I. M. and Lingane, J. C., eds. New York, Interscience Publishers, 1952, Vol. 1-2.
—and Shikata, M. 1925. *As cited in* Instrumental Methods of Analysis. 3rd ed. Princeton, New Jersey, D. Van Nostrand Co., Inc., 1958.
Hoffman, B. F. and Suckling, E. E. 1956. The effect of several cations on the transmembrane potentials of cardiac muscle. Amer. J. Physiol., 186:317-324.
—and Cranefield, P. F. 1960. Electrophysiology of the Heart. New York, McGraw-Hill Book Company, p. 157.
Hill, D. K. 1948. Oxygen tension and respiration of resting frog's muscle. J. Physiol. (London), 107:479-495.
Katz, L. N., Katz, A. M., and William, F. L. 1955. Metabolic adjustments to alterations of cardiac work in hypoxemia. Amer. J. Physiol., 181:539-549.
Kolmer, W., and Fleischmann, W. 1927. Über den sauerstoffverbrauch der Purkinjeschen faden. Pflügers Arch. Ges. Physiol., 218:530-531.
Kolthoff, I. M., and Laitinen, H. A. 1940. The voltametric determination of oxygen. Science, 92:152-154.
Krogh, A. 1918. The rate of diffusion of gases through animal tissues, with some remarks on the coefficient of invasion. J. Physiol. (London), 52:391-408.
Lange, N. A. 1941. Handbook of Chemistry. 10th Ed. Sandusky, Ohio, Handbook Publishers Inc.
Larrabee, M. G. 1958. Oxygen consumption of excised sympathetic ganglia at rest and in activity. J. Neurochem., 2:81-101.
Lee, K. S. 1953. A new technique for the simultaneous recording of oxygen consumption and contraction of muscle: The effect of ouabain on cat papillary muscle. J. Pharmacol. Exp. Ther., 109:304-312.
Ling, G., and Gerard, R. W. 1949. The normal membrane potential of frog sartorious fibers. J. Cell. Comp. Physiol., 34:383-396.

Lorber, V. 1953. Energy metabolism of the completely isolated mammalian heart in failure. Circ. Res., 1:298-311.

McKeever, W. P., Gregg, D. E. and Canney, P. C. 1958. Oxygen uptake of the nonworking left ventricle. Circ. Res., 6:612-623.

Monnier, A. M. 1952. The damping factor as a functional criterion in nerve physiology. Cold Spring Harbor Symposium on Quantitative Biology, 17:69-95.

Murray, J. A. 1954. Oxygen uptake of atrioventricular conducting tissue of beef heart. Amer. J. Physiol., 177:463-466.

Muus, J., Weiss, S., and Hasting, A. B. 1939. Tissue metabolism in vitamin deficiencies. II. Effect of thiamin deficiency. J. Biol. Chem., 129:303-307.

Olson, R. E., Pearson, O. H., Miller, O. N., and Stare, F. J. 1948. The effect of vitamin deficiencies upon the metabolism of cardiac muscle in vitro. I. The effect of thiamin deficiency in rats and ducks. J. Biol. Chem., 175:489-501.

Pearson, O. H., Hasting, A. B., and Bunting, H. 1949. Metabolism of cardiac muscle: Utilization of carbon-14 labeled pyruvate and acetate by rat heart slices. Amer. J. Physiol., 158:251-268.

Ranson, V. R., and Loomis, T. A. 1952. The effect of ouabain on the respiration of isometrically contracting rat auricle. J. Pharmacol. Exp. Ther., 104:219-223.

Ringer, S. 1880-1882. Concerning the influence exerted by each of the constituents of the blood on the contractions of the ventricle. J. Physiol. (London), 3:380-393.

Ross, S. M. 1958. Isometric recorder for small muscle tension. Rev. Sci. Instrum. 29:319-320.

Sonnenblick, E. H., Ross, J. Jr., Covell, J. W., Kaiser, G. A., and Braunwald, E. 1965. Velocity of contraction as a determinant of myocardial oxygen consumption. Amer. J. Physiol., 209:919-927.

Villee, C. A. 1953. The metabolism of human placenta in vitro. J. Biol. Chem., 205:113-123.

—1960. The Placenta and Fetal Membranes. Baltimore, The Williams and Wilkins Co.

Wagner, M. L., Lazzara, R., Weiss, R. M., and Hoffman, B. F. 1966. Specialized conducting fibers in the interatrial band. Circ. Res., 18:502-518.

Wearn, J. T. 1928. The extent of the capillary bed of the heart. J. Exp. Med., 47:273-292.

Webb, J. L., Saunders, P. R., and Nakamura, K. 1951. The metabolism of the heart in relation to drug action. VI. Metabolic actions of quinidine on rat heart muscle. J. Pharmacol. Exp. Ther., 101:287-295.

Weidman, S. 1952. The electrical constants of Purkinje fibers. J. Physiol. (London), 118:348-360.

Whalen, W. J. 1957. Oxygen consumption and tension of isolated heart muscle during rest and activity using a new technique. Circ. Res., 5:556-561.

Index